The Prevention, Treatment, and Complications of Diabetes Mellitus

The Prevention, Treatment, and Complications of Diabetes Mellitus

Editor

Manuel Aguilar-Diosdado

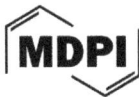

Basel • Beijing • Wuhan • Barcelona • Belgrade • Novi Sad • Cluj • Manchester

Editor
Manuel Aguilar-Diosdado
School of Medicine of Cadiz
University
Cádiz
Spain

Editorial Office
MDPI
St. Alban-Anlage 66
4052 Basel, Switzerland

This is a reprint of articles from the Special Issue published online in the open access journal *Journal of Clinical Medicine* (ISSN 2077-0383) (available at: https://www.mdpi.com/journal/jcm/special_issues/Prevention_Treatment_Complications_Diabetes_Mellitus).

For citation purposes, cite each article independently as indicated on the article page online and as indicated below:

Lastname, A.A.; Lastname, B.B. Article Title. *Journal Name* **Year**, *Volume Number*, Page Range.

ISBN 978-3-0365-9544-3 (Hbk)
ISBN 978-3-0365-9545-0 (PDF)
doi.org/10.3390/books978-3-0365-9545-0

© 2023 by the authors. Articles in this book are Open Access and distributed under the Creative Commons Attribution (CC BY) license. The book as a whole is distributed by MDPI under the terms and conditions of the Creative Commons Attribution-NonCommercial-NoDerivs (CC BY-NC-ND) license.

Contents

Ana I. Arroba and Manuel Aguilar-Diosdado
Special Issue "The Prevention, Treatment, and Complications of Diabetes Mellitus"
Reprinted from: *J. Clin. Med.* **2022**, *11*, 5305, doi:10.3390/jcm11185305 1

Alexandra-Cristina Scutca, Delia-Maria Nicoară, Monica Mărăzan, Giorgiana-Flavia Brad and Otilia Mărginean
Neutrophil-to-Lymphocyte Ratio Adds Valuable Information Regarding the Presence of DKA in Children with New-Onset T1DM
Reprinted from: *J. Clin. Med.* **2023**, *12*, 221, doi:10.3390/jcm12010221 5

Isabel Leiva-Gea, Cristina Antúnez Fernández, Roque Cardona-Hernandez, Marta Ferrer Lozano, Pilar Bahíllo-Curieses, Javier Arroyo-Díez, et al.
Increased Presentation of Diabetic Ketoacidosis and Changes in Age and Month of Type 1 Diabetes at Onset during the COVID-19 Pandemic in Spain
Reprinted from: *J. Clin. Med.* **2022**, *11*, 4338, doi:10.3390/jcm11154338 15

Sol Batule, Analía Ramos, Alejandra Pérez-Montes de Oca, Natalia Fuentes, Santiago Martínez, Joan Raga, et al.
Comparison of Glycemic Variability and Hypoglycemic Events in Hospitalized Older Adults Treated with Basal Insulin plus Vildagliptin and Basal–Bolus Insulin Regimen: A Prospective Randomized Study
Reprinted from: *J. Clin. Med.* **2022**, *11*, 2813, doi:10.3390/jcm11102813 23

Lidia Carvajal-Moreno, Manuel Coheña-Jiménez, Irene García-Ventura, Manuel Pabón-Carrasco and Ana Juana Pérez-Belloso
Prevention of Peripheral Distal Polyneuropathy in Patients with Diabetes: A Systematic Review
Reprinted from: *J. Clin. Med.* **2022**, *11*, 1723, doi:10.3390/jcm11061723 31

Mari Lukka, Vallo Tillmann and Aleksandr Peet
Decreased Need for Correction Boluses with Universal Utilisation of Dual-Wave Boluses in Children with Type 1 Diabetes
Reprinted from: *J. Clin. Med.* **2022**, *11*, 1689, doi:10.3390/jcm11061689 59

Daniel J. Rubin, Preethi Gogineni, Andrew Deak, Cherie Vaz, Samantha Watts, Dominic Recco, et al.
The Diabetes Transition of Hospital Care (DiaTOHC) Pilot Study: A Randomized Controlled Trial of an Intervention Designed to Reduce Readmission Risk of Adults with Diabetes
Reprinted from: *J. Clin. Med.* **2022**, *11*, 1471, doi:10.3390/jcm11061471 67

Almudena Lara-Barea, Begoña Sánchez-Lechuga, Álvaro Vidal-Suárez, Ana I. Arroba, Fernando Bugatto and Cristina López-Tinoco
Blood Pressure Monitoring and Perinatal Outcomes in Normotensive Women with Gestational Diabetes Mellitus
Reprinted from: *J. Clin. Med.* **2022**, *11*, 1435, doi:10.3390/jcm11051435 77

Enric Sánchez, Esther Sapiña-Beltrán, Ricard Gavaldà, Ferran Barbé, Gerard Torres, Ariadna Sauret, et al.
Prediabetes Is Associated with Increased Prevalence of Sleep-Disordered Breathing
Reprinted from: *J. Clin. Med.* **2022**, *11*, 1413, doi:10.3390/jcm11051413 89

Ashot Mkrtumyan, Alexander Ametov, Tatiana Demidova, Anna Volkova,
Ekaterina Dudinskaya, Arkady Vertkin, et al.
A New Approach to Overcome Insulin Resistance in Patients with Impaired Glucose Tolerance:
The Results of a Multicenter, Double-Blind, Placebo-Controlled, Randomized Clinical Trial of
Efficacy and Safety of Subetta
Reprinted from: *J. Clin. Med.* **2022**, *11*, 1390, doi:10.3390/jcm11051390 . . . . **101**

Fátima Cano-Cano, Laura Gómez-Jaramillo, Pablo Ramos-García, Ana I. Arroba and
Manuel Aguilar-Diosdado
IL-1β Implications in Type 1 Diabetes Mellitus Progression: Systematic Review and
Meta-Analysis
Reprinted from: *J. Clin. Med.* **2022**, *11*, 1303, doi:10.3390/jcm11051303 . . . . **115**

Isabel Leiva-Gea, Maria F. Martos-Lirio, Ana Gómez-Perea, Ana-Belen Ariza-Jiménez,
Leopoldo Tapia-Ceballos, Jose Manuel Jiménez-Hinojosa, et al.
Metabolic Control of the FreeStyle Libre System in the Pediatric Population with Type 1
Diabetes Dependent on Sensor Adherence
Reprinted from: *J. Clin. Med.* **2022**, *11*, 286, doi:10.3390/jcm11020286 . . . . **133**

Soledad Jimenez-Carmona, Pedro Alemany-Marquez, Pablo Alvarez-Ramos,
Eduardo Mayoral and Manuel Aguilar-Diosdado
Validation of an Automated Screening System for Diabetic Retinopathy Operating under Real
Clinical Conditions
Reprinted from: *J. Clin. Med.* **2022**, *11*, 14, doi:10.3390/jcm11010014 . . . . **141**

Miguel Ángel González-Moles and Pablo Ramos-García
State of Evidence on Oral Health Problems in Diabetic Patients: A Critical Review of the
Literature
Reprinted from: *J. Clin. Med.* **2021**, *10*, 5383, doi:10.3390/jcm10225383 . . . . **157**

Rocio Porcel-Chacón, Cristina Antúnez-Fernández, Maria Mora Loro, Ana-Belen
Ariza-Jimenez, Leopoldo Tapia Ceballos, Jose Manuel Jimenez Hinojosa, et al.
Good Metabolic Control in Children with Type 1 Diabetes Mellitus: Does Glycated Hemoglobin
Correlate with Interstitial Glucose Monitoring Using FreeStyle Libre?
Reprinted from: *J. Clin. Med.* **2021**, *10*, 4913, doi:10.3390/jcm10214913 . . . . **181**

Ana María Gómez-Perez, Miguel Damas-Fuentes, Isabel Cornejo-Pareja
and Francisco J. Tinahones
Heart Failure in Type 1 Diabetes: A Complication of Concern? A Narrative Review
Reprinted from: *J. Clin. Med.* **2021**, *10*, 4497, doi:10.3390/jcm10194497 . . . . **189**

Shota Okutsu, Yoshifumi Kato, Shunsuke Funakoshi, Toshiki Maeda, Chikara Yoshimura,
Miki Kawazoe, et al.
Effects of Weight Gain after 20 Years of Age and Incidence of Hyper-Low-Density Lipoprotein
Cholesterolemia: The Iki Epidemiological Study of Atherosclerosis and Chronic Kidney Disease
(ISSA-CKD)
Reprinted from: *J. Clin. Med.* **2021**, *10*, 3098, doi:10.3390/jcm10143098 . . . . **205**

Felix Aberer, Daniel A. Hochfellner, Harald Sourij and Julia K. Mader
A Practical Guide for the Management of Steroid Induced Hyperglycaemia in the Hospital
Reprinted from: *J. Clin. Med.* **2021**, *10*, 2154, doi:10.3390/jcm10102154 . . . . **213**

Hideyuki Fujii, Shunsuke Funakoshi, Toshiki Maeda, Atsushi Satoh, Miki Kawazoe,
Shintaro Ishida, et al.
Eating Speed and Incidence of Diabetes in a Japanese General Population: ISSA-CKD
Reprinted from: *J. Clin. Med.* **2021**, *10*, 1949, doi:10.3390/jcm10091949 . . . . **229**

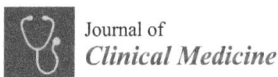

Editorial

Special Issue "The Prevention, Treatment, and Complications of Diabetes Mellitus"

Ana I. Arroba [1,2] and Manuel Aguilar-Diosdado [1,2,3,*]

1. Research Unit, Biomedical Research and Innovation Institute of Cadiz (INiBICA), 11009 Cádiz, Spain
2. Department of Endocrinology and Metabolism, Hospital Puerta del Mar, 11009 Cádiz, Spain
3. School of Medicine, Cadiz University (UCA), Ana de Viya 21, 11009 Cadiz, Spain
* Correspondence: manuel.diosdado@uca.es

Diabetes mellitus (DM) is a world health problem of global repercussion. It is expected that, in the next 20 years, the number of patients with DM will increase to 642 million people [1]. Type 1 diabetes mellitus (T1DM) responds to a multifactorial pathogenesis essentially linked to an autoimmune aggression mediated by T cells and autoantibodies that generate a progressive loss of insulin producing cells in the pancreas [2]. On the other hand, the pathogenesis of type 2 diabetes mellitus (T2DM) is essentially linked to the development of a state of resistance to the actions of insulin [3]. Both types are the consequence of an interaction of environmental, epigenetic, and genetic factors [4]. Genetic factors promote a special susceptibility to the development of the disease and epigenetics is considered as the link between the environment and genetics, altering gene and protein expression that could affect in autoimmunity and in the vulnerability of beta cells of pancreatic islets to the external factors.

In fact, clinical practice guidelines state that good metabolic—glycemic—control contributes to the reduction of complications associated with T1DM [5] and with T2DM [6] and that the best parameter to define the degree of glycemic control is glycosylated hemoglobin (HbA1c) which provides the average blood glucose levels in the last 2–3 months [5,6]. In addition, the development of new technologies to improve the management of DM, such as continuous glucose monitoring systems (CGMS) that measure glucose in interstitial fluid, show that they are the best way to monitor glucose levels to avoid hypoglycemia and to reduce glucose excursions. In fact, different studies have shown that these devices significantly reduce the number and intensity of hypoglycemia and improve HbA1c levels in both T1DM [7] and T2DM patients receiving insulin therapy [8].

However, the main challenge to clinicians is to reduce morbidity and mortality linked to DM, since complications associated with DM progression can arise both in the short and long term of the disease evolution. Hyperglycemia is a frequent finding in both hospitalized [9] and outpatients [10] and the management of glucose levels is the target on the most clinical trials. The use of modern insulin pumps offer a great variety of possibilities to which is added the incorporation of sensors-augmented insulin-pump, thus allowing its regulation and a higher and better level of safety in the device [11]. In T2DM, the treatment with non-insulin agents [12] contributes to improve the efficiency of insulin on glycemia levels and reflects the need to find a specific and personalized therapies for the profile of each patient. Actually, there is an increasing need to identify and provide evidence about the efficiency and safety of new therapy modalities and some of them have been included in this Special Issue.

DM is a life-threatening disease that causes complications and is considered as a serious disorder that doubles the risk of premature death [13]. Some aspects related with different fields into the DM progression have also been addressed in this Special Issue, such as the obstructive sleep apnea due to hypoxia implications [14], microvascular [15] and macrovascular [16] complications, elevated low-density lipoprotein (LDL) and cholesterol [17], and different oral processes [18]. A specifically complication associated with gestational diabetes mellitus (GDM) is the increased risk of hypertensive disorders; in this regard, new models based on biomarker parameters allow us to detect patients with GDM and these disorders and start earlier preventive strategies [19].

Upon the improvement of DM management, the scientific knowledge of the different underlying processes is very important. The implication of molecular mechanisms that could justify an adequate treatment option or the optimal technologies for an early diagnosis have to be included into the structural organigram of the study and follow-up of DM. The potential new biochemical targets, such as IL-1 in T1DM [20] or insulin receptor in T2DM [21], involve a deep analysis of the intracellular signaling and its potential implication in the physiopathology of the disease.

The prevention of complications of DM is relevant and requires an early diagnosis together with adequate treatment and follow-up of the patient. The most effective preventive strategy to avoid and/or delay the onset and development of DM complications is early diagnosis and early intervention aimed at mitigating symptoms and reducing sequelae and costs.

Author Contributions: Writing—original draft preparation, M.A.-D. and A.I.A.; writing—review and editing, M.A.-D. All authors have read and agreed to the published version of the manuscript.

Funding: This research received no external funding.

Conflicts of Interest: The authors declare no conflict of interest.

References

1. IDF Diabetes Atlas. 2022 International Diabetes Federation. Available online: https://diabetesatlas.org/ (accessed on 21 August 2022).
2. Gillespie, K.M. Type 1 diabetes: Pathogenesis and prevention. *Can. Med. Assoc. J.* **2006**, *175*, 165–170. [CrossRef] [PubMed]
3. DeFronzo, R.A. Pathogenesis of type 2 diabetes mellitus. *Med. Clin. N. Am.* **2004**, *88*, 787–835. [CrossRef] [PubMed]
4. Diedisheim, M.; Carcarino, E.; Vandiedonck, C.; Roussel, R.; Gautier, J.-F.; Venteclef, N. Regulation of inflammation in diabetes: From genetics to epigenomics evidence. *Mol. Metab.* **2020**, *41*, 101041. [CrossRef] [PubMed]
5. Nathan, D.M.; DCCT/EDIC Research Group. The diabetes control and complications trial/epidemiology of diabetes interventions and complications study at 30 years: Overview. *Diabetes Care* **2014**, *37*, 9–16. [CrossRef] [PubMed]
6. UK Prospective Diabetes Study Group. Intensive blood glucose control with sulphonylureas or insulin compared with conventional treatment and risk of complications in patients with type 2 diabetes (UKPDS 33). *Lancet* **1998**, *352*, 837–853. [CrossRef]
7. Bolinder, J.; Antuna, R.; Geelhoed-Duijvestijn, P.; Kröger, J.; Weitgasser, R. Novel glucose-sensing technology and hypoglycaemia in type 1 diabetes: A multicentre, non-masked, randomised controlled trial. *Lancet* **2016**, *388*, 2254–2263. [CrossRef]
8. Beck, R.W.; Riddlesworth, T.D.; Ruedy, K.; Ahmann, A.; Haller, S.; Kruger, D.; McGill, J.B.; Polonsky, W.; Price, D.; Aronoff, S.; et al. Continuous Glucose Monitoring Versus Usual Care in Patients With Type 2 Diabetes Receiving Multiple Daily Insulin Injections: A Randomized Trial. *Ann. Int. Med.* **2017**, *167*, 365–374. [CrossRef] [PubMed]
9. Kodner, C.; Anderson, L.; Pohlgeers, K. Glucose Management in Hospitalized Patients. *Am. Fam. Physician* **2017**, *96*, 648–654. [PubMed]
10. Rubin, D.J.; Shah, A.A. Predicting and Preventing Acute Care Re-Utilization by Patients with Diabetes. *Curr. Diab. Rep.* **2021**, *21*, 34. [CrossRef] [PubMed]
11. Bergenstal, R.M.; Tamborlane, W.V.; Ahmann, A.; Buse, J.B.; Dailey, G.; Davis, S.N.; Joyce, C.; Peoples, T.; Perkins, B.A.; Welsh, J.B.; et al. Effectiveness of Sensor-Augmented Insulin-Pump Therapy in Type 1 Diabetes. *N. Engl. J. Med.* **2010**, *363*, 311–320. [CrossRef] [PubMed]
12. Siegel, K.R.; Ali, M.K.; Zhou, X.; Ng, B.P.; Jawanda, S.; Proia, K.; Zhang, X.; Gregg, E.W.; Albright, A.L.; Zhang, P. Cost-effectiveness of Interventions to Manage Diabetes: Has the Evidence Changed Since 2008? *Diabetes Care* **2020**, *43*, 1557–1592. [CrossRef] [PubMed]
13. World Health Organization. Global Health Estimates (2000–2019). Available online: https://www.who.int/data/global-health-estimates (accessed on 21 August 2022).
14. Sánchez, E.; Sapiña-Beltrán, E.; Gavaldà, R.; Barbé, F.; Torres, G.; Sauret, A.; Dalmases, M.; López-Cano, C.; Gutiérrez-Carrasquilla, L.; Bermúdez-López, M.; et al. Prediabetes Is Associated with Increased Prevalence of Sleep-Disordered Breathing. *J. Clin. Med.* **2022**, *4*, 1413. [CrossRef] [PubMed]
15. Jimenez-Carmona, S.; Alemany-Marquez, P.; Alvarez-Ramos, P.; Mayoral, E.; Aguilar-Diosdado, M. Validation of an Automated Screening System for Diabetic Retinopathy Operating under Real Clinical Conditions. *J. Clin. Med.* **2022**, *11*, 14. [CrossRef] [PubMed]
16. Gómez-Perez, A.M.; Damas-Fuentes, M.; Cornejo-Pareja, I.; Tinahones, F.J. Heart Failure in Type 1 Diabetes: A Complication of Concern? A Narrative Review. *J. Clin. Med.* **2021**, *10*, 4497. [CrossRef] [PubMed]

17. Funakoshi, S.; Maeda, T.; Yoshimura, C.; Kawazoe, M.; Satoh, A.; Yokota, S.; Tada, K.; Takahashi, K.; Kenji Ito, K.; Yasuno, T.; et al. Effects of Weight Gain after 20 Years of Age and Incidence of Hyper-Low-Density Lipoprotein Cholesterolemia: The Iki Epidemiological Study of Atherosclerosis and Chronic Kidney Disease (ISSA-CKD). *J. Clin. Med.* **2021**, *10*, 3098.
18. González-Moles, M.Á.; Ramos-García, P. State of Evidence on Oral Health Problems in Diabetic Patients: A Critical Review of the Literature. *J. Clin. Med.* **2021**, *10*, 5383. [CrossRef] [PubMed]
19. Lara-Barea, A.; Sánchez-Lechuga, B.; Campos-Caro, A.; Córdoba-Doña, J.A.; de la Varga-Martínez, R.; Arroba, A.I.; Bugatto, F.; Aguilar-Diosdado, M.; López-Tinoco, C. Angiogenic Imbalance and Inflammatory Biomarkers in the Prediction of Hypertension as Well as Obstetric and Perinatal Complications in Women with Gestational Diabetes Mellitus. *J. Clin. Med.* **2022**, *11*, 1514. [CrossRef] [PubMed]
20. Cano-Cano, F.; Gómez-Jaramillo, L.; Ramos-García, P.; Arroba, A.I.; Aguilar-Diosdado, M. IL-1 Implications in Type 1 Diabetes Mellitus Progression: Systematic Review and Meta-Analysis. *J. Clin. Med.* **2022**, *11*, 1303. [CrossRef] [PubMed]
21. Mkrtumyan, A.; Ametov, A.; Demidova, T.; Volkova, A.; Dudinskaya, E.; Vertkin, A.; Vorobiev, S. A New Approach to Overcome Insulin Resistance in Patients with Impaired Glucose Tolerance: The Results of a Multicenter, Double-Blind, Placebo-Controlled, Randomized Clinical Trial of Efficacy and Safety of Subetta. *J. Clin. Med.* **2022**, *11*, 1390. [CrossRef] [PubMed]

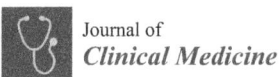

Article

Neutrophil-to-Lymphocyte Ratio Adds Valuable Information Regarding the Presence of DKA in Children with New-Onset T1DM

Alexandra-Cristina Scutca [1,2], Delia-Maria Nicoară [1,*], Monica Mărăzan [2], Giorgiana-Flavia Brad [1,2] and Otilia Mărginean [1,2,3]

1 Department of Pediatrics, University of Medicine and Pharmacy "Victor Babes", 300040 Timisoara, Romania
2 Department of Pediatrics I, Children's Emergency Hospital "Louis Turcanu", 300011 Timisoara, Romania
3 Department XI Pediatrics, Discipline I Pediatrics, Disturbances of Growth and Development in Children–BELIVE, 300011 Timisoara, Romania
* Correspondence: nicoara.delia@umft.ro

Abstract: Diabetic ketoacidosis (DKA) is an acute life-threatening complication occurring mainly at the onset of type 1 diabetes mellitus. The neutrophil-to-lymphocyte ratio (NLR), a marker for systemic inflammation, has recently generated increasing interest in many chronic diseases. The aim of this cross-sectional study was to determine the value of the neutrophil-to-lymphocyte ratio (NLR) in association with DKA severity across these cases. A total of 155 children with new-onset type 1 DM from one large center were included in the study. Total and differential leukocyte counts were measured upon admission and calculation of the NLR was performed. Patients were classified into four groups: without DKA, mild, moderate, and severe DKA at disease onset. Total WBCs, neutrophils, and monocytes increased with DKA severity (p-value < 0.005), while eosinophils displayed an inverse relationship (p-value < 0.001). Median NLR scores increased from those without ketoacidosis (1.11) to mild (1.58), moderate (3.71), and severe (5.77) ketoacidosis groups. The statistical threshold value of the NLR in predicting DKA was 1.84, with a sensitivity of 80.2% and a specificity of 80%. Study findings indicate that a higher NLR score adds valuable information regarding the presence of DKA in children with new-onset T1DM.

Keywords: new-onset T1DM; diabetic ketoacidosis; children; NLR score

1. Introduction

Diabetic ketoacidosis (DKA) is an acute life-threatening complication occurring mainly at the onset of type 1 diabetes mellitus [1,2], with an incidence rate that spans from 13 to 80% [3–5]. Being a form of systemic inflammatory state [6,7], inflammatory markers such as blood leukocytes and C-reactive protein (CRP) play a key role in the pathogenesis [8,9]. Although complete blood counts (CBCs) are a part of the routine evaluation in diabetic patients, white blood cell (WBC) fractions did not receive significant attention from diabetes specialists in the past [10]. In recent years, however, there has been growing interest regarding the neutrophil-to-lymphocyte ratio (NLR) as a marker of systemic inflammation in cardiac diseases, neoplasms, and obesity, as well as in diabetes-related complications such as diabetic foot ulcers and retinopathy [11–14]. Against this background, our aim was to study the association between the NLR and DKA severity among children with new-onset T1DM.

2. Materials and Methods

2.1. Patient Recruitment

This cross-sectional study included data from one of the largest Romanian reference centers for pediatric T1DM. We reviewed 181 consecutive T1DM patients charts from the

Pediatric Emergency Hospital "Louis Turcanu" in Timisoara, Romania, between 1 January 2015 to 30 June 2022, in accordance with the principles of the Declaration of Helsinki (1975, revised in 2013). Ethical approval was obtained from the ethics committee.

Inclusion criteria for cases were noted as new-onset T1DM in children aged 0 to 18 years, with or without diabetic ketoacidosis. Diagnosis of type 1 DM was established according to the American Diabetes Association (ADA) criteria of 2021. Exclusion criteria were as follows: infectious states, any other medical conditions that could alter hematological parameters, and patients with other types of diabetes.

Patients with DKA had a plasma glucose level > 11 mmol/L, a urine ketone level defined as moderate to high (+ to +++), and an arterial pH value < 7.30 at the time of admission. The ADA (American Diabetes Association) criteria for DKA severity were used: mild DKA, $7.20 \leq pH < 7.30$; moderate DKA, $7.10 \leq pH < 7.20$; and severe DKA, $pH < 7.10$ [15].

2.2. Biochemical Assays

Laboratory tests, including routine biochemistry tests and arterial gas analysis, were performed in the hospital laboratory. Blood samples were drawn at admission before the initial therapy, to avoid posttreatment changes in CBC parameters, and collected for differential WBC counts in tubes with EDTA and processed using a Sysmex XN-550 (Sysmex Corporation, Kobe, Japan) automatic blood counting system. Glycated Hb (HbA1c) was measured using a high-performance liquid chromatography kit supplied by Cobas E 411–Roche, Japan. Peptide C was evaluated using automated chemiluminescent assay (Cobas E 411–Roche, Tokyo, Japan). Neutrophil-to-lymphocyte ratios (NLR) were calculated.

2.3. Statistical Analysis

All data analysis was performed using the standard computer program Statistical Package for the Social Sciences (SPSS) for Windows, version 28 (SPSS Inc., Chicago, IL, USA) and GraphPad Prism9. The Shapiro–Wilk test was used to test the normality of the data distribution. Normally distributed variables were expressed as mean ± standard deviation (SD) and non-normally distributed variables were expressed as medians with interquartile ranges. Intergroup comparisons were performed by using an independent-sample t test and one-way ANOVA for normally distributed continuous data and Chi-Square tests for categorical variables. Non-normally distributed data were compared among multiple groups using the Kruskal–Wallis test. GraphPad Prism version 9 was used for univariate analysis with a post hoc procedure regarding NLR scores in DKA patients. Multiple regression analysis was performed to evaluate the association between the NLR or WBC parameters and the occurrence of DKA in T1DM patients. Receiver operating characteristic (ROC) curve analysis was plotted to compare the discrimination performance of HbA1c, C peptide, and CBC parameters in predicting DKA severity. The optimal threshold values were obtained using Youden's index (sensitivity + specificity − 1, ranging from 0 to 1) and the maximized area under the curve (AUC). A p value (two-tailed) < 0.05 was considered statistically significant.

3. Results

3.1. Patient Characteristics Stratified by DKA Grade

Following the retrospective revision of T1DM electronic charts, there were 181 newly diagnosticated children. We excluded 26 patients due to concomitant acute infections. The study group included 155 children (76 males, 79 females), with a mean age of 9.00 ± 4.39 years (range 0–18 years).

According to the onset characteristics, fasting blood glucose, islet autoantibodies, serum C-peptide, ketone bodies, and blood gas analysis results [16], children with new-onset T1DM were divided into four groups: the non-DKA ($n = 35$), mild DKA ($n = 25$), moderate DKA ($n = 33$), and severe DKA ($n = 62$) group.

There were no significant differences in terms of age among the four groups. Regarding gender, there were more female patients in the severe DKA group. HbA1c levels were approximately equal in the four groups (mean = 11.40 ± 2.01).

3.2. Differential WBC Counts

As shown in Table 1, there was a significant difference in the total and differential WBC counts regarding the four groups, especially regarding total WBCs, neutrophils, and monocytes which increased with DKA severity ($p < 0.0005$). Eosinophiles displayed an inverse relationship to DKA severity (p-value < 0.001), decreasing with DKA severity. Lymphocytes were statistically lower in severe DKA patients compared to those with mild and moderate DKA.

Table 1. Demographic data and laboratory findings of all patients.

Parameters	Non-DKA (n = 35)	Mild DKA (n = 25)	Moderate DKA (n = 33)	Severe DKA (n = 62)	p
Age (years)	10 (5–13)	9 (6.5–13)	7.00 (3.50–11)	9.00 (5–12)	0.381
Males% (n)	42 (15)	76 (19)	48 (16)	41 (26) [b]	0.028
HbA1c (%)	11.37 ± 1.95	11.68 ± 1.94	11.37 ± 2.16	11.52 ± 2.04	0.931
C-peptide (ng/mL)	0.639 (0.41–0.94)	0.481 (0.35–0.67)	0.533 (0.29–0.77)	0.330 (0.18–0.47) [a, c]	<0.001
Blood pH	7.36 (7.34–7.37)	7.28 (7.23–7.29)	7.17 (7.13–7.20) [a]	6.97 (6.89–7.03) [a, b, c]	0.000
WBCs ($\times 10^3/mm^3$)	8.53 (6.64–10.13)	8.12 (6.68–8.90)	12.27 (9.92–15.47) [a, b]	18.78 (14.06–24.52) [a, b, c]	<0.001
Neutrophils ($\times 10^3/mm^3$)	3.79 (2.99–5.24)	4.58 (3.38–5.21)	8.97 (6.24–12.6) [a, b]	14.63 (11.06–18) [a, b, c]	0.000
Lymphocytes ($\times 10^3/mm^3$)	2.92 (2.50–4.66)	2.71 (1.96–3.49)	2.86 (2.04–3.96)	2.33 (1.59–3.2) [a]	0.003
Thrombocytes ($\times 10^3/mm^3$)	299 (229–327)	259 (223–344)	347 (283–405) [a]	342 (388–422) [a, b]	<0.001
Monocytes ($\times 10^3/mm^3$)	0.60 (0.49–0.74)	0.68 (0.51–0.77)	0.87 (0.70–1.39) [a]	1.71 (1.15–2.40) [a, b, c]	<0.001
Eosinophiles ($\times 10^3/mm^3$)	0.12 (0.05–0.22)	0.09 (0.03–0.13)	0.06 (0.02–0.20)	0.00 (0–0.02) [a, b]	<0.001
NLR	1.11 (0.80–1.80)	1.58 (1.17–1.93)	3.71 (1.98–4.85) [a, b]	5.77 (4.04–9.63) [a, b, c]	0.000

One-way ANOVA, Kruskal–Wallis H-test, and Chi-Square test. Data are expressed as mean ± standard deviation, median (interquartile range, IQR) or percentage (n, %). ICU, Intensive Care Unit; HbA1c, glycated hemoglobin; WBC, white blood cell count; NLR, neutrophil-to-lymphocyte ratio. Statistically significant differences, with a probability value of $p < 0.05$, are represented in bold. Compared with the non-DKA group, [a] $p < 0.05$. Compared with the mild DKA group, [b] $p < 0.05$. Compared with the moderate DKA group, [c] $p < 0.05$.

3.3. NLR Score

A Kruskal–Wallis H test was performed to determine if there were significant differences in NLR scores between children without ketoacidosis and those with mild, moderate, or severe ketoacidosis. The distributions of NLR scores were not similar for all groups, as assessed by visual inspection of a boxplot. Median NLR scores increased from those without ketoacidosis (1.11) to mild (1.58), moderate (3.71), and severe (5.77) ketoacidosis groups (Figure 1). The distributions of NLR scores were significantly different between groups: $X^2(3) = 97.681$, $p = 0.000$. Subsequently, multiple comparisons were performed through post hoc analysis using Dunn's (1964) procedure with a Bonferroni correction. Adjusted p-values are presented. This post hoc analysis revealed statistically significant differences in median NLR scores between those with severe DKA and those with moderate ($p = 0.002$), mild ($p = 0.000$), or no DKA ($p = 0.000$); between mild and moderate DKA ($p = 0.012$), but not between those with mild DKA and no DKA ($p = 1.000$).

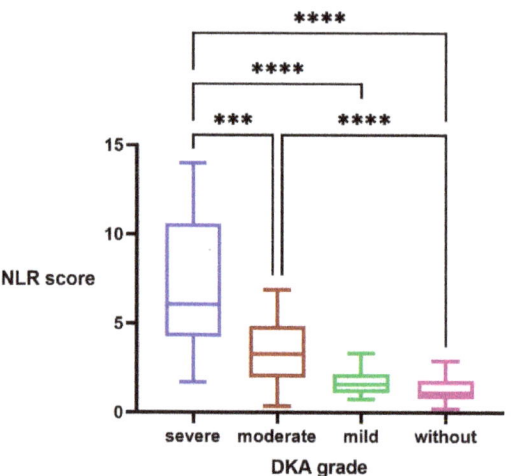

Figure 1. Univariate analysis with post hoc procedure regarding NLR scores in DKA patients; **** $p = 0.000$, *** $p = 0.002$.

3.4. Correlation and Regression Analyses

A multiple regression analysis was performed to determine the correlation between blood pH and age, gender, HbA1c, C peptide, and NLR. The multiple regression model was statistically associated with blood pH: $F(5, 130) = 41.485$, $p < 0.001$, adj. $R^2 = 0.600$. NLR score and age added significantly to the association, $p < 0.001$. Regression coefficients and standard errors are listed in Table 2.

Table 2. Linear regression analysis of factors related to blood pH in new-onset T1DM patients.

pH	B	95% CI for B		SE B	ß	R^2	ΔR^2
		LL	UL				
Model						0.654	0.640
Age	0.010 ***	0.004	0.015	0.003	0.239 ***		
Gender	0.003	−0.036	0.042	0.020	0.007		
HbA1c	0.001	−0.009	0.011	0.005	0.008		
C peptide	0.074 *	−0.014	0.135	0.030	0.145 *		
NLR	−0.038 ***	−0.044	−0.032	0.003	−0.770 ***		

B = unstandardized regression coefficient; CI = confidence interval; LL = lower limit; UL = upper limit; SE B = standard error of the coefficient; ß = standardized coefficient; R^2 = coefficient of determination; ΔR^2 = adjusted R^2. * $p < 0.05$, *** $p < 0.001$.

3.5. Receiver Operating Characteristics (ROC) Curve Analysis

The diagnostic ability of HbA1c, C peptide, WBCs, monocytes, and NLR in predicting DKA was analyzed by the ROC curve (Figures 2 and 3). The AUCs and cut-off values were calculated according to their specificity and sensitivity as predictive factors. The most influential indicators for DKA patients were WBCs (AUC 0.800; 95% CI: 0.723–0.877, $p < 0.000$), monocytes (AUC 0.815; 95% CI: 0.742–0.887, $p < 0.000$), NLR (AUC = 0.903; 95% CI: 0.854–0.952, $p < 0.000$), and, to a lesser extent, C peptide (AUC = 0.690; 95% CI: 0.591–0.789, $p = 0.001$), as opposed to HbA1c (Table 2).

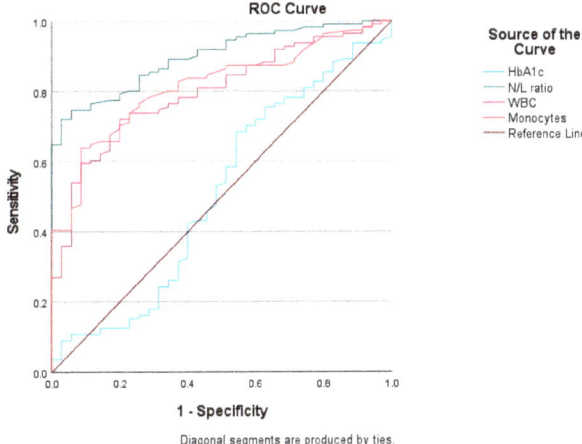

Figure 2. ROC curve analysis of HbA1c, WBCs, monocytes, and NLR; ROC, receiver operating characteristic. Significant differences were found ($p < 0.000$, respectively, for NLR, WBCs, and monocytes).

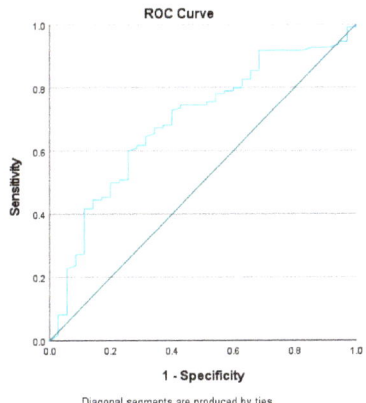

Figure 3. ROC curve analysis of C peptide; ROC, receiver operating characteristic.

The statistical threshold value of the NLR in predicting DKA was 1.84, with a sensitivity of 80.2% and a specificity of 80% (Table 3).

Table 3. ROC curve area and cut-off Values for predicting DKA. AUC = area under the curve; S.E. = standard error; CI = confidence interval.

Variable	AUC	S.E.	95% CI	Cut-Off	Sensitivity %	Specificity %
HbA1c	0.504	0.060	0.386–0.622	11.38	49.5	51.4
C peptide	0.690	0.050	0.591–0.789	0.554	68.2	60.0
WBC	0.800	0.039	0.723–0.877	8.860	79.2	57.1
Monocytes	0.815	0.037	0.742–0.887	0.675	80.2	62.9
NLR	0.903	0.051	0.854–0.952	1.84	80.2	80.0

4. Discussion

Type 1 diabetes mellitus (T1DM) represents one of the most frequent chronic illnesses affecting children [17]. Previous studies [16–23] have indicated an increase in both the frequency and severity of DKA cases in recent years. In our research, 81% of cases with T1DM presented with DKA, almost half of which were severe.

WBC counts, fractions, and indices, among which the NLR has received attention in recent years, were correlated with inflammation-associated diseases such as systemic hypertension [24], intracranial atherosclerosis [25], neoplasia [26], obesity [14], and type 2 diabetes [27–29].

The shifts in the percentage formula of white blood cells (increase in total WBCs, neutrophils, and monocytes; decrease in lymphocytes and eosinophiles) were similar to those cited in the literature [17,30].

Aside from systemic inflammation [31–33], the NLR, a well-characterized systemic inflammatory response marker [34], can also reflect both innate and adaptive immune (dys)function [9,35,36]. This simple ratio, which combines the predictive power of both increased neutrophil and decreased lymphocyte counts, has the advantage of being ubiquitous, cost effective, and also more stable compared with the absolute count [9,30,37]. Results from the present study are consistent with previous publications [10,30,38], in that WBC count and the NLR were found to be higher in patients with DKA.

Median NLR scores in our case were significantly different between groups, increasing from those without ketoacidosis (1.11; 0.80–1.80) to mild (1.58; 1.17–1.93), moderate (3.71; 1.98–4.85), and severe (5.77; 4.04–9.63) ketoacidosis groups. Our results regarding pediatric patients are consistent with a previous study addressing adults with DKA, which regards the NLR as a possible marker of the underlying severity of acute systemic inflammation in uninfected DKA patients [6]. Aside from the obvious effect of hemoconcentration on the NLR, the potential relationship between hyperglycemia and an increased NLR has been addressed in previous studies [39]. One possible explanation is that WBCs that are activated by advanced glycation end-products produce pro-inflammatory cytokines [29]. However, our study did not reveal statistical differences among the four groups in terms of mean HbA1c levels. This is consistent with some studies regarding children with DKA [40–42], and in opposition with other studies [17]. Another explanation is the fact that, in DKA, acute hyperglycemia promotes the accumulation of reactive oxygen species (ROS) which can damage peripheral blood lymphocytes' DNA. This in turn may cause the apoptosis of lymphocytes and affect their proliferation [6,43,44].

In the present study, with new-onset T1DM children grouped according to blood pH, multivariate logistic regression analysis was performed in order to assess whether confounding exists between age, sex, HbA1c, C peptide, and NLR regarding blood pH. The NLR displayed a good discriminatory power regarding association with DKA, through correlation with blood pH.; age at onset, and, to a lesser extent, C peptide added statistically significantly to the prediction. This is consistent with a previous published study regarding adult T1DM patients [10] but, to our knowledge, was not yet reported in children. An upside to examining children is their lack of many confounding factors that can affect NLR levels, such as common medications and comorbidities present in adult patients with diabetes.

Assessing the ROC curve, the presence of DKA in our study lot was associated with an elevated NLR, monocytes, and WBCs. The area under the curve was largest for the NLR, with values above 1.84 being most frequently present in children with DKA (sensitivity of 80.2% and specificity of 80%). Regarding C peptide, plasma values were negatively correlated with the presence of DKA, mainly values below 0.690 ng/mL (sensitivity of 68.2% and specificity of 60%).

There were some limitations in the present study. Firstly, the sample size was relatively small, which could limit the power of the analyses. Secondly, our patients are only from one hospital, so that selection bias cannot be ruled out. Additionally, only one measurement of CBC and subsequent NLR calculation were used in the analysis: those upon admission.

As such, there was no monitoring of the dynamic trend of the NLR. We look forward to additional multicenter studies with large samples.

5. Conclusions

This study adds complementary laboratory data regarding children with DKA at onset of T1DM [10,45]. It underlines the fact that higher NLR levels were associated with an increased prevalence of DKA in children with new-onset T1DM, and positively correlated with the DKA grade.

To the authors' knowledge, it represents the first study to evaluate the NLR based on DKA severity in children with new-onset T1DM. This finding has clinical significance, especially in pre-hospital settings, where blood gas analysis is usually not part of routine investigations, because it may improve the early diagnosis of DKA in children with elevated glucose level and thereby facilitate proper care.

Author Contributions: Conceptualization, A.-C.S., D.-M.N. and O.M.; methodology, A.-C.S., D.-M.N. and G.-F.B.; software, D.-M.N.; validation, A.-C.S. and D.-M.N.; formal analysis, A.-C.S. and G.-F.B.; investigation, A.-C.S., D.-M.N. and M.M.; resources, A.-C.S. and M.M.; data curation A.-C.S. and D.-M.N.; writing—original draft preparation, D.-M.N. and G.-F.B.; writing—review and editing, A.-C.S. and O.M.; visualization, A.-C.S., D.-M.N., M.M., G.-F.B. and O.M; supervision, A.-C.S., D.-M.N. and O.M. All authors have read and agreed to the published version of the manuscript.

Funding: This research received no specific grant from any funding agency in the public, commercial, or not-for-profit sectors.

Institutional Review Board Statement: The study was conducted according to the guidelines of the Declaration of Helsinki and was approved by the Ethics Committee for Research of "Victor Babes" University of Medicine and Pharmacy, Timisoara (approval number 21264/17.11.2022).

Informed Consent Statement: Patient consent for further use of data was waived by the Ethics Committee for Research of "Victor Babes" University of Medicine and Pharmacy, Timisoara, due to the retrospective design of the study and the use of anonymized datasets.

Data Availability Statement: The data are not publicly available due to reasons of privacy.

Conflicts of Interest: The authors declare no conflict of interest.

References

1. Alfayez, O.M.; Aldmasi, K.S.; Alruwais, N.H.; Bin Awad, N.M.; Al Yami, M.S.; Almohammed, O.A.; Almutairi, A.R. Incidence of Diabetic Ketoacidosis Among Pediatrics with Type 1 Diabetes Prior to and During COVID-19 Pandemic: A Meta-Analysis of Observational Studies. *Front. Endocrinol.* **2022**, *13*, 856958. [CrossRef] [PubMed]
2. Duca, L.M.; Wang, B.; Rewers, M.; Rewers, A. Diabetic Ketoacidosis at Diagnosis of Type 1 Diabetes Predicts Poor Long-term Glycemic Control. *Diabetes Care* **2017**, *40*, 1249–1255. [CrossRef]
3. Dhatariya, K.K.; Glaser, N.S.; Codner, E.; Umpierrez, G.E. Diabetic Ketoacidosis. *Nat. Rev. Dis. Prim.* **2020**, *6*, 1–20. [CrossRef] [PubMed]
4. Umpierrez, G.E.; Kitabchi, A.E. Diabetic Ketoacidosis: Risk Factors and Management Strategies. *Treat. Endocrinol.* **2003**, *2*, 95–108. [CrossRef] [PubMed]
5. Saydah, S.H.; Shrestha, S.S.; Zhang, P.; Zhou, X.; Imperatore, G. Medical Costs among Youth Younger than 20 Years of Age with and without Diabetic Ketoacidosis at the Time of Diabetes Diagnosis. *Diabetes Care* **2019**, *42*, 2256–2261. [CrossRef]
6. Cheng, Y.; Yu, W.; Zhou, Y.; Zhang, T.; Chi, H.; Xu, C. Novel predictor of the occurrence of DKA in T1DM patients without infection: A combination of neutrophil/lymphocyte ratio and white blood cells. *Open Life Sci.* **2021**, *16*, 1365–1376. [CrossRef]
7. Dalton, R.R.; Hoffman, W.H.; Passmore, G.G.; Martin, S.L. Plasma C-reactive protein levels in severe diabetic ketoacidosis. *Ann. Clin. Lab. Sci.* **2003**, *33*, 435–442.
8. Gosmanov, A.R.; Gosmanova, E.O.; Kitabchi, A.E. Hyperglycemic Crises: Diabetic Ketoacidosis and Hyperglycemic Hyperosmolar State. [Updated 2021 May 9]. In *Endotext*; Feingold, K.R., Anawalt, B., Boyce, A., Eds.; MDText.com, Inc.: South Dartmouth, MA, USA, 2000; Available online: https://www.ncbi.nlm.nih.gov/books/NBK279052 (accessed on 15 October 2022).
9. Russell, C.D.; Parajuli, A.; Gale, H.J.; Bulteel, N.S.; Schuetz, P.; de Jager, C.P.C.; Loonen, A.J.M.; Merekoulias, G.I.; Baillie, J.K. The utility of peripheral blood leucocyte ratios as biomarkers in infectious diseases: A systematic review and meta-analysis. *J. Infect.* **2019**, *78*, 339–348. [CrossRef]
10. Xu, W.; Wu, H.F.; Ma, S.G.; Bai, F.; Hu, W.; Jin, Y.; Liu, H. Correlation between peripheral white blood cell counts and hyperglycemic emergencies. *Int. J. Med. Sci.* **2013**, *10*, 758–765. [CrossRef]

11. Elsayed, A.M.; Araby, E. Neutrophil-Lymphocyte and Platelet-Lymphocyte ratios as a marker for diabetes control and complications. *Benha Med. J.* **2021**, *38*, 984–995. [CrossRef]
12. Durmus, E.; Kivrak, T.; Gerin, F.; Sunbul, M.; Sari, I.; Erdogan, O. Neutrophil-to-Lymphocyte Ratio and Platelet-to-Lymphocyte Ratio are Predictors of Heart Failure. *Arq. Bras. Cardiol.* **2015**, *105*, 606–613. [CrossRef]
13. Zhou, B.; Zhan, C.; Wu, J.; Liu, J.; Zhou, J.; Zheng, S. Prognostic Significance of Preoperative Neutrophil-to-Lymphocyte Ratio in Surgically Resectable Pancreatic Neuroendocrine Tumors. *Med. Sci. Monit.* **2017**, *23*, 5574–5588. [CrossRef]
14. Rodríguez-Rodríguez, E.; López-Sobaler, A.M.; Ortega, R.M.; Delgado-Losada, M.L.; López-Parra, A.M.; Aparicio, A. Association between Neutrophil-to-Lymphocyte Ratio with Abdominal Obesity and Healthy Eating Index in a Representative Older Spanish Population. *Nutrients* **2020**, *12*, 855. [CrossRef]
15. American Diabetes Association. Pharmacologic Approaches to Glycemic Treatment: Standards of Medical Care in Diabetes-2021. *Diabetes Care* **2021**, *44* (Suppl. 1), S111–S124. [CrossRef]
16. Ho, J.; Rosolowsky, E.; Pacaud, D.; Huang, C.; Lemay, J.A.; Brockman, N.; Rath, M.; Doulla, M. Diabetic Ketoacidosis at Type 1 Diabetes Diagnosis in Children During the COVID-19 Pandemic. *Pediatr. Diabetes* **2021**, *22*, 552–557. [CrossRef]
17. Boboc, A.A.; Novac, C.N.; Ilie, M.T.; Ieșanu, M.I.; Galoș, F.; Bălgrădean, M.; Berghea, E.C.; Ionescu, M.D. The Impact of SARS-CoV-2 Pandemic on the New Cases of T1DM in Children. A Single-Centre Cohort Study. *J. Pers. Med.* **2021**, *11*, 551. [CrossRef]
18. Kamrath, C.; Mönkemöller, K.; Biester, T.; Rohrer, T.R.; Warncke, K.; Hammersen, J.; Holl, R.W. Ketoacidosis in Children and Adolescents with Newly Diagnosed Type 1 Diabetes During the COVID-19 Pandemic in Germany. *JAMA J. Am. Med. Assoc.* **2020**, *324*, 801–804. [CrossRef]
19. Dilek, S.Ö.; Gürbüz, F.; Turan, I.; Celiloğlu, C.; Yüksel, B. Changes in the Presentation of Newly Diagnosed Type 1 Diabetes in Children During the COVID-19 Pandemic in a Tertiary Center in Southern Turkey. *J. Pediatr. Endocrinol. Metab.* **2021**, *34*, 1303–1309. [CrossRef]
20. Dżygało, K.; Nowaczyk, J.; Szwilling, A.; Kowalska, A. Increased Frequency of Severe Diabetic Ketoacidosis at Type 1 Diabetes Onset Among Children During COVID-19 Pandemic Lockdown: An Observational Cohort Study. *Pediatr. Endocrinol. Diabetes Metab.* **2020**, *26*, 167–175. [CrossRef]
21. Jacob, R.; Weiser, G.; Krupik, D.; Takagi, D.; Peled, S.; Pines, N.; Hashavya, S.; Gur-Soferman, H.; Gamsu, S.; Kaplan, O.; et al. Diabetic Ketoacidosis at Emergency Department Presentation During the First Months of the SARS-CoV-2 Pandemic in Israel: A Multicenter Cross-Sectional Study. *Diabetes Ther.* **2021**, *12*, 1569–1574. [CrossRef]
22. Lawrence, C.; Seckold, R.; Smart, C.; King, B.R.; Howley, P.; Feltrin, R.; Smith, T.A.; Roy, R.; Lopez, P. Increased Paediatric Presentations of Severe Diabetic Ketoacidosis in an Australian Tertiary Centre During the COVID-19 Pandemic. *Diabetes Med.* **2021**, *38*, e14417. [CrossRef] [PubMed]
23. McGlacken-Byrne, S.M.; Drew, S.E.V.; Turner, K.; Peters, C.; Amin, R. The SARS-CoV-2 Pandemic Is Associated with Increased Severity of Presentation of Childhood Onset Type 1 Diabetes Mellitus: A Multi-Centre Study of the First COVID-19 Wave. *Diabetes Med.* **2021**, *38*, e1464. [CrossRef] [PubMed]
24. Jhuang, Y.H.; Kao, T.W.; Peng, T.C.; Chen, W.L.; Li, Y.W.; Chang, P.K.; Wu, L.W. Neutrophil to lymphocyte ratio as predictor for incident hypertension: A 9-year cohort study in Taiwan. *Hypertens. Res.* **2019**, *42*, 1209–1214. [CrossRef] [PubMed]
25. Nam, K.W.; Kwon, H.M.; Jeong, H.Y.; Park, J.H.; Kim, S.H.; Jeong, S.M. High neutrophil to lymphocyte ratios predict intracranial atherosclerosis in a healthy population. *Atherosclerosis* **2018**, *269*, 117–121. [CrossRef] [PubMed]
26. Proctor, M.J.; McMillan, D.C.; Morrison, D.S.; Fletcher, C.D.; Horgan, P.G.; Clarke, S.J. A derived neutrophil to lymphocyte ratio predicts survival in patients with cancer. *Br. J. Cancer* **2012**, *107*, 695–699. [CrossRef]
27. Mertoglu, C.; Gunay, M. Neutrophil-Lymphocyte ratio and Platelet-Lymphocyte ratio as useful predictive markers of prediabetes and diabetes mellitus. *Diabetes Metab. Syndr.* **2017**, *11* (Suppl. 1), S127–S131. [CrossRef]
28. Imtiaz, F.; Shafique, K.; Mirza, S.S.; Ayoob, Z.; Vart, P.; Rao, S. Neutrophil lymphocyte ratio as a measure of systemic inflammation in prevalent chronic diseases in Asian population. *Int. Arch. Med.* **2012**, *5*, 2. [CrossRef]
29. Wheelock, K.M.; Saulnier, P.J.; Tanamas, S.K.; Vijayakumar, P.; Weil, E.J.; Looker, H.C.; Hanson, R.L.; Lemley, K.V.; Yee, B.; Knowler, W.C.; et al. White blood cell fractions correlate with lesions of diabetic kidney disease and predict loss of kidney function in Type 2 diabetes. *Nephrol. Dial. Transplant.* **2018**, *33*, 1001–1009. [CrossRef]
30. Ismail, N.A.; Abeer, M.; El Baky, N.E.D.A.; Kandil, M.E.; Rasshed, I.A.; Ahmed, A.N.; Ibrahim, M.H. Neutrophil-Lymphocyte Ratio, Platelet-Lymphocyte Ratio in Well Controlled and Uncontrolled Children and Adolescents with Type 1 Diabetes Mellitus. *Res. J. Pharm. Biol. Chem.* **2021**, *12*, 13. [CrossRef]
31. Chen, M.; Zhu, Y.; Wang, J.; Wang, G.; Wu, Y. The Predictive Value of Neutrophil-to-Lymphocyte Ratio and Platelet-to-Lymphocyte Ratio Levels of Diabetic Peripheral Neuropathy. *J. Pain Res.* **2021**, *14*, 2049–2058. [CrossRef]
32. Jambrik, Z.; Monti, S.; Coppola, V.; Agricola, E.; Mottola, G.; Miniati, M.; Picano, E. Usefulness of neutrophil/lymphocyte ratio as predictor of new-onset atrial fibrillation after coronary artery bypass grafting. *Am. J. Cardiol.* **2010**, *105*, 186–191. [CrossRef]
33. Tamhane, U.U.; Aneja, S.; Montgomery, D.; Rogers, E.K.; Eagle, K.A.; Gurm, H.S. Association between admission neutrophil to lymphocyte ratio and outcomes in patients with acute coronary syndrome. *Am. J. Cardiol.* **2008**, *102*, 653–657. [CrossRef]
34. Wang, J.R.; Chen, Z.; Yang, K.; Yang, H.J.; Tao, W.Y.; Li, Y.P.; Jiang, Z.J.; Bai, C.F.; Yin, Y.C.; Duan, J.M.; et al. Association between neutrophil-to-lymphocyte ratio, platelet-to-lymphocyte ratio, and diabetic retinopathy among diabetic patients without a related family history. *Diabetol. Metab. Syndr.* **2020**, *12*, 55. [CrossRef]

35. Sawant, A.C.; Adhikari, P.; Narra, S.R.; Srivatsa, S.S.; Mills, P.K.; Srivatsa, S.S. Neutrophil to lymphocyte ratio predicts short- and long-term mortality following revascularization therapy for ST elevation myocardial infarction. *Cardiol. J.* **2014**, *21*, 500–508. [CrossRef]
36. Rucker, A.J.; Rudemiller, N.P.; Crowley, S.D. Salt, Hypertension, and Immunity. *Annu. Rev. Physiol.* **2018**, *80*, 283–307. [CrossRef]
37. Prats-Puig, A.; Gispert-Saüch, M.; Díaz-Roldán, F.; Carreras-Badosa, G.; Osiniri, I.; Planella-Colomer, M.; Mayol, L.; de Zegher, F.; Ibánez, L.; Bassols, J.; et al. Neutrophil-to-lymphocyte ratio: An inflammation marker related to cardiovascular risk in children. *Thromb. Haemost.* **2015**, *114*, 727–734. [CrossRef]
38. Alamri, B.N.; Ferris, J.; Matheson, K.; De Tugwell, B. MON-638 The WBC Differential in Relation to DKA Severity. *J. Endocr. Soc.* **2020**, *4* (Suppl. 1), 638. [CrossRef]
39. Sefil, F.; Ulutas, K.T.; Dokuyucu, R.; Sumbul, A.T.; Yengil, E.; Yagiz, A.E.; Yula, E.; Ustun, I.; Gokce, C. Investigation of neutrophil lymphocyte ratio and blood glucose regulation in patients with type 2 diabetes mellitus. *J. Int. Med. Res.* **2014**, *42*, 581–588. [CrossRef]
40. Lee, H.J.; Yu, H.W.; Jung, H.W.; Lee, Y.A.; Kim, J.H.; Chung, H.R.; Yoo, J.; Kim, E.; Yu, J.; Shin, C.H.; et al. Factors Associated with the Presence and Severity of Diabetic Ketoacidosis at Diagnosis of Type 1 Diabetes in Korean Children and Adolescents. *J. Korean Med. Sci.* **2017**, *32*, 303–309. [CrossRef]
41. Khanolkar, A.R.; Amin, R.; Taylor-Robinson, D.; Viner, R.M.; Warner, J.; Gevers, E.F.; Stephenson, T. Diabetic Ketoacidosis Severity at Diagnosis and Glycaemic Control in the First Year of Childhood Onset Type 1 Diabetes-A Longitudinal Cohort Study. *Int. J. Environ. Res. Public Health* **2017**, *15*, 26. [CrossRef]
42. Peng, W.; Yuan, J.; Chiavaroli, V.; Dong, G.; Huang, K.; Wu, W.; Ullah, R.; Jin, B.; Lin, H.; Derraik, J.G.B.; et al. 10-Year Incidence of Diabetic Ketoacidosis at Type 1 Diabetes Diagnosis in Children Aged Less Than 16 Years from a Large Regional Center (Hangzhou, China). *Front. Endocrinol.* **2021**, *12*, 653519. [CrossRef] [PubMed]
43. Hu, H.; Xu, F.; Yang, W.; Ren, J.; Ge, W.; Yang, P. Apoptosis as an underlying mechanism in lymphocytes induced by riboflavin and ultraviolet light. *Transfus. Apher. Sci.* **2020**, *59*, 102899. [CrossRef] [PubMed]
44. Mirzaei, S.; Hadadi, Z.; Attar, F.; Mousavi, S.E.; Zargar, S.S.; Tajik, A.; Saboury, A.A.; Rezayat, S.M.; Falahati, M. ROS-mediated heme degradation and cytotoxicity induced by iron nanoparticles: Hemoglobin and lymphocyte cells as targets. *J. Biomol. Struct. Dyn.* **2018**, *36*, 4235–4245. [CrossRef] [PubMed]
45. Ma, S.G.; Jin, Y.; Xu, W.; Hu, W.; Bai, F.; Wu, X.J. Increased serum levels of ischemia-modified albumin and C-reactive protein in type 1 diabetes patients with ketoacidosis. *Endocrine* **2012**, *42*, 570–576. [CrossRef]

Disclaimer/Publisher's Note: The statements, opinions and data contained in all publications are solely those of the individual author(s) and contributor(s) and not of MDPI and/or the editor(s). MDPI and/or the editor(s) disclaim responsibility for any injury to people or property resulting from any ideas, methods, instructions or products referred to in the content.

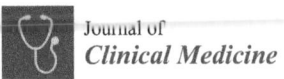

Article

Increased Presentation of Diabetic Ketoacidosis and Changes in Age and Month of Type 1 Diabetes at Onset during the COVID-19 Pandemic in Spain

Isabel Leiva-Gea [1,2], Cristina Antúnez Fernández [3], Roque Cardona-Hernandez [4,*], Marta Ferrer Lozano [5], Pilar Bahíllo-Curieses [6], Javier Arroyo-Díez [7], María Clemente León [8,9], Maria Martín-Frías [10], Santiago Conde Barreiro [11], Andrés Mingorance Delgado [12] and Jacobo Pérez Sánchez [13] on behalf of the Diabetes Group of the Spanish Pediatric Endocrinology Society (SEEP)

1. Pediatric Endocrinology, Department of Pediatrics, Hospital Regional de Málaga, 29010 Málaga, Spain
2. Instituto de Investigación Biomédica de Málaga (IBIMA), 29590 Málaga, Spain
3. Department of Pediatrics, Hospital Punta de Europa, 11207 Algeciras, Spain
4. Division of Pediatric Endocrinology, Hospital Sant Joan de Déu, Passeig Sant Joan de Déu 2, 08950 Barcelona, Spain
5. Pediatric Endocrinology, Department of Pediatrics, Hospital Universitario Miguel Servet, 50009 Zaragoza, Spain
6. Pediatric Endocrinology, Department of Pediatrics, Hospital Clínico Universitario de Valladolid, 47003 Valladolid, Spain
7. Pediatric Endocrinology, Department of Pediatrics, Hospital Universitario Materno Infantil de Badajoz, 06010 Badajoz, Spain
8. Pediatric Endocrinology, Department of Pediatrics, Institut de Recerca, Hospital Vall d'Hebron, Centre for Biomedical Research on Rare Diseases (CIBERER), 08035 Barcelona, Spain
9. Barcelona Autonomous University, 08035 Barcelona, Spain
10. Pediatric Endocrinology and Diabetes, Department of Pediatrics, Hospital Universitario Ramón y Cajal, 28034 Madrid, Spain
11. Pediatrics, Centro de Salud de Barbastro, 22300 Huesca, Spain
12. Pediatric Endocrinology, Department of Pediatrics, Hospital General Universitario de Alicante, 03010 Alicante, Spain
13. Pediatric Endocrinology, Department of Pediatrics, Consorci Coprporació Sanitaria Parc Tauli, 08208 Sabadell, Spain
* Correspondence: roque.cardona@sjd.es; Tel.: +34-93-280-40-00; Fax: +34-93-203-39-59

Abstract: **Objective**: To assess the impact of the COVID-19 pandemic and lockdown measures on the presenting characteristics (age at diagnosis, severity, monthly distribution) of newly diagnosed type 1 diabetes in Spanish children. **Research Design and Methods**: An ambispective observational multicenter study was conducted in nine Spanish tertiary-level hospitals between January 2015 and March 2021. Inclusion criteria: new cases of type 1 diabetes in children (0–14 years) recording age, sex, date of diagnosis, presence of diabetic ketoacidosis (DKA) at onset, and severity of DKA. Data were compared before and during the pandemic. **Results**: We registered 1444 new cases of type 1 diabetes in children: 1085 in the pre-pandemic period (2015–2019) and 359 during the pandemic (2020–March 2021). There was a significant increase in the group aged ≤4 years in the pandemic period (chi-squared = 10.986, df 2, p = 0.0041). In 2020–2021, cases of DKA increased significantly by 12% (95% CI: 7.2–20.4%), with a higher percentage of moderate and severe DKA, although this increase was not significant. In 2020, there was a sharp decrease in the number of cases in March, with a progressive increase from May through November, higher than in the same months of the period 2015–2019, highlighting the increase in the number of cases in June, September, and November. The first three months of 2021 showed a different trend to that observed both in the years 2015–2019 and in 2020, with a marked increase in the number of cases. **Conclusions**: A change in monthly distribution was described, with an increase in DKA at onset of type 1 diabetes. No differences were found in severity, although there were differences in the age distribution, with an increase in the number of cases in children under 4 years of age.

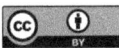

Keywords: type 1 diabetes; COVID-19; diabetes onset; DKA

1. Introduction

Epidemiological studies have an important role in type 1 diabetes, since they enable estimation of the necessary resources for its management, as well as providing insight into its etiology and risk factors.

The estimated incidence of type 1 diabetes in the Spanish population under 15 years of age is 17.69 cases/100,000 inhabitants/year [1]. In Spain, incidence figures are lower in autonomous communities located in the north of the country, and higher in the south and center of the country, suggesting that the "north–south" gradient in the incidence of the disease described in Europe does not apply [2].

On 31 January 2020, the first case of coronavirus disease 2019 (COVID-19) was diagnosed in Spain [3]. From this time onwards, the incidence of the virus skyrocketed, leading to the declaration of a state of alarm and home lockdown on 14 March 2020. An association between COVID-19 and an increase in the number of hyperglycemia or diabetes cases has been suggested based on findings from different observational studies around the world. Numerous hypotheses have been proposed, although the mechanism that links them is not clearly defined [4]. Angiotensin-converting enzyme receptor 2 (ACE2) is the binding site for SARS-CoV-1 and -2 and is strongly expressed in pancreatic endocrine cells. Therefore, some studies postulate that the exposure to SARS-CoV-2 contributes to the observed increase of cases by precipitating or accelerating the onset of type 1 diabetes [5,6]. Another suggested mechanism would be the direct action of COVID-19 on pancreatic beta cells, by increasing proinflammatory cytokines and acute phase reactants leading to inflammation and direct cell damage.

A number of studies examining the presentation of new cases of type 1 diabetes in children and adolescents after the declaration of the pandemic, reported an increase in the frequency severity of diabetes ketoacidosis (DKA) presentation [6–12]. On the other hand, some studies have described an increase in the frequency of new case presentations [6,10–16], while others reported no increase or even a decrease in the number of type 1 diabetes [9,17].

The change in the frequency and severity in type 1 diabetes forms presentation after the emergence of the pandemic, raises the hypothesis that variations in the circulation of seasonal viruses, which could have been acting as triggers for onset or the delay in diagnosis due to individuals postponing consultation because of the fear of infection, may have contributed to this new scenario [9].

The aim of the present study was to assess the impact of the COVID-19 pandemic and the resulting lockdown measures on the presenting characteristics of newly diagnosed type 1 diabetes in Spanish children with respect to age at diagnosis, severity, and monthly distribution.

2. Research Design and Methods

This was a multicenter, observational, ambispective study conducted in nine Spanish tertiary-level hospitals between January 2015 and February 2021. We included all new diagnoses of type 1 diabetes in the pediatric population (0–14 years) in each of the participating centers. Age, sex, date of diagnosis, presence of DKA at onset, and severity of DKA (blood pH, serum bicarbonate) were recorded. Data were collected in two periods and compared before the pandemic (2015–2019) and during the pandemic (2020–2021).

The study was undertaken with the approval of the Ethics Committee of the Regional Hospital of Malaga. The diagnostic criteria for type 1 diabetes were those established by the American Diabetes Association [18]. The criteria used to define the severity of DKA followed the recommendations of the International Society for Pediatric and Adolescent Diabetes (ISPAD) [19] as follows: mild if pH < 7.3 or bicarbonate < 15 mmol/L, moderate if pH < 7.2 or bicarbonate < 10 mmol/L, and severe DKA if pH < 7.1 or bicarbonate < 5 mmol/L.

The statistical analysis was performed using R Commander Version 2.7-1 software (Chapman & Hall, Boca Raton, FL, USA). To evaluate the differences between the different study years, the chi-squared test was used, with $p < 0.05$ being considered statistically significant. The resulting data are presented in tables and figures to illustrate the distribution of the data.

3. Results

We collected data from 1444 new cases of type 1 diabetes in the pediatric age group during the period 2015–2021: 1085 in the pre-pandemic period (2015–2019) and 359 during the pandemic (2020–March 2021). Regarding the distribution of cases by age, an increase in the group aged ≤4 years was evident in the pandemic period, with a chi-squared value of 10.986 with 2 degrees of freedom and a p-value of 0.0041 (Table 1), indicating that the age distribution of new cases was not the same in these periods. This significant difference was at the expense of more cases (25%) in children under 4 years of age during the pandemic rather than in the pre-pandemic period (19%). The opposite occurred in the group aged 5–9 years, where there was a higher percentage in the first period (39%) rather than in the second (30%). During the period 2015–2019, 589 boys (54%) and 494 girls (46%) presented with type 1 diabetes; meanwhile, during 2020–2021, 205 boys (57%) and 154 girls (43%) did. No differences in gender distribution were found according to the period when diabetes onset occurred (X-square 0.754, df 0.38).

Table 1. Distribution of new cases by period and by age group.

Period	Age (Years)		
	≤4 Years	5–9 Years	≥10 Years
2015–2019	204 (19%)	424 (39%)	456 (42%)
2020–2021	88 (25%)	108 (30%)	163 (45%)

During 2020–2021, the number of DKA cases increased significantly by 12% (95% CI: 7.2 to 20.4%) (Figures 1 and 2). In this period, 48% of new-onset cases presented DKA (26% mild, 38% moderate, and 36% severe), whereas during the 2015–2019 period, a lower percentage of DKA was reported, 36% (33% mild, 32% moderate, and 34% severe). A higher percentage of moderate and severe DKA cases were seen in this period, although this increase was not significant (Figure 2).

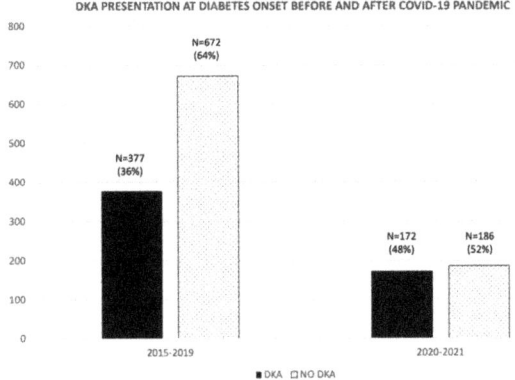

Figure 1. Percentage of DKA as a form of presentation during time periods 2015–2019 versus 2020–2021. Episodes are expressed in number and percentage (%).

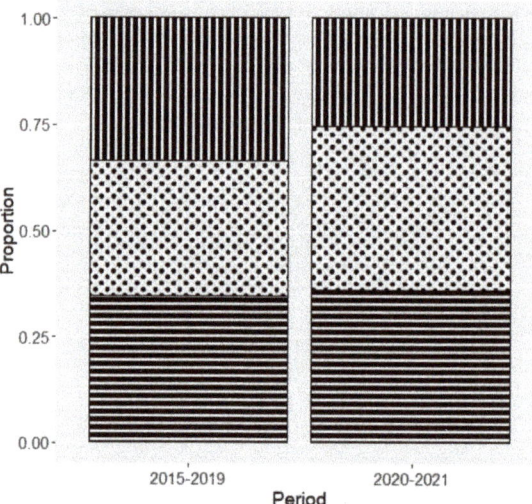

Figure 2. Proportion of cases by DKA severity during periods 2015–2019 and 2020–2021. Each square represents DKA severity cases. Squares filled with vertical black bars represent mild cases; Squares with black dots represent moderate cases. Squares filled with horizontal black bars represent severe cases.

The monthly distribution of new type 1 diabetes cases, as well as cases with DKA as a form of presentation, are shown in Figure 3. From 2015 to 2019, a dip in the number of cases from March through September was noted. In 2020, a sharp decrease in the number of cases diagnosed in March was observed, with an ulterior progressive increase from May through November, which was higher than in the same months of the period 2015–2019, with a notable increase in the number of cases during the months of June, September, and November. The first three months of 2021 showed a very different trend than the observed during the period 2015–2019 and in 2020, respectively, with a marked increase in the number of cases (Figure 3).

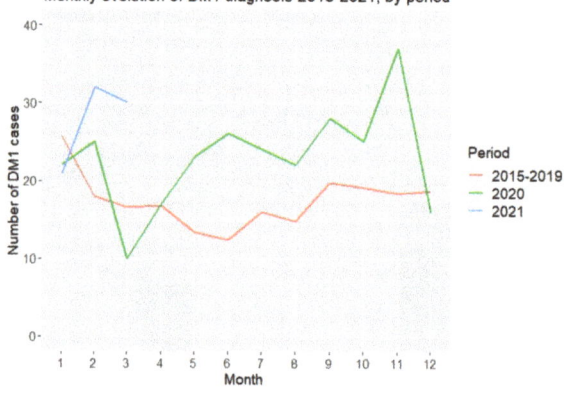

Figure 3. Monthly distribution of newly diagnosed type 1 diabetes cases by periods. Black line represents the cases by month for the period 2015–2019. Dotted line represents the cases by month during the year 2020. Dashed line represents the cases during the months of January, February, and March 2021.

4. Discussion

The COVID-19 pandemic has had a major impact on our society, generating changes that may have influenced the epidemiological situation of other diseases such as the onset of type 1 diabetes. Our study describes an increase in cases of new-onset type 1 diabetes with DKA presentation in children and adolescents under 14 years of age in the period 2020–2021, following the declaration of the COVID-19 pandemic by the WHO, compared to previous years. No differences in severity were found over the entire 2020–2021 period. This differs from observations made by other authors from Germany, Italy, Australia, and Canada during the first months after the start of the pandemic [6–13] who described an increase in moderate and severe forms of DKA. The fact that the first descriptions in this regard refer to periods immediately after lockdown may have conditioned these findings due to delayed use of health care during the beginning of the pandemic and the initial restrictions. We can speculate that this finding may lay on the fact that many patients delay or avoid visits to hospitals due to fear of getting infected with SARS-CoV-2. We can also speculate with a higher awareness of diabetes onset symptoms among primary care pediatricians from Spain that was quickly reinforced by the announcement of the International Society for Pediatric and Adolescent Diabetes (ISPAD) statement on COVID-19 and the increased risk of developing severe forms of DKA at onset [20] may have influenced this fact.

We also found significant differences in the distribution by age group, with an increase in 2020–2021 of children diagnosed under 4 years of age. A study carried out in Germany showed a significant increase in both the incidence of type 1 diabetes and severe forms of DKA, with these results being more striking in children under 6 years of age [7]. The latter leads us to consider that SARS-CoV-2 may potentially be acting as a trigger for the autoimmune destruction which accelerates the process rather than inflicting direct damage to the beta cell, as younger age groups tend to have a more rapid and intense beta cell loss [21]. In addition, we can hypothesize that a modification in the presentation pattern of other seasonal infective agents, such as syncytial respiratory virus of flu due to the pandemic, may be altering the diabetes age at diagnosis.

A study conducted by the Italian Society of Pediatric Endocrinology and Diabetes assessing the epidemiological change during the Italian lockdown (20 February to 14 April 2020), in comparison with the same period in 2019, observed a decrease in the incidence of type 1 diabetes in the confinement period, with the overall incidence being similar in both years [9]. A subsequent analysis, limited to the Lombardy region [13], which included the presentation of new-onset cases during 2020, reported an increase in the number of cases with respect to 2017 and 2018 but not 2019. An evaluation of the monthly distribution in our data shows a different distribution in both 2020 and 2021, which does not correspond to the monthly distribution of recent years in Spain. In the second quarter of 2020, coinciding with the lockdown period in Spain, there was a striking decrease in the number of cases in the months of March and April. These results are aligned with those from Germany, Italy, and Finland [9,12,17]. In contrast, there was an increase from May to November 2020. This rapid recovery of new-onset cases was both due to an interruption of the plateau of cases that usually occur during the summer months and a peak of the occurrence of new cases at the end of the year. This phenomenon has been also described more recently by Kamrath et al. in the DPV registry [22].

For the first quarter of 2021, our data show an increase in the expected number of cases in this period with respect to previous years. We cannot determine whether this increase in the actual number of cases in the first quarter of 2021 is the result of an increase in incidence or whether it is due to a change in monthly distribution as observed in previous months. We can speculate that impact that different COVID waves and associated protective measures may be having in terms of altering other seasonal infections such as flu, respiratory syncytial virus, rhinovirus, or coxsackie, would play a role in these epidemiological abnormalities observed for new diabetes cases. It is still unclear the involvement of COVID in the genesis or progression of type 1 diabetes. A recent report by the. Centers for Disease Control and Prevention (CDC) of the US reported that persons under 18 y with COVID-19 were more likely to receive a new diabetes diagnosis >30 days after the infection than were those without COVID-19 and those with pre-pandemic acute respiratory infections [23].

A limitation of our study is that we cannot provide incidence rates. The representative sample limited to nine tertiary-level hospitals in Spain showed an increase in DKA as a form of presentation, with a higher presentation in children under 4 years of age and changes in the monthly distribution. In addition, our study collects cases only under the age of 14 years old as the majority of pediatric diabetes centers in Spain take care of patients up to this age group. This might be responsible for the differences observed in the findings of other European countries such as Italy or Germany. Further studies are needed to determine whether these epidemiological changes are directly related to SARS-CoV-2, with the modification of hygiene measures, or other factors that are not being considered at the present time.

In conclusion, a change in monthly distribution was noted, as well as an increase in DKA at onset of type 1 diabetes without differences in DKA severity during the first year after the pandemic commencement. Differences in age distribution were observed with an increase in the number of cases in children under 4 years of age. The final causes of these epidemiological changes remain unknown.

Author Contributions: I.L.-G. designed the study, collected data, participated in data interpretation, and wrote the manuscript. R.C.-H. collected data, participated in data interpretation, reviewed, and edited the manuscript. J.P.S. collected data, participated in data interpretation, reviewed the manuscript, and contributed to the statistical analysis. C.A.F., M.F.L., P.B.-C., J.A.-D., M.C.L., M.M.-F., S.C.B. and A.M.D. collected cases, participated in data interpretation, and reviewed the manuscript. All coauthors approved the final version of the manuscript. I.L.-G. is the guarantor of this work and, as such, had full access to all the data in the study and takes responsibility for the integrity of the data and the accuracy of the data analysis. All authors have read and agreed to the published version of the manuscript.

Funding: This research received no external funding.

Informed Consent Statement: Patient consent was waived due to the use of anonymized data from local registries.

Acknowledgments: We are thankful for the following individuals for their support of this work: Emilio Sanchez-Cantalejo, Julia Sanchez-Cantalejo, Maria Repice, and Ines Mulero Collantes.

Conflicts of Interest: The authors declare no conflict of interest.

References

1. Barreiro, S.C.; Rodríguez, M.R.; Lozano, G.B.; Siguero, J.L.; Pelegrín, B.G.; Val, M.R.; Dea, M.L. Epidemiología de la diabetes mellitus tipo 1 en menores de 15 años en España. *An. Pediatr.* **2014**, *81*, 189.e1–189.e12.
2. Nóvoa Medina, Y. Evolución de la incidencia de la diabetes mellitus tipo 1 en edad pediátrica en España. *Endocrinol. Diabetes Nutr.* **2018**, *65*, 65–67. [CrossRef] [PubMed]
3. Spiteri, G.; Fielding, J.; Diercke, M.; Campese, C.; Enouf, V.; Gaymard, A.; Bella, A.; Sognamiglio, P.; Moros, M.J.S.; Riutort, A.N.; et al. First cases of coronavirus disease 2019 (COVID-19) in the WHO European Region, 24 January to 21 February 2020. *Eurosurveillance* **2020**, *25*, 2000178. [CrossRef] [PubMed]
4. Khunti, K.; Del Prato, S.; Mathieu, C.; Kahn, S.E.; Gabbay, R.A.; Buse, J.B. COVID-19, Hyperglycemia, and New-Onset Diabetes. *Diabetes Care* **2021**, *44*, 2645–2655. [CrossRef]
5. Boddu, S.K.; Aurangabadkar, G.; Kuchay, M.S. New onset diabetes, type 1 diabetes and COVID-19. *Diabetes Metab. Syndr. Clin. Res. Rev.* **2020**, *14*, 2211–2217. [CrossRef] [PubMed]
6. Unsworth, R.; Wallace, S.; Oliver, N.S.; Yeung, S.; Kshirsagar, A.; Naidu, H.; Kwong, R.M.W.; Kumar, P.; Logan, K.M. New-Onset Type 1 Diabetes in Children During COVID-19: Multicenter Regional Findings in the UK. *Diabetes Care* **2020**, *43*, e170–e171. [CrossRef] [PubMed]
7. Kamrath, C.; Mönkemöller, K.; Biester, T.; Rohrer, T.R.; Warncke, K.; Hammersen, J.; Holl, R.W. Ketoacidosis in Children and Adolescents with Newly Diagnosed Type 1 Diabetes during the COVID-19 Pandemic in Germany. *JAMA* **2020**, *324*, 801. [CrossRef] [PubMed]
8. Güemes, M.; Storch-de-Gracia, P.; Enriquez, S.V.; Martín-Rivada, Á.; Brabin, A.G.; Argente, J. Severity in pediatric type 1 diabetes mellitus debut during the COVID-19 pandemic. *J. Pediatr. Endocrinol. Metab.* **2020**, *33*, 1601–1603. [CrossRef]

9. Rabbone, I.; Schiaffini, R.; Cherubini, V.; Maffeis, C.; Scaramuzza, A.; The Diabetes Study Group of the Italian Society for Pediatric Endocrinology and Diabetes. Has COVID-19 Delayed the Diagnosis and Worsened the Presentation of Type 1 Diabetes in Children? *Diabetes Care* **2020**, *43*, 2870–2872. [CrossRef]
10. Lawrence, C.; Seckold, R.; Smart, C.; King, B.R.; Howley, P.; Feltrin, R.; Smith, T.A.; Roy, R.; Lopez, P. Increased paediatric presentations of severe diabetic ketoacidosis in an Australian tertiary centre during the COVID-19 pandemic. *Diabet. Med.* **2021**, *38*, e14417. [CrossRef]
11. Ho, J.; Rosolowsky, E.; Pacaud, D.; Huang, C.; Lemay, J.; Brockman, N.; Rath, M.; Doulla, M. Diabetic ketoacidosis at type 1 diabetes diagnosis in children during the COVID-19 pandemic. *Pediatr. Diabetes* **2021**, *22*, 552–557. [CrossRef]
12. Salmi, H.; Heinonen, S.; Hästbacka, J.; Lääperi, M.; Rautiainen, P.; Miettinen, P.J.; Vapalahti, O.; Hepojoki, J.; Knip, M. New-onset type 1 diabetes in Finnish children during the COVID-19 pandemic. *Arch. Dis. Child.* **2021**, *107*, 180–185. [CrossRef]
13. Mameli, C.; Scaramuzza, A.; Macedoni, M.; Marano, G.; Frontino, G.; Luconi, E.; Pelliccia, C.; Felappi, B.; Guerraggio, L.P.; Spiri, D.; et al. Type 1 diabetes onset in Lombardy region, Italy, during the COVID-19 pandemic: The double-wave occurrence. *EClinicalMedicine* **2021**, *39*, 101067. [CrossRef]
14. Vlad, A.; Serban, V.; Timar, R.; Sima, A.; Botea, V.; Albai, O.; Timar, B.; Vlad, M. Increased Incidence of Type 1 Diabetes during the COVID-19 Pandemic in Romanian Children. *Medicina* **2021**, *57*, 973. [CrossRef]
15. Gottesman, B.L.; Yu, J.; Tanaka, C.; Longhurst, C.A.; Kim, J.J. Incidence of New-Onset Type 1 Diabetes among US Children during the COVID-19 Global Pandemic. *JAMA Pediatr.* **2022**, *176*, 414. [CrossRef]
16. Kamrath, C.; Rosenbauer, J.; Eckert, A.J.; Pappa, A.; Reschke, F.; Rohrer, T.R.; Mönkemöller, K.; Wurm, M.; Hake, K.; Raile, K.; et al. Incidence of COVID-19 and Risk of Diabetic Ketoacidosis in New-Onset Type 1 Diabetes. *Pediatrics* **2021**, *148*, e2021050856. [CrossRef]
17. Tittel, S.R.; Rosenbauer, J.; Kamrath, C.; Ziegler, J.; Reschke, F.; Hammersen, J.; Mönkemöller, K.; Pappa, A.; Kapellen, T.; Holl, R.W. Did the COVID-19 Lockdown Affect the Incidence of Pediatric Type 1 Diabetes in Germany? *Diabetes Care* **2020**, *43*, e172–e173. [CrossRef]
18. American Diabetes Association Professional Practice Committee. 6. Glycemic Targets: Standards of Medical Care in Diabetes—2022. *Diabetes Care* **2022**, *45* (Suppl. S1), S83–S96. [CrossRef]
19. Wolfsdorf, J.I.; Glaser, N.; Agus, M.; Fritsch, M.; Hanas, R.; Rewers, A.; Sperling, M.A.; Codner, E. ISPAD Clinical Practice Consensus Guidelines 2018: Diabetic ketoacidosis and the hyperglycemic hyperosmolar state. *Pediatr. Diabetes* **2018**, *19*, 155–177. [CrossRef]
20. ISPAD: Summary of Recommendations Regarding COVID-19 in Children with Diabetes. Available online: https://www.ispad.org/page/COVID-19inchildrenwithdiabetesResources (accessed on 29 April 2020).
21. Leete, P.; Oram, R.A.; McDonald, T.J.; Shields, B.M.; Ziller, C.; Hattersley, A.T.; Richardson, S.J.; Morgan, N.G.; TIGI Study Team. Studies of insulin and proinsulin in pancreas and serum support the existence of aetiopathological endotypes of type 1 diabetes associated with age at diagnosis. *Diabetologia* **2020**, *63*, 1258–1267. [CrossRef]
22. Kamrath, C.; Rosenbauer, J.; Eckert, A.J.; Siedler, K.; Bartelt, H.; Klose, D.; Sindichakis, M.; Herrlinger, S.; Lahn, V.; Holl, R.W. Incidence of Type 1 Diabetes in Children and Adolescents during the COVID-19 Pandemic in Germany: Results from the DPV Registry. *Diabetes Care* **2022**. Online ahead of print. [CrossRef] [PubMed]
23. Barrett, C.E.; Koyama, A.K.; Alvarez, P.; Chow, W.; Lundeen, E.A.; Perrine, C.G.; Pavkov, M.E.; Rolka, D.B.; Wiltz, J.L.; Bull-Otterson, L. Risk for Newly Diagnosed Diabetes >30 Days after SARS-CoV-2 Infection among Persons Aged <18 Years—United States, 1 March 2020–28 June 2021. *MMWR Morb. Mortal Wkly Rep.* **2022**, *71*, 59–65. [PubMed]

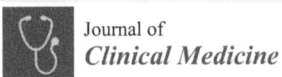

Article

Comparison of Glycemic Variability and Hypoglycemic Events in Hospitalized Older Adults Treated with Basal Insulin plus Vildagliptin and Basal–Bolus Insulin Regimen: A Prospective Randomized Study

Sol Batule [1,†], Analía Ramos [1,†], Alejandra Pérez-Montes de Oca [1], Natalia Fuentes [1], Santiago Martínez [1], Joan Raga [2], Xoel Pena [2], Cristina Tural [2], Pilar Muñoz [2], Berta Soldevila [1], Nuria Alonso [1], Guillermo Umpierrez [3] and Manel Puig-Domingo [1,*]

[1] Servicio de Endocrinología y Nutrición, Hospital Germans Trias i Pujol, 08916 Badalona, Spain; sol_batule@hotmail.com (S.B.); aeramos.germanstrias@gencat.cat (A.R.); alec148@gmail.com (A.P.-M.d.O.); natfuente@hotmail.com (N.F.); santiagomartinezag@gmail.com (S.M.); soldevila.berta@gmail.com (B.S.); nalonso32416@yahoo.es (N.A.)
[2] Servicio de Medicina Interna, Hospital Germans Trias i Pujol, 08916 Badalona, Spain; jragaa.germanstrias@gencat.cat (J.R.); xpenape.germanstrias@gencat.cat (X.P.); ctural.germanstrias@gencat.cat (C.T.); mpmunozr.germanstrias@gencat.cat (P.M.)
[3] Department of Medicine, Emory University, Atlanta, GA 30322, USA; geumpie@emory.edu
* Correspondence: mpuigd@igtp.cat; Tel.: +34-93-497-88-60
† These authors contributed equally to this work.

Abstract: Background: The basal–bolus insulin regimen is recommended in hospitalized patients with diabetes mellitus (DM), but has an increased risk of hypoglycemia. We aimed to compare dipeptidyl peptidase 4 inhibitors (DPP4-i) and basal–bolus insulin glycemic outcomes in hospitalized type 2 DM patients. Methods and patients: Our prospective randomized study included 102 elderly T2DM patients (82 ± 9 years, HbA1c 6.6% ± 1.9). Glycemic control: A variability coefficient assessed by continuous glucose monitoring (Free Style® sensor), mean insulin dose and hypoglycemia rates obtained with the two treatments were analyzed. Results: No differences were found between groups in glycemic control (mean daily glycemia during the first 10 days: 152.6 ± 38.5 vs. 154.2 ± 26.3 mg/dL; p = 0.8). The total doses Kg/day were 0.40 vs. 0.20, respectively (p < 0.001). A lower number of hypoglycemic events (9% vs. 15%; p < 0.04) and lower glycemic coefficient of variation (22% vs. 28%; p < 0.0002) were observed in the basal–DPP4-i compared to the basal–bolus regimen group. Conclusions: Treatment of inpatient hyperglycemia with basal insulin plus DPP4-i is an effective and safe regimen in old subjects with T2DM, with a similar mean daily glucose concentration, but lower glycemic variability and fewer hypoglycemic episodes compared to the basal bolus insulin regimen.

Keywords: diabetes mellitus; vildagliptin; inpatient hyperglycaemia; older adults

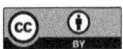

1. Introduction

Hyperglycemia is a frequent finding in hospitalized patients (12.4–25%) [1]. Remarkably, more than 30% of patients with hyperglycemia detected during a hospitalization episode do not have a previous diagnosis of diabetes mellitus (DM) [2]. Hyperglycemia in hospitalized patients was consistently associated with a poor prognosis, especially in patients without a known history of diabetes [2]. A lack of adequate control of glycemia during hospitalization leads to a longer in-hospital stay, an increased incidence of infections and more hospital complications than patients without DM [1,3], which accounts for an increased necessity of healthcare resources in these patients [4,5].

Currently, different scientific societies recommend the administration of subcutaneous insulin as the treatment of choice for glycemic control in non-critical hospitalized patients using a basal–bolus regime [4,6,7]. Treatment with oral hypoglycemic agents in this context is discouraged due to theoretical limitations regarding their effectiveness and safety. Among them, a slow onset of action and, for some oral agents, a long duration of action were found, implying an insufficient flexibility to adapt to quickly changing requirements throughout the day and to other circumstances, such as fasting requirements associated with medical therapeutic and exploratory procedures [1,8]. In addition to these potential inconveniences, there are some limitations of efficacy and safety in hospitalized patients with type 2 DM (T2DM) regarding the number of randomized studies with oral drugs, which have conditioned its full implementation as a standard of care.

Several recent randomized trials demonstrated the potential effectiveness of dipeptidyl peptidase 4 inhibitors (DPP4-i) in specific groups of hospitalized patients. DPP4-i are well-tolerated oral drugs that demonstrated their efficacy and safety in association with other oral hypoglycemic agents and/or insulin [9]. DPP4-i do not cause hypoglycemia or weight gain, nor do they present significant drug interactions, which make them a very attractive therapeutic option for the treatment of T2DM, particularly in the elderly. Among this group of antidiabetic oral agents, there is currently only one safety study in subjects older than 75 years, performed with vildagliptin to support its use in elderly patients [10].

With the aim of simplifying and facilitating the implementation of an effective and safe treatment for hospital hyperglycemia, Umpierrez et al. recently published the results of an alternative to a basal–bolus regime for patients with T2DM admitted to non-critical units (conventional hospitalization). This regime is based on the administration of a daily dose of basal insulin and a single dose of the DPP4-i sitagliptin (Sita-Hospital study) [11]. The results of the study showed a non-inferiority efficacy in relation to a full regime of insulin. Similar findings were reported in a study of non-cardiac surgical and medical patients with T2DM, in which linagliptin was used [12,13].

Glycemic variability (GV) was proposed as a novel marker of glycemic control [14,15]. A large multicenter study concluded that GV was a much stronger predictor of intensive care unit (ICU) mortality than mean glucose concentrations [16]. The coefficient of variation (CV) was also demonstrated as a strong independent index for measuring GV as it corrects for mean glucose levels [17–19].

The aim of the present study was to compare the efficacy, safety and glycemic variability outcomes of a combined basal–DPP4-i regime compared to a conventional basal–bolus insulin regimen in internal medicine patients with T2DM.

2. Materials and Methods

A prospective randomized study was set up in a tertiary university Hospital Germans Trias i Pujol, in Badalona, Spain, in which a total of 102 patients were included (Figure 1).

Patients with T2DM aged $\geq$65 years old, for whom all of the following concurrent conditions were present, were included in the study: (1) plasma glycemia on admission at less than 400 mg/dL and (2) treatment at home with any combination of oral antidiabetic drugs or with insulin therapy at a daily dose less 0.6 IU/Kg/day. Exclusion criteria were any of the following: (1) HbA1c >9%, (2) glycaemia at admission $\geq$400 mg/dL, (3) treatment with glucocorticoids (dose >5 mg/day of prednisone or equivalent), (4) previous treatment with insulin at a total daily dose $\geq$0.6 IU/Kg, and (5) any of the following active clinical situations or previous antecedents: acute myocardial infarction, acute pancreatitis, diagnosis of type 1 diabetes mellitus and/or hepatic cirrhosis. In all of the latter, the usual basal–bolus regime was administered, and the patients were not included in the study.

All participants provided written informed consent before the start of the protocol. Patients were randomly assigned to one of two treatment regimens according to the side of the room they were hospitalized in (hallway A or hallway B). The dose of insulin was started in both groups based on previous treatment of DM and capillary blood glucose (CBG) concentration at admission as indicated in Supplementary Tables S1–S3. In the basal–bolus group, half of the insulin dose was prescribed as basal insulin (glargine) once daily at bedtime and half as rapid-acting insulin (aspart) divided into three equal doses before meals. For patients in the basal–DPP4-i group, the complete calculated dose of insulin was administered as long-acting analogue once daily at bedtime, and vildagliptin dose was calculated according to GFR: 100 mg/day if GFR $\geq$50 mL/min per 1.73 m^2 and 50 mg/day if GFR <50 mL/min per 1.73 m^2.

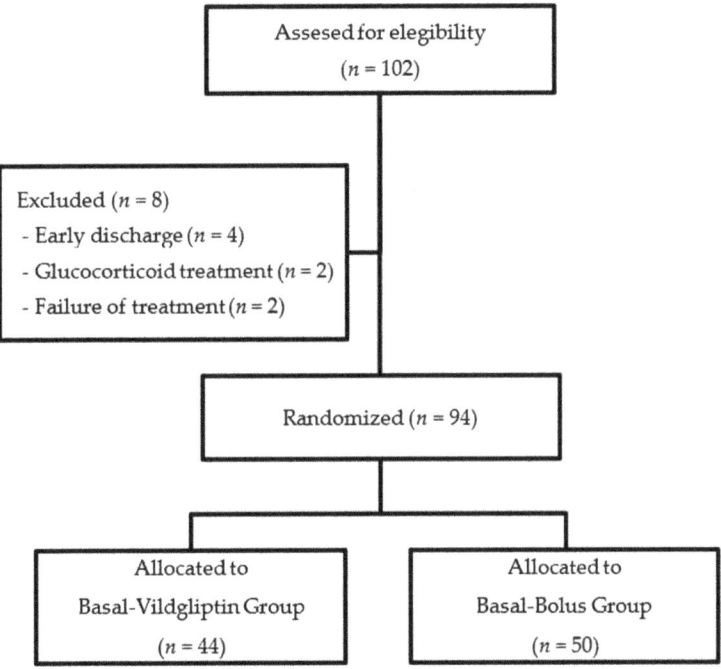

Figure 1. Flowchart of study population.

The goal of the treatment was to maintain glycemic control between 140 and 180 mg/dL. In both groups, CBG was measured before meals and bedtime. In the case of hypoglycemia (defined as grade 1 between 56 and 70 mg/dL, grade 2 < 56 mg/dL and grade 3 < 56 mg/dL plus neuroglycopenia symptoms), insulin treatment was reduced as indicated in Supplementary Tables S1 and S2. If CBG was >300 mg/dL, a correction dose of rapid-acting insulin was administered, as also indicated in Supplementary Table S1. Failure of treatment in the basal–DPP4-i group was defined as CBG > 300 mg/dL in two consecutive measures even after dose upload correction, and in these cases, the patient was switched to a basal–bolus regime.

In a subset of patients (n = 20), a FreeStyle® glycemic sensor was used to assess glycemic variability. Hypoglycemia detected by the sensor was confirmed by a CBG measurement, which was used for therapeutic decisions. The percentages of time in the various glycemic ranges were assessed according to the International Consensus on Time in Range [20] for older/high risk T2DM patients. Hyperglycemia was defined as: grade 1 (>50% of time between 181 and 250 mg/dL) and grade 2 (>10% of time >250 mg/dL). Hypoglycemia in this group was defined as a glycemic level below 70 mg/dL >1% of time. Acceptable time (time in range) in range was defined as >50% of time between 70 and 180 mg/dL.

HbA1c was measured within 24 h of randomization if the patient did not have a determination in the last 3 months. The degree of glycemic control, glycemic CV, mean insulin dose and hypoglycemia rates observed with the two therapeutic modalities were used for statistical analyses.

For the statistical analysis purpose, the first ten days of hospital stay were considered. Continuous variables are presented as mean ± standard deviations (SD). Comparisons between both therapeutic strategies were made using the Student's test for independent samples, the Fisher test or χ^2 (categorical variables). All the statistical analyses were performed with IBM SPSS Statistic software version 26 (IBM Corporation, New York, NY, USA).

3. Results

A total of 102 patients were eligible for the study. Of these, eight patients were excluded (four of them due to early discharge, two due to glucocorticoid treatment initiation after recruitment and two due to the failure of treatment). We analyzed 94 patients, 50 of which were included in the basal–bolus regime and 44 in the basal–DPP4-i regime (Figure 1).

Among all patients, the main reasons for admission were heart failure (30.8%), followed by respiratory infections (20.2%) and non-respiratory infections (16%). The causes for other patients were mostly part of geriatric syndrome and included consumptive syndrome, renal failure, confusional syndrome and falls, although none of them were significantly different regarding their frequency in both treatment arms. Those in the basal–bolus group compared to those in the basal–DPP4-i group, showed significant differences in sex (female 56% vs. 34%, $p = 0.04$, respectively) and weight (71.8 ± 16 Kg vs. 81.3 ± 18 Kg, $p = 0.008$, respectively). No significant differences were observed regarding HbA1c (6.7 ± 1.2% vs. 6.6 ± 0.9%) or any other baseline variable such as age, admission blood glucose, previous outpatient antidiabetic treatment, length of hospital stay and biochemical parameters (Table 1).

Table 1. Baseline characteristics of all the patients.

Variable	Basal–Bolus (n = 50)	Basal–DPP4-i (n = 44)	p-Value
Age (years)	78.2 ± 15	80.5 ± 7	0.35
Gender			
Male, n (%)	22 (44)	29 (66)	0.04 *
Female, n (%)	28 (56)	15 (34)	
Weight	71.8 ± 16	81.3 ± 18	0.008 *
BMI (kg/m^2)	28.53 ± 5.8	30.7 ± 6	0.05
Duration of diabetes (years)	15.4 ± 6	13.6 ± 6	0.13
Admission diabetes therapy			
1 OAD, n (%)	18 (36)	19 (43.2)	
2 or more OAD, n (%)	7 (14)	12 (27.3)	0.91
OAD + basal insulin, n (%)	11 (22)	8 (18.2)	
Basal insulin, n (%)	9 (18)	2 (4.5)	
Basal–bolus ± OAD	4 (8)	2 (4.5)	
Admission blood glucose (mg/dL)	171.9 ± 69	181.5 ± 68	0.5
HbA1c (%)	6.7% ± 1.2	6.6 ± 0.9	0.85
GFR (mL/min/1.73 m^2)	48.8 ± 24	48.1 ± 25	0.87
Length of hospital stay (days)	11.4 ± 9.3	11.9 ± 10	0.78

Abbreviations: OAD, oral antidiabetic agent; HbA1c, glycated hemoglobin, GFR, glomerular filtration rate. * Differences between groups <0.05. Data are mean ± standard deviation.

There were no statistical differences o → n any day of mean blood glucose measurements during the study period between the basal–bolus and basal–vildagliptin groups (157 ± 36.9 mg/dL vs. 145 ± 29.5 mg/dL, $p = 0.103$, respectively) (Figure 2). As expected, the mean basal insulin dose requirements were significantly higher for the basal–bolus group, and a lower number of grade 1 hypoglycemia was observed in the basal–DPP4-i group. Regarding CV, the mean was <36% in both groups, being statistically lower in the basal–vildagliptin group (Table 2).

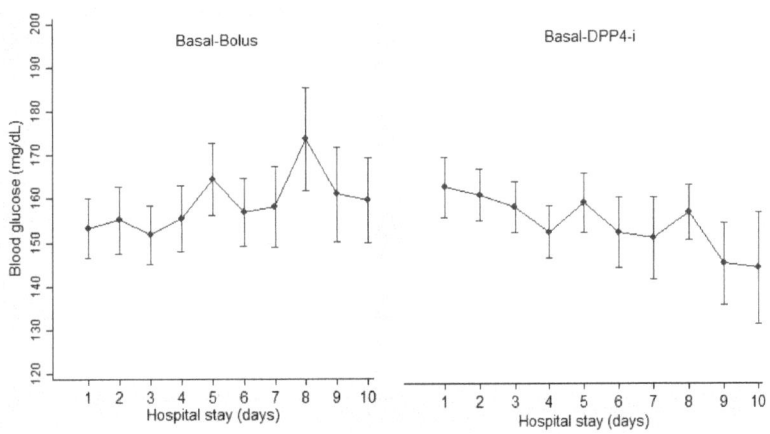

Figure 2. Mean daily blood glucose concentrations during hospital stays. Values are shown as mean ± standard deviations.

Table 2. Variables associated with glycemic control.

Variable	Basal–Bolus (n = 40)	Basal–Vildagliptin (n = 34)	p-Value
Mean CBG	157 ± 36.9	145 ± 29.5	0.103
Insulin dose			
Total mean insulin dose, IU/day	29.1 ± 11.8	15.3 ± 5.1	0.001 *
Total mean insulin dose, IU/kg/day	0.4 ± 0.17	0.2 ± 0.1	<0.001 *
Total glargine insulin dose, IU/day	14.1 ± 6	15.4 ± 5.1	0.105
Total aspart insulin dose, IU/day	14.4 ± 7.6	-	-
Hypoglycaemic events			
Patients with any blood glucose < 70 mg/dL, n (%)	8 (20)	1 (3.4)	0.023 *
Patients with any blood glucose < 54 mg/dL, n (%)	1 (2.5)	-	-
Hyperglycaemic events			
BG > 180 mg/dL, n (%)	10 (25)	5 (14.7)	0.386
CV (%)	28	22	<0.001 *

Abbreviations: CBG, capillary blood glucose; BG, blood glucose; CV, coefficient of variation. * Differences between groups <0.05. Data are mean ± standard deviation.

In patients who used the FreeStyle® glycemic sensor, when comparing the basal–bolus group with the basal–vildagliptin group, we found no statistical differences in glycemic parameters, with a mean interstitial glycemia of 157 ± 43.6 mg/dL vs. 132 ± 23.8 mg/dL (p = 0.133), time in range 74.3 ± 18.8% vs. 82.3 ± 17.7% (p = 0.341), and CV 29.2 ± 6.8% vs. 23.7 ± 3.8% (p = 0.135). In both groups, there was no grade 1 hyperglycemia. Grade 2 hyperglycemia was found in two patients in the basal–bolus group and one patient in the basal–vildagliptin group. Hypoglycemia events were present in four patients in the basal–bolus group and in two patients in the basal–vildagliptin group.

4. Discussion

The present study confirms the feasibility of implementing an easier, safer and equally effective treatment modality using basal insulin plus DPP4-i, compared to the classic basal–bolus insulin regimen for the management of hyperglycemia in hospitalized older adults. In addition to demonstrating that good glycemic control can be achieved with both treatment modalities with a mean glycemic value of about 150 mg/dL, our study indicates that the number of hypoglycemic episodes is lower, less intense and particularly fewer in absolute terms with a basal–DPP4-i combination compared to a basal–bolus regimen. Moreover, the glycemic variability was lower with basal–DPP4-i treatment.

Hypoglycemia has serious consequences in terms of hospital outcomes, in-hospital length of stay, and in general, it increases the health resources consumed in one hospital episode stay. Hypoglycemia was associated with cardiovascular events, myocardial infarction and stroke due to the impact of the sharp increase in circulating catecholamines induced by the decrease in glycemic circulating levels [21]. In addition, it has recently been confirmed that glycemic variability is a very important treatment target in every diabetic patient. Consistent data indicate that glycemic variability is associated with increased oxidative stress [22] and other deleterious biologic processes that affect general health, particularly in older adults admitted with cardiovascular or infectious episodes.

In addition to efficacy and safety issues, this alternative regime using DPP4-i is more convenient for the patient and the nursing staff who provide care in hospital conventional beds. The decrease in insulin injections per se, as well as the advantage of the non-activity of DPP4-i molecules at low–normal glycemic levels, provides comfortability and safety in old and frail patients who may be unable to complete their intake of a given hospital meal due to increased anorexia or inappetence for hospital food.

The present study has some weaknesses, including a relative low number of subjects and a small subsample of patients using continuous glucose monitoring. In addition, the group of previously studied patients had an overall good control according to the HbA1c value at hospital entry. However, as for the potential strengths of the present study, the prototype of the included patients was typical of those mostly admitted in the hospital. In this regard, it seems logical that patients with relatively well-controlled DM did not require heavy dosing with a full basal–bolus insulin regimen, which in fact may be more harmful than a single dose of long-acting insulin plus a DPP4-i for covering the prandial glycemia in a patient with an otherwise reasonable beta cell reserve. Additionally, the single-center nature of our study warranted the homogeneity of the procedures and patient inclusion.

5. Conclusions

The basal–bolus insulin therapy regimen remains a useful treatment for many inpatients, especially those with symptomatic hyperglycemia, poor glycemic control prior to admission, and those who fail to maintain glucose control with basal insulin, plus DPP4-i. However, the high rate of hypoglycemia represents a major limitation, and the active daily review of insulin dosage is mandatory, which is quite time consuming and requires certain expertise. Our results indicate that an alternative regime with the combination of basal insulin plus DPP4-I, was effective and safer than a basal–bolus regime as less hypoglycemic episodes were detected and with the added value of reduced glycemic variability in older well-controlled diabetic patients. Moreover, improved convenience for patients and the nursing staff may contribute to recommending this kind of treatment modality as the standard of care for controlling inpatient glycemia in most of adults with type 2 diabetes.

Supplementary Materials: The following supporting information can be downloaded at: https://www.mdpi.com/article/10.3390/jcm11102813/s1, Table S1: Treatment regime glargine-DPP4i group; Table S2: Treatment regim basal-bolus group and Table S3: Aspart insulin scale.

Author Contributions: S.B. and A.R. collected data, performed the statistical analysis and interpretation and drafted the manuscript. A.P.-M.d.O., N.F., S.M., J.R., X.P., C.T., P.M. and B.S. collected data, contributed to the interpretation and provided input to the manuscript. N.A., G.U. and M.P.-D. designed the study, performed the statistical analysis and interpretation, and provided input to the manuscript. All authors have read and agreed to the published version of the manuscript.

Funding: This research received no external funding.

Institutional Review Board Statement: All procedures performed in studies involving human participants were in accordance with the ethical standards of the institutional and/or national research committee (PI-19-236) and with the 1964 Helsinki declaration and its later amendments or comparable ethical standards.

Informed Consent Statement: Written informed consent was obtained from the patient(s) to publish this paper.

Data Availability Statement: The data are available from the corresponding author on request.

Conflicts of Interest: The authors declare no conflict of interest.

References

1. Clement, S.; Braithwaite, S.S.; Magee, M.F.; Ahmann, A.; Smith, E.P.; Schafer, R.G.; Hirsch, I.B.; Hirsh, I.B. American Diabetes Association Diabetes in Hospitals Writing Committee Management of Diabetes and Hyperglycemia in Hospitals. *Diabetes Care* **2004**, *27*, 553–591. [CrossRef] [PubMed]
2. Umpierrez, G.E.; Isaacs, S.D.; Bazargan, N.; You, X.; Thaler, L.M.; Kitabchi, A.E. Hyperglycemia: An Independent Marker of in-Hospital Mortality in Patients with Undiagnosed Diabetes. *J. Clin. Endocrinol. Metab.* **2002**, *87*, 978–982. [CrossRef] [PubMed]
3. Umpierrez, G.E.; Smiley, D.; Jacobs, S.; Peng, L.; Temponi, A.; Mulligan, P.; Umpierrez, D.; Newton, C.; Olson, D.; Rizzo, M. Randomized Study of Basal-Bolus Insulin Therapy in the Inpatient Management of Patients with Type 2 Diabetes Undergoing General Surgery (RABBIT 2 Surgery). *Diabetes Care* **2011**, *34*, 256–261. [CrossRef] [PubMed]
4. Moghissi, E.S.; Korytkowski, M.T.; DiNardo, M.; Einhorn, D.; Hellman, R.; Hirsch, I.B.; Inzucchi, S.E.; Ismail-Beigi, F.; Kirkman, M.S.; Umpierrez, G.E.; et al. American Association of Clinical Endocrinologists and American Diabetes Association Consensus Statement on Inpatient Glycemic Control. *Endocr. Pract.* **2009**, *15*, 353–369. [CrossRef]
5. Kyi, M.; Colman, P.G.; Wraight, P.R.; Reid, J.; Gorelik, A.; Galligan, A.; Kumar, S.; Rowan, L.M.; Marley, K.A.; Nankervis, A.J.; et al. Early Intervention for Diabetes in Medical and Surgical Inpatients Decreases Hyperglycemia and Hospital-Acquired Infections: A Cluster Randomized Trial. *Diabetes Care* **2019**, *42*, 832–840. [CrossRef]
6. Umpierrez, G.E.; Hellman, R.; Korytkowski, M.T.; Kosiborod, M.; Maynard, G.A.; Montori, V.M.; Seley, J.J.; Van den Berghe, G. Endocrine Society Management of Hyperglycemia in Hospitalized Patients in Non-Critical Care Setting: An Endocrine Society Clinical Practice Guideline. *J. Clin. Endocrinol. Metab.* **2012**, *97*, 16–38. [CrossRef]
7. Diabetes Care in the Hospital: Standards of Medical Care in Diabetes—2021. Diabetes Care. Available online: https://care.diabetesjournals.org/content/44/Supplement_1/S211 (accessed on 10 August 2021).
8. Kodner, C.; Anderson, L.; Pohlgeers, K. Glucose Management in Hospitalized Patients. *Am. Fam. Physician* **2017**, *96*, 648–654.
9. Kothny, W.; Lukashevich, V.; Foley, J.E.; Rendell, M.S.; Schweizer, A. Comparison of Vildagliptin and Sitagliptin in Patients with Type 2 Diabetes and Severe Renal Impairment: A Randomised Clinical Trial. *Diabetologia* **2015**, *58*, 2020–2026. [CrossRef]
10. Schweizer, A.; Dejager, S.; Foley, J.E.; Shao, Q.; Kothny, W. Clinical Experience with Vildagliptin in the Management of Type 2 Diabetes in a Patient Population ≥75 Years: A Pooled Analysis from a Database of Clinical Trials. *Diabetes Obes. Metab.* **2011**, *13*, 55–64. [CrossRef]
11. Pasquel, F.J.; Gianchandani, R.; Rubin, D.J.; Dungan, K.M.; Anzola, I.; Gomez, P.C.; Peng, L.; Hodish, I.; Bodnar, T.; Wesorick, D.; et al. Efficacy of Sitagliptin for the Hospital Management of General Medicine and Surgery Patients with Type 2 Diabetes (Sita-Hospital): A Multicentre, Prospective, Open-Label, Non-Inferiority Randomised Trial. *Lancet Diabetes Endocrinol.* **2017**, *5*, 125–133. [CrossRef]
12. Pérez-Belmonte, L.M.; Osuna-Sánchez, J.; Millán-Gómez, M.; López-Carmona, M.D.; Gómez-Doblas, J.J.; Cobos-Palacios, L.; Sanz-Cánovas, J.; Barbancho, M.A.; Lara, J.P.; Jiménez-Navarro, M.; et al. Glycaemic Efficacy and Safety of Linagliptin for the Management of Non-Cardiac Surgery Patients with Type 2 Diabetes in a Real-World Setting: Lina-Surg Study. *Ann. Med.* **2019**, *51*, 252–261. [CrossRef] [PubMed]

13. Pérez-Belmonte, L.M.; Gómez-Doblas, J.J.; Millán-Gómez, M.; López-Carmona, M.D.; Guijarro-Merino, R.; Carrasco-Chinchilla, F.; de Teresa-Galván, E.; Jiménez-Navarro, M.; Bernal-López, M.R.; Gómez-Huelgas, R. Use of Linagliptin for the Management of Medicine Department Inpatients with Type 2 Diabetes in Real-World Clinical Practice (Lina-Real-World Study). *J. Clin. Med.* **2018**, *7*, 271. [CrossRef] [PubMed]
14. Braithwaite, S.S. Glycemic Variability in Hospitalized Patients: Choosing Metrics While Awaiting the Evidence. *Curr. Diab. Rep.* **2013**, *13*, 138–154. [CrossRef] [PubMed]
15. Monnier, L.; Colette, C.; Owens, D.R. Glycemic Variability: The Third Component of the Dysglycemia in Diabetes. Is It Important? How to Measure It? *J. Diabetes Sci. Technol.* **2008**, *2*, 1094–1100. [CrossRef]
16. Egi, M.; Bellomo, R.; Stachowski, E.; French, C.J.; Hart, G. Variability of Blood Glucose Concentration and Short-Term Mortality in Critically Ill Patients. *Anesthesiology* **2006**, *105*, 244–252. [CrossRef]
17. Siegelaar, S.E.; Holleman, F.; Hoekstra, J.B.L.; DeVries, J.H. Glucose Variability; Does It Matter? *Endocr. Rev.* **2010**, *31*, 171–182. [CrossRef]
18. Rodbard, D. Clinical Interpretation of Indices of Quality of Glycemic Control and Glycemic Variability. *Postgrad. Med.* **2011**, *123*, 107–118. [CrossRef]
19. Mendez, C.E.; Mok, K.-T.; Ata, A.; Tanenberg, R.J.; Calles-Escandon, J.; Umpierrez, G.E. Increased Glycemic Variability Is Independently Associated with Length of Stay and Mortality in Noncritically Ill Hospitalized Patients. *Diabetes Care* **2013**, *36*, 4091–4097. [CrossRef]
20. Battelino, T.; Danne, T.; Bergenstal, R.M.; Amiel, S.A.; Beck, R.; Biester, T.; Bosi, E.; Buckingham, B.A.; Cefalu, W.T.; Close, K.L.; et al. Clinical Targets for Continuous Glucose Monitoring Data Interpretation: Recommendations From the International Consensus on Time in Range. *Diabetes Care* **2019**, *42*, 1593–1603. [CrossRef]
21. Kalra, S.; Mukherjee, J.J.; Venkataraman, S.; Bantwal, G.; Shaikh, S.; Saboo, B.; Das, A.K.; Ramachandran, A. Hypoglycemia: The Neglected Complication. *Indian J. Endocrinol. Metab.* **2013**, *17*, 819–834. [CrossRef]
22. Ceriello, A.; Novials, A.; Ortega, E.; La Sala, L.; Pujadas, G.; Testa, R.; Bonfigli, A.R.; Esposito, K.; Giugliano, D. Evidence That Hyperglycemia after Recovery from Hypoglycemia Worsens Endothelial Function and Increases Oxidative Stress and Inflammation in Healthy Control Subjects and Subjects with Type 1 Diabetes. *Diabetes* **2012**, *61*, 2993–2997. [CrossRef] [PubMed]

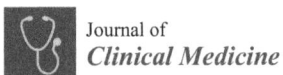

Systematic Review

Prevention of Peripheral Distal Polyneuropathy in Patients with Diabetes: A Systematic Review

Lidia Carvajal-Moreno [1], Manuel Coheña-Jiménez [1,*], Irene García-Ventura [1], Manuel Pabón-Carrasco [2] and Ana Juana Pérez-Belloso [1]

[1] Department of Podiatry, University of Seville, 41009 Seville, Spain; lidiacarvajalmoreno@gmail.com (L.C.-M.); irenepie1999@gmail.com (I.G.-V.); aperez30@us.es (A.J.P.-B.)

[2] Spanish Red Cross Nursing School, University of Seville, Avda. de la Cruz Roja, n° 1 Dpdo., 41009 Seville, Spain; mpabon@cruzroja.es

* Correspondence: mcohena@us.es; Tel.: +34-954-48-60-48

Abstract: Background: Diabetic peripheral neuropathy (DPN) is the most frequent chronic complication and is that which generates the highest disability and mortality in diabetes mellitus (DM). As it is currently the only microvascular complication of DM without a specific treatment, prevention is essential. The aim of this study was to determine the most effective preventive strategy to avoid or delay the appearance and/or development of DPN in patients with DM. Methods: A systematic search was carried out in the main health science databases (PubMed, Scopus, CINAHL, PEDro and The Cochrane Library) from 1 January 2010 to 31 August 2020. The study selection was conducted by two independent reviewers and data extraction was performed by the author. The eligibility criteria included randomized clinical trials (RCTs) and cohort studies from RCTs. Results: Eleven studies were selected that included 23,595 participants with DM. The interventions evaluated were intensive or standard glycemic control, the use of drugs to achieve glycemic control, and the promotion of a healthy lifestyle and exercise. Intensive glucose control achieved a significant reduction in the development of DPN in TIDM patients, and lifestyle modifications and exercise achieved it moderately in TIIDM patients. Conclusions: The main preventive strategy for DPN is intensive glycemic control with a target HbA1c < 6% in patients with TIDM and standard control of 7.0–7.9 in patients with TIIDM, incorporating lifestyle modifications.

Keywords: diabetes mellitus; diabetic complications; diabetic neuropathy; prevention and control; evidence; systematic review

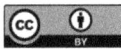

1. Introduction

Diabetic neuropathy (DN) is the most frequent chronic complication in diabetes mellitus (DM) [1–4], and is considered the most important predictor of mortality in patients with type II diabetes (TIIDM), being currently the only microvascular complication of DM without specific treatment [5]. Diabetic peripheral neuropathy (DPN) is the most common cause of diabetic foot complications, with chronic sensorimotor symptoms and signs [1]. There are several forms of DPN. The most common type is distal symmetric polyneuropathy, which causes neuropathic pain symptoms. Atypical forms of DPN include mononeuritis multiplex, radiculopathies, and treatment-induced neuropathies. Other diabetic neuropathies include autonomic neuropathies that affect the cardiovascular, gastrointestinal, and urogenital systems [5,6]. Due to the lack of treatments targeting the underlying nerve damage, prevention is the key component in this complication of DM, and for this reason it is essential to emphasize special attention paid to the feet, as these patients are at risk of injury due to a lack of sensation [6–8].

In this sense, diabetic foot is considered one of the conditions that generates more disability, economic costs in health systems and mortality [9]. It may be considered as a supercomplication of several complications. Thus, patients with DM have a high rate of lower limb amputation, which increases when DN is present, and consequently the risk of foot ulceration is three times higher in patients with DN [10–13]. This complication in the lower extremities can be life-threatening in patients with foot ulceration, and can lead to subsequent infection. In this sense, since most amputations are preceded by foot ulceration, infection must be avoided. More extensive research is necessary for determining more precisely the need for amputation. It is important to avoid non-painful foot injuries by wearing well-fitting footwear and by performing regular inspections [4,6]. Health education is essential. DPN is the most common form of DN; its presentation is slow and progressive, usually distal and symmetrical. There is a progressive loss of sensitivity as well as motor weakness of the affected muscles, and dysfunction of the peripheral nerves of the autonomic nervous system, acting mainly on the lower limbs. Patients often report a sensation of "numb" feet, have altered distal vibratory sensation as well as altered joint position and sensations of tactile pressure and abnormal reflexes [12]. Normally, none of these alterations are painful, although it is reported that up to 25% of these patients may experience symptoms of neuropathic pain. It is described as numbness, paresthesias, hyperesthesias, allodynia, loss of sensation, muscle weakness, or loss of temperature sensation, risk of the complications of diabetic ulceration and non-traumatic amputation [3]. Amputation decisions are determined by patient comorbidities, performance, imaging studies, and clinical examination results [7,8]. In this sense, more extensive research is necessary to determine more precisely the need for amputation.

The most important risk factor for the development of this complication, apart from the duration of the disease, is hyperglycemia [14]. Intensive control is associated with a reduction in the prevalence of DN and painful symptomatology, especially in patients with type I DM (TIDM). In the case of patients with type II DM (TIIDM), good glycemic control is recommended in addition to the control of cardiovascular risk factors and lifestyle modifications [15–19].

Some studies reported that screening for symptoms and signs is very important, as it allows for early diagnosis in the early stages of DN [20]. It is estimated that about half of patients with DM are undiagnosed [21], and it is also established that the group of patients with glucose intolerance and prediabetes may also develop neuropathies, mainly DPN, as this is the most common form of presentation [11]. In addition, it is stated that up to 50% of patients with DPN may be asymptomatic [8]. DPN affects at least 20% of patients with TIDM, 20 years after disease onset, and 10–15% of newly diagnosed patients with TIIDM, increasing to 50% 10 years after diagnosis [20]. Of these patients, 10–15% may develop painful DPN, and symptomatic treatment may be necessary. Painful symptoms, as well as other types of complications derived from DPN, can have a significant impact on the quality of life of these patients. In addition, patients with DM with pain have three times the expenditure on medication, so in this sense, prevention is essential [14], considering that the expenditure on medication is expensive to health systems [1,9].

On the other hand, early diagnosis, prevention and treatment of symptoms help to reduce sequelae, costs and improve the quality of life of patients with DN. Despite a large body of evidence, current medication prescribing patterns are inconsistent. Previous studies reported first-line drugs for the treatment of neuropathic pain in painful DPN, including the α-2-delta subunit voltage-gated calcium channel blockers gabapentin and pregabalin, the selective serotonin and norepinephrine reuptake inhibitors (SNRIs) duloxetine, and the tricyclic antidepressant (TCA) amitriptyline. The most studied drug, and with the most beneficial results, is pregabalin [15,22]. Thus, the American Diabetes Association (ADA) recommends starting symptomatic treatment of neuropathic pain in DM with pregabalin or duloxetine, although gabapentin can also be used, but the patient's socioeconomic status, comorbidities, and possible drug interactions must be taken into account [7]. Opioid and atypical opioid analgesics are associated with a high risk of addiction and safety concerns and numerous serious adverse effects such as abuse or mortality. To date, prevention of DN has focused primarily on glycemic control [19,22]. Although studies have been published that point out other types of preventive strategies to avoid the onset, development and evolution of this complication of DM, these lack great scientific evidence due to the poor quality of the studies, and on numerous occasions provide confusing results [7]. In this sense, this research attempts to shed light on the existing preventive alternatives for DN, not only highlighting the role of glycemic control as a preventive factor, but also revealing other options.

In view of these considerations, the aim of the present review was to determine which was the most effective preventive strategy to avoid or delay the appearance and/or development of DPN in patients with DM.

2. Materials and Methods

2.1. Protocol and Registration

This systematic review was carried out according to the general guidelines and recommendations made by the Preferred Reporting Items for Systematic Reviews and Meta-Analyses (PRISMA) and was registered in the PROSPERO database (CRD:42020206120).

2.2. Eligibility Criteria

The study population consisted of patients with DPN. Documents published up to 30 September 2021 were included. We excluded documents that did not meet the eligibility criteria and those dealing with the diagnosis of DPN, studies on gestational diabetes and on the treatment of painful DPN, and investigations related to any neuropathy other than DPN. Documents that were not published in English, Spanish, French or Portuguese were excluded. Cohort studies and RCTs carried out from 1 January 2010 to 31 August 2020, following the PICO strategy.

1. Participants: Patients with DM, aged $\geq$ 18 years.
2. Interventions: Any strategy that entailed prevention or delay of DPN onset.
3. Comparisons: Placebo substances, any other alternative or natural progression of the disease in the control group.
4. Outcomes or results: The effectiveness of the intervention in terms of the prevention of DPN at the end of the studies in patients who did not present this condition at the beginning, or the improvement of this condition if they presented it at the beginning of the study, should be evaluated. Other outcomes may include quality of life measurements, adverse events, related costs, changes in neuropathic pain symptoms, presence of foot ulcerations and/or amputations, and events that prevented continuation of clinical trials.

2.3. Sources and Search

The databases used were Scopus, Cochrane, PubMed, PEDro, EMBASE, SciELO and CINAHL. PubMed was used as a free access tool for the search in Medline and Premedline. The search and the free search were done via Mesh terms. The following search terms were used, together with the operators "OR" and "AND". According to each database, the following search strategy was used. The key words used for the search were "diabetic neuropathies", "prevention", "control", "wound", "randomized controlled trial", "diabetic nephropathy", "case control studies", "quality of life", "cerebrovascular accident", "cardiovascular disease", "diabetic nephropathies", "peripheral occlusive artery disease", "autonomic neuropathy", "coronary artery disease", "depression", "neuropathic pain", "healthcare cost", and "diabetic retinopathy". The search strategy used can be consulted in Appendix A.

2.4. Study Selection

Two blinded reviewers (XXX) (XXX) participated in each stage of the study selection. First, they screened by titles and abstracts of the references identified through the search strategy. The authors assessed whether the studies collected through the literature search met the eligibility criteria, excluding those that were irrelevant and/or whose level of methodological quality was questionable. Full reports of all potentially relevant documents were then assessed for eligibility based on the eligibility criteria of this review. Disagreements were resolved by discussion between the two evaluators, or if consensus was not possible, further opinion was sought (XXX) (XXXX).

2.5. Data Extraction and Synthesis of Results

For the data extraction process, review authors used a standardized template containing information related to the eligibility criteria of the publications and the exclusion reasons for the selection of articles, and full title, country, and year of publication. After carrying out the first evaluation of the reports, the results obtained were discussed between the investigators, as well as the inclusion or exclusion of incompatible papers and, if necessary, the intervention of a third independent investigator. Finally, a form was designed for the extraction of data from the articles ultimately selected. This task was carried out by a single researcher. The data extracted were synthesized in an evidence table (including study design and setting, population characteristics, risk of bias assessment).

2.6. Risk of Bias Assessment

The assessment of the risk of bias in the studies was carried out using the Review Manager tool (RevMan) of the Cochrane Collaboration, version 5.3.77. This software evaluates the risk of bias of individual studies as well as among the studies included in the review by generating graphs, tables and percentages from the following domains.

The risks of bias criteria are classified as: "low risk", "high risk" or "unclear risk", assessing the risks of selection, conduct, detection, attrition, reporting and other possible biases. This task was carried out by the review author and is currently the main tool used for the assessment of risk of bias in studies and for the evaluation of methodological quality [23]. Thus, studies without a high risk of bias in any category were considered to be of high quality (1++), and those with a high risk or two unclear risks were considered to be of medium quality (1+). The rest were considered low quality (1−).

In addition, the STROBE [24] and CASPe [25] checklists were used to assess the quality of cohort studies and RCTs, respectively. These two methodological quality assessment scales are expressed as a numerical score based on the number of items completed. A statistical assessment was performed by two independent assessors using the IBM SPSS Statistics 22 80 software. The data were analyzed using the intraclass correlation coefficient (ICC), the purpose of which is to assess the agreement between two or more continuous measurements carried out repeatedly in a sample. The ICC takes values between 0 and 1. A significance level of less than 0.04 would indicate poor reliability, and values above 0.75 would indicate excellent reproducibility; intermediate values are considered adequate.

3. Results

The flow diagram summarizes the study selection processes, and each stage for the studies included in this review (see for details the PRISMA flow diagram in Figure 1) [26]. In total, 11 documents were included in our systematic review. Table 1 shows the studies excluded and the reasons after the application of the quality appraisal filter.

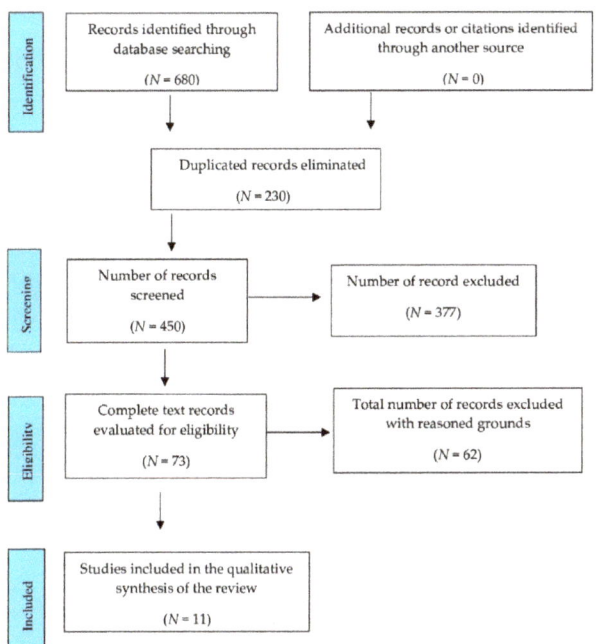

Figure 1. PRISMA flow diagram adapted with permission from the PRISMA group, 2020.

Table 1. Potential studies excluded.

Reason for Exclusion	Authors
RCTs that specifically address treatment rather than prevention of DPN	Farvid et al., 2011 [27] Song et al., 2011 [28] Rizzo et al., 2012 [29] Lavery et al., 2012 [30] Mueller et al., 2013 [31] Ulbrecht et al., 2014 [32] Dixit et al., 2016 [33] Ziegler et al., 2016 [34] Sharoni et al., 2018 [35] Venkataraman et al., 2019 [36] López-Moral et al., 2019 [37] Stubbs et al., 2019 [38] Ahmad et al., 2019 [39] Shu et al., 2019 [40] Sari et al., 2020 [41]
Cohort studies not from RCTs	Müller-Stich et al., 2013 [42] Hur et al., 2013 [43] Cho et al., 2014 [44] Ishibashi et al., 2018 [45] O'Brien et al., 2018 [46] Yang et al., 2020 [47] Cárdenas et al., 2019 [48]
Cohort studies that do not specifically address the prevention of DPN, but from RCTs	Aroda et al., 2016 [49] Gaede et al., 2016 [50] Abraham et al., 2018 [51] Braffett et al., 2020 [52]

3.1. Risk of Biases among the Studies Included

Figures 2 and 3 show the risk of biases of the study included in this systematic review.

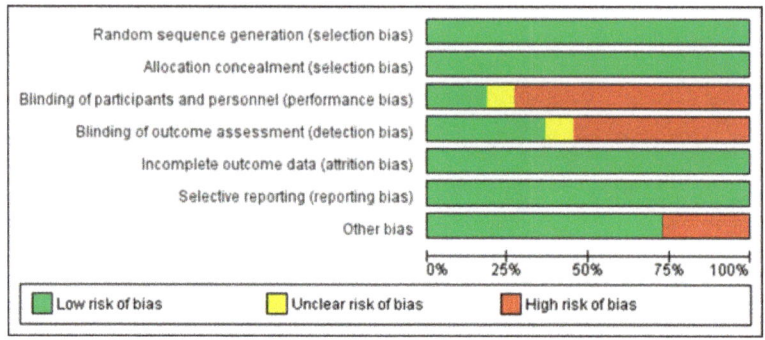

Figure 2. Risk of biases of included studies, overall analysis.

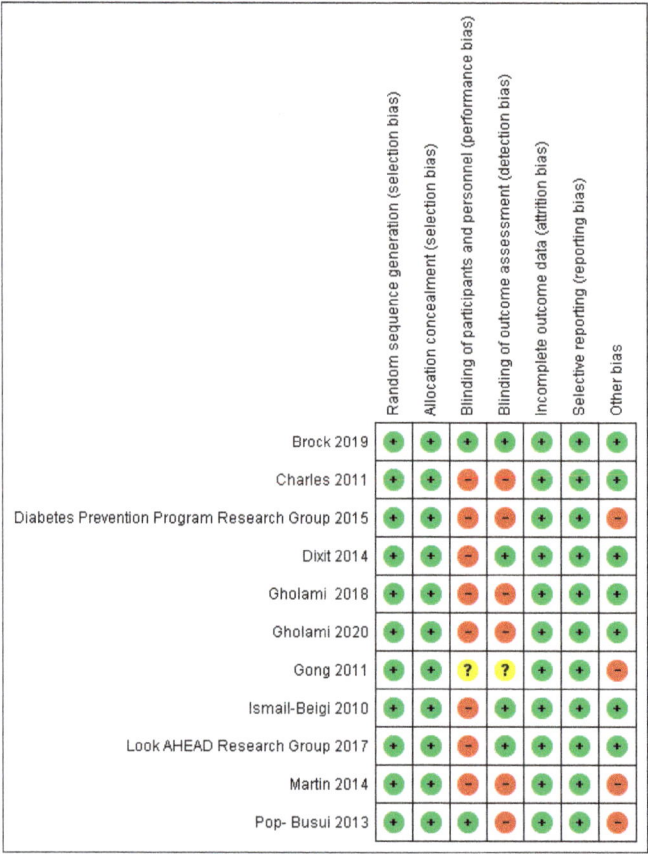

Figure 3. Risk of biases of the included studies [15,53–62], individual analysis. Green: low risk, yellow: unclear risk, red: high risk.

Allocation concealment and random sequence generation was evident in 100% of the studies. Blinding of participants and staff was present in less than 25%, and blinding of assessors was present in less than 50% of the included articles. Due to the nature of some included studies, such as cohort studies, 25% of the included studies were considered to be at high risk of other biases.

The levels of evidence evaluated according to the quality of the selected articles received a score of 1++ in 9.2% ($n = 1$) [53] qualifying it as high quality, 27.3% of the studies received a score of 1+ or medium quality ($n = 3$) [54–56], and the rest of the articles were scored as low quality, 1−, representing 63.5% ($n = 7$) [15,57–62].

3.2. Statistical Analysis of the Quality of the Included Studies

Detailed assessment ICC is summarized in Table 2. Table 3 summarizes the scores of the quality scales of the studies included in this review. The limitations of the review are summarized in Table 4.

Table 2. Intraclass correlation coefficient. Evaluation of agreement between continuous measurements.

	Intraclass Correlation [a]	95% Confidence Interval		F Test with True Value 0			
		Lower Bound	Lower Bound	Value	df1	df2	Sig.
Single Measures	0.997 [b]	0.995	0.995	687.400	10	10	0.000
Average Measures	0.999 [c]	0.995	1.000	687.400	10	10	0.000

Two-way mixed effects model where people's effects are random and measures' effects are fixed. [a] Type C intraclass correlation coefficients using a consistency definition—the between measure variance is excluded from the denominator variance. [b] The estimator is the same, whether the interaction effect is present or not. [c] This estimate is computed assuming the interaction effect is ab-sent, because it is not estimable otherwise.

Table 3. Scores of the investigators on the quality scales of the included studies.

Authors	Scale	Review 1	Review 2
Ismail-Beigi et al., 2010	CASpe	10/11	10/11
Charles et al., 2011	CASpe	6/11	6/11
Gong et al., 2011	STROBE	16/22	16/22
Pop-Busui et al., 2013	STROBE	17/22	17/22
Dixit et al., 2014	CASpe	11/11	11/11
Martin et al., 2014	STROBE	16/22	16/22
Diabetes Prevention Program Research Group et al., 2015	STROBE	17/22	17/22
Look AHEAD Research Group et al., 2017	CASpe	9/11	9/11
Gholami et al., 2018	CASpe	9/11	9/11
Brock et al., 2019	CASpe	11/11	11/11
Gholami et al., 2020	CASpe	9/11	9/11

3.3. Limitations of Included Studies

Table 4 shows some of the studies with their limitations. Some of the reasons for its limitation were the sample size, number of dropouts or that not all patients were evaluated with all the measures, among other reasons.

Table 4. Limitations of the review.

Authors	Limitations
Ismail-Beigi et al., 2010	Early termination of the RCT due to increased mortality among participants.
Charles et al., 2011	Not all patients were evaluated with all measurements. Patients in the CASE IV subgroup were younger than the rest, so microvascular complications may have been lower in this group.
Gong et al., 2011	No results were obtained for 25% of the participants who died. Low incidence of nephropathy and neuropathy due to short duration of diabetes in participants.
Pop-Busui et al., 2013	Study not designed to detect an effect of the groups on DPN. A lower incidence of neuropathy was found in the IS group; however, the authors were unable to identify whether the benefit was specific to biguanides or thiazolidinediones. Small fiber neuropathy was not evaluated, as only the Michigan Neuropathy Screening Instrument (MNSI), which evaluates large fibers, was used. Subjectivity of the MNSI.
Dixit et al., 2014	The effect of aerobic exercise to halt or interrupt the natural course of DPN was not studied. The study had a large number of dropouts.
Martin et al., 2014	Intentional exclusion at the start of Diabetes Control and Complications Trial (DDCT) of participants with severe neuropathy. Patients in the conventional insulin therapy (CON) group were switched to intensive insulin therapy (INT) group because of the benefits of intensive glycemic control in patients with T1DM.
Diabetes Prevention Program Research Group et al., 2015	The combination of three different microvascular outcomes in the aggregate microvascular outcome.
Look AHEAD Research Group et al., 2017	Relationship of biguanide use with vitamin B12 depletion and the development of DPN. Levels of this vitamin were not recorded. Diagnosis of DPN by questionnaire, MNSI physical examination and Semmes-Weinstein (SW) monofilament.
Gholami et al., 2018	Small sample size, large number of dropouts, and only male participation.
Brock et al., 2019	Severe irreversible neuropathy, more male representation.
Gholami et al., 2020	Small sample size.

3.4. Synthesis of Results

3.4.1. Studies Included

Of the 11 included studies, seven were parallel-group RCTs [59,61], of which one was placebo-controlled [53]. The remaining four studies were cohort studies from RCTs, [58,60], of which one was placebo-controlled. The total follow-up period of the studies ranged from 8 weeks to 20 years. Table 5 summarizes the characteristics of the included studies.

Table 5. Main characteristics of the studies included.

Authors	Design	Participants (N)	Groups	Diabetes Type	Average Age (Years)	Duration of the Study	Interventions	Measured Results
Brock et al. (2019)	RCT, double-blind, placebo-controlled	39	IG (Liraglutide) N = 19 CG (placebo) N = 20	TIDM	50.4	32 weeks	Liraglutide Placebo	Changes in nerve potentials, proinflammatory cytokines, autonomic function and peripheral neurophysiological tests. MNSI
Charles et al. (2011)	RCT with parallel groups	1161	Routine Care (RC) N = 459 Intensive multifactorial treatment (IT) N = 702	TIIDM	59.9	6 years	IT: Education, medication and promotion of healthy lifestyle. CR: Danish recommendations for diabetes care.	AAI Vibration detection threshold (tuning fork) Light touch (SW)
Diabetes Prevention Program Research Group et al. (2015)	Cohort study of a parallel-group placebo-controlled RCT	2776	Placebo N = 935 Metformin N = 926 Lifestyle N = 915	TIIDM	51	15 years	Metformin Placebo Lifestyle	Diagnosis of diabetes HbA1c Albuminuria (Nephropathy) Fundus evaluation (Retinopathy) SW light touch (Neuropathy)
Dixit et al. (2014)	RCT of parallel groups	87	CG N = 47 (10 lost) EG N = 40 (11 lost)	TIIDM	CG: 59.45 EG: 54.40	8 weeks	EG: Moderate aerobic exercise, foot care education, healthy diet CG: Standard medical care, education	Motor and sensory nerve conduction studies in peroneal and sural nerves MDNS

Table 5. Cont.

Authors	Design	Participants (N)	Groups	Diabetes Type	Average Age (Years)	Duration of the Study	Interventions	Measured Results
Gholami et al. (2018)	RCT of parallel groups	24	Exercise N = 12 Control N = 12	TIIDM	CG: 43 ± 6.4 EG: 42 ± 4.6	12 weeks	Exercise: Running, walking or treadmill 3 times/week for 20–45 min. Control: Maintain usual level of physical activity.	Weight, BMI, % fat HbA1c Nerve conduction velocity (NCV) and nerve action potential amplitude (APAN) peoneal, tibial and sural nerves
Gholami et al. (2020)	RCT of parallel groups	31	CG N = 15 EG N = 16	TIIDM	52.8 ± 9.6	12 weeks	EG: Cycling exercises CG: Maintaining the usual level of physical activity	HbA1c Fasting glucose Flow mediated dilation (FMD), changes in intima-media thickness and basal diameter in superficial femoral artery, MDNS
Gong et al. (2011)	Cohort study of parallel-group RCTs	577	CG = N = 136 (42 lost) EG = N = 441 (135 lost)	TIIDM	CG 66.7 ± 9.2 EG 64.7 ± 9.3	20 years	EG: diet, exercise or diet + exercise CG: Regular medical care	Plasma glucose HbA1c, oral glucose tolerance test, Examination ocular fundus Inspection extremity lower limb AAI Light touch (SW)
Ismail-Beigi et al. (2010)	RCT of parallel groups	10,251	Intensive therapy N = 5128 Standard therapy N = 5123	TIIDM	62.2 ± 6	3.5 years	Intensive therapy: HbA1c < 6.0% Standard therapy: HbA1c 7.0–7.9%	Albuminuria Creatinine Fundus examination MNSI Vibratory sensitivity (tuning fork), light touch (SW)

Table 5. *Cont.*

Authors	Design	Participants (N)	Groups	Diabetes Type	Average Age (Years)	Duration of the Study	Interventions	Measured Results
Look AHEAD Research Group et al. (2017)	RCT of parallel groups	5145	Intensive lifestyle intervention (ILI) N = 2570 Diabetes support and education (DSE) N = 2575	TIIDM	58.7	11 years	ILI: 7% weight loss, reduced caloric intake, and increased physical activity DSE: Diabetes education focused on diet and exercise	MNSI Light touch (SW)
Martin et al. (2014)	Cohort study of a parallel-group RCT	1345	Intensive insulin therapy (INT) N = 687 Conventional insulin therapy (CON) N = 688	TIDM	33.6 ± 7	14 years	INT: insulin treatment aimed at near-normal glycemia. CON: insulin treatment according to current standards	Vibratory sensitivity Light touch (SW) MNSI Nerve conduction studies HbA1c
Pop-Busui et al. (2013)	Cohort study of a parallel-group RCT	2159	Insulin-sensitizing treatments (IS) N = 1080 Insulin-providing treatments (IP) N = 1079	TIIDM	62 ± 9	4 years	Insulin-sensitizing treatments Insulin-providing treatments	HbA1c, Duration of DM, Albuminuria Retinopathy Alcohol and tobacco consumption Blood lipids, Blood pressure, MNSI Prevalence of DPN

3.4.2. Participants

The total number of participants in all studies was 23,595, with ages ranging from 33.6 ± 7 to 66.7 ± 9.2 years, including 1834 patients with TIDM and 21,761 patients with TIIDM [54–59,61,62]. All studies divided participants into two groups, except the 2015 Diabetes Prevention Program Research Group et al. [57] study, which randomized participants into two intervention groups and one control group.

3.4.3. Interventions and Comparisons

Interventions included drugs such as liraglutide [53] for the reduction in the neuroinflammatory component that appears in DPN in patients with TIDM, intensive glucose control with a glycosylated hemoglobin (HbA1c) < 6% in the case of patients with TIDM [15], or in patients with TIIDM [55,62]. Another strategy employed was the comparison of insulin-sensitizing treatments and insulin-providing treatments for standard glycemic control in patients with TIIDM [60]. Moderate aerobic exercise was evaluated in two of the included articles [54,61], as well as cycling [59]. The most employed intervention among the included studies was the promotion of a healthy lifestyle through education, medication for the control of diabetes and cardiovascular risk factors in addition to diet in patients with TIIDM [56–58]. Comparisons were made with placebo [53,57], standard recommendations for diabetes care [60,62], maintaining usual physical activity level [59,61], diabetes education focused on exercise and diet control [56].

3.4.4. Analysis of Results

The presence of DPN was mainty evaluated. Other variables were taken into account, such as ankle arm index (AAI) [58,62], albuminuria and creatinine (nephropathy), fundus examinations [58] (retinopathy), glucose levels [59], oral glucose tolerance test [58], HbA1c [62], lower limb inspection [58], weight, body mass index (BMI), fat percentage [61], diagnosis of DM [57] or changes in intima media thickness and basal diameter of the superficial femoral artery [59]. In the case of neuropathy identification, the measurements used were nerve conduction velocity (NCV) studies [15,53,54,59,61], tests for vibration detection threshold assessment with a 128 Hz tuning fork, and light touch with the SW monofilament [58,62], and questionnaires such as the Michigan Diabetic Neuropatic Score (MDNS) [54,59] or the MNSI [55,56,60]. For all the results obtained in the studies, the significance level was $p < 0.05$.

3.4.5. Summary of Results

The drug liraglutide reduced the neuroinflammatory component interleukin-6 in adults with TIDM, but did not improve established DPN [53]. Intensive glycemic control significantly reduced the development of neuropathy in patients with TIDM, but this effect was not observed in patients with TIIDM [55]. Intensive lifestyle intervention in patients with TIIDM had negative effects in two of the studies [57,58], and positive effects in one [56]. Moderate-intensity aerobic exercise had a positive outcome for the improvement of established DPN and prevention in two of the included studies [54,61], as did cycling in patients with TIIDM [59]. Glycemic control therapy with insulin sensitizers significantly reduced the incidence of DPN compared with insulin-providing therapy, with more benefits for men [60]. The effect of glycemic control therapy with insulin sensitizers in patients with TIIDM was not observed [61,62].

4. Discussion

The aim of this systematic review was to determine which is the most effective preventive strategy to avoid or delay the appearance and/or development of DPN in patients with DM. Most studies seem to indicate that glycemic control is currently the most effective preventive strategy. Our literature search identified 11 studies examining patients with the variables related to diabetic neurophaties [15,53–61]. These aims were achieved in the review.

4.1. Intensive Glycemic Control

DPN has a multifactorial origin, in which different metabolic, inflammatory, autoimmune and vascular processes take place, leading to nerve degeneration [62]., Therefore, the prevention of these alterations is fundamental, with the control of maintained hyperglycemia being the main one [63]. In this sense, large studies have been carried out in which the effect of intensive glucose control with a target HbA1c of less than 6% in patients with TIDM were evaluated [64].

The Epidemiology of Diabetes Interventions and Complications (EDIC) study was performed to record the long-term effects of therapy on the development and progression of myocardiovascular complications and cardiovascular disease. Data published in 2010 by Albers et al. [65] from the EDIC follow-up demonstrated that intensive glucose control significantly delayed the development and progression of DPN. The prevalence of neuropathy increased from 9 to 25% in the INT group and from 17 to 35% in the conventional CON insulin therapy group ($p = 0.001$) and the incidence also remained lower in the INT group (22%) relative to the CON group (28%); ($p = 0.0125$). The effect was maintained in the article included in our 2014 systematic review of Martin et al. [15] in which the prevalence and incidence of DPN and Cardiovascular autonomic neuropathy (CAN) remained significantly lower in the Diabetes Control and Complications Trial (DCCT) intensive therapy group compared to the DCCT conventional therapy group up to year 13/14 of EDIC. This is in addition to being maintained in other smaller European cohorts, such as the Oslo study [66], and the one published by Ziegler et al. [67] in 2015, as well as in the EURO-DIAB study [68]. In contrast, the results presented by Holman et al. [69] in 2008 of the 10-year follow-up of participants in the United Kingdom Prospective Diabetes Study (UKPDS) in the sulfonylureas-insulin group, relative risk reductions persisted for microvascular disease ($p = 0.04$), but this effect was not seen in the metformin group of patients with TIIDM. Along the same lines, the Steno-2 study, according to data published by Gaede et al. [70] in 2003, did not have a significant effect on the progression of DPN after a follow-up of 13.3 years in patients with microalbuminuria, although it did reduce the development of CAN by 57% (Relative risk; RR 0.37; Confidence interval, 95% CI 0.18–0.79). With similar results, the 2008 ADVANCE study [71], which included 11,140 patients with TIIDM, also with two groups, one intensive therapy and one conventional glycemic therapy, demonstrated a decrease in the incidence of combined major macrovascular and microvascular events ($p = 0.01$), as well as in major microvascular events ($p = 0.01$), mainly due to the reduction in the incidence of nephropathy ($p = 0.006$), but did not demonstrate a significant difference in the groups in terms of relative risk reduction for the occurrence of DPN.

The Action to Control Cardiovascular Risk in Diabetes (ACCORD) trial [72] was an RCT published in 2008 that studied the relationship between diabetes and cardiovascular disease, concluding that, compared with standard therapy, the use of intensive therapy to achieve target HbA1c levels for 3.5 years increased mortality and did not significantly reduce major cardiovascular events, which is why standard glycemic therapy rather than intensive therapy is advised in patients with TIIDM. In the ACCORD results for the development of microvascular complications presented in the 2010 study by Ismail-Beigi et al. [55], positive results were obtained for intensive therapy in terms of DPN prevention, but due to the increase in mortality and the number of cardiovascular events recorded, this study advises against intensive glycemic control in patients with TIIDM. Similarly, in the 2009 Veterans Affairs Diabetes Trial (VADT) RCT [73], no difference was found between the intensive or standard glucose control groups for microvascular complications of DPN after a median follow-up of 5.6 years.

In addition, the multicenter Anglo-Danish-Dutch Study of Intensive Treatment in People with Screen-Detected Diabetes in Primary Care (ADDITION-Denmark) study by Charles et al. [62] published in 2011 did not find that screening followed by intensive glycemic control intervention led to a statistically significant difference in the prevalence of DPN and peripheral arterial disease (PAD) 6 years after diagnosis. However, positive results have been obtained for intensive control in patients with TIIDM in a Japanese

RCT with a small sample size, significant improvement in NCV ($p < 0.05$) and vibration thresholds ($p < 0.05$) at 6 years from the baseline [74]. In this line, in 2013, Hur et al. [43], performed a cohort study where they identified that HbA1c levels predict nerve degeneration and regeneration of myelinated fibers in patients with TIIDM and DPN. Therefore, maintaining optimal blood glucose control is likely to be essential to prevent nerve injury. Abraham et al. [51] 2017, Ishibashi et al. [45] 2019 and Cho et al. [44] 2014 further added the importance of dyslipidemia control, as high cholesterol and triglycerides seem to be found to be related to the future development of DPN in patients with TIIDM.

In 2012, a Cochrane review and meta-analysis by Callaghan et al. [75] was published that aimed to examine the evidence for intensive glucose control in the prevention of DPN in patients with TIDM and TIIDM. Revealing a significant decrease in the relative risk of developing clinical neuropathy in those who had intensive glucose control, RR of −1.84% (95% CI −1.11 to −2.56). For patients with TIIDM, the relative risk of developing neuropathy was −0.58% (95% CI 0.01 to −1.17). Most of the secondary outcomes were significantly in favor of intensive treatment in both populations. However, both types of participants had a significant increase in serious adverse events, including hypoglycemic events.

The results of this review demonstrate that tight glycemic control is effective in preventing the development of DPN in patients with TIDM, but the data were not significant for patients with TIIDM ($p = 0.06$), although improved glucose control has been shown to significantly reduce nerve conduction and vibratory threshold abnormalities. The authors noted that this intervention significantly increases the risk of severe hypoglycemic episodes and should be taken into account when assessing risk/benefit. Buehler et al. [76], in 2013 published a systematic review and meta-analysis on the effect of tight glucose control compared to standard control, in this case in patients with TIIDM. It was determined that intensive glucose control significantly reduced the progression of retinopathy (RR 0.80; 95% CI 0.71–0.91), the incidence of DPN (RR 0.94; 95% CI 0.89–0.99), as well as the progression of nephropathy (RR 0.55; 95% CI 0.37–0.80) but had no significant effect on the incidence of nephropathy (RR 0.69; 95% CI 0.42–1.14). In agreement, Fullerton et al. [64] in 2014 conducted a systematic review in which it was observed that intensive glycemic control reduces the risk of developing microvascular complications compared to conventional treatment, in the case of neuropathy by 4.9% versus 13.9%; RR 0.35 (95% CI 0.23–0.53); $p < 0.00001$. Hasan et al. [77] in 2016 conducted a systematic review and meta-analysis evaluating the efficacy and safety of intensive control compared to standard glycemic control in preventing the development of diabetic foot. Intensive control with an HbA1c target of 6.0–7.5% was associated with a significant decrease in the relative risk of amputation (RR, 0.65; 95% CI, 0.45–0.94; I(2) = 0%). Intensive control was associated with a slower decrease in the sensitive vibration threshold (mean difference, L8, 27; 95% CI, L9, 75 to L6, 79). No effect on neuropathic changes (RR, 0.89; 95% CI, 0.75–1.05; I(2) = 32%) or ischemic changes (RR, 0.92; 95% CI, 0.67–1.26; I(2) = 0%) was found in nine RCTs of patients with TIIDM.

The management of glycemic control suggested an optimal therapeutic approach depending on the patients with TIDM and TIIDM. Despite adequate blood glucose control, patients with TIIDM are likely to develop neuropathy [72]. This is why, in patients with TIDM, glycemic control with an HbA1c target of less than 6% is advised to prevent DPN and in the case of patients with TIIDM, glycosylated hemoglobin could range from 7.0–7.9%.

4.2. Use of Drugs

Pop-Busui et al. [60], in 2013, conducted a study where it was observed that glycemic control therapy with insulin sensitizers (IS) with metformin and thiazolidinediones (TZD) significantly reduced the incidence of DPN compared to insulin-providing therapies (IP) such as sulfonylureas, meglitinide or insulin. This result could be due to the anti-inflammatory, oxidative stress, lipid profile and weight improvement effects of TZDs and metformin, which would be coupled with the reduction in glycemia. However, no other studies have been published comparing the efficacy of the different drugs used for the treatment of DM in terms of the prevention and development of DPN.

With respect to liraglutide, Brock et al. [53], did not find a significant effect in terms of DPN prevention, although a decrease in proinflammatory cytokines was observed.

4.3. Lifestyle Modification

The most important and largest study on the prevention of the development of TIIDM was the Diabetes Prevention Program (DPP) [78], where participants at high risk of developing DM were divided into two groups, and both were compared with placebo groups. One group was metformin, with an administration of 850 mg twice daily, and the other group was lifestyle modification through programs of at least 7% weight loss and 150 min of physical activity per week. The intervention reduced the incidence of DM by 58% (95% CI, 48 to 66%) in the lifestyle modification group and by 31% (95% CI 17 to 43%t) in the metformin group compared with placebo, highlighting the greater benefit of lifestyle modification.

Supporting these results, an RCT, "China Da Qing Diabetes Prevention" [79], divided participants into three subgroups: diet, exercise, and diet plus exercise. Participants in the combined intervention group obtained a 51% (hazard ratio (HR) 0.49; 95% CI 0.33–0.73) lower incidence of diabetes during the active period and 43% (0.57; 0.41–0.81) during the subsequent 20 years of follow-up.

The relationship of these interventions in terms of preventing vascular microcomplications in DM was detailed in the studies of Diabetes Prevention Program Research Group et al. [57] in 2015 and Gong et al. [58] in 2011. In both studies, negative results were obtained for the prevention of DPN development by not preventing the advancement of microvascular complications: However, in the study by Gong et al., it did decrease the incidence of severe retinopathy by 47%.

In contrast, in the case of the 2017 Look AHEAD Research Group et al. [56] study, it was determined that the intensive lifestyle intervention group demonstrated a significant decrease in DPN.

4.4. Practice of Physical Exercise

Balducci et al. [80] in 2006 examined the effects of long-term physical training on the development of DPN in patients with TIDM and TIIDM through an RCT. Significant differences were found in the improvement of nerve conduction in the peroneal and sural nerves for the group that performed physical activity, so the study suggests that long-term aerobic exercise could prevent or modify the onset of the natural history of DPN. This improvement in peroneal nerve conduction velocity and an improvement in neuropathic symptoms was observed in the longitudinal observational study by Azmi et al. [81].

Singleton et al. [82], in 2014, demonstrated increased intraepidermal nerve fiber density (IENFD) (1.5 ± 3.6 vs. -0.1 ± 3.2 fibers/mm, $p = 0.03$) of the leg in a cohort of 100 patients with DM and without neuropathy who received a weekly structured and supervised exercise program ($n = 60$) compared to patients who only received lifestyle counseling ($n = 40$), followed for 1 year.

Several RCTs have been published with positive results in terms of improved DPN with physical exercise, such as those conducted by Song et al. [28] in 2011, Mueller et al. [31] in 2013, Dixit et al. [33] in 2016, Ahmad et al. [39] in 2019, Stubbs et al. [38] in 2019, Dixit et al. [54] in 2014, Gholami et al. [61] in 2018 and Gholami et al. [59] in 2020.

However, several systematic reviews and meta-analyses have been published in favor of exercise as a preventive factor in DPN in patients with TIIDM, although it is unclear whether this effect is due to the associated decrease in HbA1c percentage, or whether other currently unidentified factors are involved.

In 2017, Villafaina et al. [83] published a systematic review determining that improved heart rate variability during exercise may be an important factor to consider as prevention in DN and associated mortality in patients with TIIDM. In the same vein, Bhati-Pooja et al. [84] in 2018 conducted a systematic review on physical exercise practice and autonomic cardiac function in patients with TIIDM ascertaining that this strategy significantly improves nerve conduction. Gu et al. [85] in 2019 observed a positive influence of aerobic exercise on nerve function. In the case of DM associated with obesity, patients with DM who have to undergo bariatric surgery show an improvement in neuropathic symptoms [86].

4.5. Limitations of the Study

The review presents several limitations. Firstly, many of the studies analyzed present heterogeneity in outcome measures, while others studies report small sample size and short duration of follow-up. The authors have found that there is little evidence, and many knowledge gaps persist in the use of preventive alternatives; this should be considered. Furthermore, the risk of detection in eight included studies. In addition, in terms of the neuropathy evaluation technique and according to the literature consulted, there is variability, which is why it should be considered as another limitation.

5. Conclusions

According to the present review, DPN cannot be cured, so preventive measures are essential, with glycemic control being the main strategy. The preventive interventions studied included intensive or standard glycemic control, the use of drugs for glycemic control, lifestyle modifications and the practice of physical exercise. In the case of patients with TIDM, a clear benefit of intensive glycemic control with an HbA1c < 6% in the prevention of microvascular complications. In patients with TIIDM, standard glycemic control with an HbA1c between 7.0 and 7.9% is recommended and lifestyle modifications based on the practice of physical exercise, dietary control and control of cardiovascular risk factors are emphasized. Intensive glycemic control with insulin-sensitizing drugs is recommended in patients with TIDM, as well as lifestyle modifications in patients with TIIDM. The practice of moderate aerobic physical exercise is emerging as an important preventive factor in the development of neuropathy. More consistent studies are needed and with unification in the evaluation techniques that allow for consolidating some aspects of the knowledge of DPN. Therefore, the main principles of treatment for peripheral neuropathy are glycemic control, foot care, and pain management.

Author Contributions: All authors have made substantial contributions to this systematic review. Conceptualization, M.C.-J., L.C.-M., I.G.-V., M.P.-C. and A.J.P.-B.; methodology, L.C.-M., A.J.P.-B., M.C.-J., I.G.-V. and M.P.-C.; software, L.C.-M., M.P.-C. and I.G.-V.; validation, L.C.-M., M.P.-C., A.J.P.-B., M.C.-J. and I.G.-V.; formal analysis, A.J.P.-B., L.C.-M. and I.G.-V.; investigation, L.C.-M., I.G.-V., M.P.-C. and M.C.-J.; resources, L.C.-M., A.J.P.-B. and M.P.-C.; data curation, L.C.-M. and M.P.-C.; writing—original draft preparation, M.P.-C., I.G.-V. and L.C.-M.; writing—review and editing, A.J.P.-B., M.P.-C., I.G.-V., M.C.-J. and L.C.-M.; visualization, A.J.P.-B., M.P.-C., I.G.-V., M.C.-J. and L.C.-M.; supervision, A.J.P.-B., M.P.-C., M.C.-J. and L.C.-M.; project administration, L.C.-M. and A.J.P.-B. All authors have read and agreed to the published version of the manuscript.

Funding: This research received no external funding.

Institutional Review Board Statement: Not applicable.

Informed Consent Statement: Not applicable.

Data Availability Statement: Details of the literature search are reported in Appendices A and B. Extracted data and details of the risk of bias assessments are available from the authors upon request.

Conflicts of Interest: The authors declare no conflict of interest.

Appendix A. Search Strategy

Appendix A.1. PubMed

Appendix A.1.1. Clinical Trials

Free search: (diabet* neuropath*) AND ("prevention" OR "control") NOT ("ulcer" OR "wound" OR "cardiovascular" OR "pain" OR "nephropath*" OR "retinopath*" OR "protocol")—Filters "Clinical trial", "10 years" and "human" were applied: 74 results were obtained.

Search by descriptors: "Diabetic Neuropathies/prevention and control" [Mesh]. Clinical trial", "10 years" and "human" filters were applied: 48 results were obtained.

Unified search: "Diabetic Neuropathies/prevention and control" [Mesh] OR [(diabet* neuropath*) AND ("prevention" OR "control") NOT ("ulcer" OR "wound" OR "cardiovascular" OR "pain" OR "nephropath*" OR "retinopath*" OR "protocol")].

The filters "Clinical trial", "10 years" and "human" were applied: In this PubMed search, we obtained a total of 122 results, and with the unified search we obtained 84, eliminating 38 duplicate records.

Appendix A.1.2. Cohort Studies

Free search: (diabet* neuropath*) AND ("prevention" OR "control") NOT ("ulcer" OR "wound" OR "cardiovascular" OR "pain" OR "netinopathy*" OR "retinopathy*" OR "systematic review" OR "meta-analysis") AND ("cohort stud*" OR "cohort analysis").

The filters "10 years" and "human" were applied: 40 results were obtained.

Search by descriptors: "Diabetic Neuropathies/prevention and control" [Mesh] AND ("cohort stud*" OR "cohort analysis").

The filters "10 years" and "human" were applied: 20 results were obtained.

Unified search: (diabet* neuropath*) AND ("prevention" OR "control") NOT ("ulcer" OR "wound" OR "cardiovascular" OR "pain" OR "netinopathy*" OR "retinopathy*" OR "systematic review" OR "meta-analysis") OR ["Diabetic Neuropathies/prevention and control" [Mesh]] AND ("cohort stud*" OR "cohort analysis").

The filters "10 years" and "human" are applied: in this search, we obtained a total of 60 results, and with the unified search 56 were obtained, so four duplicate records were eliminated.

Appendix A.2. Scopus

Free search: ("diabet* neuropath*") AND ("prevention" OR control).

This is limited to the last 5 years, from 2015 to 2020, with "article", in the "keywords" section. We limited the search to "randomized controlled trial", "Cohort Studies" and "human".

The terms "diabetic nephropathy", "case control studies", "qualitfy of life", "incidence", "cerebrovascular accident", "cardiovascular risk", "cardiovascular disease", "diabetic nephropathies", "peripheral occlusive artery disease", "child", "autonomic neuropathy", "case report", "diagnostic imaging", "coronary artery disease", "depression", "practical guideline", "neuropathic pain", "healthcare cost", "pilot study" and "diabetic retinopathy" were excluded.

Search strategy: KEY(("diabet* neuropath*") AND ("prevention" OR control)) AND DOCTYPE (ar) AND PUBYEAR > 2014 AND (LIMIT-TO (EXACTKEYWORD,"Human") OR LIMIT-TO (EXACTKEYWORD,"Cohort Studies") OR LIMIT-TO (EXACTKEYWORD," Randomized Control Trial")) AND (EXCLUDE (EXACTKEYWORD,"Case Control Study") OR EXCLUDE (EXACTKEYWORD,"Diabetic Nephropathy") OR EXCLUDE (EXACTKEYWORD,"Case-Control Studies") OR EXCLUDE (EXACTKEYWORD,"Cardiovascular Disease") OR EXCLUDE (EXACTKEYWORD,"Quality Of Life") OR EXCLUDE (EXACTKEYWORD,"Incidence") OR EXCLUDE (EXACTKEYWORD,"Cerebrovascular Accident") OR EXCLUDE (EXACTKEYWORD,"Diabetic Nephropathies") OR EXCLUDE (EXACTKEYWORD,"Peripheral Occlusive Artery Disease") OR EXCLUDE (EXACTKEYWORD,"Child") OR EXCLUDE (EXACTKEYWORD,"Autonomic Neuropathy") OR EXCLUDE (EXACTKEYWORD,"Cardiovascular Risk") OR EXCLUDE (EXACTKEYWORD,"Case Report") OR EXCLUDE (EXACTKEYWORD,"Diagnostic Imaging") OR EXCLUDE (EXACTKEYWORD,"Coronary Artery Disease") OR EXCLUDE (EXACTKEYWORD,"Depression") OR EXCLUDE (EXACTKEYWORD,"Practice Guideline") OR EXCLUDE (EXACTKEYWORD,"Neuropathic Pain") OR EXCLUDE (EXACTKEYWORD,"Health Care Cost")).

In this database, the unified search could be performed directly, since filters were added. A total of 233 results were obtained.

Appendix A.3. The Cochrane Library

Search strategy in "advanced search": "diabetic neuropathy" AND ("prevention" OR "control") NOT ("ulcer*" OR "wound*" OR "cardiovascular" OR "pain*" OR "nephropath*" OR "retinopath*" OR "treatment*" OR "protocol").

The filters from 2010 to present and "trials" are added: 154 results were obtained.

Cohort studies could not be found in this search engine, since it only indexes RCTs and systematic reviews.

In this database, we manually selected the duplicates that appeared, since it collects records from other databases, and, consequently, there were eight duplicates.

Appendix A.4. CINAHL

Appendix A.4.1. Clinical Trials

Search strategy: ("diabet* neuropath*") AND ("prevention" OR "control").

Filters applied: "Search all my search terms" "apply related words" "apply equivalent subjects", limit publication date from 2010 to 2020, publication type "clinical trial", "excludes pre-CINAHL", and gender "all": 26 results were obtained.

Appendix A.4.2. Cohort Studies

Strategy: ("diabet* neuropath*") AND ("prevention" OR "control")) AND ("cohort study" OR "cohort analysis").

Filters applied: limit publication date from 2010 to 2020, "Search all my search terms" "apply related words" "apply equivalent subjects", "exclude pre-CINAHL", and gender "all": 13 results were obtained.

Subsequently, all the references resulting from the search in all the databases were added to the bibliographic manager to eliminate possible duplicates between them, obtaining 13 more duplicates, which were eliminated. Finally, a total of 203 duplicates were eliminated.

Appendix B. Individual Characteristics of the Studies Included in the Review

- Study 1: Brock et al., 2019 [53]

Methods: Double-blind, parallel-group, placebo-controlled RCT.

Participants: Adults with T1DM and confirmed symmetrical polyneuropathy. Thirty-nine participants were randomized to receive liraglutide ($N = 19$) or placebo ($N = 20$).

Interventions: To test whether long-term treatment with liraglutide (an injectable drug used for the treatment of diabetes and obesity, acting in the same way as incretins), induces a decrease in inflammation, thus improving neuronal function, and consequently diabetic neuropathy. The duration was 6 weeks with a dose of 1.2 mg/day, continuing until 26 weeks, for a total of 32 weeks.

Results: The primary endpoint was change in latency of early brain evoked potentials. Secondary endpoints were changes in proinflammatory cytokines, cortical evoked potentials, autonomic function and peripheral neurophysiological tests. Compared to placebo, liraglutide reduced interleukin-6 ($p = 0.025$) with similar reductions in other proinflammatory cytokines. However, neuronal function was not altered at the central, autonomic or peripheral levels. Treatment was associated with 3.38 kg ($p < 0.001$) of weight loss and a decrease in urine albumin/creatinine ratio ($p = 0.02$).

Conclusions: The study concluded that treatment with liraglutide reduced interleukin-6 in adults with T1DM but did not improve established DPN. Lowering the systemic level of proinflammatory cytokines could lead to the prevention or treatment of the neuroinflammatory component in the early stages of diabetic neuropathy.

- Study 2: Charles et al., 2011 [62]

Methods: Parallel-group RCT examining the effects of early detection and intensive multifactorial treatment (IT) of patients with TIIDM in primary care on the prevalence of DPN and PAD over 6 years.

Participants: The study sample of 1161 participants was divided into two groups, the routine care group, RC ($N = 459$) and the intensive multifactorial treatment group, IT ($N = 702$).

Interventions: The interventions employed were different for the groups, consisting in the IT group of physician and patient education, medication use and promotion of healthy lifestyle, control of hyperglycemia, blood pressure and cholesterol, according to the regimen used in the Steno-2 Study [70], and in the CR group, patients received the standard pattern of diabetes care according to the Danish national recommendations.

Results: No statistically significant effect of IT on the prevalence of DPN and PAD was found compared to CR. The prevalence of an AAI ≤ 0.9 was 9.1% (95% CI 6.0–12.2) in the CR group and 7.3% (5.0–9.6) in the IT group. In participants evaluated for vibration detection threshold and light touch sensation the prevalence of at least one abnormal test was 34.8% (26.7–43.0) in the CR group and 30.1% (24.1–36.1) in the IT group.

Conclusion: It was determined that in a population with patients with type 2 diabetes screen-detected, screening followed by IT was not found to lead to a statistically significant difference in the prevalence of DPN and PAD 6 years after diagnosis. Additional information: also called "ADDITION-Denmark"study.

- Study 3: Diabetes Prevention Program Research Group et al., 2015 [57]

Methods: Study of the 3-year Diabetes Prevention Program (DPP) [87] RCT surviving cohort.

Participants: All participants were offered lifestyle training at the end of DPP. Overall, 2776 (88%) of the surviving DPP cohort were followed in the DPP Outcomes Study (DPPOS 2002–2013) and were analyzed by intention-to-treat.

Interventions: The 1996–2001 DPPOS was an RCT comparing an intensive lifestyle intervention or masked metformin with placebo in a cohort selected to be at high risk of developing diabetes. During DPPOS, the lifestyle group received a semiannual booster and the metformin group received unmasked metformin. This research aimed to determine the long-term extent of the beneficial effects of the lifestyle intervention or metformin on diabetes prevention originally demonstrated in the DPP and whether diabetes-associated microvascular complications would be reduced.

Results: During 15 years of follow-up, lifestyle intervention and metformin reduced diabetes incidence rates by 27% ($p < 0.0001$) and 18% ($p = 0.001$), respectively, compared to the placebo group. At year 15, the cumulative incidence of DM was 55%, 56% and 62%, respectively. The end-of-study prevalence of the aggregate microvascular outcome, composed of nephropathy, neuropathy and retinopathy, was not significantly different between treatment groups (11–13%) compared to the overall cohort. However, in women ($n = 1887$), the lifestyle intervention was associated with a lower prevalence (8.7%) than in the placebo (11%) and metformin (11.2%) groups, with a 21% ($p = 0.03$) and 22% ($p = 0.02$) reduction in the lifestyle group compared to placebo and metformin, respectively. Compared to participants who progressed to DM, those who did not do so had a 28% lower prevalence of microvascular complications ($p < 0.0001$).

Conclusion: This study claims that lifestyle intervention or metformin significantly reduced the development of DM over 15 years in predisposed cohorts, although there were no overall differences in aggregate microvascular outcome between treatment groups. However, those who did not progress to DM had a lower prevalence of microvascular complications than those who did.

- Study 4: Dixit et al., 2014 [54]

Methods: Parallel group RCT. The authors proposed evaluating the effect of moderate-intensity aerobic exercise (40–60% of heart rate reserve) on DPN. Participants: Patients with TIIDM and clinical neuropathy, defined with a minimum score of 7 on the Michigan

Diabetic Neuropathy Scale (MDNS). An experimental group ($N = 47$) and a control group ($N = 40$) were included.

Interventions: The experimental group ($N = 47$) received guidelines for moderate-intensity aerobic exercise, accompanied by standard medical care, foot care education and individual dietary recommendations. The control group ($N = 40$) received only standard medical care, foot care education and dietary recommendations.

Results: The groups suffered losses of 10 and 11 participants, respectively. Measurements were performed at baseline and at 8 weeks, including nerve conduction studies in the peroneal motor and sural sensory nerve, as well as the MDNS score. For the peroneal nerve, regarding nerve conduction velocity there was a significant difference in the two groups at 8 weeks ($p = 0.03$). This difference was also observed at 8 weeks in the sural sensory nerve, ($p = 0.00$). Significant differences were observed in the mean MDNS scores in the two groups at 8 weeks ($p < 0.05$).

Conclusion: It was established that moderate-intensity aerobic exercise may play a valuable role in interrupting the normal progression of MDNS in patients with TIIDM.

- Study 5: Gholami et al., 2018 [61]

Methods: Parallel group RCT. The study set out to examine the effects of aerobic training on nerve conduction velocity and action potential amplitude in lower limbs.

Participants: Men patients with TIIDM and DPN, 24 volunteers randomized into two groups: exercise group ($N = 12$) and control group ($N = 12$).

Interventions: Aerobic training consisted of 20–45 min walking or running at 50–70% of the heart rate reserve in three sessions per week for 12 weeks. Before and 48 h after the experimental period, nerve conduction studies were performed and blood samples were taken to analyze HbA1c, and fasting and 2 h postprandial glucose concentration.

Results: Sural nerve sensory conduction velocity (SNV) in the exercise group was significantly increased (from 35.2 ± 4.3 m/s to 37.3 ± 6.2 m/s) compared to the control group ($p = 0.007$). Changes in motor NCV in peroneal and tibial nerves and action potential amplitude (APAN) in all nerves studied were not significant between groups ($p > 0.05$). In addition, HbA1c decreased to a greater extent in the exercise group compared to the control ($p = 0.014$).

Conclusion: It was determined that aerobic exercise training may have the potential to hinder DPN progression by improving NCV. Given the scarce evidence in this domain, related to exercise, the mechanisms should be studied in the future.

- Study 6: Gholami et al., 2020 [59]

Methods: Parallel-group RCT. In relation to the previous study, in this case, the investigators evaluated the effect of physical training on superficial femoral artery (SFA) measurements and neuropathic symptoms in patients with DPN to observe the relationship of DPN with PAD.

Participants: Thirty-one volunteers with established DPN randomly assigned to the experimental ($N = 16$) and control ($N = 15$) groups.

Interventions: The experimental group performed cycling exercise (50–70% of heart rate reserve, 30–45 min, three sessions/week) for 12 weeks. Before and 48 h after the experimental period a 5-min flow-mediated dilation (FMD) response, changes in intima media thickness and basal diameter in SFA using color Doppler ultrasound and neuropathic score in MDNS were assessed as primary outcomes, and fasting glucose level, HbA1c and neuropathic score as secondary outcomes.

Results: The FMD percentage increased significantly in the experimental group (from $3.2 \pm 1.1\%$ to $5.7 \pm 1.2\%$) compared to the control condition ($p = 0.0001$). However, there were no significant alterations in the basement membrane diameter and intima media thickness ($p < 0.05$). Significant improvements in fasting glucose, HbA1c and Michigan diabetic neuropathy score (MDNS) after exercise intervention (all $p < 0.05$) were also observed. Linear regression analysis indicated that the change in MDNS was significantly associated with change in HbA1c ($p = 0.001$) and FMD ($p = 0.001$).

Conclusion: This finding may be clinically of great importance, as metabolic and vascular factors have been indicated to be involved in the development of DPN.

- Study 7: Gong et al., 2011 [58]

Methods: Cohort study of participants in a parallel-group RCT. A 20-year follow-up study of the original participants was conducted to compare the incidence of microvascular complications in the combined intervention group versus the control group.

Participants: The original RCT involving 577 adults with impaired glucose tolerance (IGT) who were randomly assigned to a control group or the lifestyle intervention group (divided into three subgroups: diet, exercise, and diet plus exercise). Follow-up information was obtained on 542 (94%) of the original 577 participants.

Interventions: The aim of the diet intervention was to increase vegetable intake and reduce alcohol and sugar consumption of the participants and, in those who were overweight or obese, to reduce total calorie intake in order to lose weight. In the case of the exercise intervention, this consisted of increasing leisure time physical activity. The interventions were carried out over 6 years.

Results: The cumulative incidence of severe retinopathy was 9.2% in the combined intervention group and 16.2% in the control group ($p = 0.03$). After clinical and age adjusting, the incidence of severe retinopathy was 47% lower in the intervention group than in the control group ($p = 0.048$). No significant differences were found in the incidence of severe nephropathy ($p = 0.96$) or in the prevalence of neuropathy ($p = 0.89$) among survivors after 20 years.

Conclusion: Lifestyle intervention over 6 years in persons with IGT was associated with a 47% reduction in the incidence of severe vision-threatening retinopathy over a 20-year interval, mainly due to the lower incidence of diabetes in the intervention group. However, no similar benefits were observed for nephropathy or neuropathy. Additional information: also called "China Da Qing Diabetes Prevention Outcome Study".

- Study 8: Ismail-Beigi et al., 2010 [55]

Methods: A parallel-group RCT, called the Action to Control Cardiovascular Risk in Diabetes (ACCORD) study [72], aimed to determine whether lowering blood glucose levels reduced the rate of microvascular complications in patients with TIIDM.

Participants: Patients with DM and with high HbA1c concentrations (>7.5%) and cardiovascular disease (or two or more cardiovascular risk factors) were randomized by central randomization to the intensive (target HbA1c of <6.0%) or standard (7.0–7.9%) glycemic control group. 10,251 patients were randomized, ($N = 5128$) to the intensive glycemic control group and ($N = 5123$) to the standard group.

Interventions: Intensive glycemic control compared with standard glycemic therapy. In this analysis, the predefined composite outcomes were: dialysis or renal transplantation, high serum creatinine (>291.7 μmol/L) or retinal photocoagulation or vitrectomy (first composite outcome), or peripheral neuropathy plus the first composite outcome (second composite outcome). Thirteen secondary measures of renal, ocular, and peripheral nerve function were also assessed. Investigators and participants were aware of the treatment group assignment. An analysis was performed for all patients who were evaluated for the microvascular outcome on the basis of the treatment assignment, regardless of treatments received or adherence to therapies.

Results: Intensive therapy was discontinued before the end of the study due to higher mortality in that group, and patients transitioned to standard therapy. At transition, the first composite outcome was recorded in 443 of 5107 patients in the intensive group versus 444 of 5108 in the standard group (HR 1.00, 95% CI 0.88–1.14; $p = 1.00$), and the second composite outcome was observed in 1591 of 5107 versus 1659 of 5108 (0.96, 0.89–1.02; $p = 0.19$). The results were similar at the end of the study, first composite outcome 556 of 5119 vs. 586 of 5115 (HR 0.95, 95% CI 0.85–1.07, $p = 0.42$); and the second 1956 of 5119 vs. 2046 of 5115, respectively (0.95, 95% CI 0.89–1.01, $p = 0.12$)). Intensive therapy did not reduce the risk of microvascular outcomes, but delayed the onset of albuminuria. Six secondary end-of-study measures favored intensive therapy ($p < 0.05$).

Conclusion: The research concludes that the microvascular benefits of intensive therapy must be weighed against increased total and cardiovascular disease-related mortality, weight gain, and high risk of severe hypoglycemia, so as ACCORD proved, intensive glycemic control therapy does not provide significant benefits in patients with TIIDM.

- Study 9: Look AHEAD Research Group et al., 2017 [56]

Methods: The study Look AHEAD (Action for Health in Diabetes) [88] was a parallel-group RCT. It examined whether the intensive lifestyle intervention weight loss decreased cardiovascular morbidity and mortality in overweight or obese adults with TIIDM. Due to the nature of the study, patients and center investigators were not blinded. In addition, the coordinating center staff members responsible for data management and statistical analysis were also not blinded.

Participants: Beginning in 2001, a total of 5145 overweight and obese individuals with TIIDM were randomized to intensive intervention (ILI) ($N = 2570$) or diabetes support and education (DSE) control group ($N = 2575$) using a web-based management system at the study coordinating center at Wake Forest School of Medicine (Winsto-Salem, NC, USA). Randomization was stratified by clinical center and was not disclosed to clinical staff responsible for obtaining data on study outcomes.

Interventions: Intensive intervention (ILI) or diabetes support and education (DSE) control group. Interventions ended in September 2012, 9–11 years after randomization, but both groups continued to be followed for primary and secondary outcomes. Neuropathy assessments included MNSI completed at baseline in all participants, 5145 (ILI $N = 2570$; DSE $N = 2575$) and repeated annually thereafter, as well as SW monofilament testing performed in 3775 participants (ILI $N = 1905$, DSE $N = 1870$) at 1 and 2.3 years after intervention discontinuation.

Results: At baseline, the MNSI questionnaire scores were 1.9 ± 0.04 and 1.8 ± 0.04 in the ILI and DSE groups, respectively (difference not statistically significant). After 1 year, when weight loss was maximal in the ILI group ($8.6 \pm 6.9\%$) compared with DSE ($0.7 \pm 4.8\%$), the respective MNSI scores were 1.7 ± 0.04 and 2.0 ± 0.04 ($p \leq 0.001$). Subsequently, scores increased gradually in both groups, but remained significantly lower in the ILI group during the first 3 years and at the end of follow-up. In both groups, there was a significant association between the MNSI scores and changes in body weight, HbA1c and plasma lipids. There was no significant difference between groups in participants with MNSI physical examination scores ≥ 2.5, considered indicative of DN. Light tactile sensation measured separately in the right and left great toes did not differ between ILI and DSE, but when the data were combined for both toes, a light touch was better preserved in the ILI group.

Conclusion: It was determined that the ILI group had a significant decrease in DPN based on questionnaire diagnosis, which was associated with the magnitude of weight loss. In both the ILI and DSE groups, changes in MNSI score were also associated with changes in HbA1c and lipids. There were no significant effects of ILI on DPN physical examination measures performed 1–2.3 years after completion of the active intervention, except for light touch sensation, which was significantly better in the ILI group when measures were combined for both toes.

- Study 10: Martin et al., 2014 [15]

Methods: Surviving cohort study from the RCT Diabetes Control and Complications Trial and its follow-up study Epidemiology of Diabetes Interventions and Complications (DCCT/EDIC) [87,88]. The authors described the development and progression of neuropathy and related findings among patients with TIDM at 14 years after intervention.

Participants: Patients with TIDM. There were a total of 1441 (100%) DCCT participants, of whom 1375 (95.4%) agreed to participate in EDIC, of whom 1274 (92.7%) were active in year 13 in EDIC, of whom 1226 (96.2%) were evaluated for CAN and 1186 (93.1%) for DPN [89].

Interventions: Intensive glycemic control vs. standard control. The primary outcome of DPN was assessed by clinical symptoms, signs and results of nerve conduction studies during DCCT and repeated in EDIC in year 13/14. CAN was assessed by the R-R response to stimulated breathing, Valsalva ratio and blood pressure response during years 13/14 and 16/17. In addition, symptoms reflecting neuropathic pain and autonomic function (including hypoglycemia awareness) were collected annually in EDIC using standardized questionnaires; peripheral neuropathy was also assessed annually using the MDNS. Genitourinary function assessments were collected in EDIC year 10.

Results: Intensive therapy during DCCT significantly reduced the risk of DPN and CAN at the end of DCCT (64% and 45%, respectively, $p < 0.01$). The prevalence and incidence of DPN and CAN remained significantly lower in the intensive therapy DCCT group compared to the conventional therapy DCCT group until year 13/14 of EDIC [90].

Conclusion: It was established that the persistent effects of prior intensive therapy on neuropathy measures over 14 years of EDIC largely mirror those observed for other complications of DM. DCCT/EDIC provides important information on the influence of glycemic control and the clinical course of DN and, most importantly, on how to prevent neuropathy in patients with TIDM.

- Study 11: Pop-Busui et al., 2013 [60]

Methods: Cohort study from the parallel-group RCT Bypass Angioplasty Revascularization Investigation 2 Diabetes (BARI 2D) [91] published in 2009. This trial demonstrated similar long-term clinical effectiveness of insulin-sensitizing (IS) versus insulin-providing (IP) treatments for patients with TIIDM on cardiovascular outcomes in a cohort with documented coronary artery disease.

Participants: A total of 2159 participants with TIIDM with documented coronary artery disease. IS ($N = 1080$), IP ($N = 1079$).

Interventions: Randomized glycemic control strategy of insulin-sensitizing (IS) versus insulin-providing (IP) treatments for TIIDM on the prevalence and incidence of DPN. DPN (defined as Michigan Neuropathy Screening Questionnaire (MNSI) > 2 clinical examination score) was assessed at baseline and annually for 4 years. Prevalence and incidence of DPN were compared by intention-to-treat models using generalized estimating equations logistic models for prevalence and Kaplan–Meier estimates and Cox regression models for incidence rates.

Results: The results were obtained for 2159 participants in the BARI 2D study (70% male) with baseline values and at least one follow-up MNSI score (mean age 62 ± 9 years, mean HbA1c $7.7 \pm 1.6\%$, duration of diabetes 10 ± 9 years). There was no difference in the prevalence of DPN between the IS and IP groups during the 4 years of follow-up. In 1075 BARI 2D study participants without DPN at baseline, the 4-year cumulative incidence rate of DPN was significantly lower in the IS (66%) than in the IP strategy group (72%) ($p = 0.02$), which remained significant after adjusting for HbA1c ($p = 0.04$). In subgroup analyses, the IS strategy had a greater benefit in men (Hazard Ratio 0.75 [99% 95% CI 0.58–0.99], $p < 0.01$).

Conclusion: Among patients with TIIDM followed for up to 4 years in BARI 2D, a glycemic control therapy with IS significantly reduced the incidence of DPN compared to IP therapy and may provide more benefits for men.

References

1. Crespo, C.; Brosa, M.; Soria-Juan, A.; López-Alba, A.; López-Martínez, N.; Soria, B. Costes directos de la diabetes mellitus y de sus complicaciones en España (Estudio SECCAID): Spain estimated cost Ciberdem-Cabimer in diabetes). *Av. Diabetol.* **2015**, *29*, 182–189. [CrossRef]
2. García-Soidán, F.J.; Villoro, R.; Merino, M.; Hidalgo-Vega, A.; Hernando-Martín, T.; González-Martín-Moro, B. Estado de salud, calidad de vida y utilización de recursos sanitarios de los pacientes con diabetes mellitus en España. *Semergen* **2017**, *43*, 416–424. [CrossRef]

3. Smith, S.C.; Lamping, D.L.; Maclaine, G.D.H. Measuring health-related quality of life in diabetic peripheral neuropathy: A systematic review. *Diabetes Res. Clin. Pract.* **2012**, *96*, 261–270. [CrossRef]
4. Botas-Velasco, M.; Cervell-Rodríguez, D.; Rodríguez-Montalbán, S.; Jiménez, V.A.I.; Fernández-de-Valderrama-Martínez, I. Actualización en el diagnóstico, tratamiento y prevención de la neuropatía diabética periferica. *Angiología* **2017**, *69*, 174–181. [CrossRef]
5. Feldman, E.L.; Callaghan, B.C.; Pop-Busui, R.; Zochodne, D.W.; Wright, D.E.; Bennett, D.L.; Bril, V.; Russell, J.W.; Viswanathan, V. Diabetic neuropathy. *Nat. Rev. Dis. Primers.* **2019**, *5*, 41. [CrossRef]
6. Boulton, A.J.M.; Vinik, A.I.; Arezzo, J.C.; Bril, V.; Feldman, E.L.; Freeman, R.; Malik, R.A.; Maser, R.E.; Sosenko, J.M.; Ziegler, D.; et al. Diabetic neuropathies: A statement by the American Diabetes Association. *Diabetes Care* **2005**, *28*, 956–962. [CrossRef]
7. Pop-Busui, R.; Boulton, A.J.M.; Feldman, E.L.; Bril, V.; Freeman, R.; Malik, R.A.; Sosenko, J.M.; Ziegler, D. Diabetic neuropathy: A position statement by the American diabetes association. *Diabetes Care* **2017**, *40*, 136–154. [CrossRef]
8. Tesfaye, S.; Boulton, A.J.M.; Dyck, P.J.; Freeman, R.; Horowitz, M.; Kempler, P.; Lauria, G.; Malik, R.A.; Spallone, V.; Vinik, A.; et al. Diabetic neuropathies: Update on definitions, diagnostic criteria, estimation of severity, and treatments. *Diabetes Care* **2010**, *33*, 2285–2293. [CrossRef]
9. Petrakis, I.; Kyriopoulos, I.J.; Ginis, A.; Athanasakis, K. Losing a foot versus losing a dollar; a systematic review of cost studies in diabetic foot complications. *Expert. Rev. Pharm. Outcomes Res.* **2017**, *17*, 165–180. [CrossRef] [PubMed]
10. Narres, M.; Kvitkina, T.; Claessen, H.; Droste, S.; Schuster, B.; Morbach, S.; Rümenapf, G.; Van-Acker, K.; Icks, A. Incidence of lower extremity amputation in the diabetic compared to the non-diabetic population: A systematic review protocol. *PLoS ONE* **2017**, *12*, e0182081. [CrossRef]
11. Barrett, E.J.; Liu, Z.; Khamaisi, M.; King, G.L.; Klein, R.; Klein, B.E.K.; Hughes, T.M.; Craft, S.; Freedman, B.I.; Bowden, D.W.; et al. Diabetic microvascular disease: An endocrine society scientific statement. *J. Clin. Endocrinol. Metab.* **2017**, *102*, 4343–4410. [CrossRef] [PubMed]
12. Cabezas-Cerrato, J. The prevalence of clinical diabetic polyneuropathy in Spain: A study in primary care and hospital clinic groups. *Diabetología* **1998**, *41*, 1263–1269. [CrossRef] [PubMed]
13. Moreira-Do-Nascimento, O.J.; Castelo-Branco-Pupe, C.; Boiteux-Uchoa-Cavalcanti, E. Diabetic neuropathy. Neuropatia diabética. *Rev. Dor. São Paulo* **2016**, *17*, 46–51.
14. Fatela, V.; Gutiérrez, A.; Martínez-Salio, A.; Ayan, S.; Rodríguez-Sánchez, S.; Vidal-Fernández, J. Manejo del paciente con neuropatía periférica. *Rev. Clin. Esp.* **2007**, *207*, 14–22.
15. Martin, C.L.; Albers, J.W.; Pop-Busui, R.; DCCT/EDIC Research Group. Neuropathy and related findings in the diabetes control and complications trial/epidemiology of diabetes interventions and complications study. *Diabetes Care* **2014**, *37*, 31–38. [CrossRef] [PubMed]
16. American Diabetes Association 11. Microvascular complications and foot care: Standards of medical care in diabetes 2019. *Diabetes Care* **2019**, *42*, 124–138. [CrossRef] [PubMed]
17. Diabetes Canada Clinical Practice Guidelines Expert Committee; Bril, V.; Breiner, A.; Perkins, B.A.; Zochodne, D. Neuropathy. *Can. J. Diabetes* **2018**, *42*, 217–221. [CrossRef] [PubMed]
18. Vázquez-San-Miguel, F.; Mauricio-Puente, D.; Viadé-Juliá, J. Neuropatía diabética y pie diabético. *Medicine* **2016**, *12*, 971–981. [CrossRef]
19. Veves, A.; Giurini, J.M.; LoGerfo, F.W. *The Diabetic Foot*, 2nd ed.; Humana Press: Totowa, NJ, USA, 2006.
20. Maffi, P.; Secchi, A. The Burden of Diabetes: Emerging Data. *Dev. Ophthalmol.* **2017**, *60*, 1–5. [CrossRef]
21. Cho, N.H.; Shaw, J.E.; Karuranga, S.; Huang, Y.; Da-Rocha-Fernandes, J.D.; Ohlrogge, A.W.; Malanda, B. IDF Diabetes Atlas: Global estimates of diabetes prevalence for 2017 and projections for 2045. *Diabetes Res. Clin. Pract.* **2018**, *138*, 271–281. [CrossRef]
22. Bowker, J.H.; Pfeifer, M.A. *The Diabetic Foot*, 7th ed.; Elsevier: Barcelona, Spain, 2008.
23. Manual Cochrane de Revisiones Sistemáticas de Intervenciones, Versión 5.1.0. Available online: https://es.cochrane.org/es (accessed on 1 January 2019).
24. Von-Elm, E.; Altman, D.G.; Egger, M.; Pocock, S.J.; Gøtzsche, P.C.; Vandenbroucke, J.P. Declaración de la iniciativa STROBE (Strengthening the Reporting of Observational Studies in Epidemiology): Directrices para la comunicación de estudios observacionales. *Rev. Esp. Salud Pública* **2008**, *82*, 251–259. [CrossRef]
25. CASPE. Guías CASPe de Lectura Crítica de la Literatura Médica. 2005. Available online: http://www.redcaspe.org/ (accessed on 5 January 2019).
26. Moher, D.; Liberati, A.; Tetzlaff, J.; Altman, D.; The PRISMA Group. Preferred Reporting Items for Systematic Reviews and Meta-Analyses: The PRISMA Statement. *PLoS Med.* **2009**, *2*, 1–2. [CrossRef]
27. Farvid, M.S.; Homayouni, F.; Amiri, Z.; Adelmanesh, F. Improving neuropathy scores in type 2 diabetic patients using micronutrients supplementation. *Diabetes Res Clin. Pract.* **2011**, *93*, 86–94. [CrossRef]
28. Song, C.H.; Petrofsky, J.S.; Lee, S.W.; Lee, K.J.; Yim, J.E. Effects of an exercise program on balance and trunk proprioception in older adults with diabetic neuropathies. *Diabetes Technol. Ther.* **2011**, *13*, 803–811. [CrossRef] [PubMed]
29. Rizzo, L.; Tedeschi, A.; Fallani, E.; Coppelli, A.; Vallini, V.; Iacopi, E.; Piaggesi, A. Custom-made orthesis and shoes in a structured follow-up program reduces the incidence of neuropathic ulcers in high-risk diabetic foot patients. *Int. J. Low. Extrem. Wounds* **2012**, *11*, 59–64. [CrossRef] [PubMed]

30. Lavery, L.A.; LaFontaine, J.; Higgins, K.R.; Lanctot, D.R.; Constantinides, G. Shear-reducing insoles to prevent foot ulceration in high-risk diabetic patients. *Adv. Skin Wound Care* **2012**, *25*, 519–524. [CrossRef]
31. Mueller, M.J.; Tuttle, L.J.; Lemaster, J.W.; Strube, M.J.; McGill, J.B.; Hastings, M.K.; Sinacoreet, D.R. Weight-bearing versus nonweight-bearing exercise for persons with diabetes and peripheral neuropathy: A randomized controlled trial. *Arch. Phys. Med. Rehabil.* **2013**, *94*, 829–838. [CrossRef]
32. Ulbrecht, J.S.; Hurley, T.; Mauger, D.T.; Cavanagh, P.R. Prevention of recurrent foot ulcers with plantar pressure-based in-shoe orthoses: The CareFUL prevention multicenter randomized controlled trial. *Diabetes Care* **2014**, *37*, 1982–1989. [CrossRef]
33. Dixit, S.; Maiya, A.; Shastry, B.A.; Guddattu, V. Analysis of postural control during quiet standing in a population with diabetic peripheral neuropathy undergoing moderate intensity aerobic exercise training: A single blind, randomized controlled trial. *Am. J. Phys. Med. Rehabil.* **2016**, *95*, 516–524. [CrossRef]
34. Ziegler, D.; Low, P.A.; Freeman, R.; Tritschler, H.; Vinik, A.I. Predictors of improvement and progression of diabetic polyneuropathy following treatment with α-lipoic acid for 4 years in the NATHAN 1 trial. *J. Diabetes Complicat.* **2016**, *30*, 350–356. [CrossRef]
35. Sharoni, S.K.A.; Rahman, H.A.; Minhat, H.S.; Shariff-Ghazali, S.; Ong, M.H.A. The effects of self-efficacy enhancing program on foot self-care behaviour of older adults with diabetes: A randomised controlled trial in elderly care facility, Peninsular Malaysia. *PLoS ONE* **2018**, *13*, 1–23. [CrossRef]
36. Venkataraman, K.; Tai, B.C.; Khoo, E.Y.H.; Tavintharan, S.; Chandran, K.; Hwang, S.W.; Phua, M.S.L.A.; Wee, H.L.; Koh, G.C.H.; Tai, E.S. Short-term strength and balance training does not improve quality of life but improves functional status in individuals with diabetic peripheral neuropathy: A randomised controlled trial. *Diabetologia* **2019**, *62*, 2200–2210. [CrossRef]
37. López-Moral, M.; Lázaro-Martínez, J.L.; García-Morales, E.; García-Álvarez, Y.; Alvaro-Afonso, F.J.; Molines-Barroso, R.J. Clinical efficacy of therapeutic footwear with a rigid rocker sole in the prevention of recurrence in patients with diabetes mellitus and diabetic polineuropathy: A randomized clinical trial. *PLoS ONE* **2019**, *14*, 1–14. [CrossRef]
38. Stubbs, E.B.; Fisher, M.A.; Miller, C.M.; Jelinek, C.; Butler, J.; McBurney, C.; Collins, E.G. Randomized controlled trial of physical exercise in diabetic veterans with length-dependent distal symmetric polyneuropathy. *Front. Neurosci.* **2019**, *13*, 13–51. [CrossRef]
39. Ahmad, I.; Noohu, M.M.; Verma, S.; Singla, D.; Hussain, M.E. Effect of sensorimotor training on balance measures and proprioception among middle and older age adults with diabetic peripheral neuropathy. *Gait Posture* **2019**, *74*, 114–120. [CrossRef]
40. Shu, W.; Liao, Z.; Liu, R.; Du, T.; Zhu, H. Effects of cilostazol tablets combined with epalrestat tablets on serum inflammatory response, oxidative stress, and nerve conduction velocity in elderly patients with type 2 diabetic peripheral neuropathy. *Acta Med. Mediterr.* **2019**, *35*, 2185–2189. [CrossRef]
41. Sari, A.; Altun, Z.A.; Karaman, C.A.; Kaya, B.B.; Durmus, B. Does vitamin D affect diabetic neuropathic pain and balance? *J. Pain Res.* **2020**, *13*, 171–179. [CrossRef]
42. Müller-Stich, B.P.; Fischer, L.; Kenngott, H.G.; Gondan, M.; Senft, J.; Clemens, G.; Nickel, F.; Fleming, T.; Nawroth, P.P.; Büchler, M.W. Gastric bypass leads to improvement of diabetic neuropathy independent of glucose normalization—Results of a prospective cohort study (DiaSurg 1 Study). *Ann. Surg.* **2013**, *258*, 760–766. [CrossRef]
43. Hur, J.; Sullivan, K.A.; Callaghan, B.C.; Pop-Busui, R.; Feldman, E.L. Identification of factors associated with sural nerve regeneration and degeneration in diabetic neuropathy. *Diabetes Care* **2013**, *36*, 4043–4049. [CrossRef]
44. Cho, Y.N.; Lee, K.O.; Jeong, J.; Park, H.J.; Kim, S.M.; Shin, H.Y.; Hong, J.M.; Ahn, C.W.; Choi, Y.C. The role of insulin resistance in diabetic neuropathy in Koreans with type 2 diabetes mellitus: A 6-year follow-up study. *Yonsei Med. J.* **2014**, *55*, 700–708. [CrossRef]
45. Ishibashi, F.; Taniguchi, M.; Kosaka, A.; Uetake, H.; Tavakoli, M. Improvement in neuropathy outcomes with normalizing HbA1c in patients with type 2 diabetes. *Diabetes Care* **2019**, *42*, 110–118. [CrossRef] [PubMed]
46. O'Brien, R.; Johnson, E.; Haneuse, S.; Coleman, K.J.; Connor, P.J.O.; Fisher, D.P.; Sidney, S.; Bogart, A.; Theis, M.K.; Anau, J.; et al. Microvascular outcomes in patients with diabetes after bariatric surgery versus usual-care: A matched cohort study. *Ann. Int. Med.* **2018**, *169*, 300–310. [CrossRef] [PubMed]
47. Yang, C.Y.; Su, P.F.; Hung, J.Y.; Ou, H.T.; Kuo, S. Comparative predictive ability of visit-to-visit HbA1c variability measures for microvascular disease risk in type 2 diabetes. *Cardiovasc. Diabetol.* **2020**, *19*, 1–10. [CrossRef] [PubMed]
48. Cardenas, A.; Hivert, M.F.; Gold, D.R.; Hauser, R.; Kleinman, K.P.; Lin, P.D.; Fleisch, A.F.; Calafat, A.M.; Ye, X.; Webster, T.F.; et al. Associations of perfluoroalkyl and polyfluoroalkyl substances with incident diabetes and microvascular disease. *Diabetes Care* **2019**, *42*, 1824–1832. [CrossRef] [PubMed]
49. Aroda, V.R.; Edelstein, S.L.; Goldberg, R.B.; Knowler, W.C.; Marcovina, S.M.; Orchard, T.J.; Bray, G.A.; Schade, D.S.; Temprosa, M.G.; White, N.H.; et al. Long-term metformin use and vitamin B12 deficiency in the diabetes prevention program outcomes study. *J. Clin. Endocrinol. Metab.* **2016**, *101*, 1754–1761. [CrossRef] [PubMed]
50. Gæde, P.; Oellgaard, J.; Carstensen, B.; Rossing, P.; Lund-Andersen, H.; Parving, H.H.; Pedersen, O. Years of life gained by multifactorial intervention in patients with type 2 diabetes mellitus and microalbuminuria: 21 years follow-up on the Steno-2 randomised trial. *Diabetologia* **2016**, *59*, 2298–2307. [CrossRef] [PubMed]
51. Abraham, A.; Barnett, C.; Katzberg, H.D.; Lovblom, L.E.; Perkins, B.A.; Bril, V. Nerve function varies with hemoglobin A1c in controls and type 2 diabetes. *J. Diabetes Complicat.* **2018**, *32*, 424–428. [CrossRef] [PubMed]

52. Braffett, B.H.; Gubitosi-Klug, R.A.; Albers, J.W.; Feldman, E.L.; Martin, C.L.; White, N.H.; Orchard, T.J.; Lopes-Virella, M.; Lachin, J.M.; Pop-Busui, R.; et al. Risk factors for diabetic peripheral neuropathy and cardiovascular autonomic neuropathy in the Diabetes Control and Complications Trial/Epidemiology of Diabetes interventions and Complications (DCCT/EDIC) study. *Diabetes Care* **2020**, *69*, 1000–1010. [CrossRef] [PubMed]
53. Brock, C.; Hansen, C.S.; Karmisholt, J.; Møller, H.J.; Juhl, A.; Farmer, A.D.; Drewes, A.M.; Riahi, S.; Lervang, H.H.; Jakobsen, P.E.; et al. Liraglutide treatment reduced interleukin-6 in adults with type 1 diabetes but did not improve established autonomic or polyneuropathy. *Br. J. Clin. Pharmacol.* **2019**, *85*, 2512–2523. [CrossRef]
54. Dixit, S.; Maiya, A.G.; Shastry, B.A. Effect of aerobic exercise on peripheral nerve functions of population with diabetic peripheral neuropathy in type 2 diabetes: A single blind, parallel group randomized controlled trial. *J. Diabetes Complicat.* **2014**, *28*, 332–339. [CrossRef]
55. Ismail-Beigi, F.; Craven, T.; Banerji, M.; Basile, J.; Calles, J.; Cohen, R.; Cuddihy, R.; Cushman, W.C.; Genuth, S.; Grimm, R.H., Jr.; et al. Effect of intensive treatment of hyperglycaemia on microvascular outcomes in type 2 diabetes: An analysis of the ACCORD randomised trial. *Lancet* **2010**, *376*, 419–430. [CrossRef]
56. The Look AHEAD Research Group. Effects of a long-term lifestyle modification programme on peripheral neuropathy in overweight or obese adults with type 2 diabetes: The Look AHEAD study. *Diabetologia* **2017**, *60*, 980–988. [CrossRef] [PubMed]
57. Diabetes Prevention Program Research Group; Nathan, D.M.; Barret-Connor, E.; Crandall, J.P.J.; Edelstein, S.L.; Goldberg, R.B.R.; Horton, E.S.; Knowler, W.C.; Mather, K.J.; Orchard, T.J.; et al. Long-term effects of lifestyle intervention or metformin on diabetes development and microvascular complications: The DPP outcomes study. *Lancet Diabetes Endocrinol.* **2015**, *3*, 866–875. [CrossRef]
58. Gong, Q.; Gregg, E.W.; Wang, J.; An, Y.; Zhang, P.; Yang, W.; Li, H.; Li, H.; Jiang, Y.; Shuai, Y.; et al. Long-term effects of a randomised trial of a 6-year lifestyle intervention in impaired glucose tolerance on diabetes-related microvascular complications: The China da Qing Diabetes Prevention Outcome Study. *Diabetologia* **2011**, *54*, 300–307. [CrossRef] [PubMed]
59. Gholami, F.; Nazari, H.; Alimi, M. Cycle training improves vascular function and neuropathic symptoms in patients with type 2 diabetes and peripheral neuropathy: A randomized controlled trial. *Exp. Gerontol.* **2020**, *131*, 110799. [CrossRef] [PubMed]
60. Pop-Busui, R.; Lu, J.; Brooks, M.M.; Albert, S.; Althouse, A.D.; Escobedo, J.; Green, J.; Palumbo, P.; Perkins, B.A.; Whitehouse, F.; et al. Impact of glycemic control strategies on the progression of diabetic peripheral neuropathy in the bypass angioplasty revascularization investigation 2 diabetes (BARI 2D) Cohort. *Diabetes Care* **2013**, *36*, 3208–3215. [CrossRef]
61. Gholami, F.; Nikookheslat, S.; Salekzamani, Y.; Boule, N.; Jafari, A. Effect of aerobic training on nerve conduction in men with type 2 diabetes and peripheral neuropathy: A randomized controlled trial. *Neurophysiol. Clin.* **2018**, *48*, 195–202. [CrossRef] [PubMed]
62. Charles, M.; Ejskjaer, N.; Witte, D.R.; Borch-Johnsen, K.; Lauritzen, T.; Sandbaek, A. Prevalence of neuropathy and peripheral arterial disease and the impact of treatment in people with screen-detected type 2 diabetes: The ADDITION-Denmark study. *Diabetes Care* **2011**, *34*, 2244–2249. [CrossRef] [PubMed]
63. Veves, A.; Backonja, M.; Malik, R.A. Painful diabetic neuropathy: Epidemiology, natural history, early diagnosis, and treatment options. *Pain Med.* **2008**, *9*, 660–674. [CrossRef] [PubMed]
64. Fullerton, B.; Jeitler, K.; Seitz, M.; Horvath, K.; Berghold, A.; Siebenhofer, A. Intensive glucose control versus conventional glucose control for type 1 diabetes mellitus. *Cochrane Database Syst. Rev.* **2014**, *2*, CD009122. [CrossRef]
65. Albers, J.W.; Herman, W.H.; Pop-Busui, R.; Feldman, E.L.; Martin, C.L.; Cleary, P.A.; Waberski, B.H.; Lachin, J.M.; Diabetes Control and Complications Trial/Epidemiology of Diabetes Interventions and Complications Research Group. Effect of prior intensive insulin treatment during the Diabetes Control and Complications Trial (DCCT) on peripheral neuropathy in type 1 diabetes during the Epidemiology of Diabetes Interventions and Complications (EDIC) study. *Diabetes Care* **2010**, *33*, 1090–1096. [CrossRef] [PubMed]
66. Dahl-Jørgensen, K.; Brinchmann-Hansen, O.; Hanssen, K.; Ganes, T.; Kierulf, P.; Smeland, E.; Sandvik, L.; Aagenaes, Ø. Effect of near normoglycaemia for two years on progression of early diabetic retinopathy, nephropathy, and neuropathy: The Oslo study. *Br. Med. J. (Clin. Res. Ed.)* **1986**, *293*, 1195–1199. [CrossRef] [PubMed]
67. Ziegler, D.; Behler, M.; Schroers-Teuber, M.; Roden, M. Near-normoglycaemia and development of neuropathy: A 24-year prospective study from diagnosis of type 1 diabetes. *BMJ Open* **2015**, *24*, e006559. [CrossRef] [PubMed]
68. Charles, M.; Soedamah-Muthu, S.S.; Tesfaye, S.; Fuller, J.H.; Arezzo, J.C.; Chaturvedi, N.; Witte, D.R.; EURODIAB Prospective Complications Study Investigators. Low peripheral nerve conduction velocities and amplitudes are strongly related to diabetic microvascular complications in type 1 diabetes: The EURODIAB prospective complications study. *Diabetes Care* **2010**, *33*, 2648–2653. [CrossRef] [PubMed]
69. Holman, R.R.; Paul, S.K.; Bethel, M.A.; Matthews, D.R.; Neil, H.A.W. 10-Year follow-up of intensive glucose control in type 2 Diabetes. *N. Engl. J. Med.* **2008**, *359*, 1577–1589. [CrossRef] [PubMed]
70. Gæde, P.; Vedel, P.; Larsen, N.; Jensen, G.; Parving, H.H.; Pedersen, O. multifactorial intervention and cardiovascular disease in patients with type 2 Diabetes. *N. Engl. J. Med.* **2003**, *348*, 383–393. [CrossRef] [PubMed]
71. ADVANCE Collaborative Group; Patel, A.; MacMahon, S.; Chalmers, J.; Neal, B.; Billot, L.; Woodward, M.; Marre, M.; Cooper, M.; Glasziou, P.; et al. Intensive blood glucose control and vascular outcomes in patients with type 2 Diabetes Mellitus. *N. Engl. J. Med.* **2008**, *358*, 2560–2572. [CrossRef] [PubMed]

72. Action to Control Cardiovascular Risk in Diabetes Study Group; Gerstein, H.C.; Miller, M.E.; Byington, R.P.; Goff, D.C., Jr.; Bigger, J.T.; Buse, J.B.; Cushman, W.C.; Genuth, S.; Ismail-Beigi, F.; et al. Effects of intensive glucose lowering in type 2 diabetes. *N. Engl. J. Med.* **2008**, *358*, 2545–2559. [CrossRef] [PubMed]
73. Duckworth, W.; Abraira, C.; Moritz, T.; Reda, D.; Emanuele, N.; Reaven, P.D.; Zieve, F.J.; Marks, J.; Davis, S.N.; Hayward, R.; et al. Glucose control and vascular complications in veterans with type 2 Diabetes. *N. Engl. J. Med.* **2009**, *360*, 129–139. [CrossRef] [PubMed]
74. Ohkubo, Y.; Kishikawa, H.; Arak, E.; Miyataa, T.; Isami, S.; Motoyoshi, S.; Kojima, Y.; Furuyoshi, N.; Shichiri, M. Intensive insulin therapy prevents the progression of diabetic microvascular complications in Japanese patients with non-insulin-dependent diabetes mellitus: A randomized prospective 6-year study. *Diabetes Res. Clin. Pract.* **1995**, *28*, 103–117. [CrossRef]
75. Callaghan, B.C.; Little, A.A.; Feldman, E.L.; Hughes, R.A. Enhanced glucose control for preventing and treating diabetic neuropathy. *Cochrane Database Syst. Rev.* **2012**, *6*, CD007543. [CrossRef] [PubMed]
76. Buehler, A.M.; Cavalcanti, A.B.; Berwanger, O.; Figueiro, M.; Laranjeira, L.N.; Zazula, A.D.; Kioshi, B.; Bugano, D.G.; Santucci, E.; Sbruzzi, G.; et al. Effect of tight blood glucose control versus conventional control in patients with type 2 diabetes mellitus: A systematic review with meta-analysis of randomized controlled trials. *Cardiovasc. Ther.* **2013**, *31*, 147–160. [CrossRef] [PubMed]
77. Hasan, R.; Firwana, B.; Elraiyah, T.; Domecq, J.P.; Prutsky, G.; Nabhan, M.; Prokop, L.J.; Henke, P.; Tsapas, A.; Montori, V.M.; et al. A systematic review and meta-analysis of glycemic control for the prevention of diabetic foot syndrome. *J. Vasc. Surg.* **2016**, *63*, 22S–28S. [CrossRef] [PubMed]
78. Knowler, W.C.; Barrett-Connor, E.; Fowler, S.E.; Hamman, R.F.; Lachin, J.M.; Walker, E.A.; Nathan, D.M.; Diabetes Prevention Program Research Group. Reduction in the incidence of type 2 diabetes with lifestyle intervention or metformin. *N. Engl. J. Med.* **2002**, *346*, 393–403. [CrossRef] [PubMed]
79. Li, G.; Zhang, P.; Wang, J.; Gregg, E.W.; Yang, W.; Gong, Q.; Li, H.; Li, H.; Jiang, Y.; An, Y.; et al. The long-term effect of lifestyle interventions to prevent diabetes in the China Da Qing Diabetes Prevention Study: A 20-year follow-up study. *Lancet* **2008**, *371*, 1783–1789. [CrossRef]
80. Balducci, S.; Iacobellis, G.; Parisi, L.; Di-Biase, N.; Calandriello, E.; Leonetti, F.; Fallucca, F. Exercise training can modify the natural history of diabetic peripheral neuropathy. *J. Diabetes Complicat.* **2006**, *20*, 216–223. [CrossRef] [PubMed]
81. Azmi, S.; Jeziorska, M.; Ferdousi, M.; Petropoulos, I.N.; Ponirakis, G.; Marshall, A.; Alam, U.; Asghar, O.; Atkinson, A.; Jones, W.; et al. Early nerve fibre regeneration in individuals with type 1 diabetes after simultaneous pancreas and kidney transplantation. *Diabetologia* **2019**, *62*, 1478–1487. [CrossRef]
82. Singleton, J.R.; Marcus, R.L.; Jackson, J.E.K.; Lessard, M.; Graham, T.E.; Smith, A.G. Exercise increases cutaneous nerve density in diabetic patients without neuropathy. *Ann. Clin. Transl. Neurol.* **2014**, *1*, 844–849. [CrossRef]
83. Villafaina, S.; Collado-Mateo, D.; Fuentes, J.P.; Merellano-Navarro, E.; Gusi, N. Physical exercise improves heart rate variability in patients with type 2 diabetes: A systematic review. *Curr. Diab. Rep.* **2017**, *17*, 11. [CrossRef]
84. Bhati, P.; Shenoy, S.; Hussain, M.E. Exercise training and cardiac autonomic function in type 2 diabetes mellitus: A systematic review. *Diabetes Metab. Syndr. Clin. Res. Rev.* **2018**, *12*, 69–78. [CrossRef]
85. Gu, Y.; Dennis, S.M.; Kiernan, M.C.; Harmer, A.R. Aerobic exercise training may improve nerve function in type 2 diabetes and pre-diabetes: A systematic review. *Diabetes Metab. Res. Rev.* **2019**, *35*, e3099. [CrossRef] [PubMed]
86. Adam, S.; Azmi, S.; Ho, J.H.; Liu, Y.; Ferdousi, M.; Siahmansur, T.; Kalteniece, A.; Marshall, A.; Dhage, S.S.; Iqbal, Z.; et al. Improvements in diabetic neuropathy and nephropathy after bariatric surgery: A prospective cohort study. *Obes. Surg.* **2021**, *31*, 554–563. [CrossRef] [PubMed]
87. The Diabetes Prevention Program (DPP) Research Group. The Diabetes Prevention Program (DPP): Description of lifestyle intervention. *Diabetes Care* **2002**, *25*, 2165–2171. [CrossRef] [PubMed]
88. Look AHEAD Research Group; Wing, R.R.; Bolin, P.; Brancati, F.L.; Bray, G.A.; Clark, J.M.; Coday, M.; Crow, R.S.; Curtis, J.M.; Egan, C.M.; et al. Cardiovascular effects of intensive lifestyle intervention in type 2 Diabetes. *N. Engl. J. Med.* **2013**, *369*, 145–154. [CrossRef] [PubMed]
89. Epidemiology of Diabetes and Complications (EDIC) Research Group. Epidemiology of Diabetes Interventions and Complications (EDIC): Design, implementation, and preliminary results of a long-term follow-up of the diabetes control and complications trial cohort. *Diabetes Care* **1999**, *22*, 99–111. [CrossRef] [PubMed]
90. Nathan, D.M.; DCCT/EDIC Research Group. The diabetes control and complications trial/epidemiology of diabetes interventions and complications study at 30 years: Overview. *Diabetes Care* **2014**, *37*, 9–16. [CrossRef]
91. Chaitman, B.R.; Hardison, R.M.; Adler, D.; Gebhart, S.; Grogan, M.; Ocampo, S.; Sopko, G.; Ramires, J.A.; Schneider, D.; Frye, R.L.; et al. The BARI 2D randomized trial of different treatment strategies in type 2 diabetes mellitus with stable ischemic heart disease. Impact of treatment strategy on cardiac mortality and myocardial infarction. *Circulation* **2009**, *120*, 2529–2540. [CrossRef]

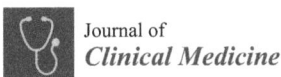

Article

Decreased Need for Correction Boluses with Universal Utilisation of Dual-Wave Boluses in Children with Type 1 Diabetes

Mari Lukka [1,2,*], Vallo Tillmann [1,2] and Aleksandr Peet [1,2]

[1] Department of Paediatrics, Institute of Clinical Medicine, University of Tartu, 50406 Tartu, Estonia; vallo.tillmann@kliinikum.ee (V.T.); aleksandr.peet@kliinikum.ee (A.P.)
[2] Children's Clinic of Tartu University Hospital, 51014 Tartu, Estonia
* Correspondence: mari.lukka@kliinikum.ee

Abstract: Insulin pumps offer standard (SB), square and dual-wave boluses (DWB). Few recommendations exist on how to use these dosing options. Several studies suggest that the DWB is more effective for high-fat or high-carbohydrate meals. Our objective was to test whether time in range (TIR) improves in children with type 1 diabetes (T1D) using the universal utilization of the dual-wave boluses for all evening meals regardless of the composition of the meal. This was a 28-day long prospective randomized open-label single-center crossover study. Twenty-eight children with T1DM using a Medtronic 640G pump and continuous glucose monitoring system were randomly assigned to receive either DWB or SB for all meals starting from 6:00 p.m. based solely on the food carbohydrate count. DWB was set for 50/50% with the second part extended over 2 h. After two weeks patients switched into the alternative treatment arm. TIR (3.9–10 mmol/L), time below range (TBR) (<3.9 mmol/L) and time above range (TAR) (>10 mmol/L) and sensor glucose values were measured and compared between the groups. Twenty-four children aged 7–14 years completed the study according to the study protocol. There were no statistically significant differences in mean TIR (60.9% vs. 58.8%; $p = 0.3$), TBR (1.6% vs. 1.7%; $p = 0.7$) or TAR (37.5 vs. 39%; $p = 0.5$) between DWB and SB groups, respectively. Subjects in the DWB treatment arm administered significantly less correction boluses between 6 p.m. and 6 a.m. compared to those in the SB group (1.2 ± 0.8 vs. 1.7 ± 0.8, respectively; $p < 0.01$). DWB for evening meals in which insulin is calculated solely on the food carbohydrate content did not improve TIR compared to standard bolus in children with T1D. However, DWB enabled to use significantly less correction boluses to achieve euglycemia by the morning compared to the SB.

Keywords: type 1 diabetes; insulin pump therapy; CGM; meal bolus; dual wave bolus; standard bolus

Citation: Lukka, M.; Tillmann, V.; Peet, A. Decreased Need for Correction Boluses with Universal Utilisation of Dual-Wave Boluses in Children with Type 1 Diabetes. *J. Clin. Med.* **2022**, *11*, 1689. https://doi.org/10.3390/jcm11061689

Academic Editor: Manuel Aguilar-Diosdado

Received: 12 February 2022
Accepted: 16 March 2022
Published: 18 March 2022

Publisher's Note: MDPI stays neutral with regard to jurisdictional claims in published maps and institutional affiliations.

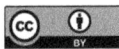

Copyright: © 2022 by the authors. Licensee MDPI, Basel, Switzerland. This article is an open access article distributed under the terms and conditions of the Creative Commons Attribution (CC BY) license (https://creativecommons.org/licenses/by/4.0/).

1. Introduction

Despite of the wide use of modern diabetes technology among the pediatric population in the last decade [1] metabolic control still remains suboptimal in many cases [2]. One of the main obstacles preventing the achievement of treatment goals is controlling postprandial hyperglycemia. Information about how to manage glycemic excursions after meals is relatively limited. It is well known that the timing of the meal boluses is essential [3], but when high-fat or high-carbohydrate meals are consumed, optimal postprandial glycaemia is still hard to achieve [4].

Modern insulin pumps offer a variation of preprogrammed boluses: standard bolus (SB) square and dual-wave boluses (DWB). However, only few recommendations exist on how to benefit from the use of different bolus administration types [5]. The International Society for Pediatric and Adolescent Diabetes states that the impact of dietary fat and protein should be considered when determining the insulin bolus dose and delivery [5], but the optimal insulin bolus dose for meals high in fat and protein is undefined [4].

The use of a fat-protein unit has been previously proposed [6], but the method seems too complex for everyday use for most patients and was associated with a higher rate of hypoglycemia [7]. According to previous research the prolonged bolus administration methods might have certain advantages for high-fat or high-carbohydrate meals [3,8–11]. For example, Jones et al. showed that the 8-h DWB was superior compared to the single wave bolus and provided the best glycemic control after a pizza meal [9]. Chase et al. demonstrated that the dual wave option where 70% is administered as a standard bolus and 30% as a square-wave over 2 h provided the most effective method of insulin administration for a meal high in carbohydrates, fat and protein [10]. O'Connell et al. confirmed the superiority of the dual-wave bolus (50% and 50% over 2 h) for low glycemic index foods as well [11]. These data suggest the DWB utilization might be the preferred insulin delivery mode as it resembles the physiologic postprandial biphasic insulin secretion described first by Curry et al. [12]. Optimal distribution of the DWB parts and duration of the extended part seems to be dependent on specific food content. Lopez et al. proposed that meals with a high fat and protein content require at least 60% of the total insulin upfront to control the initial postprandial glucose rise [13]. To our best knowledge there have been no controlled randomized studies investigating the benefit of one bolus type over the other in a real-life setting over an extended period. Previous studies have been mostly conducted in hospital-based settings and limited to analyze the effect of specific foods on postprandial hyperglycemia in very few individuals [8–10].

Therefore, we decided to perform a randomized controlled crossover study comparing SB to the DWB in a real-world setting. Considering that carb counting is difficult to master for many of our patients and substantial inter-individual differences exist in insulin dose requirements for fat and protein [14–16], high glycemic index and low glycemic index carbs [4], we decided to calculate the insulin dose solely based on the carbohydrate content in the food. Therefore, we decided to use DWB with a 50%/50% proportion with the second part extended for 2 h in order to achieve optimal insulin coverage for a typical Western type meal consumed for dinner. The main objective of the study was to test the hypothesis that the universal utilization of the DWB for all meals starting from 6:00 p.m. for 2 weeks improves time in range (TIR) in children with type 1 diabetes (T1D) compared to the SB use. The decision to limit the intervention period only to evening meals was carried out from the practical reason as this is the time when parents could supervise their children and follow the study plan.

2. Materials and Methods

This was a 28-day long prospective randomized open-label single-center crossover clinical study with a 14-day long run-in phase. Recruitment was carried out during an outpatient visit. All subjects and parents signed an informed consent form approved by the Research Ethics Committee of The University of Tartu before entering the study. The trial was registered in ClinicalTrial.gov under the identifier: NCT04668612. We used the following inclusion criteria: age 7–18 years, T1D duration over a one year, CGM and insulin pump treatment for at least 3 months prior to the recruitment, estimated HbA1c based on the 14-days CGM report below 8.5%, and a daily insulin dose of more than 0.5 international units per kilogram. A power-analysis was conducted and according to Rigby et al. the minimum sample size to demonstrate a clinically relevant change in TIR (10%) would have been 16 subjects [17]. All patients used the Medtronic MiniMed 640G pump with the Enlite sensors, because this system was most commonly used in our diabetic center at that time and equipped with the basal insulin auto suspend before low function. This was turned on in all study participants at the same level: insulin administration was temporarily suspended when the blood sugar of 3.9 mmol/L was predicted. Subjects with known diabetes complications or with elevated tissue transglutaminase IgA antibodies in the last two years and children who developed acute viral infections during the week preceding the recruitment were excluded. During the first study visit, which was the only on-site visit, we collected clinical data of subjects (age, gender, height, body weight, body mass index, pubertal stage according to Tanner scale) and evaluated the eligibility for the study. We titrated insulin doses, set up a bolus wizard in their pump and instructed patients accordingly. After the first study visit patients entered the run-in phase for two weeks. During the run-in period we optimized treatment as much as possible and titrated insulin doses twice, based on the patients CGM reports of the preceding week sent to us via e-mail. Thereafter patients were re-evaluated for eligibility according to the study inclusion and exclusion criteria. We implemented two additional exclusion criteria: patients with a basal insulin proportion of more than 55% or who developed an acute viral infection during the run-in phase, were excluded.

After that, patients were randomly assigned into DWB or SB arms. After 14 days subjects switched into the alternative treatment arm. The study structure is shown in Figure 1. In the subsequent 2 weeks subjects received either DWB (50% of the insulin delivered as a bolus 10–15 min prior to the meal and 50% delivered over two hours) or a SB (100% of the insulin delivered as a bolus 10–15 min prior to the meal) for every meal after 06:00 p.m. Repeated meals were allowed provided mealtimes took place at least two hours apart. Eating with a shorter interval was only allowed in case of hypoglycemia <3.9 mmol/L. In case of hyperglycemia above 12 mmol/L for longer than 2 h after the start of the food bolus administration a correction bolus via standard bolus for both arms was recommended to the target value of 7.0 mmol/L. Prior to the study participants were not provided with specific instructions about CGM arrow trend management. Participants were encouraged to stick to their regular meal schedule and typical diet during the different treatment periods. During the 28-day long intervention period patients and parents were discouraged to change their basal doses on their own.

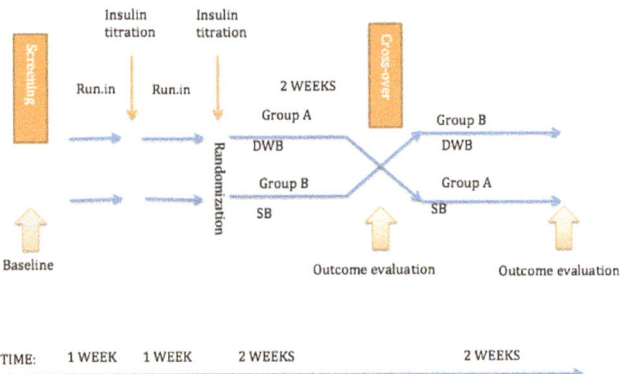

Figure 1. The structure of the study. DWB (dual-wave bolus); SB (Standard bolus).

The use of temporary basal was not recommended during 06:00 p.m. to 06:00 a.m. Within the intervention period correction bolus doses and food bolus coefficients were not modified, basal rate was adjusted only in the case of definite necessity as judged by the patient's physician. After receiving two weeks of SB or DWB CGM data from the pump were downloaded at home and sent to the investigators. Time in range (TIR), (>3.9 mmol/L and below 10 mmol/L), time below range (TBR) (<3.9 mmol/L) and time above range (TAR) (>10 mmol/L) range were recorded from the pump after finishing 2 weeks of each bolus type. Compliance to the study terms was evaluated before the data analysis. Data of the study subject was only included to our analysis if at least 80% of boluses were administered according to the bolus type the patient was randomized to CGM data were analyzed with the Care Link Professional software, which is provided by the manufacturer for the Medtronic system users. Comparison of TIR, TBR and TAR between the two groups was performed using Student's t–test. p-value 0.05 or less was considered as significant. The mean area under the curve (AUC) for the period from the first evening meal bolus after 6:00 p.m until 6:00 a.m. was calculated by the trapezoidal method [18]. The Statistical analysis was performed with R version 4.1.0 for Windows.

3. Results

Out of the screened 32 patients, 31 were enrolled and gave written consent, 1 did not meet the inclusion criteria. In total 31 participants entered the run-in-period, 3 patients had problems uploading sensor data at home and thus 28 patients completed the run-in and underwent randomization. Four participants cancelled the study's active arm due to the failure of following the study plan. Twenty-four patients (10 boys) with T1D, 7–14 years completed the study and their data was included into the analysis. The average age of the study subjects was 10.8 ± 2.0 years (Table 1). Before the run-in period, estimated HbA1c provided by the sensor CGM report was $7.6 \pm 0.7\%$. Mean basal insulin proportion was $37.8 \pm 10.7\%$ at study entry. The average daily insulin dose per kilogram of the participants was 0.8 ± 0.1 IU/kg/d. After run-in and before randomization the estimated HbA1c of the study participants reduced to the $7.4 \pm 0.5\%$ (57.4–5.2 mmol/mol) and average basal insulin proportion remained almost unchanged on the level of $39 \pm 10.5\%$. Mean TIR, mean TBR and mean TAR was not significantly different between the treatment arms as shown in Figure 2. The mean AUC calculated for the period from the first evening meal bolus after 6:00 p.m. until 6:00 a.m. was not statistically different between the SB and DWB study groups (98.73 ± 12.4 mmol/L $\times$ h vs. $101{,}63 \pm 14.8$ mmol/L $\times$ h, respectively; $p = 0.243$). Mean estimated HbA1c after two weeks of DWB or SB usage did not differ either and was $7.4 \pm 0.5\%$ for both treatment arms.

Table 1. Clinical characteristics of study subjects [1].

	Number of Study Subjects = 24
Gender (boys/girls)	10/14
Age (years)	10.8 ± 2.0
Weight (kg)	44.2 ± 12.6
BMI (kg/m^2)	18.7 ± 3.4
Predicted glycated hemoglobin A1c (%)	7.6 ± 0.7
Mean sensor glucose (mmol/L)	9.5 ± 1.1
Daily insulin dose per kg (IU/kg/d)	0.8 ± 0.1
Basal insulin (%)	37.8 ± 10.7
Bolus insulin (%)	62.2 ± 10.7

[1] Data is given as mean $\pm$ standard deviation.

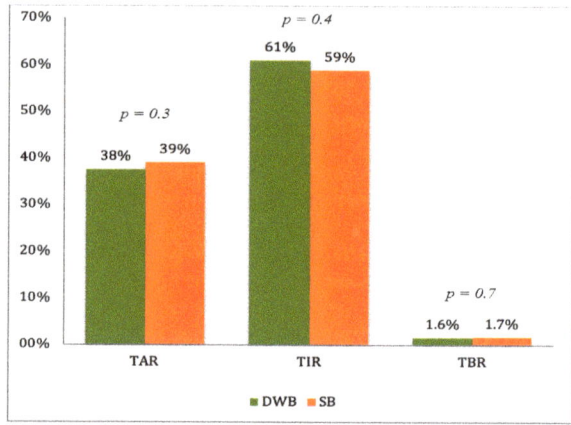

Figure 2. Comparison of mean TIR (Time in Range), TAR (Time above Range) and TBR (Time Below Range) between the treatment arms. DWB (dual-wave bolus); SB (Standard bolus).

Patients in the DWB treatment arm administered significantly less correction boluses between 6 p.m. and 6 a.m. than in the SB arm (1.2 ± 0.8 vs. 1.7 ± 0.8; $p < 0.01$). Eight patients in the SB had to use at least 2 correction boluses during the night, whereas in the DWB group only four. The mean glucose profiles in both treatment arms are shown in Figure 3. The only statistically significant difference in mean glucose levels was seen 1 h after administering the bolus when it was significantly higher in the DWB arm compared to the SB arm (9.8 ± 1.6 mmol/L vs. 8.9 ± 1.8 mmol/L; $p = 0.01$), but with no differences at 2–6 h after the bolus. The mean number of basal suspension episodes from 6:00 PM to 06:00 AM did not differ between the DWB and SB treatment arms (0.99 ± 0.5 vs. 1 ± 0.6, respectively $p = 0.89$), neither were different the mean cumulative duration of suspension (2 h 27 min vs. 2 h 28 min, respectively; $p = 0.887$). Four patients in the DWB treatment arm improved their TIR be 14% to 23% whereas two patients increased their TIR by 13% and 14% in the SB treatment arm.

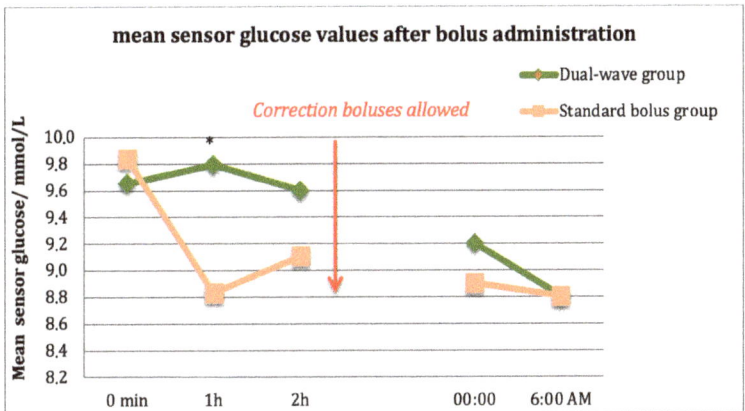

Figure 3. Comparison of mean sensor glucose values after main evening meal bolus administration between treatment arms. * Statistically relevant difference in sensor glucose between treatment arms, $p = 0.01$.

4. Discussion

We described the effect of the systematic use of the DWB on the TIR, TBR and TAR parameters in pediatric T1D patients in a real-life setting. This study was not able to demonstrate the direct benefit of such universal usage of the DWB instead of the SB for the evening meals. These results might indicate the non-superiority of one bolus type compared with the other, but could also derive from the small effect of the evening boluses on the TIR, which is affected by other glycemic and bolusing events during the day as well. In order to identify the preferred bolus type we also calculated the mean AUC for postprandial blood sugar excursions, but this was not different between the treatment arms. However, it should be taken into an account that in the current study design where additional meals and correction boluses were allowed and used 2 h after the main evening meal the mean AUC is also not an ideal parameter to compare treatment arms. In this study we showed a significantly reduced need for correction boluses in the DWB treatment arm.

Many authors have proposed that postprandial hyperglycemia is controlled more effectively when the insulin dose is calculated for both the carbohydrates and fat-protein nutrients [4–7] yet calculating the fat protein unit has not become standard practice since today although suggested a while ago. The main cause for this might be the complexity of this calculation and unwillingness of the patients to use this formulation for their prandial insulin dose. Until today the specific instructions are lacking for the accurate fat-protein adjustments and therefore we did not cover fat and proteins in our study. We hypothesized that the DWB, when calculated solely on the carbohydrate content of food, might be more effective than a SB in controlling late postprandial hyperglycemia, because it also covers the late effects of fats and proteins on blood sugar [4]. Several previously published studies support our suggestion, showing that postprandial hyperglycemia is more effectively controlled, when prolonged methods of insulin administration are used instead of the SB [8–10,13]. However, these conclusions are largely based on blood glucose analyses in very few individuals after single meal analysis in relatively controlled settings and the long-term benefit of the prolonged bolus types' utilization has not been demonstrated. Bell et al. proposed that to achieve target glucose control following a high fat and high protein meal in adults a 30%/70% split over 2.4 h is required [14]. Lopez et al., when studying different split variations after a meal high in carbohydrates, calories and fat, demonstrated that a SB controlled the blood glucose excursion for the first 120 min only, after which there was a progressive rise in glucose level [13]. We also found that the SB provides significantly better control over the first hour of postprandial hyperglycemia, but in contrast to some previous studies [6,12], no difference in sensor glucose level was evident between the treatment arms at 2–6 h after the main evening meal bolus. Bell et al. showed that the optimal combination bolus split to maintain postprandial glycemia for a high-fat and high-protein meal was 60/40% or 70/30% delivered over 3 h [14], therefore our 50/50% split choice over 2 h might explain these differences in the results. Still in our study late hyperglycemia might have been controlled more effectively in the DWB arm, because they required a significantly lower number of correction boluses compared to the SB treatment arm to achieve normoglycemia by the morning. The difference in the number of correction boluses could be explained by the direction of CGM trend arrows 2 h after main evening meal. Patients in the SB treatment arm saw a mean blood sugar value of 9.1 mmol/L with a trend arrow up and therefore probably did a decision in favor to give an additional correction bolus whereas those in the DWB treatment arm saw a mean blood sugar value of 9.0 mmol/L with the trend arrow down and therefore decided to delay or skip the correction bolus. We can only speculate about the possible late postprandial blood sugar rise in SB treatment arm without additional corrections and actual late postprandial blood sugar control in the DWB group in the case of more active usage of correction boluses. Campell et al. also clearly showed that an additional 30% insulin administered 3 h after the high fat and protein meal provided additional benefit to the postprandial glucose control and made it comparable with a meal without any fat [19]. Future studies may reveal if universal utilization of the DWB with a higher initial insulin proportion as for example 70 percent initially and 30 as a extended bolus may provide better coverage for the first hour of postprandial hyperglycaemia as well as for late hyperglycaemia. Four patients benefitted from the DWB scheme for the dinner as their TIR improved more than 10% during the two weeks of DWB administration whereas in the SB arm there were two patients who improved their TIR more than 10%. Such result may be related to some unidentified random factors, but could also indicate, that personal food content preferences might play a role in this. The analysis of food content and its relation to postprandial glucose excursion in relation to different bolus types was beyond the scope of the current work as we attempted to prove the superiority of the dual-wave bolus regardless of food composition. However, it seems that the universal utilization of only one bolus type is not justified and that the choice of the bolus type should be based on the fat and protein content in the food. Nevertheless, the universal use of DWB did not increase the incidence of hypoglycemia as TBR, basal insulin suspension duration and frequency did not differ between the treatment arms. This can be postulated with a reservation as the data about prevention of hypoglycaemia by additional food was lacking, but the systematic use of the DWB for dinner seems to be a safe option in patient using insulin pump with auto suspension function.

The major limitation of our study is the small number of participants for the randomized trial and the risk for type 1 error, when making conclusions. However, to our best knowledge this is the only randomized trial comparing different types of boluses in real-life settings. Many confounders could have influenced the change in TIR and the need for correction boluses, but their impact of the confounders was diminished due to the randomized design of our study. Another significant limitation is the absence of a meal composition analysis, which should significantly influence the pattern of postprandial hyperglycemia, but this was beyond the scope of our study. Meal content analysis could have given addition insight into the benefits and disadvantages of one or the other bolus type, but our intention was to test whether the DWB is suitable for all meals typical for a Western diet [20].

5. Conclusions

In conclusion, the present study demonstrated that the universal DWB utilization for evening meals in which insulin is calculated solely on the food carbohydrate content did not improve TIR compared to standard bolus. The DWB did not result in lower late postprandial hyperglycemia, but DWB users used fewer correction boluses to achieve euglycemia by the morning. Future studies are needed to find the most effective bolusing type for optimal postprandial blood sugar control.

Author Contributions: A.P. conceived the idea for the study; A.P. is responsible for funding acquisition; A.P., V.T. and M.L. worked on the methodology for the study; M.L. and A.P. conducted the study; M.L. is responsible for the formal analysis. Original draft preparation was carried out by M.L. All authors have read and agreed to the published version of the manuscript.

Funding: This research was funded by the by the grants of the Estonian Reaserch Cauncil PSG287 and PRG 1428.

Institutional Review Board Statement: The study was conducted according to the guidelines of the Declaration of Helsinki, and approved by the Research Ethics Committee of the University of Tartu (protocol code 307/T-17 and the date of approval was 20 April 2020).

Informed Consent Statement: All subjects provided informed consent to participate in the study.

Data Availability Statement: The trial was registered in https://clinicaltrials.gov/ct2/show/NCT04668612 under the identifier: NCT04668612.

Conflicts of Interest: The authors declare no conflict of interest. The funders had no role in the design of the study; in the collection, analyses, or interpretation of data; in the writing of the manuscript, or in the decision to publish the results.

References

1. Prahalad, P.; Tanenbaum, M.; Hood, K.; Maahs, D.M. Diabetes technology: Improving care, improving patient-reported outcomes and preventing complications in young people with Type 1 diabetes. *Diabet. Med.* **2018**, *35*, 419–429. [CrossRef] [PubMed]
2. Foster, N.C.; Beck, R.W.; Miller, K.M.; Clements, M.A.; Rickels, M.R.; DiMeglio, L.A.; Maahs, D.M.; Tamborlane, W.V.; Bergenstal, R.; Smith, E.; et al. State of Type 1 Diabetes Management and Outcomes from the T1D Exchange in 2016–2018. *Diabetes Technol. Ther.* **2019**, *21*, 66–72. [CrossRef] [PubMed]
3. Pańkowska, E.; Szypowska, A.; Lipka, M.; Szpotańska, M.; Błazik, M.; Groele, L. Application of novel dual wave meal bolus and its impact on glycated hemoglobin A1c level in children with type 1 diabetes. *Pediatr. Diabetes* **2009**, *10*, 298–303. [CrossRef] [PubMed]
4. Bell, K.J.; Smart, C.E.; Steil, G.M.; Brand-Miller, J.C.; King, B.; Wolpert, H.A. Impact of Fat, Protein, and Glycemic Index on Postprandial Glucose Control in Type 1 Diabetes: Implications for Intensive Diabetes Management in the Continuous Glucose Monitoring Era. *Diabetes Care* **2015**, *38*, 1008–1015. [CrossRef] [PubMed]
5. Smart, C.E.; Annan, F.; Higgins, L.A.; Jelleryd, E.; Lopez, M.; Acerini, C.L. ISPAD Clinical Practice Consensus Guidelines 2018: Nutritional management in children and adolescents with diabetes. *Pediatr. Diabetes* **2018**, *19*, 136–154. [CrossRef] [PubMed]
6. Piechowiak, K.; Dżygało, K.; Szypowska, A. The additional dose of insulin for high-protein mixed meal provides better glycemic control in children with type 1 diabetes on insulin pumps: Randomized cross-over study. *Pediatr. Diabetes* **2017**, *18*, 861–868. [CrossRef] [PubMed]
7. Pańkowska, E.; Błazik, M.; Groele, L. Does the Fat-Protein Meal Increase Postprandial Glucose Level in Type 1 Diabetes Patients on Insulin Pump: The Conclusion of a Randomized Study. *Diabetes Technol. Ther.* **2012**, *14*, 16–22. [CrossRef] [PubMed]
8. Lee, S.W.; Cao, M.; Sajid, S.; Hayes, M.; Choi, L.; Rother, C.; De León, R. The dual-wave bolus feature in continuous subcutaneous insulin infusion pumps controls prolonged post-prandial hyperglycaemia better than standard bolus in Type 1 diabetes. *Diabetes Nutr. Metab.* **2004**, *17*, 211–216. [PubMed]
9. Jones, S.M.; Quarry, J.L.; Caldwell-McMillan, M.; Mauger, D.T.; Gabbay, R.A. Optimal Insulin Pump Dosing and Postprandial Glycemia Following a Pizza Meal Using the Continuous Glucose Monitoring System. *Diabetes Technol. Ther.* **2005**, *7*, 233–240. [CrossRef] [PubMed]
10. Chase, H.P.; Saib, S.Z.; MacKenzie, T.; Hansen, M.M.; Garg, S.K. Post-prandial glucose excursions following four methods of bolus insulin administration in subjects with type 1 diabetes. *Diabet. Med.* **2002**, *19*, 317–321. [CrossRef] [PubMed]

11. O'Connell, M.A.; Gilbertson, H.R.; Donath, S.M.; Cameron, F.J. Optimizing Postprandial Glycemia in Pediatric Patients With Type 1 Diabetes Using Insulin Pump Therapy. *Diabetes Care* **2008**, *31*, 1491–1495. [CrossRef] [PubMed]
12. Curry, D.L.; Morris, J.G.; Rogers, Q.R.; Stern, J.S. Dynamics of insulin and glucagon secretion by the isolated perfused cat pancreas. *Comp. Biochem. Physiol. Part A Physiol.* **1982**, *72*, 333–338. [CrossRef]
13. Lopez, P.E.; Smart, C.E.; McElduff, P.; Foskett, D.C.; Price, D.A.; Paterson, M.A.; King, B.R. Optimising the combination insulin bolus split for a high fat, high protein meal in children and adolescents using insulin pump therapy. *Diabet. Med.* **2017**, *34*, 1380–1384. [CrossRef] [PubMed]
14. Bell, K.J.; Toschi, E.; Steil, G.M.; Wolpert, H.A. Optimized Mealtime Insulin Dosing for Fat and Protein in Type 1 Diabetes: Application of a Model-Based Approach to Derive Insulin Doses for Open-Loop Diabetes Management. *Diabetes Care* **2016**, *39*, 1631–1634. [CrossRef] [PubMed]
15. Wolpert, H.A.; Atakov-Castillo, A.; Smith, S.A.; Steil, G.M. Dietary fat acutely increases glucose concentrations and insulin requirements in patients with type 1 diabetes: Implications for carbohydrate-based bolus dose calculation and intensive diabetes management. *Diabetes Care* **2013**, *36*, 810–816. [CrossRef] [PubMed]
16. Neu, A.; Behret, F.; Braun, R.; Herrlich, S.; Liebrich, F.; Loesch-Binder, M.; Schneider, A.; Schweizer, R. Higher glucose concentrations following protein- and fat-rich meals-the Tuebingen Grill Study: A pilot study in adolescents with type 1 diabetes. *Pediatr. Diabetes* **2014**, *16*, 587–591. [CrossRef] [PubMed]
17. Rigby, A.S.; Vail, A. Statistical methods in epidemiology. II: A commonsense approach to sample size estimation. *Disabil. Rehabil.* **1998**, *20*, 405–410. [CrossRef] [PubMed]
18. Purves, R.D. Optimum numerical integration methods for estimation of area-un-der-the-curve (AUC) and area-under-the-moment-curve (AUMC). *J. Pharmacokinet. Biopharm.* **1992**, *20*, 211–227. [CrossRef] [PubMed]
19. Campbell, M.D.; Walker, M.; King, D.; Gonzalez, J.T.; Allerton, D.; Stevenson, E.J.; Shaw, J.A.; West, D.J. Carbohydrate Counting at Meal Time Followed by a Small Secondary Postprandial Bolus Injection at 3 Hours Prevents Late Hyperglycemia, Without Hypoglycemia, After a High-Carbohydrate, High-Fat Meal in Type 1 Diabetes. *Diabetes Care* **2016**, *39*, e141–e142. [CrossRef] [PubMed]
20. Taber's Medical Dictionary. Available online: https://medical-dictionary.thefreedictionary.com/Western+diet#:~{}:text=A%20diet%20with%20inadequate%20fruits,snacks%2C%20eggs%2C%20and%20butter (accessed on 10 February 2022).

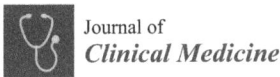

Article

The Diabetes Transition of Hospital Care (DiaTOHC) Pilot Study: A Randomized Controlled Trial of an Intervention Designed to Reduce Readmission Risk of Adults with Diabetes

Daniel J. Rubin [1,*], Preethi Gogineni [1], Andrew Deak [2], Cherie Vaz [1], Samantha Watts [2], Dominic Recco [2], Felicia Dillard [2], Jingwei Wu [3], Abhijana Karunakaran [1], Neil Kondamuri [1], Huaqing Zhao [4], Mary D. Naylor [5], Sherita H. Golden [6] and Shaneisha Allen [1]

[1] Section of Endocrinology, Diabetes, and Metabolism, Lewis Katz School of Medicine, Temple University, Philadelphia, PA 19140, USA; gpreethi7@gmail.com (P.G.); cherielisa.vaz@tuhs.temple.edu (C.V.); abhijanakaru@gmail.com (A.K.); nkondamuri@gmail.com (N.K.); shaneisha.allen@tuhs.temple.edu (S.A.)

[2] Lewis Katz School of Medicine, Temple University, Philadelphia, PA 19140, USA; andrew.deak@temple.edu (A.D.); samanthawatts0711@gmail.com (S.W.); dprecco@bidmc.harvard.edu (D.R.); felicia.dillard@temple.edu (F.D.)

[3] Department of Epidemiology and Biostatistics, College of Public Health, Temple University, Philadelphia, PA 19140, USA; tug30693@temple.edu

[4] Department of Biomedical Education and Data Science, Lewis Katz School of Medicine, Temple University, Philadelphia, PA 19140, USA; zhao@temple.edu

[5] School of Nursing, University of Pennsylvania, Philadelphia, PA 19104, USA; naylor@nursing.upenn.edu

[6] Division of Endocrinology, Diabetes, and Metabolism, Department of Medicine, Welch Center for Prevention, Epidemiology, and Clinical Research, Johns Hopkins University School of Medicine, Baltimore, MD 21205, USA; sahill@jhmi.edu

* Correspondence: daniel.rubin@tuhs.temple.edu

Abstract: Hospital readmission within 30 days of discharge (30-day readmission) is a high-priority quality measure and cost target. The purpose of this study was to explore the feasibility and efficacy of the Diabetes Transition of Hospital Care (DiaTOHC) Program on readmission risk in high-risk adults with diabetes. This was a non-blinded pilot randomized controlled trial (RCT) that compared usual care (UC) to DiaTOHC at a safety-net hospital. The primary outcome was all-cause 30-day readmission. Between 16 October 2017 and 30 May 2019, 93 patients were randomized. In the intention-to-treat (ITT) population, 14 (31.1%) of 45 DiaTOHC subjects and 15 (32.6%) of 46 UC subjects had a 30-day readmission, while 35.6% DiaTOHC and 39.1% UC subjects had a 30-day readmission or ED visit. The Intervention–UC cost ratio was 0.33 (0.13–0.79) 95%CI. At least 93% of subjects were satisfied with key intervention components. Among the 69 subjects with baseline HbA1c >7.0% (53 mmol/mol), 30-day readmission rates were 23.5% (DiaTOHC) and 31.4% (UC) and composite 30-day readmission/ED visit rates were 26.5% (DiaTOHC) and 40.0% (UC). In this subgroup, the Intervention–UC cost ratio was 0.21 (0.08–0.58) 95%CI. The DiaTOHC Program may be feasible and may decrease combined 30-day readmission/ED visit risk as well as healthcare costs among patients with HbA1c levels >7.0% (53 mmol/mol).

Keywords: rehospitalization; transition care; pilot study; prospective randomized trial

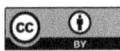

1. Introduction

Hospital readmission within 30 days of discharge (30-day readmission) is a high-priority quality measure and cost target [1]. People living with diabetes are at higher 30-day readmission risk than those without diabetes [2–4]. Several interventions have shown promise for reducing the readmission risk of diabetes patients in mostly observational studies [4]. Selecting patients at high readmission risk for intervention may enable a more efficient use of resources than applying interventions broadly without regard to readmission risk. No previously published randomized controlled trials (RCTs) have tested an intervention designed to reduce readmission risk in patients with diabetes and high readmission risk as predicted by a validated tool. We previously reported on the development and validation of the Diabetes Early Readmission Risk Indicator (DERRI^{TM}) [5–7], which predicts 30-day readmission risk in diabetes patients. The aim of the current pilot RCT was to explore the feasibility and potential efficacy of a novel, multi-component intervention, the Diabetes Transition of Hospital Care (DiaTOHC) Program, on 30-day readmission risk in adult patients with diabetes at high risk based on the DERRI^{TM}.

2. Materials and Methods

2.1. Study Design, Setting, and Ethics

This was a non-blinded pilot RCT with two parallel arms that compared usual care (UC) to the DiaTOHC Program (Intervention) at Temple University Hospital, an urban, academic, safety-net hospital in Philadelphia, PA. The protocol was registered in the National Clinical Trials Registry (NCT03243383) and approved by the Temple University Institutional Review Board (#24306). This study was carried out in accordance with the Declaration of Helsinki. Written informed consent was obtained from all subjects. The study was registered on ClinicalTrials.gov (NCT03243383), where the protocol is accessible.

2.2. Participants and Randomization

Inclusion criteria were an established diagnosis of diabetes, defined by preadmission use of a diabetes-specific medication and/or documentation of the diagnosis in the medical record, age ≥ 18 years, high predicted risk of 30-day readmission ($\geq 27\%$) based on the DERRI^{TM} [6], and hospital admission to a non-critical care unit. Exclusion criteria were pregnancy, binge drinking (at least 5 alcoholic drinks for males or 4 alcoholic drinks for females on the same day), drug abuse within 3 months before admission, receiving palliative care during the hospitalization, participation in another readmission risk reduction program, planned or actual transfer to another hospital or subacute facility, discharge expected within 12 h, lack of access to a phone, living more than 30 miles away from the hospital, HbA1c <5.7% (39 mmol/mol), and inability to speak English. After enrollment, subjects were excluded upon transfer to another hospital or subacute facility, discharge to hospice or a long-term care facility, signing out against medical advice, or inpatient death. We screened a computer-generated list of patients who were admitted to non-critical care units with orders for routine point-of-care blood glucose testing. If the primary hospital team approved, then potentially eligible patients were approached in their hospital room for further screening and informed consent.

Subjects were randomly assigned with a computer-generated randomization scheme 1:1 in randomly permuted blocks of 2, 4, or 6 to receive either the Intervention or UC. The study statistician (H.Z.) generated the random allocation sequence. Group assignments were placed in sealed envelopes and revealed sequentially as subjects were randomized. Study coordinators enrolled participants and assigned them to interventions based on the allocation sequence.

2.3. Usual Care and Intervention

Subjects in the UC group received the standard discharge instructions, education, medication reconciliation, and follow-up according to routine practice. Discharge instructions were generated using the Epic Hyperspace® (Verona, WI, USA) electronic health record (EHR), which is integrated between the inpatient and outpatient settings. Education was provided by bedside nurses and hospital providers at their discretion using stock materials in the EHR (ExitCare Clinical References). Subjects received training by a bedside nurse on using a glucometer and insulin as needed. Diabetes therapy upon discharge was determined by the primary team. Discharge instructions were routinely sent to the primary care provider (PCP) either by fax or EHR. Subjects received a phone call within 4 days after discharge from a hospital-employed community health worker that included checking on the health of the subject, confirming follow-up appointments and access to medications, and answering questions. Problems were referred to a nurse navigator, all of whom had a nurse practitioner degree, for further management. A transition-of-care appointment was scheduled for all patients with a PCP within 10 days of discharge. This appointment focused on medication reconciliation, review of discharge instructions, and updating care needs since hospital discharge.

Subjects in the Intervention group received the DiaTOHC Program in addition to the UC described above. The DiaTOHC Program has three components: (1) patient-centered discharge education, (2) HbA1c-based adjustment of diabetes therapy upon discharge, and (3) post-discharge support.

2.3.1. Patient-Centered Discharge Education

The education consisted of two parts delivered by one of three study team navigators over the phone before discharge or 1 to 3 days after discharge according to subject availability. The first part was focused, customizable, diabetes discharge instructions and education using a 19-page booklet based on American Diabetes Association (ADA) guidelines that includes information on diet, physical activity, and self-care guidance, such as how to recognize and treat hypoglycemia and hyperglycemia [8]. The instructions addressing post-discharge use of diabetes medications were adapted from previously published work [9]. All the concepts tested in the revised Diabetes Knowledge Test (DKT2) are covered in the booklet [10]. Subjects who had not completed a formal outpatient diabetes education program in the prior 12 months were referred to a Diabetes Care and Education Specialist at the Temple Diabetes Center. The second part of discharge education was a comprehensive review of the discharge plan. A navigator reviewed the discharge plan with subjects, covering the treatment plan, how to take medications, reasons for and importance of follow-up appointments and testing, and how to reach post-hospital providers.

2.3.2. HbA1c-Based Adjustment of Diabetes Therapy upon Discharge

Diabetes therapy upon hospital discharge was determined by a study endocrinologist (C.V. or D.R.) using an algorithm based on previously published work and ADA guidelines (Supplementary Table S1) [8,11]. For subjects with baseline HbA1c <7.0% (53 mmol/mol), the preadmission treatment regimen was continued unless adjustments were needed for safety. For subjects with baseline HbA1c >7.0% (53 mmol/mol), preadmission non-insulin diabetes therapy was optimized, defined as using the next higher dose up to the maximum tolerated dose. Only FDA-approved diabetes therapies were used in the study. Metformin was started in subjects with Type 2 Diabetes who did not have a contraindication to using it. Depending on the baseline HbA1c level, insulin was adjusted or added to the preadmission regimen.

2.3.3. Post-Discharge Support

One to three days after discharge, a navigator called subjects to assess their status, confirm receipt of and compliance with medications, verify follow-up appointments, assess barriers to following the discharge plan, determine the need for a community health worker, and review BG levels. Similar phone calls were made weekly for four weeks following discharge or until the first unplanned readmission. Subjects who were discharged on non-insulin regimens were asked to check their BG levels at least once a day, and subjects discharged on insulin at least twice a day. If a subject reported BG levels <70 or >240 mg/dL (3.9 or 13.3 mmol/L), then the navigator notified a study physician, who contacted the subject by phone to adjust diabetes therapy per protocol (Supplementary Tables S2 and S3). In addition, all intervention subjects received a referral for a nursing visit in the home to assess medical needs for support at home. Referral to a community health worker was made if subjects were found to have non-medical needs and/or obstacles to maintaining self-care and attending follow-up appointments, including transportation, food, housing, financial, and legal issues.

2.4. Data Collection, Measures, and Sample Size

The primary outcome was all-cause unplanned hospital readmission within 30 days of discharge. Secondary outcomes assessed at 30 days after discharge were rate of any emergency department (ED) visit not associated with a hospital admission, composite rate of unplanned readmission or ED visit, cost of post-discharge acute care and the intervention (details below), daily frequency of self-monitored blood glucose (SMBG) testing, and three categories of hypoglycemia defined as any SMBG level <70, <54, or <40 mg/dL (3.9, 3, or 2.2 mmol/L, Intervention group only). Data on hypoglycemia in the Intervention group were obtained during the follow-up navigator phone calls. Because the UC group did not receive navigator calls, comparable data on hypoglycemia were not available. Baseline characteristics were recorded based on self-report and review of the medical record.

Approximately 5 weeks after discharge, a study coordinator called subjects in both groups to assess readmissions, ED visits, and the frequency of SMBG testing. In addition, a novel patient experience questionnaire was administered to Intervention subjects. Subjects were asked to respond to each of the following statements with either Agree, Neutral, or Disagree: (1) "I understood my discharge instructions," (2) "The diabetes teaching in the booklet was helpful," and (3) "I was happy with the support I got after leaving the hospital." Healthcare encounters were confirmed in the EHR, which is integrated with several other healthcare systems in the region by Epic Care Everywhere. Readmissions that could not be confirmed in the EHR were confirmed by obtaining discharge records. Change in HbA1c level from baseline (hospital admission) was assessed 3 months after discharge.

The cost of post-discharge acute care was based on the sum of the estimated cost of all planned and unplanned readmissions and ED visits within 30 days of discharge. The cost of each readmission was based on the observed length of stay and a unit cost of USD 3045 per hospital day in 2017 among patients with diabetes [12]. The cost of each ED visit was based on a unit cost of USD 1110 [12]. The cost of the intervention was based on the value of time spent by the navigators and study physicians. Based on the average annual income of a navigator working 2000 h per year, navigator time was valued at USD 58 per hour. Similarly, based on the fiscal year 2018 median income of an assistant professor in endocrinology working 2300 h per year in the United States, physician time was valued at USD 101 per hour [13].

A target of 60 subjects per group was the largest deemed feasible. The last date of enrollment was determined by navigator availability. As a pilot trial, this study is not powered to detect statistically significant differences in outcomes.

2.5. Analysis

Distributions of the data were assessed by descriptive statistical and graphical methods. Summary statistics are reported as mean ± standard deviation or median (interquartile range). Because of skewed distributions, the ratio of estimated costs between groups was calculated using log-transformed gamma regression [14]. The primary analyses for all outcomes were performed in the intention-to-treat (ITT) population, defined as having been randomly assigned to a study group and not meeting post-enrollment exclusion criteria. In prespecified analyses, outcomes were assessed in the ITT subgroup of subjects with a baseline HbA1c >7.0% (53 mmol/mol). No statistical testing was performed for this pilot trial.

3. Results

3.1. Participant Flow

Between 16 October 2017 and 30 May 2019, a total of 3915 patients were assessed for eligibility and 3822 were excluded (Figure 1). The remaining 93 patients were randomized, and 47 were allocated to Intervention, 46 to UC. Because two subjects withdrew consent, the analyzed ITT cohort had 45 Intervention subjects and 46 UC subjects.

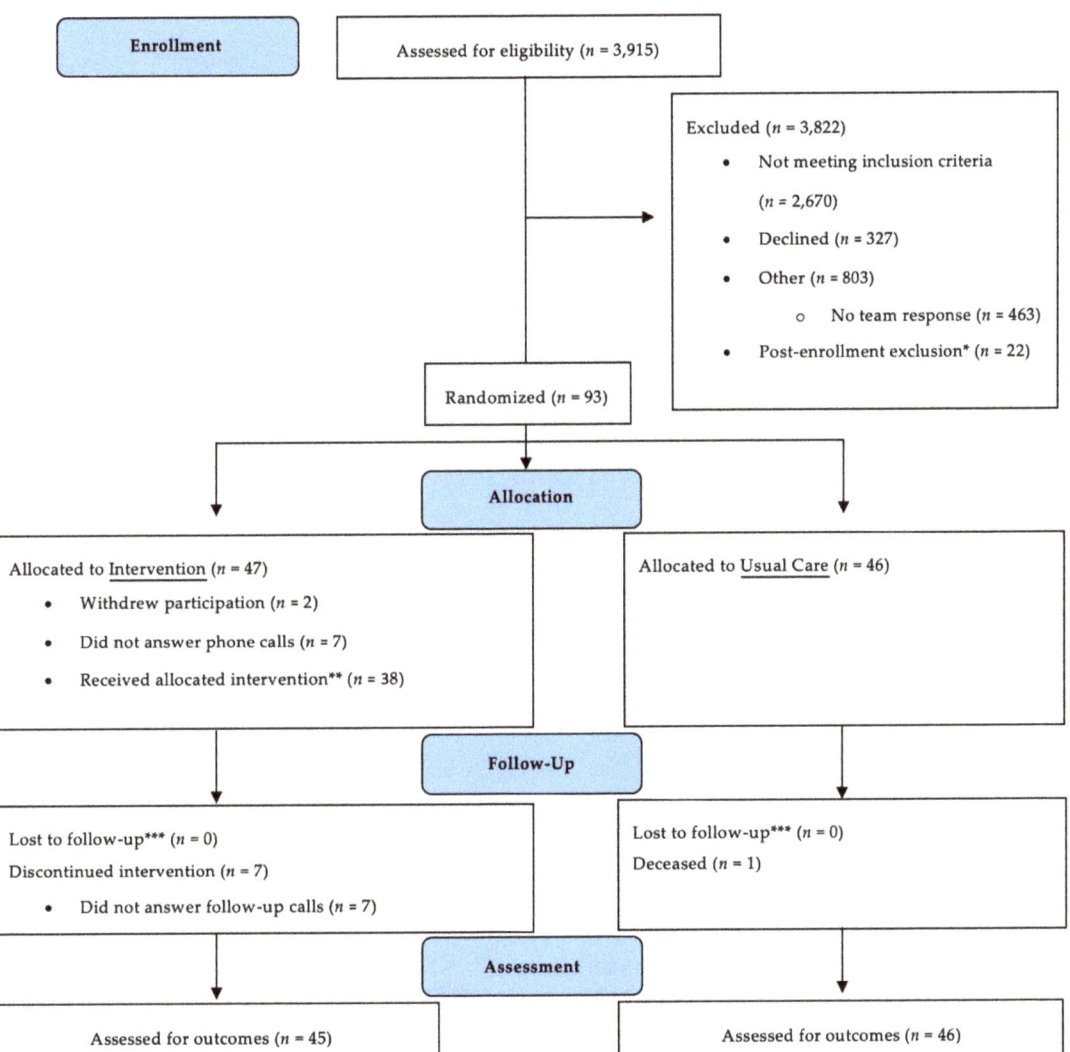

Figure 1. Flow of patients in trial. * Post-enrollment exclusion criteria were transfer to another hospital or subacute facility, discharge to hospice or a long-term care facility, signing out against medical advice, or inpatient death; ** Subject received education, adjustment of diabetes therapy upon discharge, and at least 1 follow-up phone call; *** Electronic health record used for follow-up if subject could not be contacted.

3.2. Baseline Characteristics

Mean age was 58.7 ± 12.7 years, duration of diabetes 15.1 ± 10.0 years, and median HbA1c 8.7% (7.1–10.6%), 72 mmol/mol (54–92 mmol/mol) (Table 1). The cohort was 71% Black, 28% White, 14% Hispanic and mostly low-income (86%). Most patients (95%) had Type 2 Diabetes. Predicted 30-day readmission risk was similar between groups (38.4 ± 7.6% Intervention, 37.5 ± 7.5% UC).

Table 1. Baseline characteristics of Intervention and Usual Care groups.

Variable	All Patients N = 91	Intervention n = 45	Usual Care n = 46
Age, years	58.7 ± 12.7	58.5 ± 13.7	58.9 ± 11.7
Female	47 (51.6)	21 (46.7)	26 (56.5)
Income, USD			
Less than $12,060	25 (27.5)	9 (20.0)	16 (34.8)
$12,060–$16,239	16 (17.6)	8 (17.8)	8 (17.4)
$16,240–$24,599	15 (16.5)	9 (20.0)	6 (13.0)
$24,600–$49,999	22 (24.2)	11 (24.4)	11 (23.9)
$50,000 or more	13 (14.3)	8 (17.8)	5 (10.9)
Race			
Black	65 (71.4)	29 (64.4)	36 (78.3)
Other	1 (1.1)	0 (0.0)	1 (2.2)
White	25 (27.5)	16 (35.6)	9 (20.0)
Hispanic	13 (14.3)	9 (20.0)	4 (8.7)
Education, years	12.6 ± 2.5	13.0 ± 3.0	12.1 ± 1.8
Employment Status			
Disabled	64 (70.3)	32 (71.1)	32 (69.6)
Employed	1 (1.1)	1 (2.2)	0 (0.0)
Retired	16 (17.6)	6 (13.3)	10 (21.7)
Unemployed	10 (11.0)	6 (13.3)	4 (8.7)
Insurance			
Medicaid only	16 (18.0)	9 (20.9)	7 (15.2)
Medicare and Medicaid	17 (19.1)	9 (20.9)	8 (17.4)
Medicare only	24 (27.0)	10 (23.3)	14 (30.4)
None	3 (3.4)	2 (4.7)	1 (2.2)
Private	29 (32.6)	13 (30.2)	16 (34.8)
Smoking			
Current smoker	18 (19.8)	9 (20.0)	9 (19.6)
Former smoker	40 (44.0)	20 (44.4)	20 (43.5)
Never	33 (36.3)	16 (35.6)	17 (37.0)
Body mass index (kg/m^2)	35.2 ± 10.9	36.2 ± 11.7	34.2 ± 10.0
Type of Diabetes			
Type 1	5 (5.5)	3 (6.7)	2 (4.3)
Type 2	86 (94.5)	42 (93.3)	44 (95.7)
Diabetes duration, years	15.1 ± 10.0	13.6 ± 8.5	16.6 ± 11.2
A1c at admission	8.7 (7.1–10.6)	8.9 (7.2–11.1)	8.5 (7.1–10.0)
A1c at admission >7.0% (53 mmol/mol)	69 (76.7)	34 (77.3)	35 (76.1)
Preadmission Home Medication Route			
Insulin only	52 (57.1)	27 (60.0)	25 (54.3)
No medications	7 (7.7)	1 (2.2)	6 (13.0)
Oral & insulin	19 (20.9)	13 (28.9)	6 (13.0)
Oral only	11 (12.1)	3 (6.7)	8 (17.4)
Other	2 (2.2)	1 (2.2)	1 (2.2)
Preadmission sulfonylurea use	8 (8.8)	3 (6.7)	5 (10.9)
Preadmission metformin use	19 (20.9)	9 (20.0)	10 (21.7)
Preadmission insulin use	73 (80.2)	42 (93.3)	31 (67.4)
Preadmission statin use	64 (70.3)	28 (62.2)	36 (78.3)
Preadmission glucocorticoid use	18 (19.8)	8 (17.8)	10 (21.7)
Preadmission blood pressure medications			
None	14 (15.4)	9 (20.0)	5 (10.9)
ACE-i or ARB and Non-ACE/ARB	25 (27.5)	13 (28.9)	12 (26.1)
Only ACE-i or ARB	23 (25.3)	6 (13.3)	17 (37.0)
Only non-ACE or ARB	29 (31.9)	17 (37.8)	12 (26.1)
History of severe hypoglycemia	34 (37.8)	17 (37.8)	17 (37.8)
Current or prior DKA or HHS	9 (9.9)	5 (11.1)	4 (8.7)

Table 1. Cont.

Variable	All Patients N = 91	Intervention n = 45	Usual Care n = 46
Microvascular complications			
0	35 (38.5)	15 (33.3)	20 (43.5)
1	35 (38.5)	20 (44.4)	15 (32.6)
2	15 (16.5)	7 (15.6)	8 (17.4)
3	6 (6.6)	3 (6.7)	3 (6.5)
Macrovascular complications			
0	25 (27.5)	13 (28.9)	12 (26.1)
1	38 (41.8)	20 (44.4)	18 (39.1)
2	21 (23.1)	9 (20.0)	12 (26.1)
3	6 (6.6)	2 (4.4)	4 (8.7)
4	1 (1.1)	1 (2.2)	0 (0.0)
Anemia diagnosis	62 (68.1)	33 (73.3)	29 (63.0)
Discharged within 90 days before index admission	81 (89.0)	45 (100.0)	36 (78.3)
ED visit within 90 days before index admission	24 (30.4)	10 (26.3)	14 (34.1)
Admission priority			
Emergent	75 (82.4)	37 (82.2)	38 (82.6)
Planned	4 (4.4)	2 (4.4)	2 (4.3)
Urgent	12 (13.2)	6 (13.3)	6 (13.0)
Home zip code within 5 miles of hospital	78 (85.7)	40 (88.9)	38 (82.6)
Discharge status			
Against medical advice	1 (1.1)	0 (0.0)	1 (2.2)
Home with nursing care	28 (30.8)	14 (31.1)	14 (30.4)
Home without additional services	56 (61.5)	29 (64.4)	27 (58.7)
Subacute facility (rehabilitation or skilled nursing)	5 (5.5)	2 (4.4)	3 (6.5)
No discharge within prior year	1 (1.1)	0 (0.0)	1 (2.2)
Predicted risk of readmission within 30 days, %	38.4 ± 7.6	39.2 ± 7.8	37.5 ± 7.5
Admission blood glucose, mg/dL	208.1 ± 107.7	188.7 ± 95.6	227.1 ± 116.4
Admission blood glucose, mmol/L	11.6 ± 6.0	10.5 ± 5.3	12.6 ± 6.5
Admission serum sodium, mmol/L	136.0 ± 4.9	136.3 ± 4.9	135.7 ± 5.0
Admission serum potassium, mmol/L	4.3 ± 0.8	4.3 ± 0.9	4.2 ± 0.7
Admission serum creatinine, mg/dL	1.7 (1.1–3.2)	2.0 (1.1–3.2)	1.5 (1.1–3.2)
Admission eGFR, mL/min	39.8 ± 20.6	39.8 ± 20.5	39.8 ± 20.9
Admission hematocrit, %			
High	2 (2.2)	2 (4.4)	0 (0.0)
Low	69 (75.8)	30 (66.7)	39 (84.8)
Normal	20 (22.0)	13 (28.9)	7 (15.2)
Brief Health Literacy Screen Score	11.9 ± 2.9	12.3 ± 3.0	11.6 ± 2.7
PHQ-2 Score	1.0 (0.0–2.0)	1.0 (0.0–2.0)	2.0 (1.0–3.0)
Diabetes Knowledge Test Score	57.3 ± 15.6	59.1 ± 15.7	55.5 ± 15.5
Problem Areas in Diabetes Score	30.6 ± 24.3	36.3 ± 25.1	25.1 ± 22.4
Predicted risk of readmission within 30 days, % *	38.4 ± 7.6	39.2 ± 7.8	37.5 ± 7.5

Values are mean ± SD, median (IQR), or n (%) unless otherwise stated. * Predicted risk based on Diabetes Early Readmission Risk Indicator (DERRI™). IQR (interquartile range), ACE-i (angiotensin-converting enzyme inhibitors), ARB (angiotensin II receptor blockers), DKA (diabetic ketoacidosis), HHS (hyperosmolar hyperglycemic state), eGFR (estimated glomerular filtration rate), PHQ (patient health questionnaire).

3.3. Outcomes

The 30-day readmission rate was 31.1% in the Intervention group and 32.6% in the UC group (Table 2). The combined 30-day readmission or ED visit rate was 35.6% in the Intervention group and 39.1% in the UC group. The number of SMBG tests was 2.4 ± 1.6 per day in the Intervention group and 1.8 ± 1.4 per day in the UC group. Costs in the Intervention group were 33% of the costs in the UC group. Only 11% of Intervention participants reported having at least one BG level <70 mg/dL (3.9 mmol/L) during follow-up. Change in HbA1c was similar at 3 months between the two groups. Among survey respondents in the Intervention group, 97% understood their discharge instructions, 93%

believed the diabetes teaching was helpful, and 93% were happy with the support they received after leaving the hospital.

Table 2. Outcomes in Intervention and Usual care groups.

Intention-to-Treat Cohort			
Variable [a]	All Patients N = 91	Intervention n = 45	Usual Care n = 46
Readmission	29 (31.9)	14 (31.1)	15 (32.6)
ED visit	8 (8.8)	4 (8.9)	4 (8.7)
Readmission or ED visit	34 (37.4)	16 (35.6)	18 (39.1)
Costs, USD	−	5542 ± 10,970	6657 ± 16,969
Costs, USD	−	172 (127–5546)	0 (0–5667)
Costs, Intervention:Usual Care ratio [b] (95%CI)		0.33 (0.13–0.79)	
Hypoglycemia			
-Blood glucose <70 mg/dL (3.9 mmol/L)	−	5 (11)	−
-Blood glucose <54 mg/dL (3.0 mmol/L)	−	2 (4)	−
-Blood glucose <40 mg/dL (2.2 mmol/L)	−	1 (2)	−
Number of daily SMBG tests	2.1 ± 1.5	2.4 ± 1.6	1.8 ± 1.4
Change in HbA1c at 3 months, %	−0.9 (−1.6–0.2)	−1.0 (−1.6–0.2)	−0.9 (−1.4–0.2)
Change in HbA1c at 3 months, mmol/mol	−10 (−18–2)	−11 (−18–2)	−10 (−15–2)
Subgroup with baseline HbA1c >7.0%	All Patients N = 69	Intervention n = 34	Usual Care n = 35
Readmission	19 (27.5)	8 (23.5)	11 (31.4)
ED visit	7 (10.1)	3 (8.8)	4 (11.4)
Readmission or ED visit	23 (33.3)	9 (26.5)	14 (40.0)
Costs, USD	−	3657 ± 8230	6967 ± 18,863
Costs, USD	−	154 (126–1246)	0 (0–5661)
Costs, Intervention:Usual Care ratio [b] (95%CI)		0.21 (0.08–0.58)	
Hypoglycemia			
-Blood glucose <70 mg/dL (3.9 mmol/L)	−	5 (14.7)	−
-Blood glucose <54 mg/dL (3.0 mmol/L)	−	2 (5.9)	−
-Blood glucose <40 mg/dL (2.2 mmol/L)	−	1 (2.9)	−
Number of daily SMBG tests	2.2 ± 1.6	2.5 ± 1.6	2.0 ± 1.5
Change in HbA1c at 3 months, %	−1.0 (−2.2–0.0)	−1.1 (−2.2–0.0)	−0.9 (−2.3–0.1)
Change in HbA1c at 3 months, mmol/mol	−11 (−24–0)	−12 (−24–0)	−10 (−25–1)

Values are mean ± SD, median (IQR), or n (%) unless otherwise stated. IQR, interquartile range; CI, confidence interval. [a] Within the 30 days after hospital discharge. [b] Costs of 30-day readmissions, ED visits, and the intervention. SMBG, self-monitored blood glucose.

3.4. Ancillary Analysis

Among the 69 subjects with baseline HbA1c >7.0% (53 mmol/mol), the 30-day readmission rate was 23.5% in the Intervention group and 31.4% in the UC group (Table 2). The combined 30-day readmission or ED visit rate was 26.5% in the Intervention group and 40.0% in the UC group. Among the Intervention participants, 15% reported having at least one BG level <70 mg/dL (3.9 mmol/L) during follow-up. The number of SMBG tests was 2.5 ± 1.6 per day in the Intervention group and 2.0 ± 1.5 per day in the UC group. Costs in the Intervention group were 21% of the costs in the UC group. Change in HbA1c was similar at 3 months between the two groups.

4. Discussion

This pilot RCT suggests the DiaTOHC intervention, with which participants were overwhelmingly satisfied, may be feasible at an urban, academic, safety-net hospital. Readmission rates in the Intervention and UC groups were similar. However, the trial raises the possibility that the intervention may decrease readmission/ED visit risk among patients with a baseline HbA1c >7.0% (53 mmol/mol). In this subgroup, Intervention subjects experienced a 34% relative risk reduction in readmission/ED visit risk and absolute risk reduction of 13.5%. Additionally, costs were substantially lower in the Intervention group. Furthermore, hypoglycemia during the intervention was uncommon, with 11% of Intervention participants reporting any SMBG <70 mg/dL (3.9 mmol/L). Other trials with similar HbA1c-based discharge treatment algorithms reported post-discharge hypoglycemia rates of 23–29% [11,15].

Several mostly observational studies have investigated the effect of various interventions on readmission risk in diabetes patients [4], categorizable as inpatient diabetes education only, inpatient diabetes management by a dedicated service, and multi-component programs consisting of education, transition-of-care support, and/or outpatient follow-up. The relative risk reductions of these interventions vary considerably from 0 to 71%, with most studies showing benefit.

The current study adds to the small number of related published RCTs with a novel approach: combining multi-component intervention with selection of high-risk patients using a validated tool. This pilot study, however, is limited by lacking power for detecting differences between groups. Because observation of the UC group was limited, we were unable to compare hypoglycemia rates or office visits between groups. Given the nature of the intervention, blinding was not feasible. In addition, the statisticians were not blinded. Lastly, the findings may not generalize to other sites and settings.

In conclusion, the possible reduction in 30-day readmission/ED visit risk in the higher HbA1c subgroup merits further investigation in a larger, multi-center RCT.

Supplementary Materials: The following supporting information can be downloaded at: https://www.mdpi.com/article/10.3390/jcm11061471/s1, Table S1: HbA1c-based adjustment of diabetes therapy; Table S2: Outpatient basal insulin dose adjustment; Table S3: Outpatient prandial/pre-meal insulin dose adjustment based on subsequent mealtime/HS BG values [16].

Author Contributions: D.J.R. conceived of the study and wrote the manuscript. S.W., C.V., D.R., F.D., A.K., N.K. and S.A. collected data. A.D. collected data and edited the manuscript. P.G. wrote the manuscript. M.D.N. and S.H.G. contributed to study design, discussion, and reviewed/edited the manuscript. H.Z. and J.W. conducted statistical analyses. All authors have read and agreed to the published version of the manuscript.

Funding: This research was funded by the National Institutes of Health, grant numbers K23DK102963 and R01DK122073. The content is solely the responsibility of the authors and does not necessarily represent the official views of the National Institutes of Health.

Institutional Review Board Statement: The study was conducted in accordance with the Declaration of Helsinki and approved by the Institutional Review Board of Temple University (protocol code 24306, approved on 24 May 2017).

Informed Consent Statement: Informed consent was obtained from all subjects involved in the study.

Data Availability Statement: Data are available on request due to restrictions on sharing of protected health information.

Acknowledgments: This study was published in abstract form at the ADA 79th Scientific Sessions in 2019.

Conflicts of Interest: D.R. received unrelated research funding from AstraZeneca. S.G. is a member of the Medtronic, Inc. Health Equity Advisory Board and ADA National Board of Directors. The other authors declare no conflict of interest. The funder had no role in the design of the study; in the collection, analyses, or interpretation of data; in the writing of the manuscript, or in the decision to publish the results.

References

1. Benbassat, J.; Taragin, M. Hospital readmissions as a measure of quality of health care: Advantages and limitations. *Arch. Intern. Med.* **2000**, *160*, 1074–1081. [CrossRef] [PubMed]
2. Rubin, D.J. Hospital Readmission of Patients with Diabetes. *Curr. Diabetes Rep.* **2015**, *15*, 17. [CrossRef] [PubMed]
3. Enomoto, L.M.; Shrestha, D.P.; Rosenthal, M.B.; Hollenbeak, C.S.; Gabbay, R.A. Risk factors associated with 30-day readmission and length of stay in patients with type 2 diabetes. *J. Diabetes Complicat.* **2017**, *31*, 122–127. [CrossRef] [PubMed]
4. Rubin, D.J.; Shah, A.A. Predicting and Preventing Acute Care Re-Utilization by Patients with Diabetes. *Curr. Diabetes Rep.* **2021**, *21*, 34. [CrossRef] [PubMed]
5. Rubin, D.J.; Handorf, E.A.; Golden, S.H.; Nelson, D.B.; McDonnell, M.E.; Zhao, H. Development and Validation of a Novel Tool to Predict Hospital Readmission Risk Among Patients With Diabetes. *Endocr. Pract.* **2016**, *22*, 1204–1215. [CrossRef] [PubMed]
6. Rubin, D.J. The Diabetes Early Readmission Risk Indicator (DERRI^{TM}). 2016. Available online: https://redcap.templehealth.org/redcap/surveys/?s=3XCPCAMKWE (accessed on 23 August 2020).
7. Rubin, D.J.; Recco, D.; Turchin, A.; Zhao, H.; Golden, S.H. External Validation of the Diabetes Early Re-Admission Risk Indicator (DERRI^{TM}). *Endocr. Pract.* **2018**, *24*, 527–541. [CrossRef] [PubMed]
8. ADA. Standards of Medical Care in Diabetes—2016. *Diabetes Care* **2016**, *39* (Suppl. 1), S52–S58.
9. Lauster, C.D.; Gibson, J.M.; DiNella, J.V.; DiNardo, M.; Korytkowski, M.T.; Donihi, A.C. Implementation of standardized instructions for insulin at hospital discharge. *J. Hosp. Med.* **2009**, *4*, E41–E42. [CrossRef] [PubMed]
10. Fitzgerald, J.T.; Funnell, M.M.; Anderson, R.M.; Nwankwo, R.; Stansfield, R.B.; Piatt, G.A. Validation of the Revised Brief Diabetes Knowledge Test (DKT2). *Diabetes Educator.* **2016**, *42*, 178–187. [CrossRef] [PubMed]
11. Umpierrez, G.E.; Reyes, D.; Smiley, D.; Hermayer, K.; Khan, A.; Olson, D.E.; Pasquel, F.; Jacobs, S.; Newton, C.; Peng, L.; et al. Hospital Discharge Algorithm Based on Admission HbA$_{1c}$ for the Management of Patients With Type 2 Diabetes. *Diabetes Care* **2014**, *37*, 2934–2939. [CrossRef] [PubMed]
12. ADA. Economic Costs of Diabetes in the U.S. in 2017. *Diabetes Care* **2018**, *41*, 917–928. [CrossRef] [PubMed]
13. MGMA. *MGMA 2019 Academic Total Compensation (by Rank)*; Medical Group Management Association: Englewood, CO, USA, 2019.
14. Blough, D.K.; Ramsey, S.D. Using Generalized Linear Models to Assess Medical Care Costs. *Health Serv. Outcomes Res. Methodol.* **2000**, *1*, 185–202. [CrossRef]
15. Gianchandani, R.Y.; Pasquel, F.J.; Rubin, D.J.; Dungan, K.M.; Vellanki, P.; Wang, H.; Anzola, I.; Gomez, P.; Hodish, I.; Lathkar-Pradhan, S.; et al. The Efficacy and Safety of Co-Administration of Sitagliptin with Metformin in Patients with Type 2 Diabetes at Hospital Discharge. *Endocr. Pract.* **2018**, *24*, 556–564. [CrossRef] [PubMed]
16. Eldridge, S.M.; Chan, C.L.; Campbell, M.J.; Bond, C.M.; Hopewell, S.; Thabane, L.; Lancaster, G.A.; on behalf of the PAFS consensus group. CONSORT 2010 statement: Extension to randomised pilot and feasibility trials. *BMJ* **2016**, *355*, i5239. [CrossRef] [PubMed]

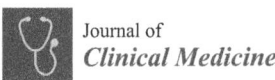

Article

Blood Pressure Monitoring and Perinatal Outcomes in Normotensive Women with Gestational Diabetes Mellitus

Almudena Lara-Barea [1,2], Begoña Sánchez-Lechuga [1], Álvaro Vidal-Suárez [1], Ana I. Arroba [1,2], Fernando Bugatto [2,3,4] and Cristina López-Tinoco [1,2,5,*]

1 Endocrinology and Nutrition Department, Hospital Universitario Puerta del Mar, 11009 Cadiz, Spain; almlarbar@gmail.com (A.L.-B.); bsanchezle@gmail.com (B.S.-L.); alvarovidal1992@gmail.com (Á.V.-S.); anaarroba@gmail.com (A.I.A.)
2 Biomedical Research and Innovation Institute of Cádiz (INiBICA), Hospital Universitario Puerta del Mar, 11009 Cadiz, Spain; fgbugatto@yahoo.com
3 Obstetric and Gynecology Department, Puerta del Mar Hospital, 11009 Cadiz, Spain
4 Area of Obstetrics and Gynaecology, Department of Child and Mother Health and Radiology, Medical School, Cadiz University (UCA), 11003 Cadiz, Spain
5 Department of Medicine, Cadiz University (UCA), 11003 Cadiz, Spain
* Correspondence: cristinalopeztinoco@gmail.com; Tel.: +34-956-003-095

Abstract: Alterations in ambulatory blood pressure detected by monitoring (ABPM) have been associated with perinatal complications in hypertensive pregnant women. Aim: To establish the relationships between the blood pressure (BP) profiles detected by ABPM and adverse perinatal outcomes in normotensive women with gestational diabetes mellitus (GDM). Methods: A prospective study of normotensive women in whom 24 h ABPM was performed at 28–32 weeks of pregnancy. The obstetric and perinatal outcomes were evaluated. Results: Two hundred patients were included. Thirty-seven women with GDM and obesity had significantly higher mean systolic BP (SBP) and nocturnal SBP and diastolic BP (DBP) compared to women with only GDM ($n = 86$). Nocturnal SBP (OR = 1.077; $p = 0.015$) and obesity (OR = 1.131; $p = 0.035$) were risk factors for the development of hypertensive disorders of pregnancy (HDPs). Mothers of newborns with neonatal complications ($n = 27$) had higher nocturnal SBP (103.8 vs. 100 mmHg; $p = 0.047$) and DBP (62.7 vs. 59.4; $p = 0.016$). Women who delivered preterm ($n = 10$) had higher BP and a non-dipper pattern ($p = 0.005$). Conclusions: Nocturnal SBP was a predictor of HDPs in normotensive women with obesity or GDM. Alterations in ABPM in these patients were associated with poor obstetric and perinatal outcomes.

Keywords: gestational diabetes mellitus; ambulatory blood pressure monitoring; hypertensive disorders of pregnancy; perinatal outcomes

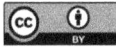

1. Introduction

Hypertensive disorders of pregnancy (HDPs) imply an increase in maternal and neonatal morbidity and mortality as well as an increased risk of obstetric and perinatal complications [1–3]. HDPs include [3] gestational hypertension, defined as hypertension (systolic blood pressure (SBP) $\geq$ 140 mmHg and/or diastolic blood pressure (DBP) $\geq$ 90 mmHg) after the 20th week of gestation in women who were normotensive at baseline, and whose BP return to normal by 12 weeks after delivery; preeclampsia, the new onset of hypertension after the 20th week of gestation and develops proteinuria or end-organ dysfunction; chronic hypertension, defined as documented prepregnancy hypertension, use of antihypertensive medication before pregnancy or hypertension before 20 weeks of gestation and persisting 12 weeks after delivery; and preeclampsia over chronic hypertension, when preeclampsia appears in women with pre-existing chronic hypertension. These disorders affect 5–10% of pregnancies worldwide [4,5], and the presence of some comorbidities, such as gestational diabetes mellitus (GDM), can increase the risk of developing HDPs [6]. Furthermore, the prevalence of GDM has been increasing worldwide; this is related to the current obesity epidemic [7]. Therefore, it is necessary to design specific models that allow us to detect the development of HDPs in patients with GDM early in order to start preventive strategies in these women who are at increased risk.

Although isolated office blood pressure (BP) measurement remains the most commonly used method to detect hypertension in pregnancy in clinical practice, ambulatory blood pressure monitoring (ABPM) provides more reliable records and informs clinicians about BP variability over a 24 h period and the circadian rhythm [8]. In a healthy population, nocturnal BP physiologically falls by 10–20% compared to daytime BP values, which is known as a dipper pattern. The absence of this nocturnal BP fall (known as a non-dipper pattern) [9] and nocturnal hypertension have been associated with the development of HDPs in pregnant women [10–12]. These observations have led some authors, such as Salazar et al. [12,13], to recommend using ABPM in high-risk pregnancies (including women with pregestational diabetes) to detect early BP profile alterations in patients who subsequently develop HDPs. In pregnant women with GDM, there is insufficient evidence, but in a previously published study, we reported that high nocturnal SBP levels increase the risk of developing HDPs in pregnant women with GDM [14].

Previous studies have described an association between BP profile alterations in hypertensive pregnant women and obstetric and perinatal complications, such as preterm delivery, lower birth weight, and fetal growth restriction (FGR) [15–17]. However, few studies have related maternal and neonatal outcomes to BP variability in normotensive pregnant women [18,19].

The aim of the present study was to analyze the relationships between BP profiles (detected by ABPM) in normotensive pregnant women and risk factors for HDPs such as GDM and adverse obstetric and perinatal outcomes.

2. Materials and Methods

2.1. Study Design and Study Population

We conducted a prospective observational study of 255 normotensive pregnant women attending a joint Endocrinology and Obstetrics clinic of the Puerta del Mar University Hospital (Cadiz, Spain), who were selected consecutively between August 2014 and December 2018. Women with GDM were divided according to their pregestational BMI (with or without obesity) and compared to non-diabetic women with normal weight (control group) and women with only obesity (without GDM). Only women with singleton pregnancies who delivered at the Puerta del Mar University Hospital were included. The following exclusion criteria were applied: women with pre-existing chronic hypertension or taking antihypertensive drugs at the time of recruitment, with a diagnosis of placental insufficiency, prepregnancy diabetes, morbid obesity (body mass index (BMI) > 40 kg/m^2), smoking, and underlying chronic or acute systemic disease. The study protocol was approved by the Ethics Committee of the hospital (code number 1507-N-16) and conformed to the principles of the Declaration of Helsinki. Informed consent was obtained from all the participants.

Pregnant women at high risk of preeclampsia were advised to take 100 mg of aspirin daily from 12 weeks until 37 weeks, according to our hospital protocol based on NICE guidelines [20]. ASA prophylaxis was indicated in women at high risk with any of the following high-risk factors: hypertensive disease during a previous pregnancy, chronic kidney disease, autoimmune disease such as systemic lupus erythematosus or antiphospholipid syndrome, type 1 or type 2 diabetes, and chronic hypertension. ASA prophylaxis was also indicated in pregnant women with more than one moderate risk factor for preeclampsia: first pregnancy, age of 40 years or older, pregnancy interval of more than 10 years, BMI $\geq$ 35 kg/m^2 at first visit, family history of preeclampsia, and multi-fetal pregnancy. Obesity was designated as having a prepregnancy BMI $\geq$ 30 Kg/m^2. GDM was defined according to the criteria of the National Diabetes Data Group [21], and women with GDM were initially managed with diet. The glycemic targets during pregnancy were fasting glucose < 95 mg/dL and postprandial glucose at 1 h < 140 mg/dL. If blood glucose targets were not achieved with dieting in two weeks, insulin therapy was initiated. None of the women received oral hypoglycemic drugs.

Between 28 and 32 weeks of pregnancy, ABPM was performed on the nondominant arm during a 24 h period using a Spacelabs 90207 monitor (Spacelabs, Redmond, WA, USA). Measurements were scheduled every 20 min during the day and every 30 min at night. Patients were instructed to maintain normal daily activities, and sleep time was defined as the period between going to bed and rising the next morning. Only ABPMs with at least 66% successful measurements and at least one record per hour were considered valid. The following ABPM circadian patterns were established: the dipper pattern (BP decrease between 10–20% in the nocturnal period compared to the daytime period) and the non-dipper pattern (BP decrease < 10% in the nocturnal period compared to the daytime period).

On the day of the insertion of the ABPM device, fasting blood samples were collected at that moment for biochemical analysis, and maternal clinical data, method of conception, and obstetric history (including parity, previous history of GDM or macrosomia, history of gestational hypertension and/or preeclampsia) were obtained. Office BP was measured with an automated BP monitor (Omron HEM-7200-E (Kyoto, Japan)) in a sitting position twice on the same day and before ABPM.

The following obstetric and perinatal data were recorded after delivery: gestational age at delivery (gestational age was determined by first trimester crown–rump length measurements and was corrected in the case of a discrepancy of ±3 days with the last menstrual period), type of delivery, delivery route (eutocic, instrumental extraction, or cesarean section) delivery complications, birthweight, and the Apgar score. We documented complications of pregnancy such as HDPs, gestational hypertension (BP > 140/90 mmHg after the 20th week of gestation and return to normal BP levels in the postpartum period), preeclampsia (BP > 140/90 mmHg associated with proteinuria >300 mg/24 h or end-organ dysfunction), miscarriage, and intrauterine fetal death. Preterm delivery was considered as a delivery that occurred before 37 gestational weeks. FGR was defined as a birthweight less than the 5th percentile on a customized pediatric curve, small for gestational age (SGA) was designated as a birthweight below the 10th percentile, and large for gestational age (LGA) was when birthweight was greater than the 90th percentile for gestational age. Neonatal composite adverse outcomes were defined by the presence of hypoglycemia, hyperbilirubinemia, congenital malformations, or admission to the neonatal intensive care unit.

2.2. Statistical Analysis

Data were processed and analyzed using IBM SPSS version 24.0 software for MS Windows. Descriptive statistics of the variables measured are presented as the mean and standard deviation (SD) for quantitative variables, and frequencies and percentages for the qualitative variables. We used the Shapiro–Wilk test to monitor the normality of the distributions. The X2 test (or Fisher's exact test, as required) was used to compare qualitative variables, which does not allow us to specify the statistical significance between the four groups. The magnitude of association was calculated using the odds ratio (OR) with the precision described by the 95% confidence interval (95% CI).

Comparisons between quantitative variables and groups were performed with the Student's t-test and one-way analysis of variance (ANOVA) for the parametric variables. Bonferroni post hoc tests were used to identify significant differences between specific groups in case of a significant F value from an ANOVA. Correlations among variables were evaluated using Pearson's correlation test.

A multivariate analysis was performed using non-conditional logistic regression. The stepwise technique was used to select the independent variables introduced into the model. The goodness of fit of the final model was assessed using the Hosmer–Lemeshow test. p values less than 0.05 were considered statistically significant.

3. Results

Two hundred and fifty-five pregnant women were recruited, and fifty-five women were excluded: 11 who gave birth elsewhere and 44 with ABPM readings that were not valid. We observed no significant difference in maternal age at enrollment, maternal pre-pregnancy BMI or gestational age between women who had valid ABPM data and completed the study when compared with the 55 women lost to follow-up. The remaining 200 women were divided into four groups (Figure 1): Group 1 (n = 37) were women with GDM and obesity, Group 2 (n = 86) were women with GDM without obesity, Group 3 (n = 13) were women with obesity without GDM, and Group 4 (n = 64) were women with neither obesity nor GDM (control group).

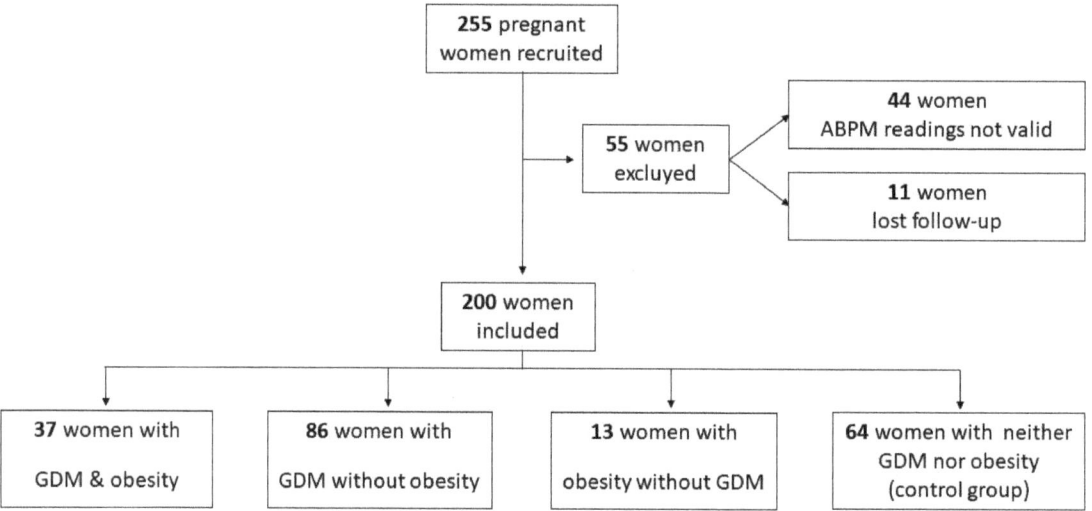

Figure 1. Study flow chart: algorithm for the identification and classification of eligible women. ABPM: ambulatory blood pressure monitoring; and GDM: gestational diabetes mellitus.

Baseline clinical characteristics and laboratory features from each group are shown in Table 1. Maternal age was significantly higher in women with GDM. There was no significant difference in the family history of diabetes mellitus or hypertension, method of conception, history of polycystic ovarian syndrome, parity, or obstetric history (including antecedent of miscarriage, previous macrosomia, history of gestational hypertension, and/or preeclampsia) between groups.

Concerning the characteristics of pregnancy, office SBP and DBP were significantly greater in the group of women with GDM and obesity than in the group of women with only GDM, but there were no significant differences compared to women with obesity without GDM or between the other groups (Table 1). In relation to the laboratory variables, women with GDM and obesity showed higher levels of triglycerides and HbA1c. The rest of the measured variables were not significantly different between groups.

Table 1. Demographic, clinical, and laboratory variables, and ABPM parameters according to presence of GDM and/or obesity.

Variables	GDM and Obesity (n = 37)	GDM without Obesity (n = 86)	Obesity without GDM (n = 13)	Control (n = 64)	p-Value
Maternal age (y)	33.97 ± 3.956	34.96 ± 4.182	30.85 ± 5.414	33.36 ± 4.876	0.009 [a]
Prepregnancy BMI (kg/m^2)	33.81 ± 2.51	24.27 ± 3.02	32.97 ± 3.15	23.80 ± 2.79	<0.001 [b]
Family history DM	19 (51.45%)	38 (44.2%)	6 (46.2%)	22 (34.4%)	0.4
Family history AHT	16 (43.2%)	38 (44.2%)	5 (38.5%)	23 (35.9%)	0.8
Parity					0.5
Nulliparous	16 (43.2%)	33 (38.4%)	7 (53.8%)	28 (43.8%)	
Multiparous	21 (56.8%)	53 (61.6%)	6 (46.2%)	36 (56.2%)	
Previous history of GDM	9 (24.3%)	21 (24.4%)	0	5 (7.8%)	0.01
Office SBP (mmHg)	114.7 ± 12.2	107.6 ± 15.6	116.2 ± 12.4	110.6 ± 11.3	0.02
Office DBP (mmHg)	70.9 ± 8.8	65.2 ± 8.6	67.6 ± 7.7	65.2 ± 8.5	0.005 [c]
Total cholesterol (mmol/L)	6.13 ± 1.21	6.47 ± 1.22	6.27 ± 1.33	6.46 ± 0.99	0.5
LDL-cholesterol (mmol/L)	3.75 ± 1.48	3.77 ± 1.28	3.29 ± 1.15	3.46 ± 0.97	0.5
HDL-cholesterol (mmol/L)	1.91 ± 0.55	1.92 ± 0.43	1.89 ± 0.47	1.99 ± 0.54	0.9
Triglycerides (mmol/L)	2.55 ± 1.15	2.16 ± 0.72	2.46 ± 0.88	2.01 ± 0.7	0.012 [d]
HbA1c (mmol/mol)	33.3 ± 2.62	30.4 ± 2.03	29.3 ± 2.03	29.2 ± 1.87	<0.001 [e]
24 h SBP (mmHg)	109.19 ± 9.61	104.27 ± 8.46	108.15 ± 7.58	104.19 ± 7.45	0.009 [f]
24 h DBP (mmHg)	66.73 ± 5.45	64.53 ± 6.66	64.38 ± 4.42	64.69 ± 5.45	0.3
Daytime SBP (mmHg)	110.89 ± 9.51	106.64 ± 9.15	109.15 ± 8.57	106.55 ± 8.04	0.06
Daytime DBP (mmHg)	68.54 ± 5.53	66.97 ± 6.90	65.77 ± 5.31	66.97 ± 5.86	0.46
Nocturnal SBP (mmHg)	105.84 ± 10.90	99.15 ± 8.68	105.31 ± 7.67	98.39 ± 7.60	<0.001 [g]
Nocturnal DBP (mmHg)	62.70 ± 7.04	59.28 ± 7.08	60.38 ± 5.63	59.03 ± 5.49	0.034 [h]
Non-dipper pattern	22 (59.5%)	42 (48.8%)	9 (69.2%)	20 (31.3%)	0.01

Values are expressed as means ± standard deviation. Categorical variables are given as the number of subjects (n) with the percentage in parenthesis. GDM = gestational diabetes mellitus; BMI = body mass index; DM = diabetes mellitus; AHT = Arterial hypertension; SBP = systolic blood pressure; DBP = diastolic blood pressure; LDL = low-density lipoprotein; HDL = high-density lipoprotein; and HbA1c = glycated hemoglobin. [a] GDM without obesity vs. Obesity without GDM p = 0.01. [b] GDM and obesity vs. GDM without obesity p < 0.001; GDM with obesity vs. control p < 0.001; Obesity without GDM vs. GDM without obesity p < 0.001; Obesity without GDM vs. control p < 0.001. [c] GDM and obesity vs. GDM without obesity p = 0.005; GDM and obesity vs. control p = 0.009. [d] GDM and obesity vs. control p = 0.01. [e] GDM and obesity vs. GDM without obesity p = 0.001; GDM and obesity vs. Obesity without GDM p = 0.007; GDM with obesity vs control p < 0.001. [f] GDM and obesity vs. GDM without obesity p = 0.018; GDM and obesity vs. control p = 0.02. [g] GDM and obesity vs. GDM without obesity p = 0.001; GDM and obesity vs. control p < 0.001. [h] GDM and obesity vs. GDM without obesity p = 0.05; GDM and obesity vs. control p = 0.04.

With regard to ABPM parameters, there were some significant differences between groups (Table 1). The GDM with obesity group had significantly higher mean SBP, nocturnal SBP and DBP than women in the GDM without obesity group. We observed a significantly positive correlation between BMI and ABPM parameters (24 h SBP and nocturnal SBP and DBP), as shown in Figure 2.

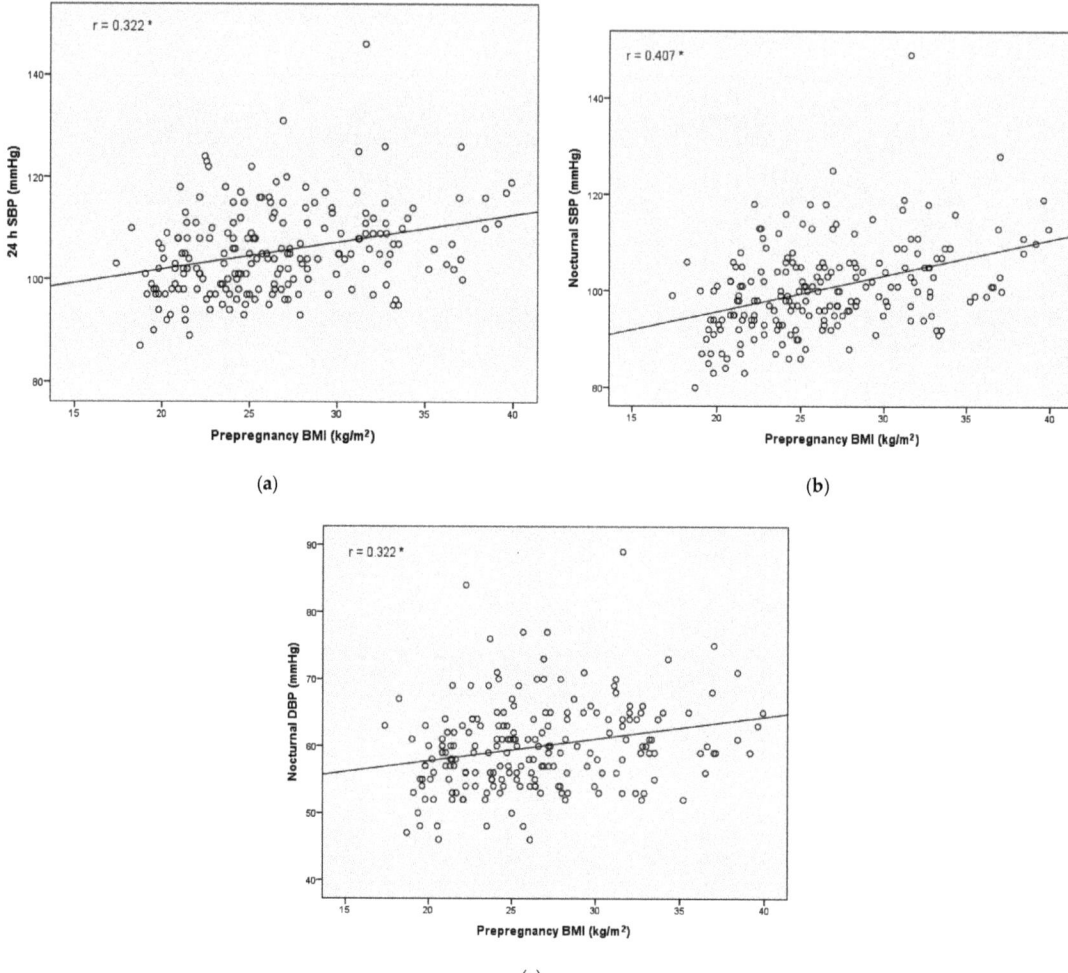

Figure 2. (a) Correlation between 24 h SBP and prepregnancy BMI. (b) Correlation between nocturnal SBP and prepregnancy BMI. (c) Correlation between nocturnal DBP and prepregnancy BMI. Linear correlation between ABPM parameters and prepregnancy BMI. Correlations were evaluated using Spearman's correlation test r. * $p < 0.01$. ABPM: ambulatory blood pressure monitoring; SBP: systolic blood pressure; DBP: diastolic blood pressure; and BMI: body mass index.

Table 2 shows the pregnancy and obstetric and perinatal outcomes data. Among women with GDM (n = 123), the use of insulin therapy was higher in women with obesity (59.5% vs. 41.5%), but the total insulin doses were similar between the two groups (20.95 ± 17.06 vs. 19.92 ± 14.21 UI). All the other women with GDM were controlled with diet and lifestyle modifications. Prophylaxis with ASA was higher in patients with obesity, particularly those with added GDM.

Table 2. Characteristics of pregnancy and obstetric and perinatal outcomes according to the presence of GDM and/or obesity.

Variables	GDM and Obesity (n = 37)	GDM without Obesity (n = 86)	Obesity without GDM (n = 13)	Control (n = 64)	p-Value
GDM treatment					0.05
Diet only	15 (40.5%)	50 (58.1%)	-	-	
Diet + insulin	22 (59.5%)	36 (41.9%)	-	-	
Total doses insulin (UI)	20.95 ± 17.06	19.92 ± 14.21			0.8
ASA prophylaxis	11 (29.7%)	7 (8.1%)	3 (23.1%)	3 (4.7%)	0.001
Development of HDPs	6 (16.2%)	5 (5.8%)	3 (23.1%)	2 (3.1%)	0.02
Preeclampsia	2 (5.4%)	2 (2.3%)	0	1 (1.6%)	0.6
Gestational hypertension	6 (16.2%)	5 (5.8%)	3 (23.1%)	1 (1.6%)	0.007
Gestational age at delivery (week)	38.47 ± 1.30	36.16 ± 1.37	40.12 ± 0.92	39.54 ± 1.23	<0.001 [a]
Preterm delivery < 37 week	4 (10.8%)	6 (7.0%)	0	0	0.06
Weight gain (kg)	7.30 ± 4.32	8.40 ± 4.17	9.15 ± 5.05	10.86 ± 4.29	0.001 [b]
Instrumental delivery	10 (27%)	25 (29.1%)	1 (7.7%)	12 (18.8%)	0.1
Cesarean section	14 (37.8%)	19 (22.1%)	6 (46.2%)	16 (25%)	0.1
Childbirth complications	25 (67.6%)	39 (45.3%)	6 (46.2%)	22 (34.4%)	0.015
Birthweight (g)	3212 ± 615	3188 ± 465	3391 ± 421	3313 ± 475	0.3
FGR	3 (8.1%)	5 (5.8%)	1 (7.7%)	5 (7.8%)	0.9
SGA	7 (18.9%)	9 (10.5%)	2 (15.4%)	8 (12.5%)	0.6
LGA	5 (13.5%)	8 (9.3%)	0	8 (12.5%)	0.5
Neonatal adverse outcomes	8 (21.6%)	12 (14.2%)	2 (15.4%)	5 (7.8%)	0.3

Values are expressed as means ± standard deviation. Categorical variables are given as the number of subjects (n) with the percentage in parenthesis. GDM = gestational diabetes mellitus; ASA = acetylsalicylic acid; HDPs = hypertensive disorders of pregnancy; FGR = fetal growth restriction; SGA = small-for gestational age; and LGA = large-for-gestational age. [a] GDM and obesity vs. GDM without obesity $p = 0.044$; GDM and obesity vs. Obesity without GDM $p = 0.001$; GDM with obesity vs. control $p = 0.001$. [b] GDM and obesity vs. control $p = 0.001$; GDM without obesity vs. control $p = 0.006$.

Regarding the development of HDPs (including gestational hypertension and preeclampsia), the subgroup analysis showed no significant difference between the GDM and non-GDM groups (68.8% vs. 31.3%; $p = 0.5$). However, HDPs were higher in groups with obesity (56.3% vs. 43.8%; $p = 0.005$).

In the analysis of obstetric and perinatal outcomes (Table 2), delivery occurred earlier in diabetic groups, and the mean gestational age at delivery was lower in the GDM without obesity group. Weight gain was higher in non-GDM women, particularly those without obesity. No statistically significant differences were found in birthweight or neonatal composite adverse outcomes (hyperbilirubinemia, hypoglycemia, congenital malformations, or admission to the intensive care unit for any reason). Conversely, the rate of global delivery complications (including cesarean section during labor, instrumental delivery, and perineal tear) was significantly higher in GDM women with obesity than in the other groups.

To evaluate the relationship between the ABPM parameters and the development of HDPs, bivariate analysis was conducted, and the results are shown in Table 3. Pregnant women who developed HDPs had higher SBP (mean, daytime and nocturnal) and daytime DBP than normotensive women. Concerning the neonatal composite adverse outcomes, the nocturnal averages were significantly higher in women whose newborns had neonatal complications, as outlined in Table 3. We also identified a non-dipper pattern, and ABPM parameters of BP were significantly higher in women with preterm delivery than in mothers who had a term pregnancy. The remaining variables analyzed for obstetric and perinatal outcomes were not significantly different (results not shown).

Table 3. Bivariate analysis of the association between BP parameters, analyzed by ABPM, and develop of HDP, preterm delivery and the presence neonatal composite adverse outcomes.

Variables	Development of HDPs		Preterm Delivery		Neonatal Adverse Outcomes	
	Yes (n = 16)	No (n = 184)	Yes (n = 10)	No (n = 190)	Yes (n = 27)	No (n = 173)
24 h SBP (mmHg)	113.1 ± 13.5 *	104.7 ± 7.6 *	114.5 ± 14.5 *	104.9 ± 7.8 *	107.9 ± 11.1	105 ± 7.9
24 h DBP (mmHg)	68.8 ± 8.9	64.6 ± 5.5	72.1 ± 8.1 *	64.6 ± 5.6 *	67.0 ± 7.9	64.6 ± 5.5
Daytime SBP (mmHg)	115.6 ± 12.5 *	106.9 ± 8.2 *	115.9 ± 13.6	107.1 ± 8.4	109.7 ± 10.8	107.2 ± 8.5
Daytime DBP (mmHg)	71.1 ± 8.1 *	66.8 ± 5.9 *	73.6 ± 7.8 *	66.8 ± 5.9 *	68.9 ± 8.0	66.9 ± 5.9
Nocturnal SBP (mmHg)	107.8 ± 16.7 *	99.9 ± 7.9 *	112.0 ± 17.4 *	99.9 ± 8.1 *	103.8 ± 13.2 *	100 ± 8.3 *
Nocturnal DBP (mmHg)	62.9 ± 11.4	59.6 ± 5.9	68.9 ± 9.8 *	59.4 ± 6.1 *	62.7 ± 8.6 *	59.4 ± 6.1 *
Non-dipper pattern	7 (43.8%)	86 (46.7%)	9 (90.0%) *	84 (44.2%) *	15 (55.6%)	78 (45.1%)

Values are expressed as means ± standard deviation. Categorical variables are given as the number of subjects (n) with the percentage in parenthesis. * $p < 0.05$. HDPs = hypertensive disorders of pregnancy; SBP = systolic blood pressure; and DBP = diastolic blood pressure.

Multivariate analysis used the development of HDPs as the independent variable and all the variables that were statistically significant in the univariate model were used as dependent variables, with some independent variables considered as having possible clinical significance. Table 4 summarizes the results of these analyses in the final model. The outcomes indicated nocturnal SBP (OR = 1.077) and BMI (OR = 1.131) as risk factors for the development of HDPs.

Table 4. Final model of the multivariable regression analysis for the risk prediction of HDP. B: Beta; Exp (B): beta exponent; 95% CI for Exp (B): 95% confidence interval for beta exponent. GDM = gestational diabetes mellitus; BMI = body mass index; and SBP = systolic blood pressure.

Variables	B	p-Value	Exp (B)	95% CI for Exp (B)
Nocturnal SBP	0.074	0.015	1.077	1.015–1.143
Prepregnancy BMI	0.123	0.035	1.131	1.009–1.268
Dipper pattern	0.990	0.112	2.691	0.793–9.130
GDM	0.077	0.902	1.080	0.316–3.685
Age	−0.033	0.601	0.967	0.854–1.096

4. Discussion

In the present study, we found higher BP levels detected by ABPM in pregnant women who subsequently developed HDPs as well as adverse obstetric and perinatal outcomes. Our results suggest that ABPM could have clinical utility in the prediction of the risk for HDPs in pregnant women with comorbidities, such as GDM and prepregnancy obesity. To our knowledge, this is the largest sample size study on ABPM performed in women with GDM, and furthermore, we have included a group of patients with only obesity, without GDM, due to the close relationship between obesity and GDM [7] and the possibility that some of the results could be attributed to the presence of obesity, independently of the metabolic alterations present in GDM.

GDM and prepregnancy obesity are independent risk factors for maternal and neonatal complications [22–26]. In our cohort, the incidence of HDPs was 8% (n = 16), and no significant differences between groups were found with respect to the presence of GDM. However, obesity was observed to be an independent risk marker for developing HDPs, which is consistent with previous studies [23,27,28]. Moreover, when obesity is associated with GDM, the risk for HDPs increases compared to pregnant women with GDM without obesity, in agreement with other investigators [24,25,29,30]. On the other hand, while some authors found that the development of HDPs was even more frequent in pregnant women with obesity without GDM [24], others have not observed the same feature [30]. Either way, prepregnancy BMI seems to have a stronger influence than GDM on the development of HDPs [26].

Currently, there are no specific recommendations regarding the use of ABPM in pregnancy, except for the differentiation between true hypertension and the white-coat effect [31,32]. However, some authors recommend its usefulness in high-risk pregnancies [13]. In fact, Salazar et al. found a higher rate of masked hypertension (defined as a mean BP > 130/80 mmHg with normal office BP levels) and nocturnal hypertension in normotensive women with high-risk pregnancy, regarding these variables as predictors of the development of HDPs. In our cohort, we found higher 24 h, daytime, and nocturnal SBP and daytime DBP levels in pregnant women who developed HDPs. Furthermore, multivariate analysis identified nocturnal SBP as an independent risk factor for the development of HDPs, coinciding with the data published in relation to pregnant women with chronic hypertension or high-risk pregnancy [10,12]. In a cohort of normotensive pregnant women with GDM, we also observed that higher nocturnal SBP increased the risk of developing HDPs [14]. In addition, in this study, we found that patients in the GDM with obesity group had higher mean SBP, nocturnal SBP, and DBP than pregnant women with GDM without obesity. These data show that ABPM could have specific utility in this group with double risk, obesity and GDM. In this group, we also observed higher levels of triglycerides, in agreement with some authors [33,34], and postulated that this atherogenic profile could be related to endothelial dysfunction causing subclinical BP alterations, as has been described in subjects with type 1 diabetes mellitus [35]. Pregnant women with obesity and GDM also had higher HbA1c levels and received insulin therapy more frequently than GDM women without obesity, similar to findings reported by other investigators [24,29], but in our cohort, there was no difference in the total dose of insulin used between the two groups. Weight gain during pregnancy was significantly lower in the GDM groups than in the control group, which can be explained by specific dietary management and better compliance to recommendations in diabetic women. Nevertheless, inadequate weight gain has been related to the development of HDPs by other authors [29] as well as poor obstetric and perinatal outcomes [36].

In our study, the non-dipper pattern was more prevalent in the obesity groups, whereas women without obesity more frequently had a dipper circadian pattern. Although a significant relationship between the non-dipper pattern and the diagnosis of GDM in normotensive pregnant women has been described [14,37], these works do not analyze the influence of pre-pregnancy obesity as an independent factor in the ABPM pattern. In fact, there was a significant correlation between prepregnancy BMI and mean SBP and nocturnal SBP levels detected by ABPM (Figure 2) but not with blood glucose levels. These findings are consistent with the previous hypothesis reported [22,24,26] that considers prepregnancy obesity to have a more important role in the development of HDPs than GDM.

The incidence of HDPs in our patients was lower than expected, but it was higher in pregnant women with prepregnancy obesity even though ASA use was greater in this population. A possible explanation for these findings could be the use of low doses of ASA according to current recommendations in clinical practice guidelines [20,31] to reduce the risk of preeclampsia, preterm delivery, FGR, and miscarriage in pregnant women with chronic hypertension or risk factors for preeclampsia.

As described in the literature, gestational age at delivery was lower in pregnant women with GDM, probably due to the higher frequency of indications for induction in these patients compared to women with obesity without GDM. Most patients who had a preterm delivery showed a non-dipper pattern in ABPM, according to the data published by other authors, in pregnant women who develop gestational hypertension [16] and preeclampsia [38]. Furthermore, we observed significantly higher mean and nocturnal BP, both systolic and diastolic, and daytime SBP levels in these women compared to those with delivery at term, similar to that described previously in patients with preterm delivery associated with gestational hypertension [17].

The rate of delivery complications was higher in pregnant women with GDM and obesity, in agreement with other publications [24], but we did not find any differences with respect to birthweight, Apgar score, the rate of cesarean section, FGR, SGA, LGA or perinatal complications (composite variable) between the different groups. An association between the presence of FGR or SGA and circadian variation in BP in both normotensive and hypertensive pregnant women has been described in the literature [15,16,18,19]. In our study, BP values in ABPM were higher in women who had FGR, but these findings were not statistically significant. Nevertheless, we detected nocturnal SBP and DBP values that were significantly higher in pregnant women whose newborns had neonatal complications (hypoglycemia, hyperbilirubinemia, congenital malformations or admissions to the intensive care unit), as has been reported by some authors in women who subsequently developed gestational hypertension [17,39].

The principal limitation of our study was the small size of the obesity group without GDM (13 women), which could have influenced our ability to detect any differences from the other groups, and the inclusion of more patients could have provided greater precision for our results. However, the sample size was adequate to detect statistically significant and clinically relevant results.

Nevertheless, the most important strength is that this study is the largest sample size study evaluating the relationship between ABPM parameters and obstetric and perinatal outcomes in pregnant women with GDM considering obesity, and the inclusion of non-diabetic women both with and without obesity.

5. Conclusions

We concluded that normotensive pregnant women with GDM and obesity have a high risk of maternal and perinatal complications, with a presumably greater impact of obesity than GDM. Subclinical alterations in the BP profile in women with preterm delivery and neonatal complications have been described, and nocturnal SBP predicts the development of HDPs. Thus, ABPM may be useful for identifying women at higher risk of adverse obstetric and perinatal outcomes who could benefit from preventive actions. Studies with larger sample sizes would be necessary to confirm our results and allow us to find greater differences.

Author Contributions: Conceptualization and study design C.L.-T. and F.B.; data acquisition and data analysis and interpretation, A.L.-B., B.S.-L. and Á.V.-S.; validation and formal analysis, A.L.-B. and B.S.-L.; writing—original draft preparation, A.L.-B. and C.L.-T.; writing—review and editing, A.I.A. All authors have read and agreed to the published version of the manuscript.

Funding: This research was funded by the Instituto de Salud Carlos III, grant number "PI16/00370" (co-funded by the European Regional Development Fund, ERDF), and the Biomedical Research and Innovation Institute of Cádiz (INiBICA).

Institutional Review Board Statement: This study was conducted in accordance with the Declaration of Helsinki, and was approved by the Institutional Review Board of Hospital Universitario Puerta del Mar, Cádiz, Spain (code number 1507-N-16, on 21 December 2016).

Informed Consent Statement: Informed consent was obtained from all subjects involved in the study.

Conflicts of Interest: The authors declare no conflict of interest. The funders had no role in the design of the study; in the collection, analyses, or interpretation of data; in the writing of the manuscript; or in the decision to publish the results.

References

1. Ananth, C.V.; Basso, O. Impact of pregnancy-induced hypertension on stillbirth and neonatal mortality. *Epidemiology* **2010**, *21*, 118–123. [CrossRef] [PubMed]
2. Li, X.; Zhang, W.; Lin, J.; Liu, H.; Yang, Z.; Teng, Y.; Huang, J.; Peng, Q.; Lin, X.; Zhang, J.; et al. Hypertensive disorders of pregnancy and risks of adverse pregnancy outcomes: A retrospective cohort study of 2368 patients. *J. Hum. Hypertens.* **2021**, *35*, 65–73. [CrossRef] [PubMed]
3. Khedagi, A.M.; Bello, N.A. Hypertensive Disorders of Pregnancy. *Cardiol. Clin.* **2021**, *39*, 77–90. [CrossRef] [PubMed]
4. Hutcheon, J.A.; Lisonkova, S.; Joseph, K.S. Epidemiology of pre-eclampsia and the other hypertensive disorders of pregnancy. *Best Pract. Res. Clin. Obstet. Gynaecol.* **2011**, *25*, 391–403. [CrossRef] [PubMed]

5. American College of Obstetricians; Task Force on Hypertension in Pregnancy. Hypertension in pregnancy. Report of the American College of Obstetricians and Gynecologists' Task Force on Hypertension in Pregnancy. *Obstet. Gynecol.* **2013**, *122*, 1122–1131.
6. Roberts, C.L.; Ford, J.B.; Algert, C.S.; Antonsen, S.; Chalmers, J.; Cnattingius, S.; Gokhale, M.; Kotelchuck, M.; Melve, K.K.; Langridge, A.; et al. Population-based trends in pregnancy hypertension and pre-eclampsia: An international comparative study. *BMJ Open* **2014**, *1*, e000101. [CrossRef]
7. Sathyapalan, T.; Mellor, D.; Atkin, S.L. Obesity and gestational diabetes. *Semin. Fetal Neonatal Med.* **2010**, *15*, 89–93. [CrossRef]
8. Gorostidi, M.; Banegas, J.R.; de la Sierra, A.; Vinyoles, E.; Segura, J.; Ruilope, L.M. Ambulatory blood pressure monitoring in daily clinical practice—The Spanish ABPM Registry experience. *Eur. J. Clin. Investig.* **2016**, *46*, 92–98. [CrossRef]
9. Parati, G.; Stergiou, G.; O'Brien, E.; Asmar, R.; Beilin, L.; Bilo, G.; Clement, D.; De La Sierra, A.; De Leeuw, P.; Dolan, E.; et al. European society of hypertension practice guidelines for ambulatory blood pressure monitoring. *J. Hypertens.* **2014**, *32*, 1359–1366. [CrossRef]
10. Bhide, A.; Sankaran, S.; Moore, J.; Khalil, A.; Furneaux, E. Ambulatory blood pressure measurements in mid-pregnancy and development of hypertensive pregnancy disorders. *Hypertens. Pregnancy* **2014**, *33*, 159–167. [CrossRef]
11. Saremi, A.T.; Shafiee, M.-A.; Montazeri, M.; Rashidi, N.; Montazeri, M. Blunted Overnight Blood Pressure Dipping in Second Trimester; A Strong Predictor of Gestational Hypertension and Preeclampsia. *Curr. Hypertens. Rev.* **2018**, *15*, 70–75. [CrossRef] [PubMed]
12. Salazar, M.R.; Espeche, W.G.; Leiva Sisnieguez, C.E.; Leiva Sisnieguez, B.C.; Balbín, E.; Stavile, R.N.; March, C.; Olano, R.D.; Soria, A.; Yoma, O.; et al. Nocturnal hypertension in high-risk mid-pregnancies predict the development of preeclampsia/eclampsia. *J. Hypertens.* **2019**, *37*, 182–186. [CrossRef] [PubMed]
13. Salazar, M.R.; Espeche, W.G.; Sisnieguez, B.C.L.; Balbín, E.; Sisnieguez, C.E.L.; Stavile, R.N.; March, C.E.; Grassi, F.; Santillan, C.; Cor, S.; et al. Significance of masked and nocturnal hypertension in normotensive women coursing a high-risk pregnancy. *J. Hypertens.* **2016**, *34*, 2248–2252. [CrossRef] [PubMed]
14. Sánchez-Lechuga, B.; Lara-Barea, A.; Córdoba-Doña, J.A.; Montero Galván, A.; Abal Cruz, A.; Aguilar-Diosdado, M.; López-Tinoco, C. Usefulness of blood pressure monitoring in patients with gestational diabetes mellitus. *Endocrinol. Diabetes Nutr. (Engl. Ed.)* **2018**, *65*, 394–401. [CrossRef]
15. Brown, M.A.; Davis, G.K.; McHugh, L. The prevalence and clinical significance of nocturnal hypertension in pregnancy. *J. Hypertens.* **2001**, *19*, 1437–1444. [CrossRef]
16. Ilic, A.; Ilic, D.J.; Tadic, S.; Stefanovic, M.; Stojsic-Milosavljevic, A.; Pavlovic, K.; Redzek, A.; Velicki, L. Influence of non-dipping pattern of blood pressure in gestational hypertension on maternal cardiac function, hemodynamics and intrauterine growth restriction. *Pregnancy Hypertens.* **2017**, *10*, 34–41. [CrossRef]
17. Liro, M.; Gąsowski, J.; Wydra, D.; Grodzicki, T.; Emerich, J.; Narkiewicz, K. Twenty-four-hour and conventional blood pressure components and risk of preterm delivery or neonatal complications in gestational hypertension. *Blood Press.* **2009**, *18*, 36–43. [CrossRef]
18. Tranquilli, A.L.; Giannubilo, S.R. Blood pressure is elevated in normotensive pregnant women with intrauterine growth restriction. *Eur. J. Obstet. Gynecol. Reprod. Biol.* **2005**, *122*, 45–48. [CrossRef]
19. Prefumo, F.; Muiesan, M.L.; Perini, R.; Paini, A.; Bonzi, B.; Lojacono, A.; Agabiti-Rosei, E.; Frusca, T. Maternal cardiovascular function in pregnancies complicated by intrauterine growth restriction. *Ultrasound Obstet. Gynecol.* **2008**, *31*, 65–71. [CrossRef]
20. National Institute for Health and Care Excellence (NICE). *Hypertension in Pregnancy: The Management of Hypertensive Disorders during Pregnancy*; RCOG Press: London, UK, 2010.
21. National Diabetes Data Group. Classification and diagnosis of diabetes mellitus and other categories of glucose intolerance. *Diabetes* **1979**, *28*, 1039–1057. [CrossRef]
22. Catalano, P.M.; McIntyre, H.D.; Cruickshank, J.K.; McCance, D.R.; Dyer, A.R.; Metzger, B.E.; Lowe, L.P.; Trimble, E.R.; Coustan, D.R.; Hadden, D.R.; et al. The hyperglycemia and adverse pregnancy outcome study: Associations of GDM and obesity with pregnancy outcomes. *Diabetes Care* **2012**, *35*, 780–786. [CrossRef] [PubMed]
23. Di Benedetto, A.; D'anna, R.; Cannata, M.L.; Giordano, D.; Interdonato, M.L.; Corrado, F. Effects of prepregnancy body mass index and weight gain during pregnancy on perinatal outcome in glucose-tolerant women. *Diabetes Metab.* **2012**, *38*, 63–67. [CrossRef] [PubMed]
24. Huet, J.; Beucher, G.; Rod, A.; Morello, R.; Dreyfus, M. Joint impact of gestational diabetes and obesity on perinatal outcomes. *J. Gynecol. Obstet. Hum. Reprod.* **2018**, *47*, 469–476. [CrossRef] [PubMed]
25. Roman, A.S.; Rebarber, A.; Fox, N.S.; Klauser, C.K.; Istwan, N.; Rhea, D.; Saltzman, D. The effect of maternal obesity on pregnancy outcomes in women with gestational diabetes. *J. Matern. Neonatal Med.* **2011**, *24*, 723–727. [CrossRef]
26. Ricart, W.; López, J.; Mozas, J.; Pericot, A.; Sancho, M.A.; González, N.; Balsells, M.; Luna, R.; Cortázar, A.; Navarro, P.; et al. Body mass index has a greater impact on pregnancy outcomes than gestational hyperglycaemia. *Diabetologia* **2005**, *48*, 1736–1742. [CrossRef]
27. Callaway, L.K.; Prins, J.B.; Chang, A.M.; Mcintyre, H.D. Australian obstetric population. *Med. J. Aust.* **2006**, *184*, 56–59. [CrossRef]
28. Athukorala, C.; Rumbold, A.R.; Willson, K.J.; Crowther, C.A. The risk of adverse pregnancy outcomes in women who are overweight or obese. *BMC Pregnancy Childbirth* **2010**, *10*, 1–8. [CrossRef]
29. Scifres, C.; Feghali, M.; Althouse, A.D.; Caritis, S.; Catov, J. Adverse Outcomes and Potential Targets for Intervention in Gestational Diabetes and Obesity. *Obstet. Gynecol.* **2015**, *126*, 316–325. [CrossRef]

30. Wahabi, H.A.; Fayed, A.A.; Alzeidan, R.A.; Mandil, A.A. The independent effects of maternal obesity and gestational diabetes on the pregnancy outcomes. *BMC Endocr. Disord.* **2014**, *14*, 47. [CrossRef]
31. Williams, B.; Mancia, G.; Spiering, W.; Agabiti Rosei, E.; Azizi, M.; Burnier, M.; Clement, D.L.; Coca, A.; de Simone, G.; Dominiczak, A.; et al. 2018 ESC/ESH Guidelines for the management of arterial hypertension. *Eur. Heart J.* **2018**, *39*, 3021–3104. [CrossRef]
32. Brown, M.A. Is there a role for ambulatory blood pressure monitoring in pregnancy? *Clin. Exp. Pharmacol. Physiol.* **2014**, *41*, 16–21. [CrossRef] [PubMed]
33. Murmu, S.; Dwivedi, J. Second-Trimester Maternal Serum Beta-Human Chorionic Gonadotropin and Lipid Profile as a Predictor of Gestational Hypertension, Preeclampsia, and Eclampsia: A Prospective Observational Study. *Int. J. Appl. Basic Med. Res.* **2020**, *10*, 49–53. [CrossRef] [PubMed]
34. Adank, M.C.; Benschop, L.; Peterbroers, K.R.; Smak Gregoor, A.M.; Kors, A.W.; Mulder, M.T.; Schalekamp-Timmermans, S.; Roeters Van Lennep, J.E.; Steegers, E.A.P. Is maternal lipid profile in early pregnancy associated with pregnancy complications and blood pressure in pregnancy and long term postpartum? *Am. J. Obstet. Gynecol.* **2019**, *221*, 150.e1–150.e3. [CrossRef] [PubMed]
35. Mateo-Gavira, I.; Vílchez-López, F.J.; García-Palacios, M.V.; Carral-San Laureano, F.; Visiedo-García, F.M.; Aguilar-Diosdado, M. Early blood pressure alterations are associated with pro-inflammatory markers in type 1 diabetes mellitus. *J. Hum. Hypertens.* **2017**, *31*, 151–156. [CrossRef] [PubMed]
36. Li, C.; Liu, Y.; Zhang, W. Joint and independent associations of gestational weight gain and pre-pregnancy body mass index with outcomes of pregnancy in Chinese women: A retrospective cohort study. *PLoS ONE* **2015**, *10*, e0136850. [CrossRef] [PubMed]
37. Soydinc, H.E.; Davutoglu, V.; Sak, M.E.; Ercan, S.; Evsen, M.S.; Kaya, H.; Oylumlu, M.; Buyukaslan, H.; Sari, I. Circadian variation of blood pressure is impaired in normotensive pregnant women with gestational diabetes mellitus. *Clin. Exp. Hypertens.* **2013**, *35*, 128–133. [CrossRef]
38. Zhong, L.; Deng, W.; Zheng, W.; Yu, S.; Huang, X.; Wen, Y.; Chiu, P.C.N.; Lee, C.L. The relationship between circadian blood pressure variability and maternal/perinatal outcomes in women with preeclampsia with severe features. *Hypertens. Pregnancy* **2020**, *39*, 405–410. [CrossRef]
39. Lv, L.J.; Ji, W.J.; Wu, L.L.; Miao, J.; Wen, J.Y.; Lei, Q.; Duan, D.M.; Chen, H.; Hirst, J.E.; Henry, A.; et al. Thresholds for Ambulatory Blood Pressure Monitoring Based on Maternal and Neonatal Outcomes in Late Pregnancy in a Southern Chinese Population. *J. Am. Heart Assoc.* **2019**, *8*, e012027. [CrossRef]

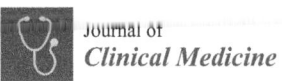

Article

Prediabetes Is Associated with Increased Prevalence of Sleep-Disordered Breathing

Enric Sánchez [1,2,3,†], Esther Sapiña-Beltrán [3,4,5,6,†], Ricard Gavaldà [7], Ferran Barbé [3,4,5,6], Gerard Torres [3,4,5,6], Ariadna Sauret [1], Mireia Dalmases [3,4,5,6], Carolina López-Cano [1,2,3], Liliana Gutiérrez-Carrasquilla [1,2,3], Marcelino Bermúdez-López [8,9], Elvira Fernández [8,9], Francisco Purroy [3,10,11], Eva Castro-Boqué [8,9], Cristina Farràs-Sallés [12,13], Reinald Pamplona [3,14], Dídac Mauricio [15,16,17,18], Cristina Hernández [17,19,20,21], Rafael Simó [17,19,20,21,*], Albert Lecube [1,2,3,17,*] and on behalf of the ILERVAS Project Collaborators [‡]

1. Endocrinology and Nutrition Department, University Hospital Arnau de Vilanova, 25198 Lleida, Spain; esanchez@irblleida.cat (E.S.); ariadnags973@gmail.com (A.S.); karolopezc@gmail.com (C.L.-C.); liligutierrezc@gmail.com (L.G.-C.)
2. Obesity, Diabetes and Metabolism (ODIM) Research Group, Institut de Recerca Biomèdica de Lleida (IRBLleida), 25198 Lleida, Spain
3. University of Lleida, 25003 Lleida, Spain; esther.sb91@gmail.com (E.S.-B.); febarbe.lleida.ics@gencat.cat (F.B.); gtorres@gss.scs.es (G.T.); mdalmases.lleida.ics@gencat.cat (M.D.); fpurroygarcia@gmail.com (F.P.); reinald.pamplona@mex.udl.cat (R.P.)
4. Respiratory Department, University Hospital Arnau de Vilanova and Santa María, 25198 Lleida, Spain
5. Group of Translational Research in Respiratory Medicine, Institut de Recerca Biomèdica de Lleida (IRBLleida), 25198 Lleida, Spain
6. Centro de Investigación Biomédica en Red de Enfermedades Respiratorias (CIBERES), Instituto de Salud Carlos III (ISCIII), 28029 Madrid, Spain
7. Amalfi Analytics, Polytechnic University of Catalonia, 08034 Barcelona, Spain; rgavalda@irblleida.cat
8. Vascular and Renal Translational Research Group, Institut de Recerca Biomèdica de Lleida (IRBLleida), 25198 Lleida, Spain; mbermudez@irblleida.cat (M.B.-L.); efernandez@irblleida.cat (E.F.); ecastro@irblleida.cat (E.C.-B.)
9. Red de Investigación Renal, Instituto de Salud Carlos III (RedinRen-ISCIII), 28029 Madrid, Spain
10. Stroke Unit, University Hospital Arnau de Vilanova, 25198 Lleida, Spain
11. Clinical Neurosciences Group, Institut de Recerca Biomèdica de Lleida (IRBLleida), 25198 Lleida, Spain
12. Applied Epidemiology Research Group, Institut de Recerca Biomèdica de Lleida (IRBLleida), 25198 Lleida, Spain; cfarras.lleida.ics@gencat.cat
13. Lleida Research Support Unit, Jordi Gol i Gurina University Institute for Research in Primary Health Care (IDIAPJGol), 25007 Lleida, Spain
14. Department of Experimental Medicine, Institut de Recerca Biomèdica de Lleida (IRBLleida), 25198 Lleida, Spain
15. Department of Endocrinology and Nutrition, Hospital de la Santa Creu i Sant Pau, 08041 Barcelona, Spain; didacmauricio@gmail.com
16. Sant Pau Biomedical Research Institute (IIB Sant Pau), 08041 Barcelona, Spain
17. Centro de Investigación Biomédica en Red de Diabetes y Enfermedades Metabólicas Asociadas (CIBERDEM), Instituto de Salud Carlos III (ISCIII), 28029 Madrid, Spain; cristina.hernandez@vhir.org
18. Grupo de Investigación Epidemiológica en Diabetes des de Atención Primaria (DAP_Cat Group), Unitat de Suport a la Recerca de Barcelona, Jordi Gol i Gurina University Institute for Research in Primary Health Care (IDIAPJGol), 08007 Barcelona, Spain
19. Endocrinology and Nutrition Department, University Hospital Vall d'Hebron, 08024 Barcelona, Spain
20. Diabetes and Metabolism Research Unit, Vall d'Hebron Institut de Recerca (VHIR), 08024 Barcelona, Spain
21. Autonomous University of Barcelona, 08024 Barcelona, Spain
* Correspondence: rafael.simo@vhir.org (R.S.); alecube@gmail.com (A.L.); Tel.: +34-973-70-51-83 (A.L.); Fax: +34-973-70-51-89 (A.L.)
† These authors contributed equally to this work.
‡ The collaborators of the ILERVAS Project are listed in the Acknowledgements section.

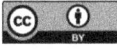

Abstract: Type 2 diabetes leads to severe nocturnal hypoxemia, with an increase in apnea events and daytime sleepiness. Hence, we assessed sleep breathing parameters in the prediabetes stage. A cross-sectional study conducted on 966 middle-aged subjects without known pulmonary disease (311 patients with prediabetes and 655 controls with normal glucose metabolism) was conducted. Prediabetes was defined by glycated hemoglobin (HbA1c), and a nonattended overnight home sleep study was performed. Participants with prediabetes ($n = 311$) displayed a higher apnea–hypopnea index (AHI: 12.7 (6.1;24.3) vs. 9.5 (4.2;19.6) events/h, $p < 0.001$) and hypopnea index (HI: 8.4 (4.0;14.9) vs. 6.0 (2.7;12.6) events/h, $p < 0.001$) than controls, without differences in the apnea index. Altogether, the prevalence of obstructive sleep apnea was higher in subjects with prediabetes than in controls (78.1 vs. 69.9%, $p = 0.007$). Additionally, subjects with prediabetes presented impaired measurements of the median and minimum nocturnal oxygen saturation, the percentage of time spent with oxygen saturations below 90%, and the 4% oxygen desaturation index in comparison with individuals without prediabetes ($p < 0.001$ for all). After adjusting for age, sex, and the presence of obesity, HbA1c correlated with the HI in the entire population ($r = 0.141$, $p < 0.001$), and the presence of prediabetes was independently associated with the AHI (B = 2.20 (0.10 to 4.31), $p = 0.040$) as well as the HI (B = 1.87 (0.61 to 3.14), $p = 0.004$) in the multiple linear regression model. We conclude that prediabetes is an independent risk factor for an increased AHI after adjusting for age, sex, and obesity. The enhanced AHI is mainly associated with increments in the hypopnea events.

Keywords: apnea; glycated hemoglobin; hypopnea; prediabetes; obstructive sleep apnea

1. Introduction

In recent years, there has been growing evidence suggesting that type 2 diabetes can lead to the development of sleep breathing disorders (SBD) [1]. The deleterious effect of type 2 diabetes on nocturnal sleep breathing includes increased nocturnal awakenings, higher sleep fragmentation through higher rates of microarousals, changes in sleep architecture, sleep quality reduction and, consequently, excessive daytime sleepiness [2–4]. Furthermore, type 2 diabetes appears to be an independent risk factor for severe hypoxemia [5]. The Sweet Sleep study characterized obstructive sleep apnea (OSA) in patients with type 2 diabetes, providing evidence that the composition of their apnea–hypopnea index (AHI) is characterized by an increase in apnea events, with no differences or even reduction in hypopnea episodes [2]. Additionally, a small interventional study with 35 patients with type 2 diabetes and OSA has recently shown how the improvement of glycemic control without significant weight loss exerts beneficial effects on sleep breathing parameters [6]. This multifaceted relationship between diabetes milieu and sleep breathing is based on several pathophysiological mechanisms that include insulin resistance, inflammatory and oxidative stress-activated signaling pathways, leptin resistance and abnormalities in the autonomic nervous system [1,7]. A recent analysis of 151,194 participants from three prospective U.S. cohorts has showed that individuals with insulin-treated diabetes had 43% higher OSA risk when compared to those without diabetes [8]. These data possibly indicate that SBD appears in established diabetes with the worst metabolic control, which requires intensive glucose lowering.

Little information exists regarding the potential nighttime respiratory dysfunction in subjects with prediabetes. This prodromal stage in the hyperglycemia continuum that exists before the clinical diagnosis of type 2 diabetes affects 34.5% of all United States adults based on their fasting glucose or glycated hemoglobin (HbA1c) level [9]. Some of the etiopathogenetic mechanisms involved in the development of SDB in type 2 diabetes, such as insulin resistance and low-grade inflammation, are also part of the prediabetes environment. In fact, data from the National Health and Nutrition Examination Survey 2005–2008 showed that self-reported markers of SDB (sleep duration, snoring, snorting, and daytime sleepiness) were associated with prediabetes [10].

On this basis, our main goal was to test the impact of prediabetes in the sleep breathing pattern in a cross-sectional study of 989 middle-aged subjects without type 2 diabetes.

2. Materials and Methods

2.1. Ethics Approval

The protocol was approved by the Arnau de Vilanova University Hospital Ethics Committee (CEIC-1410). Moreover, the trial was conducted according to the ethical guidelines of the Helsinki Declaration and Spanish legislation regarding the protection of personal information was also followed. Written informed consent was provided by all individuals when they were included in the study. Informed consent was obtained from all individual participants included in the study.

2.2. Design of the Study and Report of the Study Individuals

The ILERVAS project is an ongoing randomized intervention study to assess the prevalence of subclinical vascular disease in the province of Lleida, Spain (ClinTrials.gov Identifier: NCT03228459, 25 July 2017) [11,12]. A total of 8330 middle-aged participants were recruited from diverse primary health care centers between January 2015 and December 2018. The inclusion criteria were women aged between 50 and 70, men aged between 45 and 65, and the presence of at least one cardiovascular risk factor (dyslipidemia, hypertension, obesity, smoking and/or having a first-degree relative with premature cardiovascular disease). The exclusion criteria were medical history of cardiovascular disease, type 2 diabetes, chronic kidney disease, active neoplasia, a life expectancy less than 18 months, institutionalized population (jail and penitentiary inmates, patients at psychiatric hospitals, persons in nursing homes, and persons in boarding schools) and pregnancy.

For the present study, 2411 consecutive subjects were assessed for eligibility between March 2017 and September 2018 and invited to perform a nonattended cardiorespiratory polygraphy. We excluded 1335 for the following reasons: unwillingness to participate in the study (n = 932), unable to locate by telephone (n = 285), patients under treatment with continuous positive airway pressure (CPAP) (n = 81), previously undiagnosed type 2 diabetes (n = 15), and unknown kidney disease (n = 22). Additionally, 110 subjects with a first unsatisfactory sleep study refused to repeat it a second time. Therefore, the investigation was finally performed with nine hundred and sixty-six individuals: 311 patients with prediabetes and 655 controls with normal glucose metabolism (Supplemental Figure S1).

2.3. Diagnosis of Prediabetes

Following the present American Diabetes Association guidelines, prediabetes was defined as an HbA1c between 39 and 47 mmol/mol (5.7 to 6.4%) and a normal glucose metabolism as an HbA1c < 39 mmol/mol (<5.7%) [13]. The HbA1c test was conducted on capillary blood using a point-of-care device (Cobas B 101®, Roche Diagnostics S.L., Sant Cugat del Vallès, Spain), based on a latex agglutination inhibition immunoassay technique that meets the generally accepted performance standards for HbA1c [14].

2.4. Nighttime Respiratory Function Assessment

All participants underwent a nonattended overnight home sleep study using a cardiorespiratory polygraphy (ApneaLink™ device, Resmed, Sydney, Australia) according to standard techniques [15]. Oronasal flow, thoracoabdominal movements and pulse oximetry were recorded. Cardiorespiratory polygraph records were scored manually according to standard criteria, and records with less than 3 h of sleep time were repeated. Apnea was defined as an absence of or reduction in nasal airflow of >90% with a duration of at least 10 s. A hypopnea was defined as a reduction of 30% to 90% in oronasal airflow for at least 10 s and associated with a drop in arterial oxygen saturation (SpO2) of at least 3.0%. The AHI was defined as the sum of apneas plus hypopneas recorded during the study per h of monitoring time, and participants were classified into non-OSA (AHI < 5 events/h), mild OSA (AHI between 5 and 14.9 events/h), moderate OSA (AHI between 15 and 29.9 events/h), and severe OSA (AHI ≥ 30 events/h) [16]. Four oxygen saturation measures were considered: the median and the minimum SpO_2 level, the cumulative percentage of time spent with oxygen saturations below 90% (CT90), and the 4% oxygen desaturation index (ODI4%).

2.5. Excessive Daytime Sleepiness Assessment

Excessive daytime sleepiness was evaluated using the Epworth Sleepiness Scale (ESS), a widely used questionnaire based on one's likelihood to fall asleep unintentionally during eight daytime situations [17]. A score of 10 or more is considered sleepy. This questionnaire was completed by 80.2% of participants.

2.6. Covariates Assessment

Body weight and height were measured without shoes and slight clothing, and body mass index (BMI) was determined from kilograms divided by height in meters squared. Waist and neck circumferences were assessed using a nonstretchable tape with a precision of 0.1 cm. Waist circumference was measured midway between the iliac crest and the lowest rib on the horizontal plane with the individual in a standing position. Neck circumference was assessed in a plane as flat as possible, closely below the laryngeal prominence, while standing erect with eyes facing forward. Blood pressure was assessed in triplicate after five minutes' rest via an automated device (Omron M6 Comfort HEM-7221-E (Omron Healthcare, Kyoto, Japan)) at 2 min breaks, and the mean of the last two was calculated. Additionally, smoking habits (never, former or current smoker) were also known. Smokers who stopped smoking one or more years prior to visiting were considered former smokers.

2.7. Statistical Analysis

As the skewed distribution of all the variables was confirmed by the Shapiro–Wilk test, only nonparametric methods were used. Quantitative data were expressed as median (interquartile range) or as a percentage. The Mann–Whitney U test was used to compare continuous variables, while the Pearson's Chi-squared test was used to compare categorical records. The relationship between continuous variables was examined by the Spearman correlation test.

Three multiple linear regression models to explore the variables independently related to the AHI, the apnea index and the hypopnea index were used. Variables with a potential impact on sleep breathing function (i.e., age, sex, BMI) and the prediabetes stage were introduced in the models. The adequacy of the regression models was verified through submitting the residuals) to a normality test. All "p" values were based on a two-sided test of statistical significance. Significance was recognized at the level of $p < 0.050$. All statistical investigations were completed using the SSPS statistical package (IBM SPSS Statistics for Windows, Version 20.0. Armonk, NY, USA).

3. Results

The main clinical characteristics of the study population according to the presence of prediabetes are displayed in Table 1. Subjects with prediabetes were older and presented a higher proportion of women, obesity, and hypertension than control ones.

When the sleep breathing was assessed, participants with prediabetes displayed a significantly higher AHI (12.7 (6.1;24.3) vs. 9.5 (4.2;19.6) events/h, $p < 0.001$) than controls (Table 2). The hypopnea index was also greater among participants with prediabetes (8.4 (4.0;14.9) vs. 6.0 (2.7;12.6) events/h, $p < 0.001$), without differences in the apnea index (Figure 1). Altogether, the prevalence of OSA was higher among participants with prediabetes than in controls (78.1 vs. 69.9%, $p = 0.007$). Additionally, patients with prediabetes presented a higher CT90 and ODI4%, as well as lower median and minimum SpO$_2$ levels ($p \leq 0.001$ for all) than patients without prediabetes. No difference in the daytime sleepiness was observed between groups.

Table 1. Main clinical characteristics of the study population according to the presence of prediabetes.

	Prediabetes (n = 311)	Control Group (n = 655)	p
Age (years)	59 (54;63)	56 (52;61)	<0.001
Women, n (%)	180 (57.8)	316 (48.2)	0.004
HbA1c (mmol/mol)	40 (39;42)	36 (33;37)	<0.001
HbA1c (%)	5.8 (5.8;6.0)	5.4 (5.2;5.5)	<0.001
Hypertension, n (%)	147 (47.2)	240 (36.6)	0.001
Systolic blood pressure (mm Hg)	132 (120;143)	128 (118;139)	0.008
Diastolic blood pressure (mm Hg)	81 (75;88)	81 (74;87)	0.569
Obesity, n (%)	124 (39.8)	177 (27.0)	<0.001
BMI (Kg/m^2)	29.7 (26.9;33.2)	27.9 (24.9;31.0)	<0.001
Waist circumference (cm)	103 (96;110)	98 (92;106)	<0.001
Neck circumference (cm)	37.5 (35.0;41.0)	37.5 (34.5;41.0)	0.261
Current or former smoker, n (%)	184 (59.1)	430 (65.6)	0.050

Information is displayed as a median (interquartile range) or n (percentage). HbA1c: glycated hemoglobin; BMI: body mass index.

Table 2. Nighttime respiratory characteristics of the study population according to the presence of prediabetes.

	Prediabetes (n = 311)	Control Group (n = 655)	p
Time of evaluation (hs)	7.2 (6.4;8.0)	7.2 (6.5;8.0)	0.684
AHI (events/h)	12.7 (6.1;24.3)	9.5 (4.2;19.6)	<0.001
Apnea index (events/h)	1.6 (0.4;5.8)	1.3 (0.4;4.3)	0.159
Hypopnea index (events/h)	8.4 (4.0;14.9)	6.0 (2.7;12.6)	<0.001
OSA, n (%)	243 (78.1)	458 (69.9)	0.007
Mild OSA, n (%)	108 (34.8)	227 (34.6)	0.142
Moderate OSA, n (%)	76 (24.4)	138 (21.0)	0.060
Severe OSA, n (%)	57 (18.5)	89 (13.6)	0.010
Median SpO$_2$ level (%)	92 (91;93)	93 (92;94)	<0.001
Minimum SpO$_2$ level (%)	82 (77;85)	83 (80;87)	<0.001
CT90 (%)	14 (4;33)	6 (1;24)	<0.001
ODI4% (events/h)	14 (8;27)	11 (5;21)	0.001
Epworth Sleepiness Scale score *	4 (2;5)	3 (2;5)	0.740

Information is displayed as a median (interquartile range) or n (percentage). AHI: Apnea–hypopnea index; OSA: obstructive sleep apnea; SpO$_2$: oxygen saturation; CT90: cumulative time percentage with SpO$_2$ < 90%; ODI4%: number of 4% oxygen desaturation index; * The Epworth Sleepiness Scale was completed by 80.2% of participants.

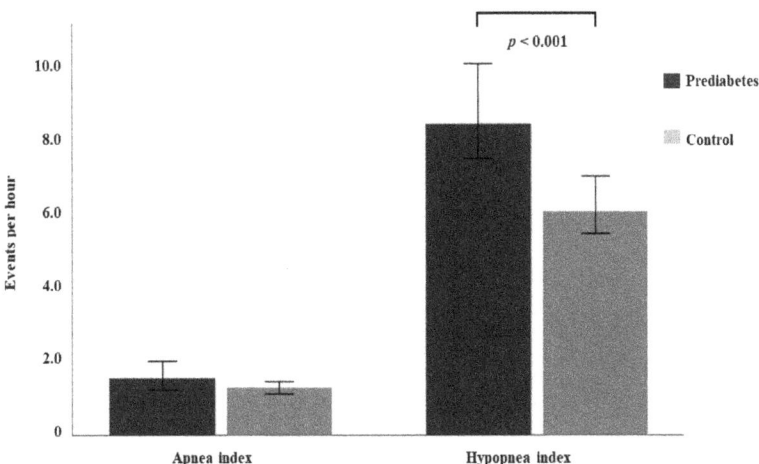

Figure 1. Plot displaying the number of apneas and hypopneas according to the presence of impaired glucose metabolism.

Both in the entire population and in those with prediabetes, HbA1c was slightly correlated with the hypopnea index (r = 0.141, $p < 0.001$ and r = 0.171, $p = 0.002$, respectively). HbA1c was also significantly correlated with others nighttime respiratory measurements in both groups (Table 3).

Table 3. Correlations of sleep respiratory measurements with glycated hemoglobin in the entire population and in participants with prediabetes.

	Prediabetes (n = 311)		Entire Population (n = 966)	
	r	p	r	p
AHI (events/h)	0.093	0.099	0.131	<0.001
Apnea index (events/h)	−0.039	0.492	0.065	0.042
Hypopnea index (events/h)	0.171	0.002	0.141	<0.001
Median SpO$_2$ level (%)	−0.166	0.003	−0.204	<0.001
Minimum SpO$_2$ level (%)	−0.126	0.025	−0.159	<0.001
CT90 (%)	0.144	0.010	0.209	<0.001
ODI4% (events/h)	0.123	0.028	0.150	<0.001
Epworth Sleepiness Scale score *	0.009	0.884	−0.035	0.322

AHI: Apnea–hypopnea index; SpO$_2$: oxygen saturation; CT90: cumulative time percentage with SpO$_2$ < 90%; ODI4%: number of 4% oxygen desaturation index; * The Epworth Sleepiness Scale was completed by 80.2% of participants.

Finally, the multiple linear regression model (Table 4) showed that there was a significant and independent association between the presence of prediabetes and the AHI (B = 2.20 (0. 10 to 4.31), $p = 0.040$) as well as the hypopnea index (B = 1.87 (0. 61 to 3.14), $p = 0.004$), but no with the apnea index.

Table 4. The multiple linear regression model for the AHI, apnea index and hypopnea index.

AHI (Events/h) R^2 = 0.12	B (95% IC)	Standardized Regression Coefficients	p
Age (Years)	0.36 (0.19 to 0.52)	0.14	<0.001
Sex (Male)	8.29 (6.23 to 10.35)	0.24	<0.001
Obesity (BMI ≥ 30 kg/m^2)	8.54 (6.44 to 10.64)	0.26	<0.001
Prediabetes (HbA1c 5.7 to 6.4%)	2.20 (0. 10 to 4.31)	0.58	0.040
Apnea index (events/h) R^2 = 0.06			
Age (Years)	0.21 (0.13 to 0.30)	0.17	<0.001
Sex (Male)	3.58 (2.55 to 4.62)	0.20	<0.001
Obesity (BMI ≥ 30 kg/m^2)	1.73 (0.67 to 2.78)	0.11	0.001
Prediabetes (HbA1c 5.7 to 6.4%)	0.16 (−0. 90 to 1.22)	0.00	0.765
Hypopnea index (events/h) R^2 = 0.12			
Age (Years)	0.13 (0.03 to 0.23)	0.11	0.013
Sex (Male)	3.81 (2.57 to 5.05)	0.15	<0.001
Obesity (BMI ≥ 30 kg/m^2)	5.94 (4.68 to 7.21)	0.29	<0.001
Prediabetes (HbA1c 5.7 to 6.4%)	1.87 (0. 61 to 3.14)	0.82	0.004

B: unstandardized beta; AHI: Apnea–hypopnea index; BMI: body mass index. The adequacy of the regression models was verified through submitting the residuals to a normality test: in all cases $p < 0.001$.

4. Discussion

To the best of our knowledge, this is the first study to provide evidence that prediabetes (after adjusting for age, sex, and presence of obesity) presents with a distinctive sleep breathing pattern, with increased hypopnea episodes but with no differences in apnea events. In our study, and together with classical risk factors for sleep disorders such as age, BMI and male sex, the presence of prediabetes is independently associated with the hypopnea events. These results suggest that the previously evidenced deleterious impact of type 2 diabetes on nocturnal sleep breathing begins in the prediabetes stage, and that any degree of disorder in glucose metabolism will influence this process. Additionally, patients with prediabetes also display a higher prevalence of OSA, as well as an impairment of nocturnal oxygen saturation. These data reinforce and extend previous reports, and run in accordance with the International Diabetes Federation, which recommends screening for OSA subjects with prediabetes [18,19].

Limited information exists on whether prediabetes increases the risk of developing OSA in the general population. A previous cross-sectional study evaluated 137 subjects with extremely obesity who underwent a portable sleep registration at home [19]. According to a standardized 2 h oral glucose tolerance test, the prevalence of OSA increased from 33% in subjects with normal glucose tolerance to 67% and 78% in patients with prediabetes and type 2 diabetes, respectively. Additionally, after adjustment for key clinical and systemic variables such as age, sex, BMI, systemic inflammation, insulin resistance, hypertension, smoking, alcohol consumption and medication, prediabetes was still associated with 3-fold increased odds of OSA compared with those subjects with normal glycaemia [19]. Our study, with a population with a mean BMI of 28.7 kg/m^2, allows us to analyze the results without the confounding factor of obesity, which directly affects OSA and glucose metabolism abnormalities. However, this study did not provide data related to the number of apneas and hypopneas added together resulting in the AHI. Therefore, our study spread these findings to a broader population with overweight and assessed the components of the AHI to better understand the impact of prediabetes on SBD.

A clear pathophysiology mechanism for the association between glucose abnormalities and sleep breathing has not yet been elucidated. However, insulin resistance, inflammation, visceral adiposity, autonomic dysfunction, and leptin resistance deserve to be commented on. In Sprague Dawley rats, *Ramadan* et al. showed the contribution of insulin resistance to apnea development. Additionally, oral treatment with metformin—an insulin-sensitizer drug—was able to avoid and reverse apnea episodes [20]. Data from 1780 men and 1785 women evaluated within the Epidemiologic Study on the Insulin Resistance Syndrome (DESIR) study showed that insulin resistance was related to a 6-year incident observed apnea during sleep [21]. The standardized odds ratios for fasting plasma insulin, HOMA-IR or triglycerides were 1.31, 1.31, and 1.24, respectively. More interestingly, the relation of insulin resistance and incident observed apnea was homogeneous across BMI classes for both men and women [21]. Similarly, women with polycystic ovary syndrome—characterized by insulin resistance—are more likely to have OSA and experience excessive daytime sleepiness than controls [22]. In addition, insulin resistance may mediate a blockage effect on the pharyngeal dilator muscle, just as the alterations in arterial muscle tone that are well recognized in prediabetes vascular disease [23,24]. Inflammatory processes associated with prediabetes might also affect the upper respiratory tract, reducing the lumen and favoring obstruction [19]. In fact, systemic inflammation measured by fibrinogen and C-reactive protein levels has been associated with nocturnal oxygen saturation parameters and the apnea–hypopnea index in snorers with compromised upper airway anatomy without type 2 diabetes [25]. In addition, other metabolic pathways that would explain the association between prediabetes and OSA have also been suggested, such as microvascular damage, lung microangiopathy, decreased muscle strength, nonenzymatic glycosylation of lung proteins, defects in the bronchiolar surfactant layer and the deficit in glucagon-like peptide 1 concentrations [1].

Our population with prediabetes exhibits a BMI near to 30.0 kg/m^2, with an increased prevalence of obesity and a higher waist circumference in comparison with control participants. Adiposity may appear as a source of proinflammatory factors as well as lead to the narrowing of the upper airways [26]. However, no differences in neck circumference between groups were observed in our study, making the second option less likely to be responsible for the higher prevalence of OSA in patients with prediabetes. As autonomic dysfunction is already present in prediabetes, both afferent and efferent motor pathway dysfunctions may influence the regulation of blood gases and oxygen delivery, contributing to a blunted ventilatory response to hypoxemia [1,27]. Finally, as leptin has been associated with prediabetes in a dose-dependent manner, pathways related to leptin resistance in type 2 diabetes could also contribute to deficiencies in central respiratory control [28].

As patients with OSA have an almost two-fold higher risk of developing cardiovascular events and all-cause mortality than controls, its increased prevalence could participate in the milieu that favors cardiovascular disease in the prediabetes stage [29,30]. In fact, in a more extensive cohort from the ILERVAS project, subjects with prediabetes presented a higher prevalence of subclinical atheromatous disease than the control group, especially in the carotid territory [31]. Furthermore, nocturnal cycling hypoxia, together with female sex and fasting plasma glucose, has been demonstrated to be independently associated with an increased density of carotid vasa vasorum, an early event in atheromatous disease [32].

Only one study has, so far, focused on weight loss intervention in subjects with both prediabetes and obstructive sleep apnea, showing that changes in SpO_2 were associated with changes in insulin sensitivity but not with weight loss [33]. Similarly, our group has demonstrated that in type 2 diabetes the improvement of metabolic control achieves a significant reduction in sleep breathing parameters not related with weigh modifications [6]. These results point out a direction for the further improvement of metabolic control in individuals with prediabetes. Whether this optimization must be conducted only with lifestyle changes or medical treatment is not known. For example, glucagon-like peptide (GLP)-1, widely used as anti-diabetic drug, may be an effective therapy for patients with prediabetes and OSA [34–36]. Similarly, the combination of metformin and dapagliflozin for 24 weeks in patients with a newly diagnosed type 2 diabetes and OSA achieved a reduction in both the AHI and daily somnolence in comparison with a control group receiving metformin plus glimepriride [37].

Sleep quality, assessed using the Pittsburgh Sleep Quality Index (PSQI), has also been evaluated in subjects with prediabetes [38]. In this way, Iyegha et al. showed how 62% of subjects with prediabetes suffered from poor sleep quality, compared with less than half of normoglycemic subjects [38]. We have no data regarding sleep quality in the ILERVAS project, but no differences in the ESS were observed between participants with and without prediabetes. Our results are in concordance with those of Renko et al., in which daytime sleepiness was not linked with using sleep medication or impaired glucose regulation [39]. Altogether, this may suggest that sleep quality is more sensitive to the prediabetes stage than daytime sleepiness.

This study has a few limitations that need to be addressed. Currently, we have diagnosed prediabetes according only to HbA1c values, one of the three possibilities accepted by the American Diabetes Association. However, as different tools identify different populations, future studies using fasting plasma glucose (impaired fasting glucose) and 2 h plasma glucose (impaired glucose tolerance) are needed. Second, we have no information about the time of appearance of prediabetes in our population, a factor that might influence our results similarly to how the known evolution time in type 2 diabetes affects the incidence of classical chronic complications. Third, the gold standard diagnosis of OSA according to the American Academy of Sleep Medicine is through polysomnograms, not cardiorespiratory polygraphs. The latter shows a lower diagnostic performance compared to polysomnography that is related to the difficulty in identifying apneas and especially hypopneas. However, population-based studies assessing sleep breathing parameters in large populations are easily performed with at-home registers. In addition, this fact amplifies the significance of our results, in which a higher prevalence of hypopnea events in patients with prediabetes compared to the control group has been detected. Fourth, we have no circulating biomarkers of insulin resistance or systemic inflammation, and therefore, their potential role in this association could not be assessed in our study. Finally, Fifth, we do not have data on psychiatric illnesses in our population, which have a direct effect on the severity of OSA. Moreover, the cross-sectional nature of the study does not allow us to establish causality with the results, as well as characteristic of the ILERVAS population (Spanish middle-aged individuals with low-to-moderate cardiovascular risk) precludes us from generalizing our results to the global population. Finally, future studies need to be designed to better evaluate the underlying mechanisms that link prediabetes with OSA and its clinical significance.

5. Conclusions

In summary, the prevalence of OSA was significantly higher in participants with prediabetes that in the control group in a large cohort study of Spanish subjects with low-to-moderate CV risk. After adjusting for age, sex, and the presence of obesity, the increased AHI in participants with prediabetes was mainly associated with increments in the hypopnea events, supporting the hypothesis that glucose abnormalities exert a lineal negative impact on SBD, from insulin resistance with normal fasting glucose to confirmed diagnosis of type 2 diabetes. Moreover, the presence of prediabetes independently predicted the AHI and the hypopnea events per hour. Additional studies to identify subjects with prediabetes more vulnerable to experiencing problems with nighttime respiratory function, and factors that accelerate its progression and severity, are needed.

Supplementary Materials: The following supporting information can be downloaded at: https://www.mdpi.com/article/10.3390/jcm11051413/s1, Figure S1: Flow chart in study population.

Author Contributions: Data curation: R.G, F.B., G.T., A.S., M.D., C.L.-C. and L.G.-C. Formal analysis: R.G., F.B., G.T., A.S., M.D., C.L.-C. and L.G.-C. Project administration: M.B.-L., E.F. and A.L. Investigation: F.P., E.C.-B. and C.F.-S. Methodology: F.P., E.C.-B. and C.F.-S. Software: F.P., E.C.-B. and C.F.-S. Resources: M.B.-L., E.F. and A.L. Supervision: R.P., D.M., C.H., R.S. and A.L. Validation: R.P., D.M., C.H., R.S. and A.L. Visualization: E.S. and E.S.-B. Writing—original draft: E.S. and E.S.-B. Writing—review and editing as well as final approval of the version to be published: all authors. All authors have read and agreed to the published version of the manuscript.

Funding: This work was supported by grants from the Lleida Provincial Council, Autonomous Government of Catalonia (2017SGR696 and SLT0021600250), Instituto de Salud Carlos III (Fondo de Investigación Sanitaria PI12/00803, PI15/00260 and PI18/00964), and European Union (European Regional Development Fund, Fondo Europeo de Desarrollo Regional, "Una manera de hacer Europa"). CIBER de Diabetes y Enfermedades Metabólicas Asociadas and CIBER de Enfermedades Respiratorias are initiatives of the Instituto de Salud Carlos III.

Institutional Review Board Statement: The study was conducted in accordance with the Declaration of Helsinki, and approved by the Ethics Committee of Arnau de Vilanova University Hospital (protocol code CEIC-1410; date approval: 2 January 2015).

Informed Consent Statement: Informed consent was obtained from all subjects involved in the study.

Data Availability Statement: The data presented in this study are available on request from the corresponding author. The data are not publicly available due to the signed consent agreements around data sharing, which only allow access to the researchers of the study following the project purposes. Requestors wishing to access the data used in this study can make a request to M.B.-L. The request will be subjected to approval and formal agreements regarding confidentiality and secure data storage being signed the data would be the provided.

Acknowledgments: The authors would like to thank Fundació Renal Jaume Arnó, IRBLleida, and the Primary Care teams from Lleida for recruiting subjects and their efforts in the accurate development of the ILERVAS project. Additionally, thanks are also due to ILERVAS project collaborators: Manuel Sanchez-de-la-Torre, Jessica González, Marta Hernández, Ferran Rius, Silvia Barril, Serafí Cambray, Gloria Arqué, Ana Vena, José Manuel Valdivielso, Montserrat Martínez-Alonso, Pere Godoy, Eva Miquel, Marta Ortega-Bravo, Mariona Jové, Manel Portero-Otin, Esmeralda Castelblanco, and Josep Franch-Nadal.

Conflicts of Interest: The authors declare no conflict of interest.

References

1. Lecube, A.; Simó, R.; Pallayova, M.; Punjabi, N.M.; López-Cano, C.; Turino, C.; Hernández, C.; Barbé, F. Pulmonary Function and Sleep Breathing: Two New Targets for Type 2 Diabetes Care. *Endocr. Rev.* **2017**, *38*, 550–573. [CrossRef] [PubMed]
2. Lecube, A.; Sampol, G.; Hernández, C.; Romero, O.; Ciudin, A.; Simó, R. Characterization of Sleep Breathing Pattern in Patients with Type 2 Diabetes: Sweet Sleep Study. *PLoS ONE* **2015**, *10*, e0119073. [CrossRef] [PubMed]
3. Lecube, A.; Romero, O.; Sampol, G.; Mestre, O.; Ciudin, A.; Sánchez, E.; Hernández, C.; Caixàs, A.; Vigil, L.; Simó, R. Sleep biosignature of Type 2 diabetes: A case-control study. *Diabet. Med.* **2016**, *34*, 79–85. [CrossRef]
4. Lecube, A.; Sánchez, E.; Gómez-Peralta, F.; Abreu, C.; Valls, J.; Mestre, O.; Romero, O.; Martinez, M.D.; Sampol, G.; CIudin, A.; et al. Global Assessment of the Impact of Type 2 Diabetes on Sleep through Specific Questionnaires. A Case-Control Study. *PLoS ONE* **2016**, *11*, e0157579. [CrossRef]
5. Lecube, A.; Sampol, G.; Lloberes, P.; Romero, O.; Mesa, J.; Hernandez, C.; Simo, R. Diabetes is an independent risk factor for severe nocturnal hypoxemia in obese patients. A case-control study. *PLoS ONE* **2009**, *4*, e4692. [CrossRef]
6. Gutiérrez-Carrasquilla, L.; López-Cano, C.; Sánchez, E.; Barbé, F.; Dalmases, M.; Hernández, M.; Campos, A.; Gaeta, A.M.; Carmona, P.; Hernández, C.; et al. Effect of Glucose Improvement on Nocturnal Sleep Breathing Parameters in Patients with Type 2 Diabetes: The Candy Dreams Study. *J. Clin. Med.* **2020**, *9*, 1022. [CrossRef] [PubMed]
7. Reutrakul, S.; Mokhlesi, B. Obstructive sleep apnea and diabetes: A state of the art review. *Chest* **2017**, *152*, 1070–1086. [CrossRef] [PubMed]
8. Huang, T.; Lin, B.M.; Stampfer, M.J.; Tworoger, S.S.; Hu, F.B.; Redline, S. A population-based study of the bidirectional association between obstructive sleep apnea and type 2 diabetes in three prospective U.S. cohorts. *Diabetes Care* **2018**, *41*, 2111–2119. [CrossRef]
9. Centers for Disease Control and Prevention. *National Diabetes Statistics Report*; Centers for Disease Control and Prevention, US Department of Health and Human Services: Atlanta, GA, USA, 2020.
10. Alshaarawy, O.; Teppala, S.; Shankar, A. Markers of Sleep-Disordered Breathing and Prediabetes in US Adults. *Int. J. Endocrinol.* **2012**, *2012*, 902324. [CrossRef]
11. Betruu, À.; Farràs, C.; Abajo, M.; Martinez-Alonso, M.; Arroyo, D.; Barbé, F.; Buti, M.; Lecube, A.; Portero, M.; Purroy, F.; et al. Randomised intervention study to assess the prevalence of subclinical vascular disease and hidden kidney disease and its impact on morbidity and mortality: The ILERVAS project. *Nefrología* **2016**, *36*, 389–396. [CrossRef]
12. Bermúdez-López, M.; Martínez-Alonso, M.; Castro-Boqué, E.; Betriu, À.; Cambray, S.; Farràs, C.; Barbe, F.; Pamplona, R.; Lecube, A.; Mauricio, D.; et al. Subclinical atheromatosis localization and burden in a low-to-moderate cardiovascular risk population: The ILERVAS study. *Rev. Esp. Cardiol.* **2021**, *74*, 1042–1053. [CrossRef] [PubMed]
13. American Diabetes Association. Classification and diagnosis of diabetes. Sec. 2. In standards of medical care in diabetes—2017. *Diabetes Care* **2017**, *40*, S11–S24.
14. Lenters-Westra, E.; Slingerland, R.J. Three of 7 hemoglobin A1c point-of-care instruments do not meet generally accepted analytical performance criteria. *Clin. Chem.* **2014**, *60*, 1062–1072. [CrossRef] [PubMed]
15. Erman, M.K.; Stewart, D.; Einhorn, D.; Gordon, N.; Casal, E. Validation of the ApneaLink™ for the screening of sleep apnea: A novel and simple single-channel recording device. *J. Clin. Sleep Med.* **2007**, *3*, 387–392. [CrossRef] [PubMed]
16. Kapur, V.K.; Auckley, D.H.; Chowdhuri, S.; Kuhlmann, D.C.; Mehra, R.; Ramar, K.; Harrod, C.G. Clinical practice guideline for diagnostic testing for adult obstructive sleep apnea: An American Academy of Sleep Medicine clinical practice guideline. *J. Clin. Sleep Med.* **2017**, *13*, 479–504. [CrossRef]
17. Johns, M.W. A new method for measuring daytime sleepiness: The Epworth Sleepiness Scale. *Sleep* **1991**, *14*, 540–545. [CrossRef]
18. Shaw, J.E.; Punjabi, N.M.; Wilding, J.P.; Alberti, K.G.; Zimmet, P.Z. International Diabetes Federation Taskforce on Epidemiology and Prevention. Sleep-disordered breathing and type 2 diabetes: A report from the International Diabetes Federation Taskforce on Epidemiology and Prevention. *Diabetes Res. Clin. Pract.* **2008**, *81*, 2–12. [CrossRef]
19. Fredheim, J.M.; Rollheim, J.; Omland, T.; Hofsø, D.; Røislien, J.; Vegsgaard, K.; Hjelmesæth, J. Type 2 diabetes and pre-diabetes are associated with obstructive sleep apnea in extremely obese subjects: A cross-sectional study. *Cardiovasc. Diabetol.* **2011**, *25*, 10–84. [CrossRef]
20. Ramadan, W.; Dewasmes, G.; Petitjean, M.; Wiernsperger, N.; Delanaud, S.; Geloen, A.; Libert, J.P. Sleep apnea is induced by a high-fat diet and reversed and prevented by metformin in non-obese rats. *Obesity* **2007**, *15*, 1409–1418. [CrossRef]
21. Balkau, B.; Vol, S.; Loko, S.; Andriamboavonjy, T.; Lantieri, O.; Gusto, G.; Meslier, N. Epidemiologic Study on the Insulin Resistance Syndrome Study Group. High baseline insulin levels associated with 6-year incident observed sleep apnea. *Diabetes Care* **2010**, *33*, 1044–1049. [CrossRef]
22. Vgontzas, A.N.; Legro, R.S.; Bixler, E.O.; Grayev, A.; Kales, A.; Chrousos, G.P. Polycystic ovary syndrome is associated with obstructive sleep apnea and daytime sleepiness: Role of insulin resistance. *J. Clin. Endocrinol. Metab.* **2001**, *86*, 517–520. [PubMed]
23. Yki-Järvinen, H.; Westerbacka, J. Vascular actions of insulin in obesity. *Int. J. Obes. Relat. Metab. Disord.* **2000**, *24* (Suppl. 2), S25–S28. [CrossRef]
24. Osman, A.M.; Carter, S.G.; Carberry, J.C.; Eckert, D.J. Obstructive sleep apnea: Current perspectives. *Nat. Sci. Sleep* **2018**, *10*, 21–34. [CrossRef] [PubMed]
25. Jahn, C.; Gouveris, H.; Matthias, C. Systemic inflammation in patients with compromised upper airway anatomy and primary snoring or mild obstructive sleep apnea. *Eur. Arch. Oto-Rhino-Laryngol.* **2016**, *273*, 3429–3433. [CrossRef]

26. Levy, P.; Bonsignore, M.R.; Eckel, J. Sleep, sleep-disordered breathing and metabolic consequences. *Eur. Respir. J.* **2009**, *34*, 243–260. [CrossRef] [PubMed]
27. Coopmans, C.; Zhou, T.L.; Henry, R.M.; Heijman, J.; Schaper, N.C.; Koster, A.; Schram, M.T.; van der Kallen, C.J.; Wesselius, A.; Engelsman, R.J.D.; et al. Both Prediabetes and Type 2 Diabetes Are Associated with Lower Heart Rate Variability: The Maastricht Study. *Diabetes Care* **2020**, *43*, 1126–1133. [CrossRef]
28. Bassi, M.; Furuya, W.; Zoccal, D.B.; Menani, J.V.; Colombari, D.; Mulkey, D.; Colombari, E. Facilitation of breathing by leptin effects in the central nervous system. *J. Physiol.* **2016**, *594*, 1617–1625. [CrossRef]
29. Bradley, T.D.; Floras, J.S. Obstructive sleep apnea and its cardiovascular consequences. *Lancet* **2009**, *373*, 82–93. [CrossRef]
30. Xie, C.; Zhu, R.; Tian, Y.; Wang, K. Association of obstructive sleep apnoea with the risk of vascular outcomes and all-cause mortality: A meta-analysis. *BMJ Open* **2017**, *7*, e013983. [CrossRef]
31. Sánchez, E.; Betriu, À.; López-Cano, C.; Hernández, M.; Fernández, E.; Purroy, F.; Bermúdez-López, M.; Farràs-Sallés, C.; Barril, S.; Pamplona, R.; et al. Characteristics of atheromatosis in the prediabetes stage: A cross-sectional investigation of the ILERVAS project. *Cardiovasc. Diabetol.* **2019**, *18*, 154. [CrossRef]
32. López-Cano, C.; Rius, F.; Sánchez, E.; Gaeta, A.M.; Betriu, À.; Fernández, E.; Yeramian, A.; Hernández, M.; Bueno, M.; Gutiérrez-Carrasquilla, L.; et al. The influence of sleep apnea syndrome and intermittent hypoxia in carotid adventitial vasa vasorum. *PLoS ONE.* **2019**, *14*, e0211742.
33. Gilardini, L.; Lombardi, C.; Redaelli, G.; Vallone, L.; Faini, A.; Mattaliano, P.; Parati, G.; Invitti, C. Glucose tolerance and weight loss in obese women with obstructive sleep apnea. *PLoS ONE.* **2013**, *8*, e61382. [CrossRef] [PubMed]
34. Reutrakul, S.; Sumritsopak, R.; Saetung, S.; Chanprasertyothin, S.; Anothaisintawee, T. The relationship between sleep and glucagon-like peptide 1 in patients with abnormal glucose tolerance. *J. Sleep Res.* **2017**, *26*, 756–763. [CrossRef] [PubMed]
35. Matsumoto, T.; Harada, N.; Azuma, M.; Chihara, Y.; Murase, K.; Tachikawa, R.; Minami, T.; Hamada, S.; Tanizawa, K.; Inouchi, M.; et al. Plasma Incretin Levels and Dipeptidyl Peptidase- 4 Activity in Patients with Obstructive Sleep Apnea. *Ann. Am. Thorac. Soc.* **2016**, *13*, 1378–1387. [CrossRef] [PubMed]
36. Blackman, A.; on behalf of the SCALE Study Group; Foster, G.D.; Zammit, G.; Rosenberg, R.; Aronne, L.; Wadden, T.; Claudius, B.; Jensen, C.B.; Mignot, E. Effect of liraglutide 3.0 mg in individuals with obesity and moderate or severe obstructive sleep apnea: The SCALE Sleep Apnea randomized clinical trial. *Int. J. Obes.* **2016**, *40*, 1310–1319. [CrossRef] [PubMed]
37. Tang, Y.; Sun, Q.; Bai, X.Y.; Zhou, Y.F.; Zhou, Q.L.; Zhang, M. Effect of dapagliflozin on obstructive sleep apnea in patients with type 2 diabetes: A preliminary study. *Nutr. Diabetes* **2019**, *9*, 32. [CrossRef]
38. Iyegha, I.D.; Chieh, A.Y.; Bryant, B.M.; Li, L. Associations between poor sleep and glucose intolerance in prediabetes. *Psychoneuroendocrinology* **2019**, *110*, 104444. [CrossRef]
39. Renko, A.K.; Hiltunen, L.; Laakso, M.; Rajala, U.; Keinänen-Kiukaanniemi, S. The relationship of glucose tolerance to sleep disorders and daytime sleepiness. *Diabetes Res. Clin. Pract.* **2005**, *67*, 84–91. [CrossRef]

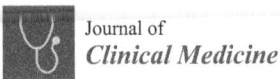

Article

A New Approach to Overcome Insulin Resistance in Patients with Impaired Glucose Tolerance: The Results of a Multicenter, Double-Blind, Placebo-Controlled, Randomized Clinical Trial of Efficacy and Safety of Subetta

Ashot Mkrtumyan [1,2,*], Alexander Ametov [3], Tatiana Demidova [4,5], Anna Volkova [6], Ekaterina Dudinskaya [7], Arkady Vertkin [8,9] and Sergei Vorobiev [10]

1. Department of Endocrinology, Moscow Clinical Scientific and Practical Center Named after A. S. Loginov, 111123 Moscow, Russia
2. Department of Endocrinology and Diabetology, A. I. Evdokimov Moscow State University of Medicine and Dentistry, 127473 Moscow, Russia
3. Department of Endocrinology, Faculty of Medicine, Medical Academy of Continuing Professional Education, 125993 Moscow, Russia; alexander.ametov@gmail.com
4. Department of Endocrinology, City Clinical Hospital Named after V. P. Demikhova, 117463 Moscow, Russia; t.y.demidova@gmail.com
5. Department of Endocrinology, Faculty of Medicine, Pirogov Russian National Research Medical University, 117997 Moscow, Russia
6. Department of Faculty Therapy, Faculty of Medicine, Pavlov First Saint Petersburg State Medical University, 197022 St. Petersburg, Russia; volkovaa@mail.ru
7. Department of Age-Related Metabolic and Endocrine Disorders, Russian Gerontological Research and Clinical Center, Pirogov Russian National Research Medical University, 129226 Moscow, Russia; katharina.gin@gmail.com
8. Department of Therapy, Clinical Pharmacology and Emergency Medicine, A. I. Evdokimov Moscow State University of Medicine and Dentistry, 127473 Moscow, Russia; kafedrakf@mail.ru
9. Department of Therapy, City Clinical Hospital Named after S.I. Spasokukotsky, 127006 Moscow, Russia
10. Department of Endocrinology, Rostov State Medical University, 344022 Rostov-on-Don, Russia; endocrinrostov@mail.ru
* Correspondence: mkrtumyan_ashot@rambler.ru; Tel.: +7-495-6096700

Abstract: Impaired glucose tolerance (IGT) is a common carbohydrate metabolism disorder worldwide. To evaluate the efficacy and safety of 12-week Subetta therapy in correcting 2-h plasma glucose in patients with IGT, a multicenter, double-blind, placebo-controlled, randomized clinical trial was performed. Derived by technological treatment of antibodies to insulin receptor β-subunit and endothelial NO synthase, Subetta increases the sensitivity of insulin receptors by activating the insulin signaling pathway. Oral glucose tolerance test (OGTT), fasting plasma glucose (FPG), and glycated hemoglobin (HbA1c) were examined at screening, after 4 and 12 weeks. In Per Protocol population, 2-h plasma glucose in the Subetta group decreased by 2.05 ± 2.11 mmol/L (versus 0.56 ± 2.55 mmol/L in the Placebo group) after 12 weeks. The difference between the two groups was 1.49 ± 2.33 mmol/L ($p < 0.0001$). After 12 weeks, 65.2% of patients had 2-h plasma glucose <7.8 mmol/L. FPG remained almost unchanged. HbA1c tended to decrease. The number of adverse events did not differ in both groups. Subetta treatment is beneficial for patients with IGT; it also prevents progression of carbohydrate metabolism disorders.

Keywords: impaired glucose tolerance; 2-h plasma glucose; glycated hemoglobin

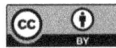

1. Introduction

Impaired glucose tolerance (IGT) is an intermediate stage of carbohydrate metabolism disorders between normal glucose tolerance (NGT) and type 2 diabetes mellitus (T2DM) [1,2]. The average transition time from IGT to T2DM is 4 years [3]. IGT can be associated with impaired fasting glucose (IFG) or normal fasting plasma glucose (FPG) [1,4,5]. IGT is considered as prediabetes, along with IFG and glycated hemoglobin (HbA1c) values in the range of 5.7–6.4% [1,2]. Progression from IGT to T2DM is associated with hyperglycemia, age, and weight [4].

The global prevalence of IGT was 7.5% of the adult population in 2019, and projected prevalence is expected to reach 8.0% in 2030, and 8.6% in 2045 [6].

The rates for the patients who have both IFG and IGT are 15.8% and 20.2% according to World Health Organization (WHO) and American Diabetes Association (ADA) data, respectively [1,5,7].

In patients with IGT, the risk of T2DM development is 6 times higher compared to people with NGT, the relative risk of mortality is 1.48 times more than in a healthy population, and frequency of fatal cardiovascular events is increased by 1.66 times [1]. According to the International Diabetes Federation, 1 in 10 adults are living with diabetes [8].

It was proposed that IGT is a manifestation of insulin resistance due to "lipid overspill from subcutaneous adipose into ectopic sites" [5] (i.e., liver, pancreas, and skeletal muscle) in individuals with a positive energy balance, excess lipid accumulation, and weight gain [9].

Intensive lifestyle/behavior change programs are the first-line interventions in patients with prediabetes for T2DM prevention [10–15]. If these approaches are insufficient to achieve weight loss and glycemic control, metformin therapy is recommended by ADA [12]. However, the U.S. Food and Drug Administration has yet to approve any medicines for diabetes prevention [12]. At the same time, in 2021 the European Medicines Agency approved liraglutide [16] and recommended the granting of marketing authorization for semaglutide [17] for weight management in patients with obesity or overweight in the presence of prediabetes and other comorbidities.

One of the approaches to overcome insulin resistance and prevent progression of the carbohydrate metabolism disorders is Subetta therapy. This drug is a biotechnological product containing two components based on affinity-purified antibodies to the β-subunit of the insulin receptor (INSR-β) and to endothelial NO synthase (eNOS). Subetta stimulates activation of the insulin receptor alone and in the presence of insulin increasing phosphorylation of INSR-β [18]. Subetta significantly enhances the insulin sensitivity of human muscle cells through stimulation of glucose transport to myocytes mediated by glucose transporter 4 [19,20].

In patients with T1DM and poor glycemic control in a basal-bolus insulin regimen, Subetta add-on therapy improved the glycemic profile without insulin dose intensification and without increasing the overall hypoglycemia rates [21].

The pharmacological activity of Subetta can be used in patients with IGT to increase the sensitivity of cells to endogenous insulin, which is reduced due to insulin resistance.

In this clinical trial, we evaluated the efficacy and safety of 12-week Subetta therapy in correcting 2-h plasma glucose in patients with IGT.

2. Materials and Methods

2.1. Study Overview

This multicenter, double-blind, placebo-controlled, randomized, parallel-group clinical trial was carried out between 10 October 2018 and 23 March 2020 in 44 medical institutions in the Russian Federation (see Supplementary Materials, Study overview). The protocol of the study and the study results are posted in the ClinicalTrials.gov results database (NCT03725033) [22].

The screening of patients was performed over 7 days, after which they were randomized into two groups and treated for 12 weeks. Patients visited medical centers three times—on day 1, after 4 weeks (visit 2), and after 12 weeks (visit 3) of the treatment, and they were examined at each visit. The observation period lasted for up to 13 weeks.

2.2. Patient Selection and Assessment

Patients of either gender, aged 18–70 years old, with prediabetes, obesity (especially visceral or abdominal obesity), dyslipidemia (with high triglycerides and/or low high-density lipoproteins), arterial hypertension, or high genetic burden of diabetes mellitus (diabetes in first-degree relatives) were considered as candidates for participation in the study.

The screening procedures included medical history, registration of concomitant conditions and diseases, physical examination, calculation of body mass index (BMI), and oral glucose tolerance test (OGTT) for measurement of FPG and 2-h plasma glucose. In addition, venous blood samples (for detection of HbA1c level and biochemical and clinical analyses) and urine samples were obtained from each patient.

All laboratory tests were carried out in the central laboratory, which provided the equipment for collection and sample preparation in the medical centers. Blood samples were collected after a night fast of no less than 10 h. A venous blood sample from the antecubital vein was drawn into two vacuum tubes for plasma and serum separation. The delivery of biological samples was performed within 6 h, in compliance with the requirements of transportation conditions. Measurement of FPG and 2-h plasma glucose was performed using the enzyme (hexokinase) method and photometry in a biochemical analyzer (ARCHITECT c16000, Abbot, Chicago, IL, USA). HbA1c was determined by a method certified in accordance with the National Glycohemoglobin Standardization Program and standardized in compliance with the reference values adopted in the Diabetes Control and Complications Trial. Hematology, blood chemistry and urinalysis were performed to assess the safety of the treatment. Blood chemistry included alkaline phosphatase, aspartate aminotransferase, alanine aminotransferase, creatinine, total cholesterol, total bilirubin, total protein, sodium, and potassium.

The inclusion criteria were as follows: plasma glucose level from 7.8 to 11.0 mmol/L two hours after a 75 g oral glucose load during an OGTT, while FPG < 7.0 mmol/L; HbA1c, 5.7–6.4%; BMI, 25.0–39.9 kg/m^2; consent to use contraceptive methods during the study (for men and women with reproductive potential).

The recommendations of the WHO and the International Diabetes Federation were used for the diagnosis of IGT and prediabetes.

One of the inclusion criterion was a BMI of 25.0–39.9 kg/m^2 (overweight, or 1/2 degree obesity). Measurement of body weight and height was carried out at the screening stage on standardized (calibrated according to the factory method) scales and a stadiometer. BMI was calculated according to the formula: weight/(height in meters)^2.

Candidates with normal BMI were not included in the study. After examination during the screening period, the presence of IGT in patients with a BMI of 25.0–39.9 kg/m^2 could be not confirmed if the parameters of carbohydrate metabolism did not meet the inclusion criteria.

The exclusion criteria were as follows: T1DM, T2DM, and other specific types of diabetes; acute disease or exacerbation/decompensation of a chronic disease; uncontrolled arterial hypertension; acute coronary syndrome, myocardial infarction, acute impairment of cerebral circulation during the previous 6 months; unstable or life-threatening arrhythmia during the previous 3 months; acute or chronic heart failure with functional class III or IV; respiratory failure; chronic kidney disease (classes C3–5 A3); hepatic insufficiency (class C according to Child–Pugh); oncology disease; an allergy/hypersensitivity to medication administered; mental illness or drug abuse; history of bariatric surgery; pregnancy, breastfeeding; childbirth less than 3 months before enrollment; use of any prohibited medications.

One of the exclusion criterion was uncontrolled arterial hypertension, defined as office systolic blood (BP) pressure $\geq$ 160 mmHg and/or diastolic BP $\geq$ 100 mm Hg (grade 2 hypertension or grade 3 hypertension according to ESH/ESC 2013 guidelines for the management of arterial hypertension). BP was measured in the office by a doctor at screening and at every visit using an automated validated upper-arm cuff BP devices based on the oscillometric technique. Measurement of BP was performed in accordance with 2017 American College of Cardiology/American Heart Association Guideline.

2.3. Randomization and Blinding

After screening, the patients were randomized into two groups to be assigned Subetta or Placebo. An interactive voice/web response randomization system (based on a random number generator) was used by physicians. Block randomization was performed in blocks of 4. A personal code documented in the chart and unchanged during the study was given to each patient in order to maintain confidentiality.

The studied drug was delivered to medical centers in boxes and packages that did not carry information regarding the active substance. Manufacturing, packaging, and labelling with unique identification codes of the double-blind medications (Subetta or placebo/identical in shape and taste tablet containing excipients) were performed by OOO NPF MMH. Neither participants nor physicians, investigators, trial centers staff, or the Sponsor's project team were aware of the treatment group assignment throughout the study and until the database lock.

2.4. Treatment

Subetta was administered for oral use, 2 tablets per intake twice a day, 15 min before a meal for 12 weeks. The tablet should be held in the mouth until complete dissolution occurred.

Each Subetta tablet contains affinity purified technologically-treated antibodies to β-subunit of the insulin receptor (6 mg) and antibodies to endothelial NO synthase (6 mg). The active substance is produced by patented technology (US Patent 8,617,555 B2) in accordance with European Pharmacopeia requirements [21].

Placebo was administered according to Subetta administration schedule.

The compliance with the study therapies was assessed at the 2nd and 3rd visits according to the count of tablets returned.

Patients were given advice on nutrition and physical activity. A pregnancy test was carried out for all fertile women.

Patients were allowed to use concomitant therapy, including agents acting on the renin-angiotensin system, beta blocking agents, and calcium channel blockers.

Blood glucose lowering drugs, insulins and analogues, corticosteroids, thyroid preparations, hormonal contraceptives, appetite stimulants, anti-obesity preparations, long-action organic nitrates, and diuretics were prohibited drugs.

2.5. Study End Points and Statistical Analysis

The primary efficacy end point was a change in 2-h plasma glucose (during OGTT) after 12 weeks of treatment. The secondary end points were as follows: percentage of patients with 2-h plasma glucose <7.8 mmol/L, change in FPG, and change in HbA1c after 12 weeks of treatment.

Statistical analysis was performed using SAS (Version 9.4) (SAS Institute, Cary, NC, USA) statistical software. Data of the full analysis set, excluding the failure to satisfy major entry criteria, were used for the intention-to-treat (ITT) analysis. The data of all patients who completed the therapy as per the study protocol without any missing scheduled visits were used for the Per-Protocol (PP) analysis of the efficacy (data are presented in square brackets).

The sample size was calculated assuming the difference in reduction of 2-h plasma glucose between Product and Placebo groups would be no less than $\varepsilon = 1.1$, while the standard deviation would be $\sigma = 3.11$. The power of statistical tests "$p = (1 - \beta)$" was assumed to be 80% (the probability of correct rejection of the null hypothesis was 0.8); the probability of a type I error "α" was allowed to be less than 0.05% (the probability of the erroneous acceptance of an alternative hypothesis was less than 0.05); the statistical criteria used were two-tailed. The minimum required size for each group was 143 patients; at least 842 patients had to be included, taking into account a dropout rate at 66% subjects (Cw = 0.66) during the study for various reasons. The dropout rate was based on the results of a blinded interim analysis.

Two interim analyses were planned and performed during the study:
(1) Blinded interim analysis to clarify population characteristics and adjust the sample size (only upward). As a result of this analysis, the sample was increased, and Version 2 of the study protocol was released.
(2) Unblinded interim analysis included data from more than 50% of the planned sample ($n = 538$). Unblinded interim analysis was planned for early trial stop due to efficacy (O'Brien–Fleming boundary) or null hypothesis acceptance (Pocock boundary).

According to O'Brien and Fleming [23], if the p-value for the primary efficacy endpoint is <0.00388 in the interim analysis of data, the study may be stopped due to evidence of efficacy.

After the inclusion of 538 patients, the study was terminated when interim analysis showed significant reduction in 2-h plasma glucose in patients of the Subetta group in comparison with placebo therapy. Interim analysis demonstrated that the result of the Subetta therapy was sufficient to stop the study due to the achievement of efficacy, because the type I error (0.0028 (<0.0001)) was below the critical value (0.00388) established by the O'Brien–Fleming rules for the interim analysis.

Analysis of continuous variables was carried out using the nonparametric Wilcoxon test and Student's t-test for normally distributed variables. Normality of variables was accessed using the Shapiro–Wilk test. Multivariate analysis was performed using analysis of variance for repeated measurements (repeated-measures ANOVA, PROC MIXED). The Holm method (PROC MULTTEST) was used as a correction for multiplicity. Fisher's exact test was used to compare the proportions.

3. Results

3.1. Patient Demographics and Baseline Characteristics

In total, 538 subjects with suspected IGT were enrolled. After passing the screening procedures, 336 subjects were excluded by the doctors as they did not meet inclusion criteria, or they met exclusion criteria. The remaining 202 subjects were randomized into two groups: 105 to the Subetta group and 97 to the Placebo group. The results of the treatment and observation of these patients ($n = 202$) were used to conduct an ITT analysis of efficacy and to assess the safety of the investigational therapy. The number of patients who received the full course of the therapy, completed all prescribed visits, and did not have significant deviations from the protocol was 174, including 92 in the Subetta group and 82 in the Placebo group. The data from these patients were used for the PP efficacy analysis. Data from 28 patients (13 patients in the Subetta group and 15 patients in the Placebo group) were not included in the PP analysis of efficacy for various reasons. Figure 1 presents the study design flow diagram.

Patients in both groups did not differ in demographic and baseline clinical characteristics, including age, gender, BMI, vital signs, and initial parameters of carbohydrate metabolism (2-h plasma glucose, FPG, and HbA1c). Baseline characteristics of the patients are presented in the Tables 1–3.

As can be seen from Table 1, the majority of the study participants were women. To assess the effect of gender on the results of the study, we conducted analysis that showed no statistical significance of gender, both in ITT and PP populations. The statistical analysis used involves mixed models for 2-h plasma glucose with gender covariate and CMH test with Breslow–Day test for percentage of patients with 2-h plasma glucose < 7.8 mmol/L after 12 weeks with gender as the main strata (see Supplementary Materials, Tables S1–S4).

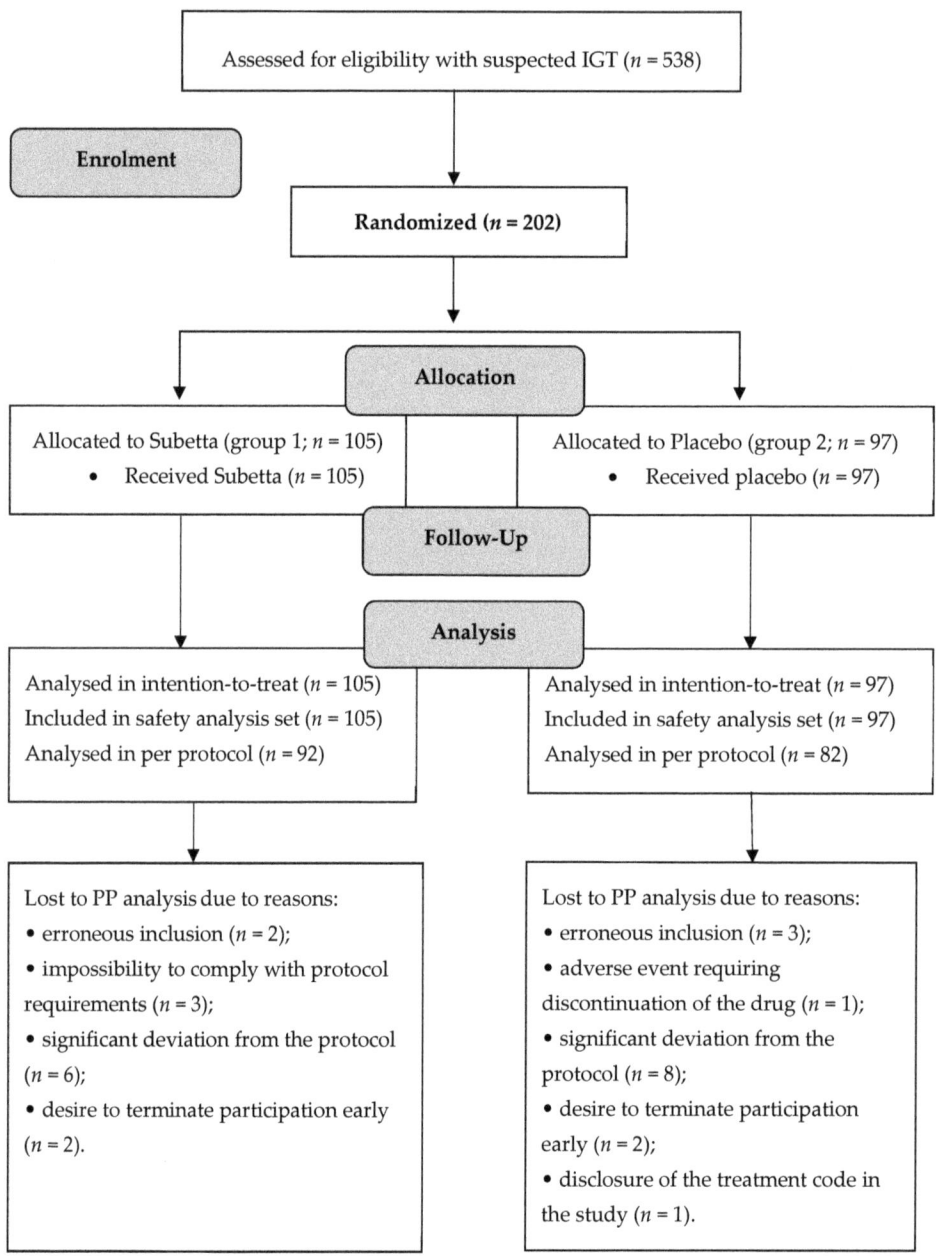

Figure 1. Study design flow diagram.

Table 1. Baseline demographic and anthropometric characteristics of the patients.

Characteristics	ITT Analysis (N = 202)		PP Analysis (N = 174)	
	Subetta	Placebo	Subetta	Placebo
Age, years				
Mean ± SD	56.6 ± 8.6	56.1 ± 8.6	57.0 ± 9.1	56.3 ± 8.6
Median	58	57	58.5	56.5
Minimum	28	33	28	38
Maximum	70	69	70	69
Q1–Q3	51–54	52–64	52.5–64	52–64
Statistics	$Z = 0.64; p = 0.52$		$Z = 0.84; p = 0.40$	
Male/female, %	25.7/74.3	22.7/77.3	27.2/72.8	25.6/74.4
	$p = 0.63$		$p = 0.86$	
Body weight, kg				
Mean ± SD	88.2±15.0	88.7±14.5	87.8±14.4	89.3 ± 14.8
Median	85	89	84.8	89
Minimum	58	62	58	62
Maximum	120	128.2	120	128.2
Q1–Q3	76.6–99.1	77–98	77.3–98.4	77–98.7
Statistics	$Z = 0.30; p = 0.76$		$Z = 0.68; p = 0.50$	
BMI, kg/m^2				
Mean ± SD	31.8 ± 4.2	32.0 ± 4.3	31.7 ± 4.0	32.0 ± 4.1
Median	31.2	32.1	31.2	31.9
Minimum	25.1	25.3	25.1	25.4
Maximum	39.7	39.5	39.7	39.5
Q1–Q3	28.4–35	28.2–35.5	28.6–34.7	28.3–35.5
Statistics	$Z = 0.28; p = 0.78$		$Z = 0.30; p = 0.77$	

Notes. Mean ± SD—mean and standard deviation. Q1–Q3—the first and third quartiles. N—number of patients. The age of the patients was analyzed using the Wilcoxon test; the result of the normality test using the Shapiro–Wilk test: ITT—Subetta—$p = 0.0003$, Placebo—$p = 0.0019$; PP—Subetta—$p = 0.0002$, Placebo—$p = 0.0030$. Gender was analyzed and compared using Fisher's exact test. The result of the normality test using the Shapiro–Wilk test: BMI—Subetta—$p = 0.0006$, Placebo—$p = 0.0017$; PP—Weight—Subetta—$p = 0.1249$, Placebo—$p = 0.2565$, BMI—Subetta—$p = 0.0055$, Placebo—$p = 0.0008$.

Table 2. Baseline blood pressure of the patients.

	ITT Analysis (N = 202)		PP Analysis (N = 174)	
	Subetta	Placebo	Subetta	Placebo
Systolic blood pressure, mm Hg				
Mean ± SD	127.5 ± 8.0	127.8 ± 8.5	127.4 ± 7.9	127.8 ± 8.3
Median	129	127	128.5	127
Minimum	100	98	100	98
Maximum	147	156	147	156
Q1–Q3	122–132	122–134	122–132	122–134
Statistics	$Z = 0.48; p = 0.63$		$Z = 0.56; p = 0.58$	
Diastolic blood pressure, mm Hg				
Mean ± SD	79.1 ± 5.6	79.4 ± 6.9	78.8 ± 5.7	79.4 ± 7.0

Table 2. Cont.

	ITT Analysis (N = 202)		PP Analysis (N = 174)	
	Subetta	Placebo	Subetta	Placebo
Median	80	80	80	80
Minimum	62	54	62	54
Maximum	90	97	90	97
Q1–Q3	75–83	75–84	74.5–83	75–84
Statistics	Z = 0.15; p = 0.88	Z = 0.41; p = 0.68	Z = 0.15; p = 0.88	Z = 0.41; p = 0.68

Notes. Mean ± SD—mean and standard deviation. Q1–Q3—the first and third quartiles. N—number of patients. Blood pressure indicators were analyzed using Student's t-test and Wilcoxon's test; the result of the normality test using the Shapiro–Wilk test: Systolic blood pressure (ITT analysis)—Subetta—$p = 0.1900$, Placebo—$p = 0.0071$; (PP analysis)—Subetta—$p = 0.1205$, Placebo—$p = 0.0019$; Diastolic blood pressure (ITT analysis)—Subetta—$p = 0.0483$, Placebo—$p = 0.2262$; (PP analysis)—Subetta—$p = 0.0489$, Placebo—$p = 0.2045$.

Table 3. Baseline parameters of carbohydrate metabolism of the patients.

Parameters	ITT Analysis (N = 193 *)		PP Analysis (N = 174)	
	Subetta	Placebo	Subetta	Placebo
2-h plasma glucose, mmol/L				
Mean ± SD	9.3 ± 0.9	9.1 ± 0.9	9.3 ± 0.8	9.1 ± 0.9
Median	9.2	9.0	9.2	9.0
Q1–Q3	8.5–9.9	8.4–9.6	8.5–9.9	8.4–9.6
95% CI	9.1–9.4	8.9–9.3	9.1–9.4	8.9–9.3
N *	101	92	92	82
Statistics	Z = 1.22; p = 0.22		Z = 1.47; p = 0.14	
Fasting plasma glucose, mmol/L				
Mean ± SD	5.8 ± 0.6	5.9 ± 0.6	5.9 ± 0.6	5.9 ± 0.6
Median	5.9	5.9	5.95	5.9
Q1–Q3	5.4–6.3	5.5–6.3	5.4–6.3	5.5–6.3
95% CI	5.7–6.0	5.7–6.0	5.7–6.0	5.7–5.9
N *	101	92	92	82
Statistics	Z = 0.29; p = 0.77		Z = 0.23; p = 0.82	
HbA1c,%				
Mean ± SD	6.0 ± 0.2	6.0 ± 0.20	6.0 ± 0.2	6.0 ± 0.2
Median	5.9	6.0	5.9	6.0
Q1–Q3	5.8–6.1	5.8–6.2	5.8–6.1	5.8–6.2
95% CI	5.9–6.0	6.0–6.0	5.9–6.00	6.0–6.0
N *	101	92	92	82
Statistics	Z = 1.92; p = 0.06		Z = 1.72; p = 0.08	

Notes. Mean ± SD—mean and standard deviation. Q1–Q3—the first and third quartiles. * N—number of patients. Blood samples were taken from 9 randomized patients (n = 4, Subetta group; n = 5, placebo group) who were fully treated and underwent all procedures according to the protocol, but the central laboratory did not provide carbohydrate metabolism values due to technical problems. Data were analyzed using the Wilcoxon test; the result of the normality test using the Shapiro–Wilk test: 2-h plasma glucose (ITT analysis)—Subetta—$p = 0.0013$, placebo—$p = 0.0034$; (PP analysis)—Subetta—$p = 0.0047$, Placebo—$p = 0.0050$; fasting plasma glucose (ITT analysis)—Subetta—$p = 0.0002$, Placebo—$p = 0.0226$; (PP Analysis)—Subetta—$p = 0.0001$, Placebo—$p = 0.0490$; HbA1c (ITT analysis)—Subetta—$p = 0.0001$, Placebo—$p = 0.0009$; (PP Analysis)—Subetta—$p = 0.0001$, Placebo—$p = 0.0011$.

Various comorbidities were found in 91.4 [91.3]% (n = 96 [n = 84]) of patients in the Subetta group and in 87.6 [89.0]% (n = 85 [n = 73]) of subjects of the Placebo group (p = 0.49 [p = 0.62]).

Sixty one percent of patients [60.9]% (n = 62 [n = 56]) in the Subetta group and 63.9 [63.4]% (n = 62 [n = 52]) of patients in the Placebo group (p = 1.00 [p = 0.76]) had metabolic and nutritional disorders (dyslipidemia, hyperlipidemia, hypertriglyceridemia, hypercholesterolemia, hyperuricemia, etc.); 57.1 [57.6]% (n = 60 [n = 53]) and 45.4 [47.6]% (n = 44 [n = 39]) of patients (p = 0.12 [p = 0.22]) had vascular diseases (arterial hypertension, atherosclerosis of vessels of various localization, chronic venous insufficiency, etc.); 40.0 [42.4]% (n = 62 [n = 56]) and 37.1 [37.8]% (n = 62 [n = 56]; p = 0.77 [p = 0.77 [p = 0.64]) had heart diseases (coronary heart disease, angina pectoris, cardiac arrhythmias, NYHA class I/II heart failure, etc.); 22.9 [25.0]% (n = 24 [n = 23]) and 22.7 [24.4]% (n = 22 [n = 20]; p = 1.00 [p = 1.00]) had diseases of muscle, skeletal, and connective tissue; 24.8 [22.8]% (n = 26 [n = 21]) and 23.7 [25.6]% (n = 23 [n = 21]; p = 0.87 [p = 1.00]) had diseases of the gastrointestinal tract; 19.0 [17.4]% (n = 20 [n = 16]) and 19.6 [18.3]% (n = 19 [n = 15]; p = 1.00 [p = 1.00]) had diseases of the liver and biliary tract; 21.0 [21.7]% (n = 22 [n = 20]) and 20.6 [20.7]% (n = 20 [n = 17]; p = 1.00 [p = 1.00]) had thyroid gland pathology. Other diseases were less common. Statistical analysis using Fisher's exact test did not reveal significant differences between groups of patients in the incidence of concomitant diseases.

Seventy two percent [71.7]% (n = 75 [n = 66]) of patients in the Subetta group and 72.2 [72.0]% (n = 70 [n = 59]) in the Placebo group received permitted concomitant therapy (p = 1.00 [p = 1.00]). Most patients in both groups took drugs for the treatment of cardiovascular diseases, including agents acting on the renin-angiotensin system (52.4 [53.3]% (n = 55 [n = 49]) in the Subetta group and 53.6 [52.4]% (n = 52 [n = 43]) in the Placebo group; p = 0.89 [p] = 1.00]), beta blocking agents (30.5 [29.3]% (n = 32 [n = 27]) and 26.8 [29.3]% (n = 26 [n = 24]); p = 0.64 [p = 1.00]), calcium channel blockers (13.3 [15.2]% (n = 14 [n = 14]) and 10.3 [9.8]% (n = 10 [n = 8]), respectively; p = 0.52 [p = 0.36]). Medications from other pharmacological groups were taken by a relatively small percentage of the study participants. Fisher's exact test did not show differences between groups for concomitant therapy.

Patients in the Subetta and the Placebo groups excluded from the PP analysis also did not differ (both among themselves and compared to patients whose data were included in the analysis) in baseline demographic, anthropometric, clinical characteristics, comorbidities, and concomitant therapy.

The adherence of patients to the therapy after 4 weeks was 100.5 ± 12.5 [99.7 ± 5.6]% in the Subetta group and 101.9 ± 13.6 [100.6 ± 4.8]% in the Placebo group, and after 12 weeks of treatment this was 98.1 ± 7.4% [98.3 ± 4.8]% and 100.5 ± 8.5 [98.8 ± 4.4]%, respectively (p = 0.76 [p = 0.72]).

3.2. Primary Efficacy Endpoint

Two-hour plasma glucose concentration in the Subetta group significantly decreased after 12 weeks of treatment. Figure 2 indicates the change from baseline of 2-h plasma glucose after 12 weeks of treatment in patients of the PP sample.

The difference in 2-h glucose level between baseline and after 12 weeks of treatment in the Subetta group was −1.9 ± 2.2 [−2.0 ± 2.1] mmol/L (versus −0.7 ± 2.2 [−0.5 ± 2.5] mmol/L in the Placebo group). The difference in the reduction of 2-h plasma glucose between the Subetta and the Placebo groups was 1.2 ± 2.3 [1.4 ± 2.3] mmol/L (p = 0.0028 [p < 0.0001]).

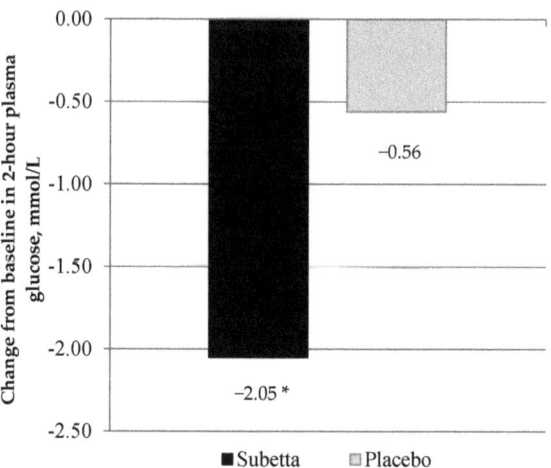

Figure 2. Change from baseline in 2-h plasma glucose after 12 weeks of treatment (PP analysis). Note. * $p < 0.0001$ vs. placebo.

3.3. Secondary Efficacy Endpoint

Figure 3 shows the percentage of patients with 2-h plasma glucose < 7.8 mmol/L after 12 weeks of treatment in patients of the PP sample, where the advantage of Subetta was 17.6% ([$p = 0.0219$]).

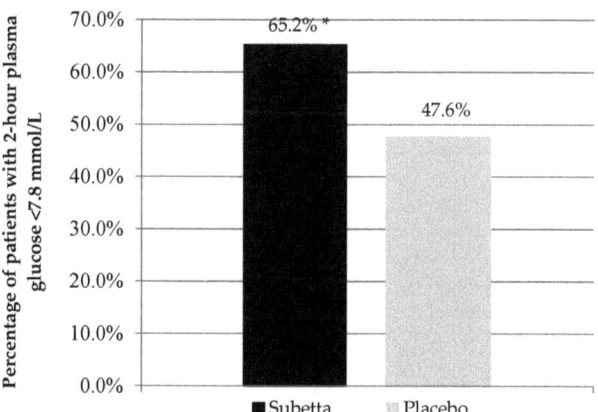

Figure 3. Percentage of patients with 2-h plasma glucose < 7.8 mmol/L after 12 weeks of treatment (PP analysis). Note. * $p = 0.0219$ vs. placebo.

The baseline FPG level was either within the normal range or slightly exceeded the normal threshold level of 6.0 mmol/L in most patients in both groups. The boundaries of the lower and upper quartiles were 5.4–6.3 [5.4–6.3] mmol/L in the Subetta group and 5.5–6.3 [5.5–6.3] mmol/L in the Placebo group ($p = 0.06$ [$p = 0.08$]).

FPG remained almost unchanged during 12 weeks of treatment in both groups. The boundaries of the lower and upper quartiles after 12 weeks were 5.4–6.5 [5.4–6.5] mmol/L and 5.4–6.4 [5.4–6.5] mmol/L in the Subetta and the Placebo group, respectively ($p = 0.99$ [$p = 0.74$]).

Within 12 weeks of treatment, there was a trend towards a decrease in HbA1c level in both groups. The boundaries of the lower and upper quartiles after 12 weeks were 5.5–6.0

[5.5–6.0]% and 5.6–6.0 [5.6–6.1]% in the Subetta and the Placebo group, respectively. This means that, after 12 weeks, 25% of patients in the Subetta group had HbA1c below 5.5%.

3.4. Safety Analysis

Subetta had no impact on the vital signs of patients, including blood pressure, heart rate, and respiratory rate. The mean values of the vital signs throughout the study were normal and well-controlled. There were no differences in these parameters during treatment between both groups.

In total, 16 adverse events (AEs) were reported in 15 (14.3%) patients of the Subetta group, and 27 AEs reported in 20 (20.6%) patients of the Placebo group (see Supplementary Table S5).

Frequency analysis (Fisher's exact test) did not reveal significant differences between the number of patients with AEs in the Subetta and the Placebo groups ($p = 0.27$).

The most frequent AEs were changes in laboratory and instrumental test results. In the Subetta group, this was an increase in the number of leukocytes in urine ($n = 1$), an increase in alanine aminotransferase (ALT) level ($n = 1$), an increase in blood pressure ($n = 1$), weight loss ($n = 1$), and in the Placebo group, an increase in the ALT ($n = 1$), an increase in aspartate aminotransferase ($n = 1$), an increase in HbA1c level ($n = 1$), an increase in blood pressure ($n = 3$), and a decrease in weight ($n = 1$).

Within 3 months, in 7 patients IGT progressed to T2DM, including 2 patients in the Subetta group and 5 patients in the Placebo group.

In the Subetta group, 13 (81.43%) AEs were mild and 3 (18.7%) were moderate. No AEs were reported with definite/possible relationship with the study drug. The frequency of distribution of AEs depending on the severity ($p = 0.42$) and the relationship with the drug ($p = 0.17$) did not differ in the two groups (see Supplementary Tables S6 and S7).

AEs classified as severe were not registered in the clinical trial. There was no evidence of drug-to-drug interaction with medications administered concomitantly with Subetta, nor were there any hypersensitivity events.

4. Discussion and Conclusions

This study demonstrated the efficacy of Subetta in patients with IGT. The therapeutic action of Subetta is manifested in the reduction of 2-h glucose, which prevents progression of disorders of carbohydrate metabolism. After 12 weeks of Subetta administration, 2-h glucose was restored to normal levels in most patients with IGT.

Administration of Subetta had no effect on FPG. On the one hand, this may indicate that the drug has (first of all) an antihyperglycemic effect, without affecting normal plasma glucose concentration. On the other hand, it was found that disorders of carbohydrate metabolism in IFG and IGT differ in development mechanisms. It is known that impaired insulin secretion and suppression of gluconeogenesis are the main mechanisms in the development of IFG [24]. Obviously, the pharmacological activity of Subetta, which consists of sensitizing the insulin receptor and increasing the sensitivity of cells to insulin, does not significantly affect the processes of hormone secretion and gluconeogenesis [20]. In this regard, the level of fasting glycemia in patients who took the study drug for 12 weeks remained unchanged, while 2-h (post-load) hyperglycemia was amenable to good correction (precisely by reducing insulin resistance).

Along with eliminating IGT in most patients, Subetta "initiated" HbA1c correction. Baseline "pre-diabetic" HbA1c values tended to decrease after 12 weeks of treatment. As is known, HbA1c is a long-term blood glucose control indicator; it reflects glucose concentration over the past 2–3 months [25]. Obviously, during the very first weeks after starting the treatment, there was no significant change in 2-h plasma glucose. Therefore, peaks of postprandial hyperglycemia in this initial treatment period contributed negatively and HbA1c was not decreased below 5.7% in most patients. However, it should be noted that 25% of patients in the Subetta group had HbA1c values below 5.5%. It is possible that the use of the drug for a longer period may normalize HbA1c in most patients with IGT.

Insulin resistance, which is leading in carbohydrate metabolism disorders in patients with IGT, is well corrected by Subetta over a 12-week course of treatment. The effect of the drug is realized by improving glucose utilization due to a decrease in insulin resistance. Obviously, longer therapy can contribute to a more significant normalization of carbohydrate metabolism and prevent the progression of disorders to T2DM.

The endothelioprotective effect of the second component of Subetta (technologically treated antibodies to eNOS) [19] is also important in therapy because vascular complications manifest already at the IGT stage [26]. The synergistic action of the two components of the drug has a positive effect on both insulin resistance and endothelial dysfunction, thereby preventing the progression of micro- and macroangiopathies.

This study has several limitations. It has a relatively small sample size due to a high drop-out rate during screening. Patients with serious concomitant diseases were not included in the study, and therefore the efficacy of Subetta in these patient categories was not investigated. Due to the short duration of treatment (12 weeks), the effects of Subetta on body weight, as well as waist circumference and lipid profile, were not evaluated. In addition, the therapeutic effects of various schemes of Subetta administration have not been evaluated.

In conclusion, the results of this study demonstrated the therapeutic potential of Subetta in patients with IGT. Obviously, longer studies need to be planned to prove the long-term effects of Subetta in patients with insulin resistance.

5. Patents

Subetta is a drug manufactured by OOO "NPF" MATERIA MEDICA HOLDING". Patents on Subetta: US 8,617,555 B2; MX 331246; RU 2509572, and RU2531048.

Supplementary Materials: The following are available online at https://www.mdpi.com/article/10.3390/jcm11051390/s1: Study overview; Table S1: Level of 2-h plasma glucose with gender covariate (ITT analysis); Table S2: Level of 2-h plasma glucose with gender covariate (PP analysis); Table S3: Percentage of patients with 2-h plasma glucose <7.8 mmol/L after 12 weeks of treatment (ITT analysis); Table S4: Percentage of patients with 2-h plasma glucose <7.8 mmol/L after 12 weeks of treatment (PP analysis); Table S5: Adverse events; Table S6: Relationship between the drug and adverse events; Table S7: Adverse events severity.

Author Contributions: Conceptualization, A.M. and A.A.; methodology, A.M.; validation, T.D., A.V. (Anna Volkova) and E.D.; formal analysis, A.M.; investigation, A.M., A.A., A.V. (Anna Volkova), E.D., A.V. (Arkady Vertkin) and S.V.; data curation, A.M.; writing—original draft preparation, A.M.; writing—review and editing, A.M. and A.A.; supervision, A.M.; project administration, A.M. All authors have read and agreed to the published version of the manuscript.

Funding: This study was sponsored by OOO "NPF" MATERIA MEDICA HOLDING" (9, 3rd Samotyochny per., 127473, Moscow, Russia).

Institutional Review Board Statement: The study was conducted according to the guidelines of the Declaration of Helsinki and approved by the Institutional Review Boards of all medical centers and the National Council for ethics of the Ministry of Health of the Russian Federation (protocol code 195 dated 9 July 2019).

Informed Consent Statement: Informed consent was obtained from all subjects involved in the study prior to enrolment.

Data Availability Statement: Study details are provided at (https://clinicaltrials.gov/ct2/show/NCT03725033 (accessed on 23 January 2022)) and can also be obtained by contacting the study sponsor OOO "NPF" MATERIA MEDICA HOLDING".

Acknowledgments: The authors thank the research staff at the participating sites. The investigators involved were Alekseeva E.V., Alpenidze D.N., Arefieva E.V., Arushanova Yu.V., Belousova O.N., Bondar I.A., Chernysheva E.V., Chizhov D.A., Chizhova O.Yu., Demicheva O.Yu., Erofeeva S.B., Ershova O.B., Gofman A.M., Gordeeva E.V., Khalimov Yu.Sh., Khmelnitsky O.K., Khromtsova O.M., Kosmacheva E.D., Kostenko V.A., Kropova O.E., Marchenkova L.A., Mekhtiev S.N., Meleshkevich T.A., Nedogoda S.V., Pavlysh E.F., Ruyatkina L.A., Rymar O.D., Schwartz Yu.G., Shunkov V.B., Smolenskaya O G., Sobolev A.A., Startseva M.A., Varvarina G.N., Verbovoy A.F., Zanozina O.V., Zhdanova E.A., Yanovskaya M.E.

Conflicts of Interest: Ashot Mkrtumyan, Alexander Ametov, Tatiana Demidova, Anna Volkova, Ekaterina Dudinskaya, Arkady Vertkin, and Sergei Vorobiev received the investigator's grant from OOO "NPF" MATERIA MEDICA HOLDING" to conduct the clinical trial. The funder had a role in the design of the study; in the collection and analyses of data; in the decision to publish the results.

References

1. World Health Organization. *Definition and Diagnosis of Diabetes Mellitus and Intermediate Hyperglycemia*; Report of WHO/IDF Consultation; World Health Organization: Geneva, Switzerland, 2006; 50p. Available online: https://www.who.int/diabetes/publications/diagnosis_diabetes2006/en/ (accessed on 23 January 2022).
2. American Diabetes Association. Classification and Diagnosis of Diabetes: Standards of Medical Care in Diabetes-2021. *Diabetes Care* **2021**, *44* (Suppl. S1), S15–S33. [CrossRef] [PubMed]
3. Gong, Q.; Zhang, P.; Wang, J.; Ma, J.; An, Y.; Chen, Y.; Zhang, B.; Feng, X.; Li, H.; Chen, X.; et al. Morbidity and mortality after lifestyle intervention for people with impaired glucose tolerance: 30-year results of the Da Qing Diabetes Prevention Outcome Study. *Lancet Diabetes Endocrinol.* **2019**, *7*, 452–461. [CrossRef]
4. International Diabetes Federation: IDF Diabetes Atlas, 10th ed.; International Diabetes Federation: Brussels, Belgium, 2021. Available online: https://www.diabetesatlas.org/en/ (accessed on 23 January 2022).
5. Yip, W.C.Y.; Sequeira, I.R.; Plank, L.D.; Poppitt, S.D. Prevalence of Pre-Diabetes across Ethnicities: A Review of Impaired Fasting Glucose (IFG) and Impaired Glucose Tolerance (IGT) for Classification of Dysglycaemia. *Nutrients* **2017**, *9*, 1273. [CrossRef] [PubMed]
6. Saeedi, P.; Petersohn, I.; Salpea, P.; Malanda, B.; Karuranga, S.; Unwin, N.; Colagiuri, S.; Guariguata, L.; Motala, A.A.; Ogurtsova, K.; et al. Global and regional diabetes prevalence estimates for 2019 and projections for 2030 and 2045: Results from the International Diabetes Federation Diabetes Atlas, 9th ed. *Diabetes Res. Clin. Pract.* **2019**, *157*, 107843. [CrossRef] [PubMed]
7. Hostalek, U. Global epidemiology of prediabetes—present and future perspectives. *Clin. Diabetes Endocrinol.* **2019**, *5*, 5. [CrossRef] [PubMed]
8. idf.org. International Diabetes Federation; c2021. Available online: https://idf.org/InternationalDiabetesFederation (accessed on 13 January 2022).
9. Saponaro, C.; Gaggini, M.; Carli, F.; Gastaldelli, A. The subtle balance between lipolysis and lipogenesis: A critical point in metabolic homeostasis. *Nutrients* **2015**, *7*, 9453–9474. [CrossRef] [PubMed]
10. Diabetes Prevention Program Research Group. Long-term effects of lifestyle intervention or metformin on diabetes development and microvascular complications over 15-year follow-up: The Diabetes Prevention Program Outcomes Study. *Lancet Diabetes Endocrinol.* **2015**, *3*, 866–875. [CrossRef]
11. Howells, L.; Musaddaq, B.; McKay, A.J.; Majeed, A. Clinical impact of lifestyle interventions for the prevention of diabetes: An overview of systematic reviews. *BMJ Open* **2016**, *6*, e013806. [CrossRef] [PubMed]
12. American Diabetes Association. Prevention or Delay of Type 2 Diabetes: Standards of Medical Care in Diabetes-2021. *Diabetes Care* **2021**, *44* (Suppl. S1), S34–S39. [CrossRef] [PubMed]
13. Selvin, E.; Steffes, M.W.; Zhu, H.; Matsushita, K.; Wagenknecht, L.; Pankow, J.; Coresh, J.; Brancati, F.L. Glycated Hemoglobin, Diabetes, and Cardiovascular Risk in Nondiabetic Adults. *N. Engl. J. Med.* **2010**, *362*, 800–811. [CrossRef] [PubMed]
14. Knowler, W.C.; Barrett-Connor, E.; Fowler, S.E.; Hamman, R.F.; Lachin, J.M.; Walker, E.A.; Nathan, D.M.; Diabetes Prevention Program. Morbidity and mortality after lifestyle intervention for people with impaired glucose tolerance: 30-year results of the Da Qing Diabetes Prevention Outcome Study Research Group. Reduction in the incidence of type 2 diabetes with lifestyle intervention or metformin. *N. Engl. J. Med.* **2002**, *346*, 393–403. [CrossRef] [PubMed]
15. Kanat, M.; DeFronzo, R.A.; Abdul-Ghani, M.A. Treatment of prediabetes. *World J. Diabetes* **2015**, *6*, 1207–1222. [CrossRef] [PubMed]
16. European Medicines Agency. Saxenda. Available online: https://www.ema.europa.eu/en/medicines/human/EPAR/saxenda (accessed on 7 December 2021).
17. European Medicines Agency. Wegovy. Available online: https://www.ema.europa.eu/en/medicines/human/summaries-opinion/wegovy (accessed on 7 December 2021).
18. Gorbunov, E.A.; Nicoll, J.; Kachaeva, E.V.; Tarasov, S.A.; Epstein, O.I. Subetta increases phosphorylation of insulin receptor β-subunit alone and in the presence of insulin. *Nutr. Diabetes* **2015**, *5*, e169. [CrossRef] [PubMed]
19. Mkrtumyan, A.M.; Yegshatyan, L.V. Subetta—A new activator of the insulin receptor. *Eff. Pharmacother.* **2019**, *15*, 12–17. [CrossRef]

20. Gorbunov, E.A.; Nicoll, J.; Myslivets, A.A.; Kachaeva, E.V.; Tarasov, S.A. Subetta Enhances Sensitivity of Human Muscle Cells to Insulin. *Bull. Exp. Biol. Med.* **2015**, *159*, 463–465. [CrossRef] [PubMed]
21. Mkrtumyan, A.; Romantsova, T.; Vorobiev, S.; Volkova, A.; Vorokhobina, N.; Tarasov, S.; Putilovskiy, M.; Andrianova, E.; Epstein, O. Efficacy and safety of Subetta add-on therapy in type 1 diabetes mellitus: The results of a multicenter, double-blind, placebo-controlled, randomized clinical trial. *Diabetes Res. Clin. Pract.* **2018**, *142*, 1–9. [CrossRef]
22. Clinicaltrials.gov. Clinical Trial of Efficacy and Safety of Subetta in the Treatment of Impaired Glucose Tolerance. Available online: https://clinicaltrials.gov/ct2/show/NCT03725033?term=Subetta&draw=2&rank=3 (accessed on 7 December 2021).
23. O'Brien, P.C.; Fleming, T.R. A multiple testing procedure for clinical trials. *Biometrics* **1979**, *35*, 549–556. [CrossRef] [PubMed]
24. Santaguida, P.L.; Balion, C.; Hunt, D.; Morrison, K.; Gerstein, H.; Raina, P.; Booker, L.; Yazdi, H. *Diagnosis, Prognosis, and Treatment of Impaired Glucose Tolerance and Impaired Fasting Glucose*; Evidence Report/Technology Assessment No. 128. (Prepared by the McMaster University Evidence-based Practice Center under Contract No. 290-02-0020). AHRQ Pub. No 05-E026-2; Agency for Healthcare Research and Quality: Rockville, MD, USA, 2005.
25. *Guideline on Clinical Investigation of Medicinal Products in the Treatment or Prevention of Diabetes Mellitus*; CPMP/EWP/1080/00 Rev. 2 Committee for Medicinal Products for Human Use (CHMP); European Medicines Agency: Amsterdam, The Netherlands, 2018; 24p.
26. Wang, H.; Wang, A.X.; Aylor, K.; Barrett, E.J. Nitric oxide directly promotes vascular endothelial insulin transport. *Diabetes* **2013**, *62*, 4030–4042. [CrossRef] [PubMed]

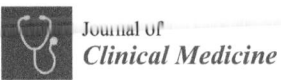

Review

IL-1β Implications in Type 1 Diabetes Mellitus Progression: Systematic Review and Meta-Analysis

Fátima Cano-Cano [1,†], Laura Gómez-Jaramillo [1,†], Pablo Ramos-García [2,*], Ana I. Arroba [1,3,*] and Manuel Aguilar-Diosdado [1,3]

1. Research Unit, Biomedical Research and Innovation Institute of Cadiz (INiBICA), Puerta del Mar University Hospital, 11009 Cadiz, Spain; canocano.fatima@gmail.com (F.C.-C.); laugomjar@gmail.com (L.G.-J.); manuel.aguilar.sspa@juntadeandalucia.es (M.A.-D.)
2. Faculty of Dentistry, University of Granada, 18011 Granada, Spain
3. Department of Endocrinology and Metabolism, University Hospital Puerta del Mar, 11009 Cadiz, Spain
* Correspondence: pabloramos@ugr.es (P.R.-G.); anaarroba@gmail.com (A.I.A.)
† These authors contributed equally to this work.

Abstract: During Type 1 Diabetes Mellitus (T1DM) progression, there is chronic and low-grade inflammation that could be related to the evolution of the disease. We carried out a systematic review and meta-analysis to evaluate whether peripheral levels of pro-inflammatory markers such as interleukin-1 beta (IL-1β) is significantly different among patients with or without T1DM, in gender, management of the T1DM, detection in several biological fluids, study design, age range, and glycated hemoglobin. We searched PubMed, Embase, Web of Science, and Scopus databases, and 26 relevant studies (2186 with T1DM, 2047 controls) were included. We evaluated the studies' quality using the Newcastle–Ottawa scale. Meta-analyses were conducted, and heterogeneity and publication bias were examined. Compared with controls, IL-1β determined by immunoassays (pooled standardized mean difference (SMD): 2.45, 95% CI = 1.73 to 3.17; $p < 0.001$) was significantly elevated in T1DM. The compared IL-1β levels in patients <18 years (SMD = 2.81, 95% CI = 1.88–3.74) was significantly elevated. The hemoglobin-glycated (Hbg) levels in patients <18 years were compared (Hbg > 7: SMD = 5.43, 95% CI = 3.31–7.56; $p = 0.001$). Compared with the study design, IL-1β evaluated by ELISA (pooled SMD = 3.29, 95% CI = 2.27 to 4.30, $p < 0.001$) was significantly elevated in T1DM patients. IL-1β remained significantly higher in patients with a worse management of T1DM and in the early stage of T1DM. IL-1β levels determine the inflammatory environment during T1DM.

Keywords: IL-1β; type 1 diabetes mellitus; chronic inflammation; systematic review; meta-analysis

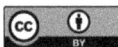

1. Introduction

Type 1 diabetes mellitus (T1DM) is an autoimmune disease often diagnosed in childhood that progresses with pancreatic β-cell destruction and life-long insulin dependence. T1DM susceptibility involves a complex interplay between genetic and environmental factors and with the participation of adaptive immunity, although there is now growing evidence for the role of innate inflammation [1].

T1DM, in the early stage of the disease, is characterized by chronic inflammation that involves pancreatic islet degeneration. The maintenance activation of the innate immune system impairs insulin secretion and action, and inflammation also contributes to diabetes complications, such as diabetic retinopathy and nephropathy. Prior to the manifestation of the disease, a pre-diabetic period may last several years and is characterized by the detection of circulating autoantibodies against beta-cell antigens [2]. There is evidence that indicates a direct pathogenic effect of IL-1β on the islet during the development of T1DM. In pancreatic samples from adult living donors, the presence of IL-β and TNF-α has been detected, mainly in macrophages and dendritic cells [3]. However, despite strong preclinical evidence demonstrating that targeting inflammatory pathways can prevent secondary complications, there are still no treatments for diabetes that target innate immune mediators [4].

In patients with T1DM, higher levels of proinflammatory cytokines have been detected that are physiological constituents of any inflammatory reaction, including interleukins (IL-1α, IL-1β, IL-10, IL-12), interferons (IFNα/β, IFNγ), transforming growth factor-β (TGF-β), tumor necrosis factors (TNFα, TNFβ), and nitric oxide (NO) [5]. The microenvironment is also enriched in anti-inflammatory cytokines including IL-4, IL-10, IL-13, and IL-22, which are generally associated with protective effects over β-cell survival [6].

The role of cytokines in the pathogenesis of autoimmune disorders, particularly T1DM, has been extensively investigated to determine their potential therapeutic value. Screening for the presence of cytokines during the early stages of T1DM can serve to identify immunological response-related soluble factors and a better diagnosis and treatment of the disease.

Interleukin 1 (IL-1) is a 17 kDa protein highly conserved through evolution and is a key mediator of inflammation [7], and it has been suggested as candidate for inducing beta-cell apoptosis in vitro and aggravating diabetes in vivo. Recently, a significant number of studies have given attention to the role of IL-1β in the pathogenesis of autoimmune and inflammatory diseases. There are numerous studies that relate the polymorphisms and gene variations in the IL-1β gene with the differences in the transcription and expression of the IL-1β gene that could correlate with the development of many autoimmune and inflammatory diseases, such as systemic lupus erythematosus [8], rheumatoid arthritis [9], and multiple sclerosis [10].

The genetic or pharmacological inhibition of IL-1 action has clinical efficacy in many inflammatory diseases, due to IL-1 acting on T-lymphocyte regulation. The adverse effects of IL-1β on human beta cells in vitro and in animal models have promoted recent clinical trials in volunteers with recent-onset type 1 diabetes, using strategies involving the systemic blockade of IL-1β or its receptors [7,11]. Genetic or pharmacological abrogation of IL-1 action reduces disease incidence in animal models of type 1 diabetes mellitus [12]. The modulating effect of IL-1 on the interaction between the innate and adaptive immune systems and the effects of IL-1 on the beta-cell point to this molecule being a potential interventional target in autoimmune diabetes mellitus.

Regarding the participation of other pro-inflammatory cytokines, such as TNF-α and IL6, in patients with T1DM, these were found to be linked to elevated level of serum IL-6 and TNF-α, on which the age, ethnicity, and disease duration [12,13] in T1DM patients had no effect on the serum IL-6 levels for promoting diabetes mellitus. The IL-1β level's modulation during different stages of T1DM could be a sensor of progression and good management of disease over time.

With this background, we conducted the first systematic review and meta-analysis to qualitatively and quantitatively evaluate the available scientific evidence on circulating IL-1β levels in T1DM. The aim of this work is to determine the modulated levels of IL-1β between patients with or without T1DM, and to explore their hypothetical influential variables (i.e., geographical area, age, sex, human tissues, biochemical parameters, research methods, and IL-1β determination techniques).

2. Material and Methods

This systematic review and meta-analysis complied with *Preferred Reporting Items for Systematic Reviews and Meta-Analyses* (PRISMA) and *Meta-analysis of Observational Studies in Epidemiology* (MOOSE) guidelines [14,15], and closely followed the criteria of the *Cochrane Handbook for Systematic Reviews of Interventions* [16].

2.1. Protocol

In order to minimize the risk of bias and improve the transparency, precision, and integrity of this study, a protocol on its methodology was a priori registered in the PROSPERO international prospective register of systematic reviews (www.crd.york.ac.uk/PROSPERO, accessed on July 2020, registration code CRD42020180062) [17]. The protocol adhered to the PRISMA-P statement to ensure a rigorous approach [18].

2.2. Search Strategy

We searched PubMed, Embase, Web of Science, and Scopus databases for studies published before the search date (upper limit = October 2020), with no lower date limit. The searches were conducted by combining thesaurus terms used by the databases (i.e., MeSH and EMTREE) with free terms (Table S1, Supplementary Materials p. 1), and built to maximize sensitivity. We also manually screened the reference lists of retrieved studies for additional relevant studies. All references were managed using Mendeley Desktop v. 1.19.4 (Elsevier, Amsterdam, The Netherlands); duplicate references were eliminated using this software.

2.3. Eligibility Criteria

Inclusion criteria: (1) original research studies without language, publication date, follow up periods, study design, geographical area, sex, or age restrictions; (2) T1DM subjects compared to no T1DM as control group; (3) IL-1β determination by enzyme-linked immunosorbent assay (ELISA), quantitative real time polymerase chain reaction (qRT-PCR) and/or flow cytometry in human samples from any anatomical origin; (4) the names and affiliations of authors, recruitment period and settings were examined to determine whether studies were conducted in the same study population. In such cases, we included the most recent study or that which published more complete data.

Exclusion criteria: (1) retracted articles, reviews, meta-analyses, case reports, clinical trials, editorials, letters, abstracts of scientific meetings, personal opinions or comments, and book chapters; (2) in vitro and animal experimental studies; (3) studies that do not report the disease of interest (i.e., T1DM), do not assess IL-1β levels, or those without a control group; (4) studies reporting insufficient data to extract or estimate mean ± standard deviation (SD); (5) overlapping populations.

2.4. Study Selection Process

The eligibility criteria were applied independently by three authors (LGJ, FCC, and AIA). Discrepancies were resolved by consensus with a fourth author (PRG). Articles were selected in two phases, first screening the titles and abstracts of the retrieved articles in an initial selection, and then reading the full text of the selected articles, excluding those that did not meet the review eligibility criteria.

2.5. Data Extraction

Three authors (LGJ, FCC, and AIA) independently extracted data from the selected articles, completing a data collection form in a standardized manner using Excel v. Microsoft Office Professional Plus 2013 (Microsoft. Redmond, WA, USA). These data were additionally cross-checked in multiple rounds, solving discrepancies by consensus. The data were gathered on the first author, publication year, study country and continent, sample size, source of sample (i.e., type of tissue), IL-1β determination (extracting means ± SD and measuring units) in T1DM and controls (i.e., patients not affected by T1DM), age, year of diagnosis, sex of patients, Hbg levels, research methods analysis technique (e.g., ELISA or qRT-PCR), and type of study (i.e., cross-sectional, case-control, or cohorts).

2.6. Evaluation of Quality and Risk of Bias

We used the Newcastle–Ottawa quality assessment scale (NOS) to assess the risk of bias [19]. The evaluation was conducted by two independent reviewers who were knowledgeable about the content and methodology. The results were compared and conflicts resolved by agreement between the two reviewers, with input from a third reviewer if necessary. The studies that received a star in each domain were considered to be of high quality. The maximum score was 8, the minimum 0. It was decided a priori that a score of

7 reflected high methodological quality (i.e., low risk of bias), a score of 5 or 6 indicated moderate quality, and a score of 4 or less indicated low quality (i.e., high risk of bias).

2.7. Statistical Analysis

Mean (±SD) IL-1β levels were extracted to compare between T1DM patients and controls. Since variations in laboratory determination methods were expected (see protocol), the standardized mean difference (SMD) was chosen as an effect size measure, estimated by Cohen's d method with their corresponding 95% confidence intervals (CI). Data expressed as order statistics (i.e., median, interquartile range and/or maximum–minimum values) were computed and transformed into means (±SD) using the methods proposed by Luo et al. and Wan et al. [20,21]. If it was desirable to combine two or more different means (±SD) from subgroups into a single group, the method provided by the Cochrane Handbook was followed [16]. When the data were only expressed graphically, they were measured and extracted using Engauge Digitizer 4.1. In the meta-analyses, SMDs with 95% CIs were pooled using the inverse-variance method under a random-effects model (based on the DerSimonian and Laird method), which accounts for the possibility that there are different underlying results among study subpopulations (i.e., IL-1β variations among tissues, linked to geographical areas, or related to the inherent heterogeneity of the wide range of experimental methods). Forest plots were constructed to graphically represent the overall effect and for subsequent visual inspection analysis ($p < 0.05$ was considered significant). The heterogeneity between studies was evaluated applying the χ^2-based Cochran's Q test (given its low statistical power, $p < 0.10$ was considered significant) and quantified using Higgins I^2 statistic (values of 50–75% were interpreted as a moderate to high degree of inconsistency across the studies), which estimates what proportion of the variance in observed effects reflects variation in true effects, rather than sampling error [22,23]. Preplanned stratifications (by geographical area, type of tissue, age, Hbg levels, study design, matching, and type of analysis) and univariable meta-regression analyses (by sex and risk of bias) were conducted to identify potential sources of heterogeneity and to explore the potential variation of IL-1β levels on these subgroups [24]. For illustrative purposes, weighted bubble plots were also constructed to graphically represent the fitted meta-regression lines. Sensitivity analyses were additionally performed to test the reliability of our results, evaluating the influence of each individual study on the pooled estimations. For this purpose, the meta-analyses were repeated sequentially, omitting one study each time (the classic "leave-one-out" method). Finally, canonical and contour-enhanced funnel plots were constructed, and the Egger regression test ($p < 0.10$ considered significant) and the non-parametric trim-and-fill method were performed to evaluate small-study effects, such as publication bias [25–28]. Stata version 16.1 (Stata Corp., College Station, TX, USA) was employed for all tests, with the commands syntax being manually typed (PRG) [29].

3. Results

3.1. Results of the Literature Search

The flow diagram (Figure 1) depicts the identification and selection process of the studies. We retrieved a total of 3143 records published before October 2020: 626 from MEDLINE/PubMed, 817 from Embase, 826 from the Web of Science, 874 from Scopus, and one [30] from the reference lists screening. After eliminating the duplicates, 1666 studies were considered potentially eligible. After screening their titles and abstracts, 59 were selected for full-text reading. After excluding studies that did not meet all eligibility criteria (all of the studies excluded and their exclusion criteria are listed in the Supplementary Materials, pp. 2–6), 26 studies were finally included in the systematic review for qualitative evaluation (all of the studies included are listed in the Supplementary Materials, pp. 7–9) and 25 studies for quantitative meta-analysis. Due to the presence of a considerable degree of clinical, methodological, and statistical heterogeneity, only plasma and serum studies were meta-analyzed to obtain results derived from more homogeneous subpopulations and more reliable results, while determinations from gingival fluid and vitreous humor were omitted from the meta-analysis.

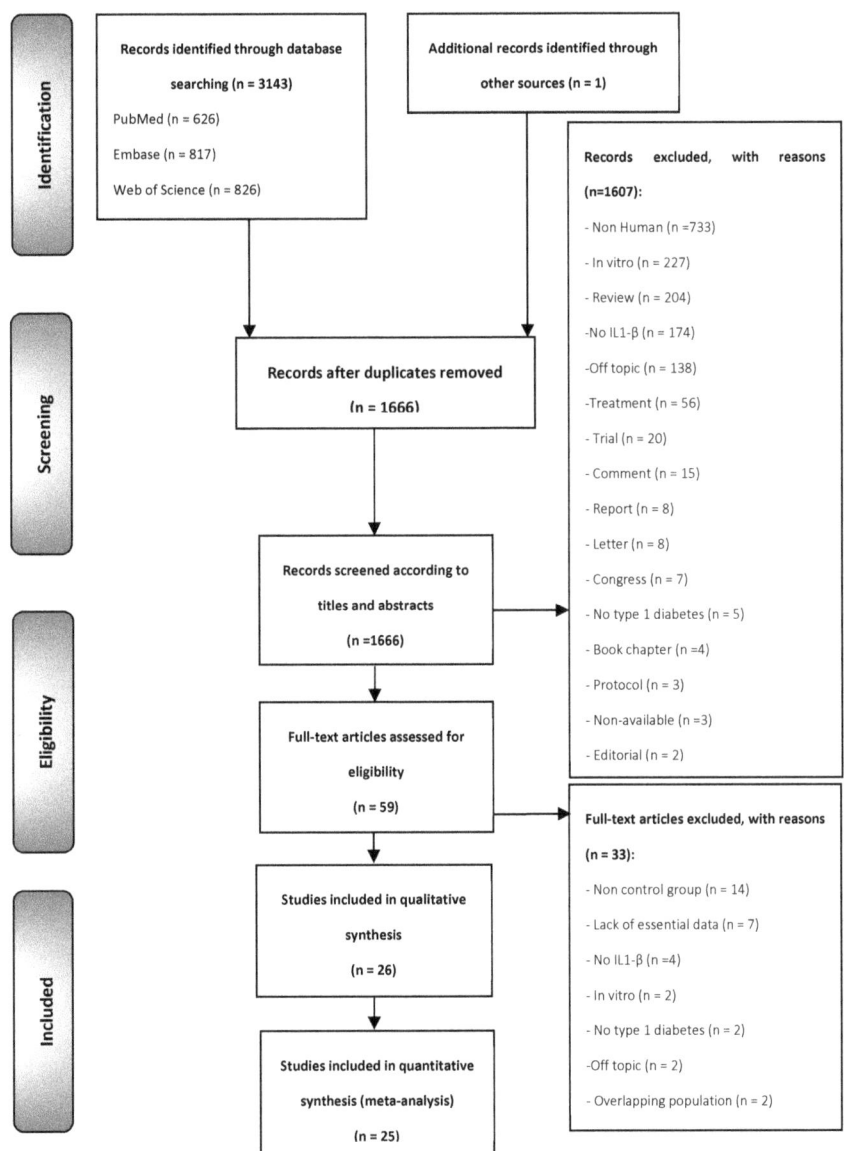

Figure 1. Flow diagram. Identification and selection process of relevant studies comparing IL-1β levels between T1DM patients and controls.

3.2. Study Characteristics

Table 1 summarizes the characteristics of the 26 selected studies comparing the changes in circulating IL-1β levels on a total of 4179 T1DM and control patients, and Table S2 (Supplementary Materials, p. 10) exhibits the variables gathered from each study in more detail. One study [31] analyzed IL-1β levels in two tissues (plasma and vitreous humor) being considered as two different analysis units (i.e., n = 27 studies/4233 patients). Sample sizes ranged between 18 and 961 subjects. The studies were conducted in all continents except for Oceania and comprised 12 in Europe, 6 in Asia, 5 in South America, 3 in Africa, and 1 in North America. IL-1β determination was performed by immunoassays in 22 studies (18 by ELISA and 4 by panels; 15 in serum, 5 in plasma, and 1 in gingival crevicular fluid (not meta-analyzed) and 1 in vitreous humor (not meta-analyzed)), flow cytometry in 3 studies (2 in serum and 1 in cord blood plasma), and 2 studies in qRT-PCR (gingival tissue and peripheral blood mononuclear cells (PBMC)).

Table 1. Summarized characteristics of reviewed studies.

Total	26 studies *
Year of publication	2004–2019
Number of patients	
Total	4179 patients *
Cases with T1DM	2186 patients
Controls	2047 patients
Sample size, range	18–961 patients
IL-1β determination	
Immunoassays	22 studies (18 by ELISA, 4 by panels)
Flow cytometry	3 studies
qRT-PCR	2 studies
Source of samples	
Serum	17 studies
Plasma	5 studies
Gingival crevicular fluid	1 study
Vitreus humour	1 study
Cord blood plasma	1 study
Gingival tissue	1 study
Peripheral blood leukocytes	1 study
Geographical region	
Europe	12 studies
Asia	6 studies
South America	5 studies
Africa	3 study
North America	1 study

*—One study (Koskela et al., 2013) analyzed IL-1β levels in two tissues (plasma and humour vitreus), being considered as two different analysis units (i.e., n total = 27 studies/4233 patients).

3.3. Qualitative Evaluation

The qualitative analysis was conducted using the Newcastle–Ottawa Scale (NOS), which evaluates potential sources of bias in eight domains (Table 2).

Table 2. Summary of risk of bias assessment based on Newcastle–Ottawa Quality Assessment Scale. Two reviewers who had content and methodological expertise independently and in duplicate assessed and graded the risk of bias for the included studies with an adapted version of the Newcastle–Ottawa scale (NOS), which has been described elsewhere [8]. The assessments were compared and conflicts resolved by agreement between the two reviewers. The maximum score was 8, the minimum score 0. It was decided a priori that a score of 7 was reflective of high methodological quality (e.g., low risk of bias), a score of 5 or 6 indicated moderate quality, and a score of 4 or less indicated low quality (e.g., high risk of bias). A filled blue star indicates that a star has been awarded, and a blank star indicates that no star has been awarded and the study has been graded as poor quality in that category [8]. Wells GA (2010) The Newcastle–Ottawa Scale (NOS) For Assessing The Quality Of Non Randomised Studies In Meta-Analyses. Ottawa (ON): Ottawa Health Research Institute.

Study	Selection			Control			Outcomes		Overall Quality
	Representativeness of the T1DM patients	Selection of the non-T1DM subjects	Properly IL1b quantification	Glycemic control	Control of confounding factors	Assessment of T1DM progression	Appropriate follow up period	Adequacy of follow up	
Pérez-Bravo et al. (2004)	★	★	★	★	★	☆	★	★	High
Lo et al. (2004)	★	★	★	★	★	☆	★	★	High
Holm et al. (2006)	★	★	★	★	★	★	★	★	High
Dogan et al. (2006)	★	★	★	☆	★	★	★	★	High
Arabi et al. (2007)	★	★	★	★	★	★	★	★	High
Duarte et al. (2007)	★	★	★	★	★	★	★	★	High
Salvi et al. (2010)	★	★	★	★	★	☆	★	★	High
Meyers et al. (2010)	★	★	★	★	★	★	★	★	High
Gabbay et al. (2012)	★	★	★	☆	★	☆	★	★	Moderate
Svensson et al. (2012)	★	★	★	☆	★	★	★	★	High
Ururahy et al. (2012)	★	★	★	★	★	★	★	★	High
Fartushok et al. (2012)	★	★	★	★	★	☆	★	★	High
Koskela et al. (2013)	★	★	★	★	★	☆	★	★	High

Table 2. *Cont.*

Study	Selection			Control		Outcomes		Overall Quality
	Representativeness of the T1DM patients	Selection of the non-T1DM subjects	Properly IL1b quantification	Glycemic control	Control of confounding factors	Assessment of T1DM progression	Appropriate follow up period	Adequacy of follow up
Allam et al. (2014)	★	★		★	★	★	★	★	High
Farhan et al. (2014)	★	★	★	☆	★	☆	★	★	Moderate
Aguilera et al. (2015)	★	★	★	★	★	★	★	☆	High
Aravindhan et al. (2015)	★	★	★	☆	★	★	★	☆	Moderate
Alnek et al. (2015)	★	★	★	★	★	★	★	★	High
Mohamed et al. (2016)	★	★	★	☆	★	★	★	★	High
Fatima et al. (2016)	★	★	★	★	★	★	★	☆	Moderate
Talaat et al. (2016)	★	★	★	★	★	★	★	★	High
Duque et al. (2017)	★	★	★	☆	★	☆	★	☆	Moderate
Abdel-Latif et al. (2017)	★	★	★	★	★	★	★	★	High
Leiva-Gea et al. (2018)	★	★	★	★	★	★	★	★	High
Ziaja et al. (2018)	★	★	★	☆	★	☆	★	☆	Moderate
Thorsen et al. (2019)	★	★	★	★	★	☆	★	★	High

The most frequent biases could be the inadequate description of patient characteristics (age, sex, etc.), failure to report the study period or place of recruitment, and the inclusion of patients outside the population of interest. In our revision, we only included studies in which the groups of diabetic patients were adequately selected and matched between conditions with their respective controls. Studies without a non-T1DM comparator group were excluded.

However, 100% of the studies showed a representativeness of the T1DM patients, selection of the non-T1DM subjects, and proper IL-1β quantification. In relation to confounding factors, the analysis revealed the use of remarkably severe criteria, and no confounding factors were found. Moreover, there were no studies without T1DM patients, improperly diagnosed patients, or insulin-treated patients. The sum of all of these criteria contributes to avoidance of the overall risk of potential bias, increasing the quality of the evidence of the results reported in this systematic review. On the other hand, there were some parameters that introduced a higher possibility of bias. The absence of suitable glycemic control introduces potential bias into our research (30% of the studies were potentially biased). Concerning T1DM progression, this was increased in 46% of the reviewed studies due to the lack of information about the years of evolution of the disease. In regard to the follow up and attrition rate, the risk of bias was elevated in 19% of the studies due to participants being lost to follow-up, which means essential data to evaluate any differences with the characteristics of the final study sample were not fully obtained.

3.4. Quantitative Evaluation (Meta-Analysis)

3.4.1. IL-1β Determination by Immunoassays

The *IL-1β* levels were significantly higher in T1DM patients than in controls (SMD = 2.45, 95% CI = 1.73 to 3.17; p < 0.001). A significant degree of heterogeneity was observed (p < 0.001; I^2 = 98.6%) (Figure 2, Table 3).

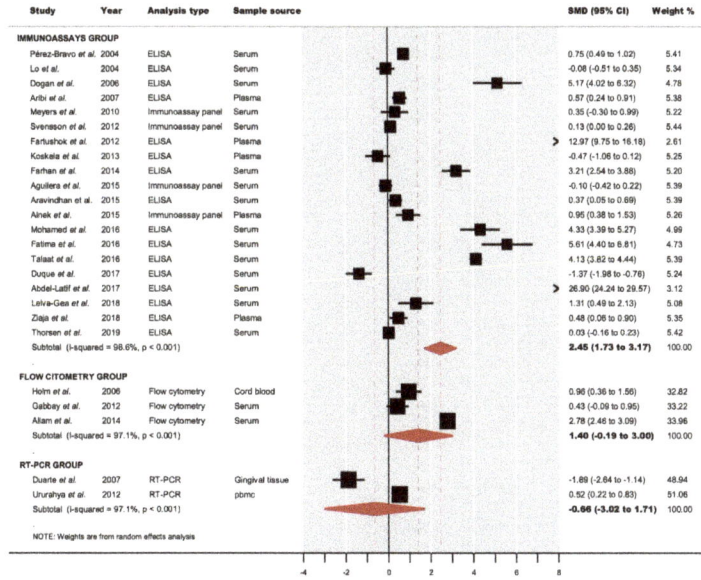

Figure 2. Forest plot graphically representing the meta-analyses evaluating the changes in circulating IL-1β levels between T1DM patients and controls (random-effects models, inverse-variance weighting based on the DerSimonian and Laird method). Standardized mean difference (SMD) was chosen as effect size measure. An SMD > 0 suggests that IL-1β levels are higher in T1DM. Diamonds indicate the overall pooled SMDs with their corresponding 95% confidence intervals (CI).

Table 3. Meta-analyses on circulating IL-1β levels in type 1 diabetes mellitus.

Meta-Analyses	No. of Studies	No. of Patients	Stat. Model	Wt	Pooled Data SMD (95% CI)	p-Value	Heterogeneity P_{het}	I^2 (%)	Supplementary Materials [a]
All [b]	20	3490	REM	D-L	2.45 (1.73 to 3.17)	<0.001	<0.001	98.6	—
Determination by immunoassays									
									Figure S1, p. 11
Subgroup analysis by geographical area [c]									
Africa	3	403	REM	D-L	10.41 (2.58 to 18.23)	0.01	<0.001	99.5	
Asia	5	885	REM	D-L	2.61 (0.56 to 4.66)	0.01	<0.001	99.0	
Europe	9	1875	REM	D-L	1.04 (0.49 to 1.59)	<0.001	<0.001	95.0	
North America	1	38	—	—	0.35 (−0.30 to 0.99)	0.29	—	—	
South America	2	289	REM	D-L	−0.29 (−2.37 to 1.79)	0.78	<0.001	97.4	Figure S2, p. 12
Subgroup analysis by age [c]									
<18 years old	14	2870	REM	D-L	2.81 (1.88 to 3.74)	<0.001	<0.001	98.9	
>18 years old	6	620	REM	D-L	1.56 (0.48 to 2.65)	0.002	<0.001	96.5	Figure S3, p. 13
Subgroup analysis by HbAc1 levels in patients <18 years old [c,d]									
<7	2	79	REM	D-L	−0.04 (−2.67 to 2.58)	0.97	<0.001	96.2	
>7	8	1138	REM	D-L	5.43 (3.31 to 7.56)	0.001	<0.001	99.1	Figure S4, p. 14
Subgroup analysis by age matching [c]									
Matched	15	3172	REM	D-L	3.06 (2.19 to 3.94)	<0.001	<0.001	98.8	
Unmatched	5	318	REM	D-L	0.90 (−0.18 to 1.97)	0.10	<0.001	94.4	Figure S5, p. 15
Subgroup analysis by sex matching [c]									
Matched	11	2379	REM	D-L	0.55 (0.19 to 0.91)	0.003	<0.001	92.9	
Unmatched	3	224	REM	D-L	0.88 (−1.15 to 2.90)	0.40	<0.001	97.5	
NA	6	887	REM	D-L	8.66 (5.37 to 11.96)	<0.001	<0.001	98.9	Figure S6, p. 16
Subgroup analysis by sample source [c]									
Serum	15	3111	REM	D-L	2.73 (1.85 to 3.61)	<0.001	<0.001	98.9	
Plasma	5	379	REM	D-L	1.34 (0.28 to 2.41)	0.01	<0.001	94.3	Figure S7, p. 17
Subgroup analysis by type of analysis [c]									
ELISA	16	2235	REM	D-L	3.29 (2.27 to 4.30)	<0.001	<0.001	98.8	
Immunoassay panel	4	1255	REM	D-L	0.25 (−0.08 to 0.58)	0.14	0.02	70.5	
Subgroup analysis by study design [c]									
Case-control	16	2447	REM	D-L	2.77 (2.00 to 3.55)	<0.001	<0.001	98.1	
Cohort	1	398	—	—	0.03 (−0.164 to 0.23)	0.74	—	—	Figure S8, p. 18

Table 3. Cont.

Meta-Analyses	No. of Studies	No. of Patients	Stat. Model	Wt	SMD (95% CI)	p-Value	P_{het}	I^2 (%)	Supplementary Materials [a]
Cross-sectional	3	645	REM	D-L	1.39 (−1.56 to 4.34)	0.36	<0.001	99.3	—
					Univariable meta-regression [e]				
Sex (% of T1DM males)	17	2928	Random-effects Meta-regression		Coef = 0.011 (−0.619 to 0.641)	0.97	—	—	Figure S9, p. 19
Risk of bias (NOS score)	20	3490	Random-effects Meta-regression		Coef = 0.195 (−3.209 to 3.598)	0.91	—	—	Figure S10, p. 20
Determination by qRT-PCR									
All [b]	2	216	REM	D-L	−0.66 (−3.02 to 1.71)	0.59	<0.001	97.1	—
Determination by Flow Citometry									
All [b]	3	455	REM	D-L	1.40 (−0.19 to 3.00)	0.08	<0.001	91.8	—

Abbreviations: Stat., statistical; Wt, method of weighting; SMD, standardized mean difference; CI, confidence intervals; REM, random-effects model; D-L, DerSimonian and Laird method; HbAc1, hemoglobin Ac1; T1DM, type 1 diabetes mellitus; NOS, Newcastle–Ottawa Scale; NA, not available. [a] More information in the Supplementary Materials; [b] meta-analyses; [c] subgroup meta-analyses; [d] the studies recruiting patients >18 years old or with missing data were excluded for this analysis; [e] effect of study covariates on circulating IL-1β levels among patients with T1DM compared with controls.

3.4.2. IL-1β Level Determination by Flow Cytometry

The *IL-1β* levels were higher in T1DM patients than in controls (SMD = 1.40, 95% CI = −0.19 to 3.00), close to significant ($p = 0.08$), and very probably underpowered (potentially yielding a non-significant result due to type II error) (n = 3 studies) (Figure 2, Table 3).

3.4.3. IL-1β mRNA Level Determination by qRT-PCR

We did not find significant differences ($p = 0.59$) between T1DM and controls (SMD = −0.66, 95% CI = −3.02 to 1.71). This result was derived from the meta-analysis of only two studies, with imprecise results (very wide confidence intervals) and the true direction of the effect is not yet estimable (Figure 2, Table 3).

3.4.4. Analysis of Subgroups

Subgroup meta-analyses were only performed for *IL-1β* determination by immunoassays, due to the considerable number of studies (n = 20) and high number of patients (n = 3490) being investigated (Table 3). The statistically significant association was maintained in the following subgroups by continents (Africa: SMD = 10.41, 95% CI = 2.58 to 18.23, $p = 0.01$; Asia: SMD = 2.61, 95% CI = 0.56 to 4.46, $p = 0.01$; Europe: SMD = 1.04, 95% CI = 0.49 to 1.59, $p < 0.001$), age (<18 years: SMD = 2.81, 95% CI = 1.88 to 3.74, $p < 0.001$; >18 years: SMD = 1.56, 95% CI = 0.48 to 2.65, $p = 0.002$), Hbg levels in patients <18 years (Hbg > 7: SMD = 5.43, 95% CI = 3.31 to 7.56, $p = 0.001$), sample source (serum: SMD = 2.73, 95% CI = 1.85 to 3.61, $p < 0.001$; plasma: SMD = 1.34, 95% CI = 0.28 to 2.41, $p = 0.01$), type of analysis (ELISA: SMD = 3.29, 95% CI = 2.27 to 4.30, $p < 0.001$), and study design variables (case-control design: SMD = 2.77, 95% CI = 2.00 to 3.55, $p < 0.001$, age matching: SMD = 3.06, 95% CI= 2.19 to 3.94, $p < 0.001$; sex matching: SMD = 0.55, 95% CI = 0.19 to 0.91, $p = 0.003$) (Table 3) (Figures S1–S8, Supplementary Materials, pp. 11–18).

3.4.5. Meta-Regression

The potential effect of sex and risk of bias on IL-1β levels determined by immunoassays was explored, but we did not find any significant association for the covariates under analysis ($p = 0.97$ and $p = 0.91$, respectively) (Table 3) (Figures S9 and S10, Supplementary Materials, pp. 19–20).

3.5. Quantitative Evaluation (Secondary Analyses)

3.5.1. Sensitivity Analysis

The general results did not substantially vary after the sequential repetition of meta-analyses, omitting one study each time. This suggests that the combined estimations reported do not depend on the influence of a particular individual study (Table S3, Supplementary Materials, p. 21).

3.5.2. Small-Study Effects Analysis

These analyses were only applied to the meta-analysis on *IL-1β* determination by immunoassays (n = 22 analysis units). The meta-analyses on *IL-1β* determination by flow cytometry (n = 3) and qRT-PCR (n = 2) harbored low sample sizes, and these methods lack statistical power when the number of primary studies is fewer than ten [28]. Egger's regression test indicates statistically significant asymmetry ($p_{Egger} = 0.014$). The funnel plot appears to be slightly asymmetric for the studies plotted at the bottom (Figure 3); however, due to a considerable degree of inter-study heterogeneity, its visual inspection analysis is complex. Consequently, a contour-enhanced funnel plot was constructed (overlaid on the "canonical" funnel plot; Figure 3) to help distinguish publication bias from other causes of asymmetry. This plot leads us to suspect that "missing" studies would be located in the symmetric counterparts with negative significance (i.e., outside of the white region), potentially ruling out publication bias. In addition, the non-parametric trim and fill method did not detect the presence of unpublished studies, confirming the reliability of our results according to the studies published, so the final estimate was not adjusted based on imputation techniques for missing studies.

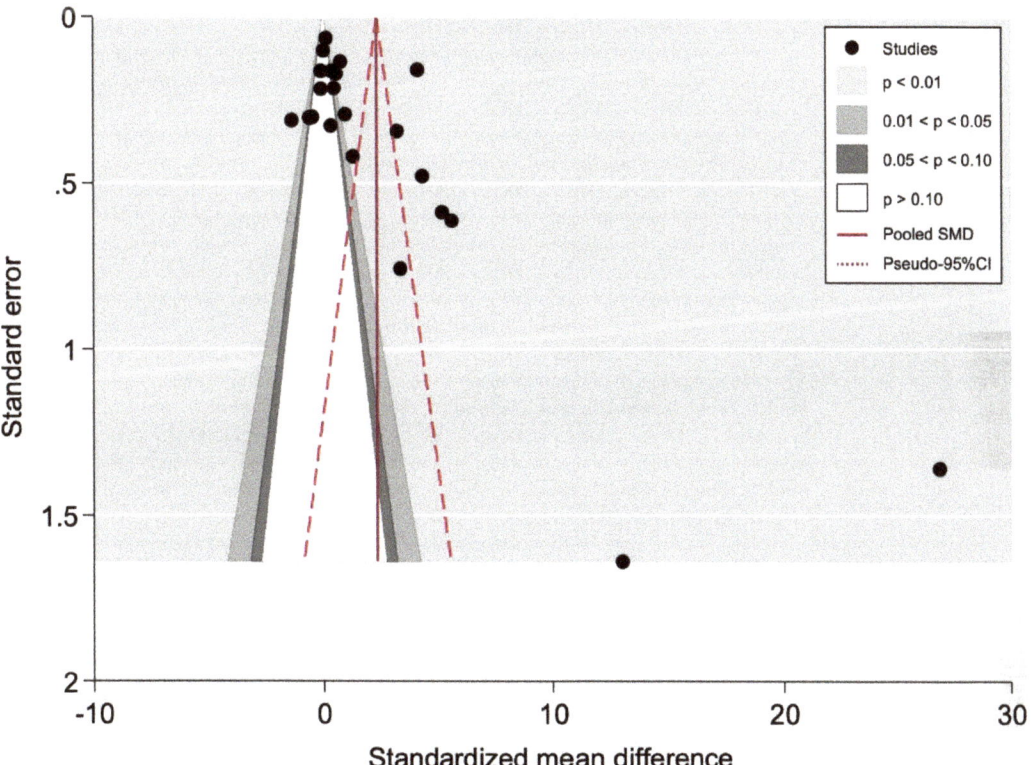

Figure 3. Canonical and contour funnel plots of the estimated circulating IL-1β levels (assessed across immunoassays) comparing type 1 diabetes mellitus and controls, expressed as standardized mean difference (SMD) against its standard error. The red vertical line corresponds to the pooled SMD estimated in the meta-analysis. The two diagonal intermittent lines represent their pseudo-95% CI. Contours represent the defined conventional levels of statistical significance (i.e., 0.01, 0.05, 0.10) accompanied by associated shaded regions. The black circles represent the 22 studies meta-analyzed.

4. Discussion

In this systematic review, significantly higher IL-1β peripheral levels in T1DM patients compared to healthy subjects were shown, according to the meta-analysis on the determination of IL-1β by immunoassays from serum or plasma (SMD = 2.45, 95% CI = 1.73 to 3.17; $p < 0.001$; n = 20 primary-level studies/3490 patients). Young T1DM patients remained significantly higher than T1DM adults. The present study determines an association between glycemic status and IL-1β peripheral levels, which is important in the methodological approach performed to determine them. Based on this window of opportunity, our meta-analysis supports further research on IL-1β as a therapeutic target in T1DM.

The increased peripheral IL-1β levels in childhood indicate a potent role during the first years of the disease, which can contribute to the cytokine storm [32] associated with the first stage of T1DM. Primary prevention strategies targeting inflammatory-mediated comorbidity may prevent secondary complications in the future for these patients [33–35]. Previous study revealed the potential therapeutic effects of anti-inflammatory treatments by reducing the peripheral levels of pro-inflammatory cytokines in T1DM-associated complications [36]. Our results suggest that the peripheral pro-inflammatory marker IL-1β is more likely to be increased in the younger population with T1DM compared to adult patients. The different levels detected between the two age ranges studied is particularly significant: child T1DM patients (<18 years old) show a higher IL-1β level than adult T1DM patients (>18 years old), which could be related to the cytokine storming associated with early events in T1DM [37]. Usually, younger T1DM patients present a shorter evolution time of disease, and the immune alterations develop at the beginning of the onset of T1DM. Moreover, in this age group, insulin sensitivity is highly variable due to growth, sexual maturation, and self-care capacity at these ages. In this regard, and supporting these data, young T1DM patients with poor glycemic control present higher IL-1β levels compared with the same age range of T1DM patients with good glycemic management. Several studies have demonstrated an association between the low presence of cytokines and better insulin secretion [12]. The analysis of demographic and geographic area indicates a significant influence of medical assistance and management of T1DM progression care on the level of IL-1β detected.

This study is the first meta-analysis focusing on IL-1β implications in T1DM, different from previous meta-analytic studies based on other cytokines and only restricted to adult patients [12,13,38]. Many previous studies examining other blood cytokine levels during T1DM, such as TNF-α and IL6 [12,13], only included adult patients and this could possibly be attributed by lack of data on IL-1β expression along the T1DM or the inadequate methodological standardization of patient characteristics.

The importance of the methodological approach used for determining IL-1β, and its biological source, has been elucidated in the present work. We found a significantly increased number of analyses performed in serum compared to other biological fluids. The easy accessibility of serum and the periodical clinical testing of it could indicate serum as the principal biological fluid for the determination of inflammatory parameters. Regarding the methodological approaches, we found that the results obtained by ELISA assay are more consistent and with homogeneous groups than other actual immunoassay techniques. The precision of ELISA or the use of only one marker could contribute to a better determination. The exact determination of IL-1β levels is a critical point for determining the clinical standard value, and the results showed in the present analysis confirm that ELISA maintained the range of determination between different studies analyzed; however, other types of immunoassays present a higher range of variability.

IL-1 is a therapeutic target in T1DM patients [11]. Different clinical trials with IL1Ra (anakinra) for adult patients or human monoclonal anti-IL-1β antibody (canakinumab) in pediatric T1DM patients have not been effective in maintaining B-cell function; however, the present meta-analysis showed a critical time point during T1DM progression that could be important to keep in mind for the administration of treatments. A significant relationship between the inflammatory index and β-cell function was not observed in the TN-14 trial. As in consonance with the TN-14 study, our results validated that pediatric onset T1DM is characterized by a more aggressive disease process compared to adult onset T1DM [39], and the relationship identified age dependency in young patients (<18 years (Figure S3)), as shown in the Cabrera et al. article [40]. It is important to note that in the majority of trials, all of the studies focused on evaluating the function of the pancreas using insulin secretion/C-peptide levels; however, in the present study, we tried to elucidate the waves in T1DM-associated IL-1β levels, and determine the relationship with glycated hemoglobin, T1DM management, and age. Usually, the younger T1DM patients present a shorter evolution time of disease, with the immune alterations developing at the beginning of the onset of T1DM. Moreover, in this age group, insulin sensitivity is highly variable due to growth, sexual maturation, and self-care capacity at these ages. In this regard, and supporting these data, the young T1DM patients with a poor glycemic control present higher IL-1β levels compared with the same age range of T1DM patients with good glycemic management. Several studies have demonstrated an association between the low presence of cytokines and better insulin secretion [12]. A positive correlation (change versus change) of plasma HbA1c and plasma IL-6, TNF-α, and IL-1β has been described in a diabetic animal model [41], and in our meta-analysis, we found an association between the glycated hemoglobin and the serum IL-1β levels detected.

According to our qualitative evaluation carried out using the Newcastle–Ottawa Scale, the included studies harbored a low overall risk of potential bias. This fact increases the quality of the evidence of the results reported in our meta-analysis [42]. We also showed that not all studies were conducted, in methodological terms, with the same rigor. Studies should more meticulously communicate the years of evolution of the disease, and control groups should be more carefully designed, being appropriately matched for age and sex. Future studies assessing the relationships between IL-1β levels among T1DM patients could consider the recommendations given in this systematic review and meta-analysis to improve and standardize future research.

Some potential limitations should also be discussed. First, our meta-analysis revealed a considerable degree of inter-study heterogeneity. Heterogeneity is a common finding in meta-analyses dealing with serum biomarkers—particularly cytokines—measured and expressed as continuous variable [12,13]. It must also be noted that a random-effects model was applied in all meta-analyses to account for heterogeneity. When considering the uses and limitations of meta-analytical techniques, a key strength is the ability to reveal patterns across the study results and identifying potential subpopulations (i.e., sources of heterogeneity) [43]. In this sense, our meta-analysis may have identified differences among geographical regions, age, Hbg levels, and analysis techniques, among other factors, that may constitute true sources of heterogeneity, potentially exerting an impact on IL-1β level variations in T1DM. Furthermore, only plasma and serum determinations were meta-analyzed to obtain results derived from more homogeneous clinical and methodological subgroups. Future studies are needed to obtain a higher quality of evidence on the determinations derived from other anatomical sites (e.g., crevicular gingival fluid or vitreous humor). Another element that can explain the heterogeneity is the lack of standardization of the assays used to measure IL-1β. Second, visual inspection analysis of the canonical funnel plot and statistical analyses detected the presence of asymmetry, pointing out small-study effects. Therefore, the random-effects model could be overestimating our results, giving more weight to the studies with a lower sample size, where sampling error may be influential [44]. Nevertheless, the enhanced-contour funnel plot and the trim and fill method allowed us to suspect that the reported asymmetry is artefactual, due to sampling variation or to chance [9], and not really to the presence of publication bias, which could be ruled out [26]. Third, another potential limitation could be related to our eligibility criteria, where clinical trials were excluded, in spite of the advantages in longitudinal associations derived from this study design. In order to meet our objectives, we first a priori designed our study protocol, and we only considered primary-level cohort studies/small case series, case control, and cross-sectional studies to be included, due to their observational study design. There are controversies on the integration of observational and interventional mixed primary-level studies in meta-analysis, particularly in the context of molecular biomarkers with clinical implications. Since our research was performed to better understand the natural history of the condition type 1 diabetes mellitus in the context of IL-1β levels, the inclusion of treatment/interventionist studies (which, by definition, try to decrease the chronic inflammation in diabetes or to eliminate risk factors) could potentially distort the reality of this disease, attenuate inflammation, modulate il-1β levels, introduce a new heterogeneity source, and, consequently, affecting the achievement of our goals. Finally, another potential limitation is the absence of an association between secondary complications, such as diabetic retinopathy, and the IL-1β levels. It was demonstrated that IL-1β increased in the diabetic mouse retina and IL-1β induced pericyte apoptosis via NF-κB activation under high glucose conditions, thereby increasing endothelial permeability in diabetic retinopathy [45]. However, we could not undertake a meta-analytical approach on the diabetic secondary complications due to the low number of articles with inclusion criteria established. Despite the above limitations, the study strengths include our careful study design, a sensitive literature search strategy, the absence of restrictions by date limits or publication language, robust qualitative recommendations for the development and design of future studies on this topic, and the comprehensive meta-analytical approach, showing powerful statistical findings across many analyses.

5. Conclusions

In conclusion, this systematic review and comprehensive meta-analysis provides a deep exploration of the possible role of IL-1β as a tool cytokine in T1DM progression and management of disease. IL-1β is significantly increased in young T1DM patients, which can be used as a marker to initiate the administration of new therapeutic approaches for IL-1β modulation. The relationship between the status of T1DM and IL-1β levels measured by ELISA corroborate the strong affinity between the inflammatory context and T1DM glycemic status, determined by Hbg levels. Further analysis and validation are needed to establish a clinical standard value for IL-1β associated with different T1DM status. The results obtained allow for the hypothesis of a potential role of IL-1β as a therapeutic target in the early stages of T1DM, where the actual treatments are focused on the pharmacological abrogation of IL-1β action and reducing T1DM progression. The evaluation of IL-1β levels in the early stages of the disease could support the finding that inflammatory status is associated with glycemic control.

Supplementary Materials: The following supporting information can be downloaded at: https://www.mdpi.com/article/10.3390/jcm11051303/s1, Table S1: Search strategy for each database, number of results, and execution date; Table S2: Variables of study; Figure S1: Geographical area; Figure S2: Age; Figure S3: HbAc1 levels in patients <18 years; Figure S4: Age matching; Figure S5: Sex matching; Figure S6: Source of sample; Figure S7: Type of analysis; Figure S8: Study design; Figure S9: Effect of the covariate Sex; Figure S10: Effect of the covariate Risk of Bias; Table S3: Sensitivity analysis.

Author Contributions: Conceptualization, F.C.-C., L.G.-J., A.I.A. and M.A.-D.; methodology, F.C.-C., L.G.-J., P.R.-G., A.I.A. and M.A.-D.; software, F.C.-C., L.G.-J., P.R.-G. and A.I.A.; validation, F.C.-C., L.G.-J., P.R.-G., A.I.A. and M.A.-D.; formal analysis, F.C.-C., L.G.-J., P.R.-G. and A.I.A.; investigation, F.C.-C., L.G.-J., P.R.-G., A.I.A. and M.A.-D.; resources, F.C.-C., L.G.-J., P.R.-G., A.I.A. and M.A.-D.; data curation, F.C.-C., L.G.-J., P.R.-G. and A.I.A.; writing—original draft preparation, F.C.-C., L.G.-J., P.R.-G. and A.I.A.; writing—review and editing, F.C.-C., L.G.-J., P.R.-G., A.I.A. and M.A.-D.; visualization, F.C.-C., L.G.-J., P.R.-G. and A.I.A.; supervision, P.R.-G., A.I.A. and M.A.-D.; project administration, M.A.-D.; funding acquisition, M.A.-D. All authors have read and agreed to the published version of the manuscript.

Funding: A.I.A. was supported by grants from Instituto de Salud Carlos III (PI18/01287), Consejería de Salud de la Junta de Andalucía (PI-0123-2018), and Convocatoria de Subvenciones para la Financiación de la Investigación y la Innovación Biomédica y en Ciencias de la Salud en el Marco de la Iniciativa Territorial Integrada 2014–2020 para la Provincia de Cádiz, Fondos ITI-FEDER (PI-0012-2019); M.A.-D. was supported by grants from Convocatoria de Subvenciones para la Financiación de la Investigación y la Innovación Biomédica y en Ciencias de la Salud en el Marco de la Iniciativa Territorial Integrada 2014–2020 para la Provincia de Cádiz, Fondos ITI-FEDER (PI-0029-2017) and from Instituto de Salud Carlos III (PI18/01287) and Consejería de Salud de la Junta de Andalucía (PI-0036-2020).

Institutional Review Board Statement: Not applicable.

Informed Consent Statement: Not applicable.

Data Availability Statement: The data that support the findings of this study are available in the Supplementary Material of this article.

Acknowledgments: Arroba's contract is supported by Servicio Andaluz de Salud-Consejería de Salud y Familias, Programa Nicolás Monardes.

Conflicts of Interest: The authors declare that the research was conducted in the absence of any commercial or financial relationships that could be construed as a potential conflict of interest.

References

1. Eizirik, D.L.; Colli, M.L.; Ortis, F. The role of inflammation in insulitis and B-cell loss in type 1 diabetes. *Nat. Rev. Endocrinol.* **2009**, *5*, 219–226. [CrossRef] [PubMed]
2. Vaarala, O. Is the origin of type 1 diabetes in the gut? *Immunol. Cell Biol.* **2012**, *90*, 271–276. [CrossRef] [PubMed]
3. Uno, S.; Imagawa, A.; Okita, K.; Sayama, K.; Moriwaki, M.; Iwahashi, H.; Yamagata, K.; Tamura, S.; Matsuzawa, Y.; Hanafusa, T.; et al. Macrophages and dendritic cells infiltrating islets with or without beta cells produce tumour necrosis factor-α in patients with recent-onset type 1 diabetes. *Diabetologia* **2007**, *50*, 596–601. [CrossRef] [PubMed]
4. Donath, M.Y.; Dinarello, C.A.; Mandrup-Poulsen, T. Targeting innate immune mediators in type 1 and type 2 diabetes. *Nat. Rev. Immunol.* **2019**, *19*, 734–746. [CrossRef] [PubMed]
5. Pankewycz, O.G.; Guan, J.-X.; Benedict, J.F. Cytokines as Mediators of Autoimmune Diabetes and Diabetic Complications. *Endocr. Rev.* **1995**, *16*, 164–176. [CrossRef]
6. Singh, B.; Nikoopour, E.; Huszarik, K.; Elliott, J.F.; Jevnikar, A.M. Immunomodulation and regeneration of islet beta cells by cytokines in autoimmune type 1 diabetes. *J. Interf. Cytokine Res.* **2011**, *31*, 711–719. [CrossRef]
7. Mandrup-Poulsen, T.; Pickersgill, L.; Donath, M.Y. Blockade of interleukin 1 in type 1 diabetes mellitus. *Nat. Rev. Endocrinol.* **2010**, *6*, 158–166. [CrossRef]
8. Mohammadoo-Khorasani, M.; Salimi, S.; Tabatabai, E.; Sandoughi, M.; Zakeri, Z.; Farajian-Mashhadi, F. Interleukin-1β (IL-1β) & IL-4 gene polymorphisms in patients with systemic lupus erythematosus (SLE) & their association with susceptibility to SLE. *Indian J. Med. Res.* **2016**, *143*, 591–596. [CrossRef]
9. Hu, S.L.; Huang, C.C.; Tseng, T.T.; Liu, S.C.; Tsai, C.H.; Fong, Y.C.; Tang, C.H. S1P facilitates IL-1β production in osteoblasts via the JAK and STAT3 signaling pathways. *Environ. Toxicol.* **2020**, *35*, 991–997. [CrossRef]
10. Malhotra, S.; Costa, C.; Eixarch, H.; Keller, C.W.; Amman, L.; Martínez-Banaclocha, H.; Midaglia, L.; Sarró, E.; Machín-Díaz, I.; Villar, L.M.; et al. NLRP3 inflammasome as prognostic factor and therapeutic target in primary progressive multiple sclerosis patients. *Brain* **2020**, *143*, 1414–1430. [CrossRef]
11. Moran, A.; Bundy, B.; Becker, D.J.; DiMeglio, L.A.; Gitelman, S.E.; Goland, R.; Greenbaum, C.J.; Herold, K.C.; Marks, J.B.; Raskin, P.; et al. Interleukin-1 antagonism in type 1 diabetes of recent onset: Two multicentre, randomised, double-blind, placebo-controlled trials. *Lancet* **2013**, *381*, 1905–1915. [CrossRef]
12. Chen, Y.L.; Qiao, Y.C.; Pan, Y.H.; Xu, Y.; Huang, Y.C.; Wang, Y.H.; Geng, L.J.; Zhao, H.L.; Zhang, X.X. Correlation between serum interleukin-6 level and type 1 diabetes mellitus: A systematic review and meta-analysis. *Cytokine* **2017**, *94*, 14–20. [CrossRef] [PubMed]
13. Qiao, Y.C.; Chen, Y.L.; Pan, Y.H.; Tian, F.; Xu, Y.; Zhang, X.; Zhao, H.L. The change of serum tumor necrosis factor alpha in patients with type 1 diabetes mellitus: A systematic review and meta-analysis. *PLoS ONE* **2017**, *12*, e0176157. [CrossRef] [PubMed]
14. Stroup, D.F.; Berlin, J.A.; Morton, S.C.; Olkin, I.; Williamson, G.D.; Rennie, D.; Moher, D.; Becker, B.J.; Sipe, T.A.; Thacker, S.B. Meta-analysis of observational studies in epidemiology: A proposal for reporting. *J. Am. Med. Assoc.* **2000**, *283*, 2008–2012. [CrossRef]
15. Moher, D.; Liberati, A.; Tetzlaff, J.; Altman, D.G. Preferred Reporting Items for Systematic Reviews and Meta-Analyses: The PRISMA Statement. *PLoS Med.* **2009**, *6*, e1000097. [CrossRef]
16. Higgins, J.P.; Green, S. *Cochrane Handbook for Systematic Reviews of Interventions: Cochrane Book Series*; Wiley: Hoboken, NJ, USA, 2008.
17. Booth, A.; Clarke, M.; Dooley, G.; Ghersi, D.; Moher, D.; Petticrew, M.; Stewart, L. The nuts and bolts of PROSPERO: An international prospective register of systematic reviews. *Syst. Rev.* **2012**, *1*, 2. [CrossRef]
18. Shamseer, L.; Moher, D.; Clarke, M.; Ghersi, D.; Liberati, A.; Petticrew, M.; Shekelle, P.; Stewart, L.A.; PRISMA-P Group. Preferred reporting items for systematic review and meta-analysis protocols (PRISMA-P) 2015: Elaboration and explanation. *BMJ* **2015**, *350*, g7647. [CrossRef]
19. Welch, V.; Tugwell, P.; Petticrew, M.; de Montigny, J.; Ueffing, E.; Kristjansson, B.; McGowan, J.; Benkhalti Jandu, M.; Wells, G.A.; Brand, K.; et al. How effects on health equity are assessed in systematic reviews of interventions. *Cochrane Database Syst. Rev.* **2010**, *2010*, MR000028. [CrossRef]
20. Luo, D.; Wan, X.; Liu, J.; Tong, T. Optimally estimating the sample mean from the sample size, median, mid-range, and/or mid-quartile range. *Stat. Methods Med. Res.* **2018**, *27*, 1785–1805. [CrossRef]
21. Wan, X.; Wang, W.; Liu, J.; Tong, T. Estimating the sample mean and standard deviation from the sample size, median, range and/or interquartile range. *BMC Med. Res. Methodol.* **2014**, *14*, 135. [CrossRef]
22. Higgins, J.P.T.; Thompson, S.G. Quantifying heterogeneity in a meta-analysis. *Stat. Med.* **2002**, *21*, 1539–1558. [CrossRef] [PubMed]
23. Higgins, J.P.T.; Thompson, S.G.; Deeks, J.J.; Altman, D.G. Measuring inconsistency in meta-analyses. *Br. Med. J.* **2003**, *327*, 557–560. [CrossRef] [PubMed]
24. Thompson, S.G.; Higgins, J.P.T. How should meta-regression analyses be undertaken and interpreted? *Stat. Med.* **2002**, *21*, 1559–1573. [CrossRef]
25. Duval, S.; Tweedie, R. A non-parametric "trim and fill" method of assessing publication bias in meta-analysis. *J. Am. Stat. Assoc.* **2000**, *95*, 89–98. [CrossRef]
26. Peters, J.L.; Sutton, A.J.; Jones, D.R.; Abrams, K.R.; Rushton, L. Contour-enhanced meta-analysis funnel plots help distinguish publication bias from other causes of asymmetry. *J. Clin. Epidemiol.* **2008**, *61*, 991–996. [CrossRef]

27. Egger, M.; Davey Smith, G.; Schneider, M.; Minder, C. Bias in meta-analysis detected by a simple, graphical test. *BMJ* **1997**, *315*, 629–634. [CrossRef]
28. Sterne, J.A.C.; Sutton, A.J.; Ioannidis, J.P.A.; Terrin, N.; Jones, D.R.; Lau, J.; Carpenter, J.; Rücker, G.; Harbord, R.M.; Schmid, C.H.; et al. Recommendations for examining and interpreting funnel plot asymmetry in meta-analyses of randomised controlled trials. *BMJ* **2011**, *343*, d4002. [CrossRef]
29. Palmer, T.M.; Sterne, J.A.C. *Meta-Analysis in Stata: An Updated Collection from the Stata Journal*, 2nd ed.; Stata Press: College Station, TX, USA, 2016.
30. Thorsen, S.U.; Pipper, C.B.; Ellervik, C.; Pociot, F.; Kyvsgaard, J.N.; Svensson, J. Association between neonatal whole blood iron content and cytokines, adipokines, and other immune response proteins. *Nutrients* **2019**, *11*, 543. [CrossRef]
31. Koskela, U.E.; Kuusisto, S.M.; Nissinen, A.E.; Savolainen, M.J.; Liinamaa, M.J. High vitreous concentration of IL-6 and IL-8, but not of adhesion molecules in relation to plasma concentrations in proliferative diabetic retinopathy. *Ophthalmic Res.* **2013**, *49*, 108–114. [CrossRef]
32. Mateo-Gavira, I.; Vílchez-López, F.J.; García-Palacios, M.V.; Carral-San Laureano, F.; Visiedo-García, F.M.; Aguilar-Diosdado, M. Early blood pressure alterations are associated with pro-inflammatory markers in type 1 diabetes mellitus. *J. Hum. Hypertens.* **2017**, *31*, 151–156. [CrossRef]
33. Zorena, K.; Raczyńska, D.; Raczyńska, K. Biomarkers in diabetic retinopathy and the therapeutic implications. *Mediat. Inflamm.* **2013**, *2013*, 193604. [CrossRef] [PubMed]
34. AboElAsrar, M.A.; Elbarbary, N.S.; Elshennawy, D.E.; Omar, A.M. Insulin-like growth factor-1 cytokines cross-talk in type 1 diabetes mellitus: Relationship to microvascular complications and bone mineral density. *Cytokine* **2012**, *59*, 86–93. [CrossRef] [PubMed]
35. Sawires, H.; Botrous, O.; Aboulmagd, A.; Madani, N.; Abdelhaleem, O. Transforming growth factor-β1 in children with diabetic nephropathy. *Pediatr. Nephrol.* **2019**, *34*, 81–85. [CrossRef]
36. Wołoszyn-Durkiewicz, A.; Myśliwiec, M. The prognostic value of inflammatory and vascular endothelial dysfunction biomarkers in microvascular and macrovascular complications in type 1 diabetes. *Pediatr. Endocrinol. Diabetes Metab.* **2019**, *25*, 28–35. [CrossRef]
37. Alexandraki, K.I.; Piperi, C.; Ziakas, P.D.; Apostolopoulos, N.V.; Makrilakis, K.; Syriou, V.; Diamanti-Kandarakis, E.; Kaltsas, G.; Kalofoutis, A. Cytokine secretion in long-standing diabetes mellitus type 1 and 2: Associations with low-grade systemic inflammation. *J. Clin. Immunol.* **2008**, *28*, 314–321. [CrossRef] [PubMed]
38. Zhou, T.; Li, H.Y.; Zhong, H.; Zhong, Z. Relationship between transforming growth factor-β1 and type 2 diabetic nephropathy risk in Chinese population. *BMC Med. Genet.* **2018**, *19*, 201. [CrossRef] [PubMed]
39. Crinò, A.; Schiaffini, R.; Manfrini, S.; Mesturino, C.; Visalli, N.; Beretta Anguissola, G.; Suraci, C.; Pitocco, D.; Spera, S.; Corbi, S.; et al. A randomized trial of nicotinamide and vitamin E in children with recent onset type 1 diabetes (IMDIAB IX) Pozzillion behalf of the IMDIAB group. *Eur. J. Endocrinol.* **2004**, *150*, 719–724. [CrossRef]
40. Cabrera, S.M.; Wang, X.; Chen, Y.G.; Jia, S.; Kaldunski, M.L.; Greenbaum, C.J.; Mandrup-Poulsen, T.; Hessner, M.J. Interleukin-1 antagonism moderates the inflammatory state associated with Type 1 diabetes during clinical trials conducted at disease onset. *Eur. J. Immunol.* **2016**, *46*, 1030–1046. [CrossRef]
41. Kazemi, F. Myostatin alters with exercise training in diabetic rats; possible interaction with glycosylated hemoglobin and inflammatory cytokines. *Cytokine* **2019**, *120*, 99–106. [CrossRef]
42. Guyatt, G.H.; Oxman, A.D.; Vist, G.E.; Kunz, R.; Falck-Ytter, Y.; Alonso-Coello, P.; Schünemann, H.J. GRADE: An emerging consensus on rating quality of evidence and strength of recommendations. *BMJ* **2008**, *336*, 924–926. [CrossRef]
43. Greenland, S. Can meta-analysis be salvaged? *Am. J. Epidemiol.* **1994**, *140*, 783–787. [CrossRef] [PubMed]
44. Lin, L. Bias caused by sampling error in meta-analysis with small sample sizes. *PLoS ONE* **2018**, *13*, e0204056. [CrossRef] [PubMed]
45. Yun, J.H. Interleukin-1β induces pericyte apoptosis via the NF-κB pathway in diabetic retinopathy. *Biochem. Biophys. Res. Commun.* **2021**, *546*, 46–53. [CrossRef] [PubMed]

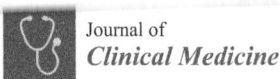

Article

Metabolic Control of the FreeStyle Libre System in the Pediatric Population with Type 1 Diabetes Dependent on Sensor Adherence

Isabel Leiva-Gea [1,2,3], Maria F. Martos-Lirio [1,3], Ana Gómez-Perea [1], Ana-Belen Ariza-Jiménez [4,*], Leopoldo Tapia-Ceballos [1,2], Jose Manuel Jiménez-Hinojosa [1] and Juan Pedro Lopez-Siguero [1,2,3]

1. Pediatric Endocrinology, Hospital Regional Materno Infantil de Málaga, 29011 Malaga, Spain; isabeleiva@hotmail.com (I.L.-G.); mariaml_huelma@hotmail.com (M.F.M.-L.); gomezpereana@gmail.com (A.G.-P.); leotapiaceb@hotmail.com (L.T.-C.); jmhinojosa@hotmail.com (J.M.J.-H.); lopez.siguero@gmail.com (J.P.L.-S.)
2. Multidisciplinary Group on Paediatric Research, Instituto de Investigación Biomédica de Málaga, 29010 Malaga, Spain
3. Pharmacology and Pediatrics Department, University of Malaga, 29016 Malaga, Spain
4. Pediatric Endocrinology, Hospital Universitario Reina Sofia, 14004 Cordoba, Spain
* Correspondence: micodemas@hotmail.com

Abstract: Aims: To evaluate the relationship between daily sensor scan rates and changes in HbA1c and hypoglycemia in children. Methods: We enrolled 145 paediatric T1D patients into a prospective, interventional study of the impact of the FreeStyle Libre 1 system on measures of glycemic control. Results: HbA1c was higher at lower scan rates, and decreased as the scan rate increased to 15–20 scans, after which it rose at higher scan rates. An analysis of the change in hypoglycemia, based on the number of daily sensor scans, showed there was a significant correlation between daily scan rates and hypoglycemia. Subjects with higher daily scan rates reduced all levels of hypoglycaemia. Conclusions: HbA1c is higher at lower scan rates, and decreases as scan rate increases. Reductions in hypoglycemia were evident in subjects with higher daily scan rates.

Keywords: flash glucose monitoring; sensor scanning; hypoglycemia

1. Introduction

The FreeStyle Libre 1 flash glucose monitoring system (Abbott Diabetes Care, Witney, UK) is an established technology that measures glucose in interstitial fluid (ISF). A sensor worn on the back of the upper arm takes a reading every minute that can be scanned using a hand-held reader or smartphone to receive a current glucose result, along with historic results with a 15-min frequency. The FreeStyle Libre sensors are calibrated in the factory and have a wear time of up to 14 days without the need for the user to perform daily calibration using finger-prick tests [1].

The FreeStyle Libre flash glucose monitoring system was proven in the IMPACT and REPLACE studies [2,3] to reduce time in hypoglycemia below 70 mg/dL by 38% (IMPACT) and 43% (REPLACE) over 26 weeks, for adults with type 1 (T1D) or type 2 diabetes (T2D) on insulin, compared with the finger-prick method for the self-monitoring of blood glucose (SMBG). Neither study showed a significant change in HbA1c observed with the flash glucose monitoring compared with SMBG. In the SELFY prospective interventional single-arm study [4], which used the FreeStyle Libre system in 76 children and adolescents with T1D, mean HbA1c was reduced from 7.9% to 7.5% over 8 weeks, compared with SMBG. Separate prospective observational and randomized control studies show that flash glucose monitoring is associated with significant improvements in HbA1c in adults with T1D [5], or with T2D on insulin [6]. Moreover, meta-analysis of up to 25 real-world clinical studies has confirmed that starting the FreeStyle Libre system is associated with a significant and sustained reduction in HbA1c for adults and children with T1D [7,8] and for adults with T2D [7]. However, none of those studies correlated these improvements with the number of scans.

Flash glucose monitoring is now included in the Portfolio of Services of the Public Health System in Spain for T1D, and Andalucia has been a pioneer region in introducing flash glucose monitoring in the paediatric population in Spain. Here, we report on the impact of flash glucose monitoring over 6 months on measures of glycaemic control in a paediatric T1D population, being treated either with multiple daily injections of insulin (MDI), or with the continuous subcutaneous infusion of insulin (CSII).

The aim of the study is to understand the association between daily sensor scan rates and changes in HbA1c and in measures of hypoglycemia, in order to be able to establish from what number of scans per day an improvement can be seen, and from what point during the follow-up period (1 month, 3 months or 6 months) we will be able to give realistic recommendations to achieve the expected effect.

2. Methods

2.1. Study Design and Participants

We enrolled 145 pediatric T1D diabetes patients into a prospective, interventional study on the impact of the continuous use of FreeStyle Libre system on HbA1c levels, and on measures of hypoglycemia. The inclusion criteria were as follows: the presence of T1D with disease duration >1 year; an age of 4–18 years at study entry. Subjects were excluded if they did not adhere with the routine clinical review, or had used the FreeStyle Libre system prior to start of the study. Baseline characteristics are shown in Table 1. Mean age ($\pm$SD) of study subjects was 11.36 ($\pm$3.06) years, and the average duration of diabetes was 5.2 ($\pm$3.2) years. Patients were treated either with MDI (n = 119) or with CSII (n = 26).

Table 1. Baseline clinical characteristics of the study population.

Parameter		n
Age (years)	11.36 $\pm$ 3.06	145
Duration of diabetes (years)	5.2 $\pm$ 3.2	145
Mean HbA1c at baseline (%)	7.11 $\pm$ 0.80	142
Mean HbA1c for subjects <7.5% at baseline	6.73 $\pm$ 0.47	102
Mean HbA1c for subjects ≥7.5% at baseline	8.09 $\pm$ 0.71	40
Treatment type	MDI	119
Treatment type	CSII	26

Values are mean $\pm$ SD unless otherwise indicated. MDI, multiple daily injections of insulin; CSII, continuous subcutaneous insulin infusion.

All study subjects underwent group training, along with their main caregivers and diabetes team, to understand the functionality of the FreeStyle Libre flash glucose monitoring system, as well as the LibreView web platform which is used to view the glycaemic data collected by the FreeStyle Libre system.

The study was carried out in accordance with the regulations published in Boletín Oficial de la Junta de Andalucía (BOJA), with resolution on 17 April 2018, from the SAS management, for the inclusion of glucose monitoring systems in the Portfolio of Services of the Public Health System of Andalusia.

Data acquisition and analysis was performed in compliance with protocols approved by the Ethical Committee of the Provincial Ethics Committee of Malaga and Andalusian Ministry of Health and Family (ethical approval number: PIGE 0533-219).

Written informed consent was obtained from all participants prior to study. All data is available through contacting the authors.

2.2. Outcomes Measures

Laboratory measurement of HbA1c was carried out at baseline, and at 1, 3, and 6 months. Measures of hypoglycemia were monitored using the LibreView® platform, (Abbott Diabetes Care, Witney, UK) using the most recent 14 days of glycaemic data at 1 month, 3 months and 6 months. Parameters measured included those accepted in international consensus guidelines for interpreting continuous glucose monitoring (CGM) data [9,10]. These were: the number of sensor scans per day; percentage of readings <70 mg/dL; number of Level 1 hypoglycemia events <70 mg/dL; number of Level 2 hypoglycemia events <54 mg/dL; percentage time in range (TIR) between 70–180 mg/dL. Across the study period, FreeStyle Libre users were divided into 4 groups based on their mean daily scan rates. These subgroups corresponded to the quartiles of the daily scan rates. These were: 0–6 scans/day; 7–8 scans/day; 9–11 scans/day; and >11 scans/day. Changes in reported glycemic measures were assessed in this context.

2.3. Statistical Analysis

Data were analysed using the established parametric method of comparing the means of normally distributed observations (paired Student's t statistic), X^2 for percentages. ANOVA was used for comparing different groups, as well as applying generalized mixed linear models, which can be more flexible in the analysis of data which incorporates multiple variables, such as metabolic control and insulin-treatment modality.

3. Results

3.1. Change in HbA1c in Relation to Daily Scan Rates with the FreeStyle Libre System

When we looked at the changes in HbA1c across the whole study group, there was a significant relationship between the change in HbA1c with the number of daily scans ($p < 0.001$), as demonstrated by the mixed linear modelling. Figure 1 shows that the change in HbA1c had a U-shaped relationship with the number of daily scans; HbA1c was higher at lower scan rates, and decreased as scan rate increased to between 15–20 scans, after which it raised at higher scan rates.

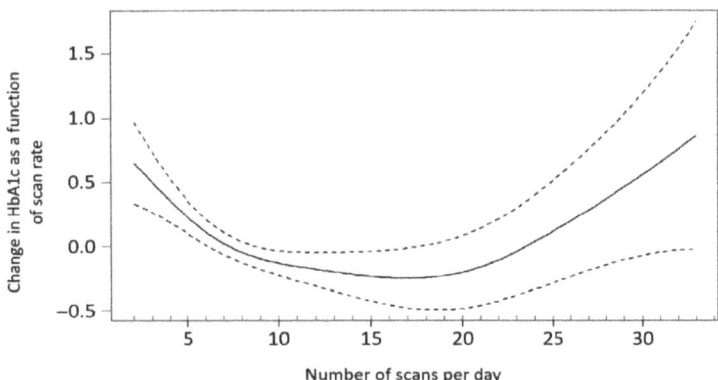

Flexible effects of the number of scans on HbA1c (The 95% confidence interval is shown as a dotted line).

Figure 1. Relationship between number of daily scans with the FreeStyle Libre system and HbA1c.

It is interesting to observe that from 15–20 scans a day glycosylated hemoglobin was negatively influenced. This fact may be related to an infective adherence, which shows repeated ineffective acts. These data had already been published with the number of capillary glycemic controls per day, where it was seen that a greater number of capillary glucose controls were related to better control measures in hemoglobin; however, from a certain number it was related to caregiver anxiety, and/or the patient, without having a favorable impact on metabolic control.

The confidence interval, represented as a dotted line in the graph, shows the dispersion of the results.

3.2. Relationship between Daily Scanning Rates and Change in Hypoglycemia

Hypoglycemia was assessed using three parameters based on FreeStyle Libre sensor data uploaded to the LibreView platform for the preceding 14 days at each study point. These were: percentage time with glucose readings <70 mg/dL; the number of clinically relevant Level 1 hypoglycemic events <70 mg/dL; the number of clinically significant Level 2 hypoglycemic events <54 mg/dL.

An analysis of change in hypoglycemia, based on the number of daily sensor scans, showed that there was a significant correlation between daily scan rates and the change in all three measures of hypoglycemia over the intervention period (Table 2). At each timepoint after starting FreeStyle Libre, there was a pattern of increasing % time <70 mg/dL, as well as an increase in events <70 mg/dL and <54 mg/dL, for groups with scan rates rising to 9–11 scans/day, then reducing for the group at >11 scans/day. With increasing time using the FreeStyle Libre system, the number of events <70 mg/dL and events <54 mg/dL decreased consistently, as scan rates increased. For the number of events <70 mg/dL, there was a significant reduction from 19.29 events/day to 12.69 events/day by 6 months ($p < 0.001$), for people with 9–11 scans/day, and from 13.57 events/day to 9.82 events/day ($p = 0.01$) for users with >11 scans/day. The number of events <54 mg/dL fell from 6.22 events/day to 3.68 events/day ($p = 0.01$) over 6 months for users with 7–8 scans/day, and from 7.50 events/day to 5.03 events/day ($p = 0.04$) for users with 9–11 scans/day. For % time <70 mg/dL, there was a significant fall from 5.8% to 3.88% ($p = 0.023$) from 1 to 6 months with scan rates of >11 scans/day.

Table 2. Relationship between daily scanning rates and change in hypoglycemia.

	% Time <70 mg/dL (±SE)			
No daily scans	Month 1	Month 3	Month 6	p value *
0–6	4.75 (0.55)	4.94 (0.37)	4.83 (0.41)	0.909
7–8	6.64 (0.69)	5.48 (0.51)	5.26 (0.41)	0.169
9–11	7.92 (0.81)	6.21 (0.47)	6.52 (0.47)	0.14
>11	5.89 (0.81)	4.53 (0.39)	3.88 (0.34)	0.03
	Number of events <70 mg/dL (±SE)			
No daily scans	Month 1	Month 3	Month 6	p value *
0–6	8.22 (0.96)	7.74 (0.50)	5.97 (0.45)	0.06
7–8	13.30 (1.15)	9.81 (0.68)	11.16 (0.60)	0.1
9–11	19.29 (1.66)	13.27 (0.71)	12.69 (0.66)	<0.001
>11	13.57 (1.34)	12.37 (0.68)	9.82 (0.55)	0.01
	Number of events <54 mg/dL (±SE)			
No daily scans	Month 1	Month 3	Month 6	p value *
0–6	1.93 (0.37)	2.73 (0.29)	2.28 (0.28)	0.455
7–8	6.22 (0.83)	3.00 (0.38)	3.68 (0.34)	0.01
9–11	7.50 (1.12)	4.54 (0.42)	5.03 (0.42)	0.04
>11	3.38 (0.65)	3.45 (0.35)	3.28 (0.32)	0.897

Data are means (±standard error) in each case. * p value for change in readings at 6 months compared to 1 month.

In the variable number of events for <70 mg/dL in the 7–8 scan group, the difference at 6 months, compared with the third, was not significant nor clinically relevant (6.21 versus 6.52), so it cannot be taken into account. This scan group (7–8) only shows significant and concordant differences in the reduction of events of less than 54 mg/dL. For scan group of

>11 scans/day there was a significant fell from 5.8% to 3.88% ($p = 0.023$) from 1 to 6 months, and for users with 9-11 scans/day fell from 7.50 events/day to 5.03 events/day ($p = 0.04$) at 6 months.

4. Discussion

This study, regarding a cohort of 145 children and young people aged 18 years or younger with T1D, shows that starting the FreeStyle Libre system is associated with improvements in glucose control for this group of people with diabetes. This includes reductions in HbA1c and improvements in hypoglycemia.

As they are part of other articles published in relation to glycosylated hemoglobin and the reduction of severe hypoglycemia, this article focuses on the role of wear time and adherence measured by the number of scans per day in metabolic control parameters.

This article has the purpose of being able to establish practical recommendations regarding the number of scans recommended to achieve the established objectives that do not enslave the patient or the caregiver, and allow realistic expectations for their use.

Moreover, we established that in case of more than 15–20 scans per day, an unfavorable impact was observed on the metabolic control valued in glycosylated hemoglobin. This may show an uneffective adherence and, it could be a diagnostic key of psycho-emotional exhaustion for those seeking positive results in the short and long term by raising the number of scans.

An important observation from our study is that there was a significant correlation between daily scan rates and the change in all three measures of hypoglycemia over the 6-month study period, including the number of hypoglycemic events < 54 mg/dL. Across the outcome timepoints after starting FreeStyle Libre, there was a pattern of decreasing % time < 70 mg/dL, as well as a decrease in events <70 mg/dL and <54 mg/dL for groups with higher daily scan rates, which emphasizes again the importance of patient education and compliance with the use of the device, and acting according to the sensor readings revealed at higher scan rates. In the absence of masked baseline measures of hypoglycemia, the simplest explanation for this trend is that the different scan rates at month 1 are diagnostic of the level of glycemic control prior to starting the FreeStyle Libre. The lowest scanning group may correlate with those with poor prior control if they were previously low SMBG testers, and could likely have the least time with low glucose. Higher scan rates can indicate a desire for good control that is revealed by more events with glucose <70 mg/dL and <54 mg/dL in the early phase of using the FreeStyle Libre system.

However, as users become more experienced with the FreeStyle Libre system, at 3 months and at 6 months, the higher-scanning patients improve their glycemic performance compared to month 1, as they learn to use the full capabilities of the system. Thus, the number of low glucose events <70 mg/dL decreases significantly from month 1 to month 6, for the groups scanning 9 times per day or more, and the % time <70 mg/dL falls significantly for people with >11 scans/day. Since there was no masked baseline for measures of hypoglycemia, the interpretation for this might be that as scan rates increased, the FreeStyle Libre device provided diagnostic feedback on glucose levels, but above 11 scans/day the users were able to make therapeutic decisions themselves to avoid hypoglycemia.

Similarly, the number of clinically significant hypoglycemic events < 54 mg/dL fell significantly across the study period for people scanning between 7 and 11 times per day. Overall, this paints a picture of how the experience and engagement by the user makes an impact, such that they are able to interpret and act on their flash glucose data more effectively. By 6 months, the higher-scanning users were able to improve on their performance of the first month. This emphasises the value of the FreeStyle Libre system as a therapeutic tool in terms of reducing hypoglycemia at higher scan rates for experienced users. This observation is aligned with a real-world analysis of associations between FreeStyle Libre sensor-scanning frequency and a range of glycaemic measures [11].

These observations are aligned with data from the AWeSoMe real-world study [12] on 71 young people, aged from 1–25 years old with T1D, who had self-funded their FreeStyle Libre system; however, this latter study did not include a masked baseline set of readings. The SELFY single-arm study in 76 children and young people did not show a significant change in % time in hypoglycemia <70 mg/dL, despite a 14-day masked baseline period of wear [4], which appeared to differ from the overall pattern that we saw in our study. However, the SELFY study was an 8-week multicentre study, compared with our single-centre 6-month real-world study, and showed a significant reduction in the number of events <70 mg/dL, in common with our observations.

Reduction in the risk of severe hypoglycemia amongst children and young people with T1D has been reported in only one other study to date, which showed a 53% reduction in the rate of severe hypoglycemia for 278 subjects after 12 months, following a switch from SMBG testing to the use of the FreeStyle Libre system [13].

Although the reduction in hypoglycemia is present in other studies on monitoring systems, ref. [12] the Flash device has one peculiarity in comparison with other monitoring devices: it is easier to manage, because it is not necessary to calibrate it.

Regarding HbA1c, it is curious that after 20 scans HbA1c increased in our sample. This could be a result of ineffective repeated impulsive behaviors. These data had already been published with the number of capillary glycemic controls per day, where it was seen that a greater number of capillary glucose controls were related to better control measures of hemoglobin [12]; however, from a certain number, this was related to caregiver anxiety, and/or the patient, without having a favorable impact on metabolic control.

A limitation of our study is that the longitudinal changes in measures of hypoglycemia were not able to include a baseline reading for those derived from the masked use of the FreeStyle Libre system, prior to users becoming aware of their sensor-glucose readings. Thus, changes in these metrics across the 6-month study period can be argued to be a study effect, as the consequence of the users becoming better educated in the day-to-day management of their diabetes was due to their participation in the study.

5. Conclusions

This prospective observational report from a single centre in Spain underlines both the value of flash glucose monitoring with the FreeStyle Libre system, and also the importance of understanding individual glycaemic profiles. In our study, we show that adherence with the FreeStyle Libre system is important to fully realize the benefits of flash glucose monitoring. Our study also indicates that additional investigation is required to identify which children and young people with T1D are most likely to benefit from use of the FreeStyle Libre system.

Author Contributions: Conceptualization, I.L.-G.; methodology, M.F.M.-L.; formal analysis, L.T.-C.; investigation, I.L.-G.; resources, J.M.J.-H.; data curation, A.G.-P.; writing—original draft preparation, J.M.J.-H.; writing—review and editing, A.-B.A.-J.; visualization, J.P.L.-S.; supervision, J.P.L.-S.; funding acquisition, I.L.-G. All authors have read and agreed to the published version of the manuscript.

Funding: Research project funded by the Andalusian Ministry of Health and Family (PIGE 0533-219).

Institutional Review Board Statement: The study was conducted according to the guidelines of the Declaration of Helsinki, and approved by the Provincial Ethics Committee of Malaga (17th April 2018).

Informed Consent Statement: Informed consent was obtained from all subjects involved in the study.

Data Availability Statement: All data is available through contacting the authors.

Acknowledgments: We thank Biostatech Advice Training & Innovation in Biostatistics, S.L. for statistical review. All individuals included in this section have consented to the acknowledgement.

Conflicts of Interest: The authors declare no conflict of interest. The funders had no role in the design of the study; in the collection, analyses, or interpretation of data; in the writing of the manuscript, or in the decision to publish the results.

References

1. Bailey, T.; Bode, B.W.; Christiansen, M.P.; Klaff, L.J.; Alva, S. The Performance and Usability of a Factory-Calibrated Flash Glucose Monitoring System. *Diabetes Technol. Ther.* **2015**, *17*, 787–794. [CrossRef] [PubMed]
2. Bolinder, J.; Antuna, R.; Geelhoed-Duijvestijn, P.; Kröger, J.; Weitgasser, R. Novel glucose-sensing technology and hypoglycaemia in type 1 diabetes: A multicentre, non-masked, randomised controlled trial. *Lancet* **2016**, *388*, 2254–2263. [CrossRef]
3. Haak, T.; Hanaire, H.; Ajjan, R.; Hermanns, N.; Riveline, J.P.; Rayman, G. Use of Flash Glucose-Sensing Technology for 12 months as a Replacement for Blood Glucose Monitoring in Insulin-treated Type 2 Diabetes. *Diabetes Ther.* **2017**, *8*, 573–586. [CrossRef] [PubMed]
4. Campbell, F.M.; Murphy, N.P.; Stewart, C.; Biester, T.; Kordonouri, O. Outcomes of using flash glucose monitoring technology by children and young people with type 1 diabetes in a single arm study. *Pediatr. Diabetes* **2018**, *19*, 1294–1301. [CrossRef] [PubMed]
5. Tyndall, V.; Stimson, R.H.; Zammitt, N.N.; Ritchie, S.A.; McKnight, J.A.; Dover, A.R.; Gibb, F.W. Marked improvement in HbA1c following commencement of flash glucose monitoring in people with type 1 diabetes. *Diabetologia* **2019**, *62*, 1349–1356. [CrossRef]
6. Yaron, M.; Roitman, E.; Aharon-Hananel, G.; Landau, Z.; Ganz, T.; Yanuv, I.; Rozenberg, A.; Karp, M.; Ish-Shalom, M.; Singer, J.; et al. Effect of Flash Glucose Monitoring Technology on Glycemic Control and Treatment Satisfaction in Patients with Type 2 Diabetes. *Diabetes Care* **2019**, *42*, 1178–1184. [CrossRef] [PubMed]
7. Evans, M.; Welsh, Z.; Ells, S.; Seibold, A. The Impact of Flash Glucose Monitoring on Glycaemic Control as Measured by HbA1c: A Meta-analysis of Clinical Trials and Real-World Observational Studies. *Diabetes Ther.* **2020**, *11*, 83–95. [CrossRef] [PubMed]
8. Gordon, I.; Rutherford, C.; Makarounas-Kirchmann, K.; Kirchmann, M. Meta-analysis of average change in laboratory-measured HbA1c among people with type 1 diabetes mellitus using the 14 day Flash Glucose Monitoring System. *Diabetes Res. Clin. Pract.* **2020**, *164*, 108158. [CrossRef] [PubMed]
9. Danne, T.; Nimri, R.; Battelino, T.; Bergenstal, R.M.; Close, K.L.; DeVries, J.H.; Garg, S.; Heinemnann, L.; Hirsch, I.; Amiel, S.A.; et al. International Consensus on Use of Continuous Glucose Monitoring. *Diabetes Care* **2017**, *40*, 1631–1640. [CrossRef] [PubMed]
10. Battelino, T.; Danne, T.; Bergenstal, R.M.; Amiel, S.A.; Beck, R.; Biester, T.; Bosi, E.; Buckingham, B.A.; Cefalu, W.T.; Close, K.L.; et al. Clinical Targets for Continuous Glucose Monitoring Data Interpretation: Recommendations From the International Consensus on Time in Range. *Diabetes Care* **2019**, *42*, 1593–1603. [CrossRef] [PubMed]
11. Dunn, T.C.; Xu, Y.; Hayter, G.; Ajjan, R.A. Real-world flash glucose monitoring patterns and associations between self-monitoring frequency and glycaemic measures: A European analysis of over 60 million glucose tests. *Diabetes Res. Clin. Pract.* **2018**, *137*, 37–46. [CrossRef] [PubMed]
12. Landau, Z.; Abiri, S.; Gruber, N.; Levy-Shraga, Y.; Brener, A.; Lebenthal, Y.; Barash, G.; Pinhas-Hamiel, O.; Rachmiel, M. Use of flash glucose-sensing technology (FreeStyle Libre) in youth with type 1 diabetes: AWeSoMe study group real-life observational experience. *Acta Diabetol.* **2018**, *55*, 1303–1310. [CrossRef] [PubMed]
13. Messaaoui, A.; Tenoutasse, S.; Crenier, L. Flash Glucose Monitoring Accepted in Daily Life of Children and Adolescents with Type 1 Diabetes and Reduction of Severe Hypoglycemia in Real-Life Use. *Diabetes Technol. Ther.* **2019**, *21*, 329–335. [CrossRef]

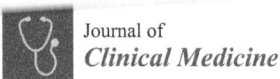

Article

Validation of an Automated Screening System for Diabetic Retinopathy Operating under Real Clinical Conditions

Soledad Jimenez-Carmona [1,*], Pedro Alemany-Marquez [1,*], Pablo Alvarez-Ramos [1], Eduardo Mayoral [2] and Manuel Aguilar-Diosdado [3]

1. Ophthalmology Department, Hospital Universitario Puerta del Mar, University of Cadiz, 11009 Cadiz, Spain; pablo.alvarez.ramos@gmail.com
2. Comprehensive Healthcare Plan for Diabetes, Regional Ministry of Health and Families of Andalusia, Government of Andalusia, 41020 Seville, Spain; eduardo.mayoral.sspa@juntadeandalucia.es
3. Biomedical Research and Innovation Institute of Cadiz (INiBICA), 11009 Cadiz, Spain; manuel.aguilar.sspa@juntadeandalucia.es
* Correspondence: Soledad.jimenez@uca.es (S.J.-C.); pedromaria.alemany@uca.es (P.A.-M.)

Abstract: Background. Retinopathy is the most common microvascular complication of diabetes mellitus. It is the leading cause of blindness among working-aged people in developed countries. The use of telemedicine in the screening system has enabled the application of large-scale population-based programs for early retinopathy detection in diabetic patients. However, the need to support ophthalmologists with other trained personnel remains a barrier to broadening its implementation. Methods. Automatic diagnosis of diabetic retinopathy was carried out through the analysis of retinal photographs using the 2iRetinex software. We compared the categorical diagnoses of absence/presence of retinopathy issued by family physicians (PCP) with the same categories provided by the algorithm (ALG). The agreed diagnosis of three specialist ophthalmologists is used as the reference standard (OPH). Results. There were 653 of 3520 patients diagnosed with diabetic retinopathy (DR). Diabetic retinopathy threatening to vision (STDR) was found in 82 patients (2.3%). Diagnostic sensitivity for STDR was 94% (ALG) and 95% (PCP). No patient with proliferating or severe DR was misdiagnosed in both strategies. The k-value of the agreement between the ALG and OPH was 0.5462, while between PCP and OPH was 0.5251 ($p = 0.4291$). Conclusions. The diagnostic capacity of 2iRetinex operating under normal clinical conditions is comparable to screening physicians.

Keywords: diabetic retinopathy; teleophthalmology; diagnostic accuracy; population-based screening; sight-threatening diabetic retinopathy

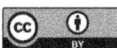

1. Introduction

In 2019, the IDF (International Diabetes Federation) estimated that 463 million adults worldwide suffered from diabetes, and projected the number to rise to 700 million by 2045 [1]. The prevalence of diabetes in Andalusia, the most populated autonomous community in the south of Spain, is higher (15.3%) than in the rest of Spain (12.5%), in close relation to lifestyle and socioeconomic factors [2].

Retinopathy is the most common microvascular complication in patients with diabetes mellitus [3]. In developed countries, diabetic retinopathy (DR) is one of the leading causes of blindness among people of working age [4]. A recent meta-analysis has calculated that in diabetic patients aged 20–79 years, the overall prevalence of any DR is 35% [5]. While the global prevalence of DR and Diabetic Macular Edema (DME; potential complication of DR), for the period 2015 to 2019 were 27.0%, and this prevalence in Europe was estimated to be 20.6%, calculated from the results of population-based studies with retinography [6]. It has been known for decades that proper treatment of DR decreases the incidence of severe visual loss when early diagnosed [7]. Telemedicine systems enable the remote analysis of digital fundus photographs, thus detecting the presence of DR lesions. Based on this technology, population-based screening programs have been developed in different countries [8]. The growing number of diabetic patients and their periodic medical monitoring entails an increase of these DR-detection digital analyses. Due to the limited number of ophthalmologists, other professionals are required to address DR screening. In particular, these range from family physicians, endocrinologists or nurses in high-income countries to trained non-medical personnel in middle-income countries [9–13].

In recent years, the research effort has focused on the development of automated diagnostic strategies that can complement or replace screening personnel, which would help reduce the workload and improve access for diabetic patients requiring early diagnosis [14,15].

The Andalusian Public Health System (APHS) provides universal health care to the 8.4 million inhabitants of Andalusia, which represent 18% of the Spanish population. The APHS encompasses an extensive network, with two levels of care (1500 primary healthcare centers and 49 hospitals) based on accessible, high-quality, patient-centered care, in a system with universal coverage and funded by taxation. The APHS, through the program for Early Detection of Diabetic Retinopathy (APDR), which is part of the Comprehensive Healthcare Plan for Diabetes (CHPD), provides a network of digital desktop fundus cameras placed in primary healthcare centers throughout the region. The screening system developed by APHS consists of two phases: in the first phase, digital fundus photographs of diabetic subjects with no previous diagnosis of DR are recorded with a non-mydriatic retinal camera (NMRC). Secondly, the primary care physicians (PCP) of each center assess these photographs, and then, both those displaying a probable DR diagnosis and inconclusive ones are sent via a specific intranet to a reference ophthalmologist for diagnostic confirmation. From January 2005 to June 2019, 888,318 examinations were performed, corresponding to 429,791 patients [2]. It should be noted that patients with a healthy retina are examined periodically, which increases the number of images under study every year.

To reduce this increasing workload of PCP performing the screening activity, the Lynch Diagnostics (Granada, Spain) (LD) computer-aided diagnostic platform, in collaboration with APHS, developed the 2iRetinex algorithm. The 2iRetinex software (Granada, Spain) lassifies the screening images according to their quality. Specifically, for the non-rejected images, it provides information on the number, type and location of the lesions and, ultimately, a final diagnostic decision.

The aim of this research study is the validation of the 2iRetinex software as a complement or substitute for the screening physician. The clinical diagnosis of the screening physician is formulated in terms of the absence or presence of DR. To perform the comparison of this categorical diagnostic strategy with the same categories provided by the algorithm, we introduced the algorithm into the APDR system. The algorithm extracted the diagnosis of the presence or absence of diabetic retinopathy from the system, obviating the additional information. The agreed diagnosis of three specialist ophthalmologists is used as the reference standard ("ground truth") to measure its clinical performance.

2. Materials and Methods

2.1. Study Participants from APDR

An analytical study of diagnostic tests was performed on the fundus images of diabetic patients regularly attending the Andalusian program for early diagnosis of diabetic retinopathy (APDR) circuit. The used protocols were approved by the Ethical Committee for Research and Clinical Trial of Hospital Puerta del Mar (Cadiz, Spain), number 62/16.

To compare the diagnostic capability of the 2iRetinex algorithm (ALG) with that of the screening PCP under usual clinical conditions, we calculated the required sample based on a previous APDR study with a prevalence of retinopathy in diabetic patients of 30% [16]. To obtain an average sensitivity of 85% and specificity of 82% for the screening PCP [16] and a sensitivity of 90% and a specificity of 93% for the ALG (internal unpublished data from the company, on a random sample of 575 patients in 2015), as well as, a type 1 and 2 error at 0.5 and at 0.2, respectively, the sample size estimated was 2421 patients. For a paired sample, the required sample size calculation was 2297 patients. Furthermore, as the rate of ungradable (UNG) images was estimated to be 10%, an additional 242 and 230 patients were added, for independent and paired samples, respectively [16].

Retinographies were obtained from all diabetic patients attending ten primary care health centers in the region of Andalusia (Spain) included in the APDR patient flow circuit using a standardized protocol previously described [16–18]. Briefly, three photographs of each eye were recorded using a retinal camera. The following camera models were used: the Topcon NW 200 (Topcon, Tokyo, Japan) in seven of the ten study centers and in the remaining three centers, the Topcon NW100 (Topcon, Tokyo, Japan), the Zeiss VISUCAM (Carl Zeiss Meditec AG, Jena, Germany) and DRS retinography, respectively. Then, the PCP analyzed the images stored on the APDR server. The images of the patients classified as UNG and those that present findings of DR are assigned, through the intranet, to the reference ophthalmologist who issued a clinical judgment of confirmation. If no DR lesions were detected (NODR) the patient continued in the screening system for future examinations.

2.2. 2iRetinex Software

The 2iRetinex software (patent number RPI201499900601833) extracted different features from the retinographies. Specifically, 2iRetinex extracted the vascular tree through the isolation of the green channel and microaneurysms and hemorrhages (which are candidates for lesions by applying structural characteristics), through analysis of the dark residual objects. In addition, the 2iRetinex software superimposed a binary mask on the green layer of the images, which made it possible to locate the optic disc. Using a filter also highlighted the bright lesions (exudates and cotton spots). Furthermore, it was able to detect the position of the macula. Finally, a topographic reference system was established to locate the lesions by coordinates. After checking that the image was suitable for analysis, the original image (Figure 1a) was transformed into the resulting image shown in Figure 1b.

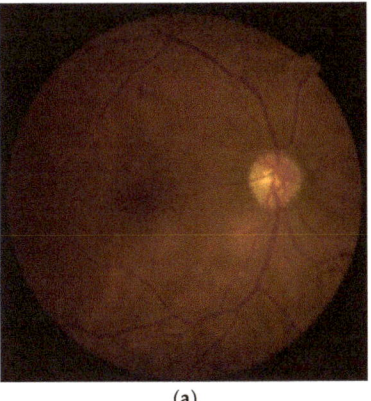
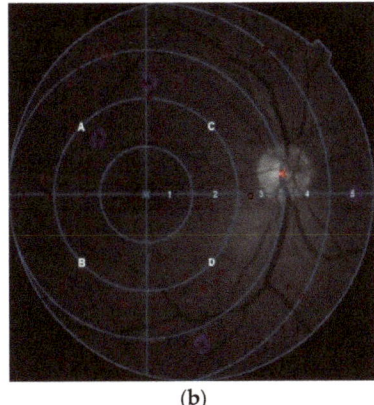

(a)   (b)

Figure 1. Software analysis 2iRetinex: (**a**) A original APDR image of fundus photography of a patient with diabetic retinopathy; (**b**) Location and type of lesions. Superimposed the coordinates system. Red lesions in red, white lesions in blue.

2.3. Source of Images and Data

In the participating centers of this study, between April 2017 and June 2018, a capture system was installed between the retinography and the APDR network. This system allowed the original images in TIFF format to be sent to the LD diagnostic platform to obtain the patient's clinical diagnosis through the 2iRetinex software (ALG) using the same diagnostic categories as the PCP. These images, but not the diagnoses, were available on a server for the ophthalmic researchers (SJC, PAM, PAD). The latter were the ones who established the reference diagnosis (OPH). Simultaneously, the images were returned to the APDR network for compression into JPG for final screening by the PCP, following the usual circuit. The PCPs were not aware of the parallel diagnostic systems. Moreover, at no time were the real graders aware of the diagnosis issued by the other study participants before issuing their clinical judgment.

To ensure that the study was double-blind, the LD platform provided an internal control code. Once the OPH and ALG diagnoses were established, the list of codes related to the original health identification was sent to the administrative management of the APDR. Likewise, the demographic data of the study sample and the PCP diagnoses were sent from the APDR for cross-checking.

For each patient, data were obtained for the categorical variables (gender and type of diabetes) and the quantitative variables (age and years of duration of the disease at the time the retinographies were taken; years from diagnosis). The database also recorded the use of pre-exploration mydriatics.

2.4. Diagnostic Criteria and Convention

For each patient, the PCP, ALG and OPH diagnosis were obtained, with the same diagnostic categories. The following criteria were used to classify the images:

If the image lacked sufficient quality to confirm or rule out diabetic lesions, it was classified as Ungradable (UNG).

If the image quality was sufficient and no diabetic retinopathy lesions were found, it was classified as No Diabetic Retinopathy (NODR)

Regardless of the quality of the image, if retinopathy lesions were observed, the image was classified as DR.

For the final diagnosis of each patient, as carried out in the APDR circuit, the following criteria were followed:

If at least one of the patient's two eyes was classified as UNG, the patient was diagnosed as UNG.

If DR lesions were detected in the images of at least one eye, the patient was diagnosed as DR.

If none of the images of the patients considered evaluable showed lesions of DR, the patient was diagnosed as NODR.

Research ophthalmologists (SJC, PAM, PAD) classified the stage of DR according to the International Clinical Diabetic Retinopathy Severity Scale [18]. This scale consists of five stages: no diabetic retinopathy (NODR), mild (MILD), moderate (MOD), and severe non-proliferative DR (SEV), and proliferative retinopathy (PROL). The diagnosis of diabetic macular edema (DME) was established by detecting the presence of any signs suggestive or evident of macular edema in at least one eye. Cases diagnosed as DME, SEV and PROL were considered as patients with sight-threatening DR lesions (STDR). If the patient had DR lesions in both eyes, the stage of diagnosis corresponded to that of the eye with the highest degree of DR.

2.5. Statistical Analyses

The study data were analyzed using descriptive statistics. Means and standard deviations were calculated for quantitative variables and proportions for qualitive ones. We used the Chi-squared test and the t-test to compare proportions and means, respectively. Sensitivity, specificity, predictive values, and likelihood ratios were used to assess the accuracy of diagnostic tests. Likewise, reliability and agreement were quantified using kappa coefficient. The kappa concordance values of each test (ALG and PCP) were established with respect to the OPH diagnosis and the similarity of the results were examined. The area of the simple ROC curve was calculated for each examiner with respect to ground truth and compared between them. Level of significance was estimated at $p < 0.05$.

Statistical analyzes performed using IBM SPSS Statistic v 24 software (Armonk, NY, USA). The sample calculation and the capacity of the diagnostic tests have been quantified using the Epidat 3.1 program (Xunta de Galicia, Galicia, Spain) (www.sergas.es/Saude-publica/EPIDAT).

3. Results

3.1. Analysis of the Original Sample. Gradable/Ungradable Concordance

During the download period, image folders of 3575 diabetic patients were obtained from the 10 primary healthcare centers. Due to duplication of files and empty downloads without files, 55 patients were removed. Therefore, the original sample consisted of 3520 image folders, of which 43,9% corresponded to women (Table 1). The average age of the patients was 64.4 ± 14.6 years and the mean of the years since the diagnosis of diabetes was 10.37 ± 7.5 years. The majority of patients (88.2%) had type 2 diabetes mellitus (DM2), while patients with type 1 diabetes mellitus (DM1) accounted for 11.4%. In contrast, a minimum proportion (0.4%) of the sample corresponded to patients either diagnosed with other categories or without detailed diagnosis (Others).

Table 1. Main characteristics of the study sample obtained from de APDR between April 2017 and June 2018. * Mean SD. DR = diabetic retinopathy. DME = diabetic macular edema. NDME = no diabetic macular edema. STDR = sight-threatening DR.

Variable of Interest			Study Sample (*n* = 3520)	
Gender (F/M)			43.9%/56.1%	(1545/1975)
Age (years)			64.4 ± 14.6 *	
Years from diagnosis			10.4 ± 7.5 *	
Mydriasis (before photograph)			97.8%	(3443)
Diabetes type	Type 2		88.2%	(3103)
	Type 1		11.4%	(402)
	Others		0.4%	(15)
Ungradable images (UNG)			11.6%	(407)
No diabetic Retinopathy (NODR)			69.9%	(2460)
Diabetic retinopathy (DR)	Mild		8.1%	(286)
	Moderate	NDME	8.1%	(285)
		DME	1.8%	(65)
	Severe	NDME	0.1%	(2)
		DME	0.2%	(8)
	Proliferative	NDME	0.1%	(3)
		DME	0.1%	(4)
STDR			2.3%	(82)

Six hundred and fifty-three patients (18,5%) had images with features of DR. Macular edema was detected in 77 patients (2.2%) and DR stage became STDR in 82 patients (2.3%). However, it was not possible to establish diagnostic criteria on the condition of the retina in 11.6% of the images (UNG).

Regarding the distribution by gender, the mean age and mean duration of diabetes were significantly higher among the diabetic females. In addition, in female patients, the proportion of DM1 was higher, and the proportion of DM2 was lower than in the male group. However, there was no significant difference in the prevalence of each stage of DR between genders (Table 2).

Table 2. Comparison of the study variables between female and male patients. DR = diabetic retinopathy. DME = macular edema diabetic. STDR = sight-threatening DR. * Results with statistically significant differences.

Variable of Interest		Female (n = 1545)	Male (n = 1975)	p-Value
Age (years)		65.4 ± 15.6	64 ± 13.8	0.0419 *
Years from diagnosis		11.1 ± 8.1	9.8 ± 7	<0.0001 *
Mydriasis		97.6%	98%	0.4196
Diabetes type	Type 2	85.8%	90%	=0.0001 *
	Type 1	13.7%	9.6%	=0.0001 *
	Others	0.5%	0.4%	0.6579
DR stage	Mild	8.1%	8.2%	0.9143
	Moderate	10%	9.9%	0.9216
	Severe	0.2%	0.4%	0.2913
	Proliferative	0.2%	0.2%	1
DME		2.1%	2.2%	0.8394
STDR		2.2%	2.4%	0.6952

Considering the gradable/non-gradable (GRAD/UNG) category of images (previously described in methods), we found that the group of patients with UNG images showed significant differences in the mean age and proportions of the types of diabetes compared to patients with GRAD images (Table 3). Specifically, our data showed that patients with UNG images were 9.3 years older than patients with GRAD images (72. 6 vs. 63. 4). We also found a statistically significantly higher proportion of type 2 diabetic patients and a lower proportion of type 1 diabetic patients, in the group of patients with UNG images (Table 3).

Table 3. Comparison of the common variables between patients with gradable and ungradable images. * Results with statistically significant differences.

Variable of Interest		Gradable	Ungradable	p-Value
Gender (F/M)		43.8%/56.2%	44.2%/55.8%	0.8785
Age (years)		63.4 ± 14.6	72.6 ± 11.8	<0.0001 *
Years from diagnosis		10.3 ± 7.3	10.9 ± 9.2	0.1450
Mydriasis		98%	96.6%	0.0678
Diabetes type	Type 2	87.2%	95.6%	<0.0001 *
	Type 1	12.4%	4.2%	<0.0001 *
	Others	0.4%	0%	0.2012

Regarding the graders used, the images of 407 patients (11.6%) were classified as UNG according to the consensus diagnosis of the OPHs (Tables 4 and 5). Likewise, the automatic analysis software considered the images of 927 patients (26.3%) as inadequate (Table 4), while the PCPs could not provide any diagnosis in 461 patients (13.1%; Table 5). A significant difference was detected in the proportions of UNG images between ALG and OPH classifier strategies and between ALG and PCP classifier strategies ($p < 0.0001$). The difference of 1.54% in the proportions of UNG images between OPH and PCP also reached the limit of significance ($p = 0.0494$).

Table 4. Number of patients in every pair of diagnostic categories comparing ALG vs. OPH.

	OPH-DR	OPH-NODR	OPH-UNG	Total
ALG-DR	455	379	33	867
ALG-NODR	80	1582	64	1726
ALG-UNG	118	499	310	927
Total	653	2460	407	3520

Table 5. Number of patients in every pair of diagnostic categories comparing PCP vs. OPH.

	OPH-DR	OPH-NODR	OPH-UNG	Total
PCP-DR	373	233	25	631
PCP-NODR	214	2005	209	2428
PCP-UNG	66	222	173	461
Total	653	2460	407	3520

The unweighted Kappa statistic was used to assess inter-rater reliability in classifying images into UNG or GRAD. The Kappa statistic shows the observed level of agreement adjusted for the level of agreement that could have occurred by simple chance. A value of 0.75–1.00 indicates an excellent agreement, 0.4–0.75 represents a moderate agreement, and lower values display the deficient agreement. We found that the kappa value was 0.3623 for the agreement between ALG and OPH classifier strategies. The agreement between PCP and OPH obtained a k-value of 0.3144. The kappa homogeneity test showed a Chi-square value of 2.7274 corresponding to a $p = 0.0986$. Therefore, the difference in agreement between the two diagnostic strategies was not statistically significant.

Description of the distribution of the diagnostic categories UNG, DR and NODR of the two diagnostic strategies compared to the criteria of the ophthalmologists:

The proportions of the GRAD/GRAD and UNG/UNG agreement categories for ALG versus OPH were 0.78 and 0.30, respectively, with a composite agreement ratio of 0.80. The proportions of the GRAD/GRAD and UNG/UNG agreement categories for PCP versus OPH were 0.84 and 0.25, respectively, with a composite ratio of 0.85.

Overall, these results demonstrated the proportion of UNG was higher in ALG, and the proportion of composite agreement was higher in PCP. It should be noted that the concordance between ALG and OPH was slightly better (0.3623 vs. 0.3144) because there was a greater coincidence when classifying UNG images (ALG 0.30 vs. PCP 0.25).

3.2. Comparison of DR/NODR Diagnostic Category in Unpaired Samples. Diagnostic Validity

The 407 patients considered as UNG by the OPHs were removed from the original sample. This new sample of 3113 patients was partially described when the comparison between GRAD vs. UNG samples was carried out (Table 3). Based on the results of Tables 4 and 5, two samples were selected. The first sample, called ALG-OPH, contained all patients considered GRAD by these two graders ($n = 2496$). The second sample, called PCP-OPH, included all patients considered GRAD by these other pairs of graders ($n = 2825$).

Our data showed that the PCP-OPH group had a mean age of 1.4 years, significantly higher than that of the ALG-OPH group ($p = 0.0003$). No significant differences were detected between the two samples for any of the other variables (Table 6).

Table 6. Comparison of the study variables ALG-OPH vs. PCP-OPH. NDME = no diabetic macular edema. DR = diabetic retinopathy. DME = diabetic macular edema. STDR = sight-threatening DR. * Results with statistically significant differences.

Variable of Interest		ALG-OPH (n = 2496)	PCP-OPH (n = 2825)	p Value
Gender (F/M)		42.9%/57.1%	43.6%/56.4%	0.6071
Age (years)		61.4 ± 14.7	62.8 ± 14.6	0.0003 *
Years from diagnosis		10.2 ± 7.3	10.3 ± 7.3	0.6522
Mydriasis		98.3% (2454)	98.6% (2785)	0.3753
Diabetes type	Type 1	14.5% (361)	12.8% (362)	0.0710
	Type 2	85.2% (2126)	86.8% (2451)	0.0928
	Others	0.3% (9)	0.4% (12)	0.5394
NODR		78.6% (1961)	79.2% (2238)	0.5924
DR		21.43% (535)	20.78 (587)	0.5619
DR stage	Mild	10.1% (251)	9.5% (267)	0.4622
	Moderate	10.9% (272) (NDME 217) (DME 55)	10.8% (305) (NDME 245) (DME 60)	0.9068
	Severe	0.3% (7) (NDME 1) (DME 6)	0.3% (9) (NDME 2) (DME 7)	1
	Proliferative	0.2% (5) (NDME 2) (DME 3)	0.2% (6) (NDME 2) (DME 4)	1
DME		2.6% (64)	2.5% (71)	0.8173
STDR		2.7% (67)	2.7% (75)	1

The frequencies of the matching of the diagnostic categories of each strategy with the criteria of the OPH and the values of indexes (sensitivity, specificity, positive and negative predictive values, likelihood ratios) that determine the validity of the diagnostic tests with the different classifier strategies are shown in Table 7. In particular, the ALG strategy showed a greater ability than the PCP to detect retinopathy in diabetic patients' retinographies (Sensitivity, 85.05 vs. 64.54). However, the PCP strategy better identified individuals without retinopathy as demonstrated by its specificity values (80.67 vs. 89.59). These results suggest that the diagnostic ability of the ALG was overall superior to that of the PCP.

Table 7. Unpaired sample. Diagnostic category pairs frequency and diagnostic validity indexes.

Variable of Interest	ALG-OPH (95% CI)	PCP-OPH (95% CI)
True Positive	455	373
False Positive	379	233
False Negative	80	214
True Negative	1582	2005
Prevalence	21.43% (19.80−23.06)	20.78% (19.26−22.29)
Sensitivity	85.05% (81.93−88.16)	63.54% (59.56−67.52)
Specificity	80.67% (78.90−82.45)	89.59% (88.30−90.88)
Positive Predictive Value	54.56% (51.12−58.00)	61.55% 57.60−65.51)
Negative Predictive Value	95.19% (94.13−96.25)	90.36% (89.11−91.61)
Likelihood Ratio +	4.40 (3.99−4.85)	6.10 (5.33−6.99)
Likelihood Ratio -	0.19 (0.15−0.23)	0.41 (0.37−0.45)

Four of the 80 DR patients classified as healthy by the ALG were positive for MOD plus DME and in the case of the PCP strategy it was 4 out of 214. The proportion of STDR patients incorrectly diagnosed was 5.9% (4/67) for the ALG and 5.3% (4/75) for the PCP. There was no statistically significant difference in the proportions of misdiagnosed patients between the two strategies (ALG vs. PCP; $p = 0.8693$). In fact, the sensitivity of the ALG strategy to diagnose STDR was 94% and that of PCP 95%. No patient with severe or proliferative retinopathy was misdiagnosed by ALG or PCP. Both strategies had a low positive predictive value (PPV; Table 7), being even lower for ALG (PPV 54.56 vs. 61.55) but a high negative predictive value (ALG 95.19 vs. PCP 90.36). The ALG strategy not only had a higher sensitivity, but also a better negative predictive value than the PCP strategy.

Likelihood ratios (LR) are another alternative for calculating the diagnostic accuracy and summarizing the information endowed in both sensitivity and specificity. The LR is the probability that a particular test result would be expected among patients with the condition diagnosed compared to the likelihood that that same result would be expected in a patient without the condition. Good diagnostic tests have LR+ > 10 and their positive result has a significant input to the diagnosis. Good diagnostic tests have LR- < 0,1. The lower the LR- the more significant contribution of the test is in ruling-out (Table 8)

Table 8. Ranges of likelihood ratio values and their impact on diagnostic accuracy.

Likelihood Ratio +	Likelihood Ratio −	Usefulness
10	<0.1	Highly relevant
5–10	5–10	Good
2–5	2–5	Fair
<2	<2	Poor

In the ALG strategy, the modification of the previous probability for positive test results was small (LH + 4.40, Table 7). In fact, we calculated the post-test probability using Fagan's nomogram and obtained that the probability of a patient having a DR changed from 21% to 55%. About 1 in 1.8 positive tests corresponded to patients with retinopathy. The subsequent probability, if the test was negative, was modified to 5%, so approximately 1 of each negative result corresponded to an individual without DR. Likewise, the modification of the previous probability in the PCP test, for positive results, was moderate (LH + 6.10), changing the probability of a patient having a DR from 21% to 62% (Fagan's nomogram). About 1 in 1.6 positive tests corresponded to patients with retinopathy. The subsequent probability, if the test is negative, was modified from 21% to 10%, so approximately 1 in 1.1 negative results corresponded to an individual without retinopathy.

To determine the discriminative power of the different classifier strategies of DR diagnosis, our results were compared using the area under the curve (AUC) of the Receiver Operating Characteristics (ROC) curve (Figure 2).

The AUC for the PCP displayed a value of 0.7657 (95% CI 0.7452 to 0.7861), while the value of AUC for ALG was 0.8286 (95% CI 0.8111 to 0.8461). We found that there was a significant difference between the two curves ($p = 0.0000$). Therefore, these power results shown in Figure 2 indicate that the ALG was more efficient than the PCP.

Finally, to assess the intergrader reliability for DR diagnosis, we used the Kappa statistic. We found that the k-value of the agreement between the ALG and OPH was 0.5462 (95% CI 0.5109 to 0.5815), while between PCP and OPH was 0.5251 (95% CI 0.4865 to 0.5636). The kappa homogeneity test showed a Chi-square value of 0.6252 corresponding to a $p = 0.4291$. Therefore, the difference in concordance between the two diagnostic strategies was not statistically significant.

3.3. Comparison of Diagnostic Tests in Paired Samples

To confirm the previous results, we studied the patients classified as GRAD by the three diagnostic strategies, removing from the original sample all patients considered UNG for any of the strategies. In Table 9, the proportions and means of the paired sample obtained were described.

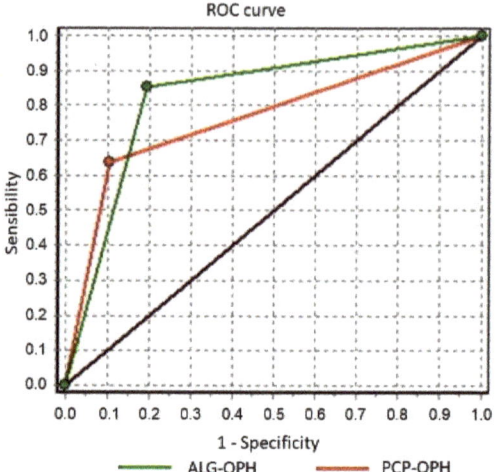

Figure 2. ROC curves comparison. Green line: Algorithm. Red line: Primary Care Physician.

Table 9. Main descriptors of the sample obtained from de APDR for the study between April 2017 and June 2018. * Mean SD. DME = diabetic macular edema. NDME = macular edema non-diabetic. STDR= sight-threatening DR.

	Variable of Interest			Study Sample (n = 2335)
	Gender (F/M)			42.7%/57.3% (997/1338)
	Age (years)			61.1 ± 14.7 *
	Years from diagnosis			10.1 ± 7.2 *
	Mydriasis (before photograph)			98.8% (2306)
Diabetes type	Type 2			85% (1984)
	Type 1			14.7% (343)
	Others			0.3% (8)
Diabetic retinopathy (DR)	No Diabetic Retinopathy (NODR)			78.9% (1842)
	DR prevalence			21.1%
	Mild			10.2% (238)
	Moderate	NDME		8.3% (194)
		DME		2.2% (51)
	Severe	NDME		0.04% (1)
		DME		0.2% (5)
	Proliferative	NDME		0.04% (1)
		DME		0.1% (3)
	STDR			2.6% (61)

The frequencies of pairs of diagnostic categories of each strategy compared to the criteria of the OPH, and the values of the diagnostic validity indexes for the sample described are displayed in Table 10.

Table 10. Paired sample. Diagnostic category pairs frequency and diagnostic validity indexes.

Variable of Interest	ALG-OPH (95% CI)	PCP-OPH (95% CI)
True Positive	418	300
False Positive	351	200
False Negative	75	193
True Negative	1491	1642
Prevalence	21.1% (19.44–22.79)	
Sensibility	84.8% (81.52–88.06)	60.9% (56.44–65.26)
Specificity	80.9% (79.12–82.77)	89.1% (87.69–90.59)
Positive Predictive Value	54.36% (50.77–57.94)	60% (55.61–64.39)
Negative Predictive Value	95.21% (94.12–96.30)	89.48% (88.05–90.91)
Likelihood Ratio +	4.45 (4.02–4.92)	5.60 (4.83–6.50)
Likelihood Ratio −	0.19 (0.15–0.23)	0.44 (0.39–0.49)

The pattern of the indexes shown in Table 10 is comparable to that found in the unpaired sample (Table 7). In fact, the prevalence of DR was the same in all the samples. In summary in the paired sample, the ALG showed a greater ability than PCP to detect DR lesions. However, PCP better identified patients without DR.

Similarly, as in the unpaired sample, we determined that the probability that an individual with a positive test would have retinopathy was small in both strategies (PPV 54.36% vs. 60%), being even lower for the ALG. Both tests presented a high negative predictive value. Therefore, for the unpaired sample, we can conclude that the 2iRetinex software is a good predictor of the absence of DR and a moderate predictor of the presence of DR. In contrast, the diagnostic utility of PCP screening is considered good for positive results and fair for negative.

The AUC for the PCP showed a value of 0.75, while for the ALG was 0.8287. We found that there was a significant difference between the two curves (Chi-square value 28.0575, $p = 0.0000$). Consequently, these results shown in Figure 3 indicate a greater diagnostic power of the ALG.

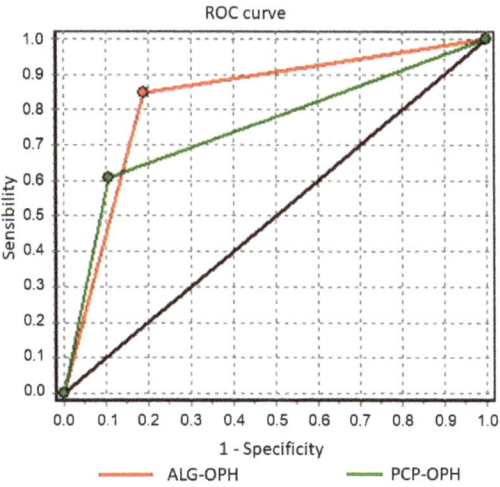

Figure 3. ROC curves comparison of the diagnostic validity. Paired sample. Red: Algorithm. Green: Primary Care Physician.

The k-value of the concordance between the ALG and OPH was 0.5455, while between PCP and OPH it was 0.4974. The homogeneity test for the difference in k-values was not significant (Chi-square 2.7898 $p = 0.949$).

4. Discussion

Digital fundus photography is considered an acceptably accurate procedure for detecting DR [13]. Image processing and interpretation in DR screening programs require initial training and ongoing updating for all personnel involved. This entails personal effort and resource consumption. Population-based screening programs for detecting DR help reduce visual loss by identifying sight-threatening cases and referring them to specialists for treatment. A recent meta-analysis of 33 studies worldwide concludes that teleophthalmology has a moderate sensitivity and high specificity for detecting the absence of DR. However, the results obtained for the diagnosis of the diseased retina show widespread variations [19]. In recent years, there has been increasing interest in applying automation processes in ophthalmic telemedicine to reduce the need for screening professionals and to homogenize diagnostic criteria regardless of the origin and composition of the sample being evaluated [20]. For that reason, in this study, we assessed the use of the 2iRetinex software as a complement or substitute for the screening physician.

In this assessment of images from 3520 patients from ten APDR primary care centers, the prevalence of any form of DR was 18.5%, while STDR cases accounted for 2.3% of the study subjects. Similar results were obtained in the first-year screening of the Scottish program, where the prevalence of DR and STDR was 19.3% and 1.9%, respectively. These values increased in the subjects reviewed one year (20.5% and 2.3%, respectively) [21]. Likewise, other studies with similar characteristics showed a percentage of STDR ranging from 2.57% to 4% [8,22,23].

According to the American Telemedicine Association Validation Level, the first phase of our APDR screening system can be classified as a category 1 program, with an on-disease/non-disease diagnostic criterion issued by the PCP [24]. Meanwhile, the second phase, characterized by the review of pathological retinographies by the referring ophthalmologist is classified as a category C2 program. The ophthalmologist establishes the stage and the time frame for the patient's review or for initiating treatment. Previous studies indicated that artifacts may be present in 3–30% of the photographs without mydriasis [25]. Of note, widespread use of tropicamide (97.8% of patients) does not pose any additional risk [26]. In this regard, the proportion of non-valuable retinal images in published studies is highly dependent on the age distribution of the sample, which in turn is related to the presence of eyelid and corneal abnormalities and especially cataracts. In our study, despite the use of tropicamide to dilate the pupil, the proportion of patients with UNG images was 11. 6%. Moreover, PCPs were unable to make a judgement on 13. 1% of patients. Likewise, the automatic analysis of the algorithm considered 26.3% to be unclassifiable. Our data are consistent with those of other studies. In particular, in a validity study, the iGrading automatic assessment system found 26.16% of 2309 patients to be ungradable [27]. The Italian multicenter study NO BLIND classified 23.4% of the telediagnostic images as "poor quality non-diagnostic images" [28]. Following this line in another study, the ratio of non-gradable patients classified by the automatic system was twice that of the human classification [22]. Indeed, in this study, 404 patients by the criteria of the automatic system were discarded, and 197 patients by the criteria of the ophthalmologist. Only in two other cases did they agree in classifying them as non-gradable [22]. Similarly, in our study, we found the same lack of diagnostic agreement in image grading between ALG and PCP with respect to OPH (k = 0.3623 and 0.3144, respectively). This suggests that the mechanisms underlying decision-making are different in algorithms and clinicians. The grading criteria of the automatic systems may have been more demanding than those of the humans, but what is evident is that their implementation is invariable and not affected by the inherent inconsistency of human subjectivity [29].

Our results on the diagnostic accuracy of screening PCP for any grade of DR showed a good mean specificity (89.6%) and a reduced sensitivity (63.5%). However, for STDR the sensitivity increased to 95%. These values are similar to those reported in other studies [8,11,26,30]. Noteworthy, our findings are consistent with a previous partial study about the diagnostic ability of screening PCP at three APDR primary care centers in a small sample of patients [17]. Similarly, the concordance in the diagnosis of DR with respect to the clinical judgment of the ophthalmologist was k = 0.408 and sensitivity was 97% and specificity 80%.

The second level of APDR development, which would make it a screening and follow-up program to monitor patients with mild and moderate retinopathy without macular edema within the program, has not yet been implemented [30]. It could be that the screening physicians want to reduce the workload of ophthalmologists at the second and third levels of care by under-diagnosing cases that do not require referral.

Regarding the results related to the diagnostic accuracy of the 2iRetinex software analysis test (ALG), an overall sensitivity of 85% was obtained for any degree of retinopathy and a specificity of 81%. For STDR cases, sensitivity increased to 94%. It should be noted that the agreement with the diagnosis of the reference ophthalmologists was similar to that of PCP and the area of the simple ROC curve (0. 8286) was slightly similar to that of PCP. Cost-effective ALG screening programs to identify DR lesions on digital images have been reported previously [31]. In particular, Fleming et al. [31] stated that this inclusion of algorithms increased the sensitivity to 100% in DR detection and reduced manual screening by more than 35%.

EyeArt, Retmaker, iGrading or IDx are commercially available systems that have been used in teleophthalmic screening programs for DR diagnosis [20]. The functionality of iGrading is comparable to that of 2iRetinex by combining an image quality system and a DR identification criterion. In the validation study conducted in Valencia [23], iGrading showed excellent sensitivity values of 97.4% and specificity values of 98.3% for patients with STDR. For its part, iGrading has been used as a level 1 grading in the Scottish screening program after extensive validation since 2010 with a sensitivity of 97.8% and specificity of 41.2% for referable DR [32]. The other two systems, Eyeart and Retmaker showed good diagnostic accuracy with a sensitivity for STDR of 94.7% and 85%, respectively [33]. These methods qualified as Automated Retinal Image Analysis System (ARIAS) have not yet developed a sufficient level of autonomy to establish a classification of the patient's damage and recommend treatment [34].

ARIAS have been changed with the development of artificial intelligence systems and Deep learning (DL), a subtype of machine learning (ML) that does not require image engineering. Early ML techniques for detecting DR used mathematical image transformation techniques and image engineering [35]. Moreover, DL develops its own pattern recognition representations after being fed raw data [36,37].

In relation to this, it is known that IDx has updated its ARIAS with an artificial intelligence system. The new version IDx-DR v2 is designed to identify DR referable to a specialist without human supervision. IDx-DR v2 achieved 100% sensitivity and 81.82% specificity for derivable DR and 100% sensitivity and 94.64% specificity for STDR in the sample examined [38]. A meta-analysis demonstrated that ML algorithms have a high diagnostic accuracy for the diagnosis of DR on color fundus photographs suggesting that they may also be ready for clinical application in screening programs [29]. However, early results published in relation to this ML had methodological inconsistencies, such as lack of external validation and the presence of biases. Most of these methods do not provide full interpretations of the relevant findings of retinal pathological signs. Furthermore, it should be noted that, at present, the full implementation of this "black box classification system" presents difficulties for acceptance by clinicians and patients [39].

The main limitation of our study is the dichotomous diagnosis made by the screening PCP. At least at this stage, the APDR screening program is not designed for PCP to classify the DR stage. Indeed, this limitation has prevented us from obtaining full diagnostic validity indexes results in patients with STDR.

The diagnostic capability for STDR stages is excellent for both diagnostic strategies (PCP and ALG). In the case of the overall diagnostic ability for any form of diabetic retinopathy with our algorithm, the 2iRetinex and PCP strategies are comparable. Moreover, their agreement with respect to the re-evaluation of ophthalmologists does not show significant differences. Therefore, the introduction of this real-time software into the APDR workflow would allow knowing whether the images taken of the patient's fundus are of sufficient quality before the patient leaves the examination center. Thus, a re-examination could be recommended if necessary. This strategy would reduce the delay of repeat examinations and consequently, less disrupt the patient's social and work activity. All this suggests that the automatic examination system could be introduced in a real way by integrating it with the screening physician in the first phase.

In this study, we have validated our DR prediction software (2iRetinex) on a sample of patients under real clinical conditions in the routine APDR circuit. Although further assessment is needed to validate the system, it has been confirmed as a tool that could be integrated into DR screening programs. This could improve the quality of screening models in the future. Due to this, studies of the combined use of algorithms and manual classification emerge as an urgent need to achieve better performance. Thereby, the workload of manual classification could be minimized. We plan to conduct studies that focus on extending the algorithm using the 2iRetinex software to detect other common comorbid eye diseases such as age-related macular degeneration (AMD) and glaucoma.

Author Contributions: S.J.-C. and P.A.-M. were responsible for all aspects of the project including conceptualization and design of the study. S.J.-C., P.A.-M. and P.A.-R. reviewed all the images and stablished the reference diagnosis; E.M. acquired and analyzed APDR data. S.J.-C. and P.A.-M. prepared figures and tables. S.J.-C. and P.A.-M. provided the first draft, prepared final figures, and discussed the results. E.M. and M.A.-D. provided critical review; S.J.-C. and P.A.-M. provided the final version and financial support for the project leading to this publication. All authors have read and agreed to the published version of the manuscript.

Funding: This research was funded by Instituto de Salud Carlos III (FIS PI1601543).

Institutional Review Board Statement: The study was conducted according to the guidelines of the Declaration of Helsinki and approved by the Research and Ethics Committee of Hospital Universitario Puerta del Mar (protocol code PI16-01543, date of approval 26 July 2016).

Informed Consent Statement: Not applicable.

Data Availability Statement: Anonymized data processed in an excel file are available on reasonable request. Restrictions apply to the availability of APDR data. These data are subject to ethical restrictions (Data Protection Act).

Acknowledgments: The authors are grateful for the commitment of the nurses and technicians involved in the appointments and photographs, and of the primary care physicians who contributed with their diagnosis and referrals, to the diabetic retinopathy screening program and this research.

Conflicts of Interest: The authors declare that there is no conflict of interests regarding the publication of this paper.

References

1. International Diabetes Federation. *IDF Diabetes Atlas*, 9th ed.; International Diabetes Federation: Brussels, Belgium, 2019.
2. Rodriguez-Acuña, R.; Mayoral, E.; Aguilar-Diosdado, M.; Rave, R.; Oyarzabal, B.; Lama, C.; Carriazo, A.; Asuncion Martinez-Brocca, M. Andalusian program for early detection of diabetic retinopathy: Implementation and 15-year follow-up of a population-based screening program in Andalusia, Southern Spain. *BMJ Open Diabetes Res. Care* **2020**, *8*, 1–8. [CrossRef] [PubMed]
3. Vithian, K.; Hurel, S. Microvascular complications: Pathophysiology and management. *Clin. Med. J. R. Coll. Phys. Lond.* **2010**, *10*, 505–509. [CrossRef] [PubMed]
4. Liew, G.; Michaelides, M.; Bunce, C. A comparison of the causes of blindness certifications in England and Wales in working age adults (16–64 years), 1999–2000 with 2009–2010. *BMJ Open* **2014**, *4*, 1999–2000. [CrossRef] [PubMed]
5. Yau, J.W.Y.; Rogers, S.; Kawasaki, R.; Lamoreux, E.L.; Kowalski, J.; Bek, T.; Chen, S.-J.; Dekker, J.M.; Fletcher, A.; Grauslund, J.; et al. Global prevalence and major risk factors of diabetic retinopathy. *Diabetes Care* **2012**, *35*, 556–564. [CrossRef]
6. Thomas, R.L.; Halim, S.; Gurudas, S.; Sivaprasad, S.; Owens, D.R. IDF Diabetes Atlas: A review of studies utilising retinal photography on the global prevalence of diabetes related retinopathy between 2015 and 2018. *Diabetes Res. Clin. Pract.* **2019**, *157*, 107840. [CrossRef]

7. Lin, K.Y.; Hsih, W.H.; Lin, Y.B.; Wen, C.Y.; Chang, T.J. Update in the epidemiology, risk factors, screening, and treatment of diabetic retinopathy. *J. Diabetes Investig.* **2021**, *12*, 1322–1325. [CrossRef]
8. Vujosevic, S.; Aldington, S.J.; Silva, P.; Hernandez, C.; Scanlon, P.; Peto, T.; Simo, R. Screening for diabetic retinopathy: New perspectives and challenges. *Lancet Diabetes Endocrinol.* **2020**, *8*, 337–347. [CrossRef]
9. Teo, Z.L.; Tham, Y.C.; Yu, M.; Cheng, C.Y.; Wong, T.Y.; Sabanayagam, C. Do we have enough ophthalmologists to manage vision-threatening diabetic retinopathy? A global perspective. *Eye* **2020**, *34*, 1255–1261. [CrossRef]
10. Cunha, L.P.; Figueiredo, E.A.; Pereira Araujo, H.; Ferreira Costa-Cunha, L.V.; Ferreira Costa, C.; de Melo Costa Neto, J.; Mota Freitas Matos, A.; de Oliveira, M.M.; Gomes Bastos, M.; Ribeiro Monteiro, M.L. Non-Mydriatic Fundus Retinography in Screening for Diabetic Retinopathy: Agreement Between Family Physicians, General Ophthalmologists, and a Retinal Specialist. *Front. Endocrinol.* **2018**, *9*, 251. [CrossRef]
11. Thapa, R.; Bajimaya, S.; Pradhan, E.; Sharma, S.; Kshetri, B.B.; Paudyal, G. Agreement on grading retinal findings of patients with diabetes using fundus photographs by allied medical personnel when compared to an ophthalmologist at a diabetic retinopathy screening program in nepal. *Clin. Ophthalmol.* **2020**, *14*, 2731–2737. [CrossRef]
12. Andonegui, J.; Zurutuza, A.; Pérez de Arcelus, M.; Serrano, L.; Eguzkiza, A.; Auzmendi, M.; Gaminde, I.; Aliseda, D. Diabetic retinopathy screening with non-mydriatic retinography by general practitioners: 2-Year results. *Prim. Care Diabetes* **2012**, *6*, 201–205. [CrossRef] [PubMed]
13. Begum, T.; Rahman, A.; Nomani, D.; Mamun, A.; Adams, A.; Islam, S.; Khair, Z.; Khair, Z.; Answar, I. Diagnostic accuracy of detecting diabetic retinopathy by using digital fundus photographs in the peripheral health facilities of Bangladesh: Validation study. *JMIR Public Health Surveill.* **2021**, *7*, 1–14. [CrossRef] [PubMed]
14. Katada, Y.; Ozawa, N.; Masayoshi, K.; Ofuji, Y.; Tsubota, K.; Kurihara, T. Automatic screening for diabetic retinopathy in interracial fundus images using artificial intelligence. *Intell. Med.* **2020**, *3–4*, 100024. [CrossRef]
15. Rogers, T.W.; Gonzalez-Bueno, J.; Garcia Franco, R.; Lopez Star, E.; Mendez Marin, D.; Vassallo, J.; Lansingh, V.C.; Trikha, S.; Jaccard, N. Evaluation of an AI system for the detection of diabetic retinopathy from images captured with a handheld portable fundus camera: The MAILOR AI study. *Eye* **2021**, *35*, 632–638. [CrossRef]
16. Mataix, B.; Ponte, B. Teleophthalmology as screening method for diabetic retinopathy. *Av. Diabetol.* **2009**, *25*, 209–212.
17. Vargas-Sánchez, C.; Maldonado-Valenzuela, J.J.; Pérez-Durillo, F.T.; González-Calvo, J.; Pérez-Milena, A. Cribado de retinopatía diabética mediante retinografía midriática en atención primaria. *Salud Pública México* **2011**, *53*, 212–219.
18. Wilkinson, C.P.; Ferris, F.L., III; Klein, R.E.; Lee, R.P.; Agardh, C.D.; Davis, M.; Dills, D.; Kampik, A.; Pararajasegaram, A.; Verdaguer, J.T.; et al. Proposed international clinical diabetic retinopathy and diabetic macular edema disease severity scales. *Ophthalmology* **2003**, *110*, 1677–1682. [CrossRef]
19. Ullah, W.; Pathan, S.H.; Panchal, A.; Anandan, S.; Saleem, K.; Sattar, Y.; Ahmad, E.; Mukhtar, M.; Nawaz, H. Cost-effectiveness and diagnostic accuracy of telemedicine in macular disease and diabetic retinopathy: A systematic review and meta-analysis. *Medicine* **2020**, *99*, e20306. [CrossRef]
20. Sim, D.A.; Keane, P.A.; Tufail, A.; Egan, C.A.; Aiello, L.P.; Silva, P.S. Automated Retinal Image Analysis for Diabetic Retinopathy in Telemedicine. *Curr. Diabetes Rep.* **2015**, *15*, 14. [CrossRef]
21. Looker, H.C.; Nyangoma, S.O.; Cromie, D.; Olson, J.A.; Leese, G.P.; Black, M.; Doig, J.; Lee, N.; Lindsay, R.S.; McKnight, J.A.; et al. Diabetic retinopathy at diagnosis of type 2 diabetes in Scotland. *Diabetologia* **2012**, *55*, 2335–2342. [CrossRef]
22. Shah, A.; Clarida, W.; Amelon, R.; Hernaez-Ortega, M.C.; Navea, A.; Morales-Olivas, J.; Dolz-Marco, R.; Verbaak, F.; Jorda, P.P.; van der Heijden, A.A.; et al. Validation of Automated Screening for Referable Diabetic Retinopathy with an Autonomous Diagnostic Artificial Intelligence System in a Spanish Population. *J. Diabetes Sci. Technol.* **2020**, *15*, 655–663. [CrossRef] [PubMed]
23. Soto-Pedre, E.; Navea, A.; Millan, S.; Hernaez-Ortega, M.C.; Morales, J.; Desco, M.C.; Perez, P. Evaluation of automated image analysis software for the detection of diabetic retinopathy to reduce the ophthalmologists' workload. *Acta Ophthalmol.* **2015**, *93*, e52–e56. [CrossRef] [PubMed]
24. Tozer, K.; Woodward, M.A.; Newman-Casey, P.A. Telemedicine and Diabetic Retinopathy: Review of Published Screening Programs. *J. Endocrinol. Diabetes* **2015**, *2*. [CrossRef]
25. Scanlon, H.; Stephen, J. The influence of age, duration of diabetes, cataract, and pupil size on image quality in digital photographic retinal screening. *Diabetes Care* **2005**, *28*, 2448–2453. [CrossRef] [PubMed]
26. Pandit, R.J.; Taylor, R. Mydriasis and glaucoma: Exploding the myth. A systematic review. *Diabetes Med.* **2000**, *17*, 693–699. [CrossRef] [PubMed]
27. Scarpa, G.; Urban, F.; Vujosevic, S.; Tessarin, M.; Gallo, G.; Vissentin, A.; Foglia, E.; Ferrario, L.; Midena, E. The Nonmydriatic Fundus Camera in Diabetic Retinopathy Screening: A Cost-Effective Study with Evaluation for Future Large-Scale Application. *J. Ophthalmol.* **2016**, *2016*, 4625096. [CrossRef]
28. Sasso, F.C.; Pafundi, P.C.; Gelso, A.; Bono, V.; Costagliola, C.; Marfella, R.; Sardu, C.; Rinaldi, L.; Galiero, R.; Acierno, C.; et al. Telemedicine for screening diabetic retinopathy: The NO BLIND Italian multicenter study. *Diabetes Metab. Res. Rev.* **2019**, *35*, e3113.
29. Wu, J.-H.; Liu, T.-Y.A.; Hsu, W.-T.; Ho, J.H.-C.; Lee, C.-C. Performance and limitation of machine learning algorithms for diabetic retinopathy screening: A meta-analysis. *J. Med. Internet Res.* **2020**, *23*, e23863. [CrossRef]
30. Oquendo, M.V.I. Programa de Detección Precoz de la Retinopatía Diabética en Andalucía. *Investig. Diabetes* **2013**, 33–37. Available online: http://www.diabetespractica.com/files/docs/publicaciones/138512840910_Iborra.pdf (accessed on 23 October 2021).

31. Fleming, A.D.; Goatman, K.A.; Phillip, S.; Williams, G.J.; Prescott, G.J.; Scotland, G.S.; McNamee, P.; Leese, G.; Wykes, W.; Sharp, P.F.; et al. The role of haemorrhage and exudate detection in automated grading of diabetic retinopathy. *Br. J. Ophthalmol.* **2010**, *94*, 706–711. [CrossRef]
32. Philip, S.; Fleming, A.D.; Goatman, K.A.; Fonseca, S.; McNamee, P.; Scotland, G.S.; Prescott, G.J.; Sharp, P.F.; Olson, J.A. The efficacy of automated 'disease/no disease' grading for diabetic retinopathy in a systematic screening programme. *Br. J. Ophthalmol.* **2007**, *91*, 1512–1517. [CrossRef] [PubMed]
33. Tufail, A.; Rudisill, C.; Egan, C.; Kapetanakis, V.V.; Salas-Vega, S.; Owen, C.G.; Lee, A.; Louw, V.; Anderson, J.; Liew, G.; et al. Automated Diabetic Retinopathy Image Assessment Software: Diagnostic Accuracy and Cost-Effectiveness Compared with Human Graders. *Ophthalmology* **2017**, *124*, 343–351. [CrossRef]
34. Abràmoff, M.D.; Leng, D.; Ting, D.S.W.; Rhee, K.; Horton, M.B.; Brady, C.J.; Chiang, M.F. Automated and Computer-Assisted Detection, Classification, and Diagnosis of Diabetic Retinopathy. *Telemed. eHealth* **2020**, *26*, 544–550. [CrossRef]
35. Wernick, M.N.; Yang, Y.; Brankov, J.G.; Yourganov, G.; Strother, S.C. Drawing conclusions from medical images. *IEEE Signal Process. Mag.* **2010**, *25*, 25–38. [CrossRef]
36. Abbas, Q.; Fondon, I.; Sarmiento, A.; Jiménez, S.; Alemany, P. Automatic recognition of severity level for diagnosis of diabetic retinopathy using deep visual features. *Med. Biol. Eng. Comput.* **2017**, *55*, 1959–1974. [CrossRef] [PubMed]
37. Esteva, A.; Robicquet, A.; Ramsundar, B.; Kuleshov, V.; DePristo, M.; Chou, K.; Cui, C.; Corrado, G.; Thrun, S.; Dean, J. A guide to deep learning in healthcare. *Nat. Med.* **2019**, *25*, 24–29. [CrossRef] [PubMed]
38. Peris-Martínez, C.; Shaha, A.; Clarida, W.; Amelon, R.; Hernáez-Ortega, M.C.; Navea, A.; Morales-Olivas, J.; Dolz-Marco, R.; Pérez-Jordá, P.; Verbraak, F.; et al. Use in clinical practice of an automated screening method of diabetic retinopathy that can be derived using a diagnostic artificial intelligence system. *Arch. Soc. Esp. Oftalmol.* **2021**, *96*, 117–126. [CrossRef]
39. Colomer, A.; Igual, J.; Naranjo, V. Detection of early signs of diabetic retinopathy based on textural and morphological information in fundus images. *Sensors* **2020**, *20*, 1005. [CrossRef] [PubMed]

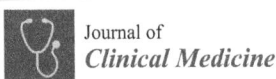 Journal of
Clinical Medicine

Review

State of Evidence on Oral Health Problems in Diabetic Patients: A Critical Review of the Literature

Miguel Ángel González-Moles [1,2,*,†] and Pablo Ramos-García [1,2]

1. School of Dentistry, University of Granada, 18010 Granada, Spain; pramos@correo.ugr.es
2. Instituto de Investigación Biosanitaria ibs.GRANADA, 18012 Granada, Spain
* Correspondence: magonzal@ugr.es
† WHO Collaborating Group for Oral Cancer.

Abstract: Diabetes mellitus (DM) is a global health problem, having recognized that in the next 20 years the number of diabetic patients in the world will increase to 642 million. DM exerts enormous repercussions on general health diabetic (especially derived from vascular, cardiac, renal, ocular, or neurological affectation). It entails in addition a high number of deaths directly related to the disease, as well as a high health care cost, estimated at $673 billion annually. Oral cavity is found among all the organs and systems affected in the course of DM. Important pathologies are developed with higher prevalence, such as periodontitis (PD), alterations in salivary flow, fungal infections, oral cancer, and oral potentially malignant disorders (OPMD). It has been proven that PD hinders the metabolic control of DM and that the presence of PD increases the possibility for developing diabetes. Despite the relevance of these oral pathologies, the knowledge of primary care physicians and diabetes specialists about the importance of oral health in diabetics, as well as the knowledge of dentists about the importance of DM for oral health of patients is scarce or non-existent. It is accepted that the correct management of diabetic patients requires interdisciplinary teams, including dentists. In this critical review, the existing knowledge and evidence-degree on the preventive, clinical, diagnosis, prognosis, and therapeutic aspects of oral diseases that occur with a significant frequency in the diabetic population are developed in extension.

Keywords: diabetes mellitus; oral health; oral medicine; oral pathology; periodontitis; dental caries; oral cancer

Citation: González-Moles, M.Á.; Ramos-García, P. State of Evidence on Oral Health Problems in Diabetic Patients: A Critical Review of the Literature. *J. Clin. Med.* **2021**, *10*, 5383. https://doi.org/10.3390/jcm10225383

Academic Editor: Manuel Aguilar-Diosdado

Received: 27 October 2021
Accepted: 13 November 2021
Published: 18 November 2021

Publisher's Note: MDPI stays neutral with regard to jurisdictional claims in published maps and institutional affiliations.

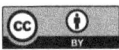

Copyright: © 2021 by the authors. Licensee MDPI, Basel, Switzerland. This article is an open access article distributed under the terms and conditions of the Creative Commons Attribution (CC BY) license (https://creativecommons.org/licenses/by/4.0/).

1. Introduction

Diabetes mellitus (DM) is a health problem of global importance that affects a large number of patients around the world. According to data reported by relevant international organizations (http://diabetesatlas.org/es/sections/worldwide-toll-of-diabetes.html, accessed on 15 December 2020), in the next 20 years, the number of worldwide diabetic patients will increase to 642 million people. DM exerts enormous repercussions on general health diabetic (especially derived from vascular, cardiac, renal, ocular, or neurological affectation). It entails in addition a high number of deaths directly related to the disease, as well as a high health care cost, estimated at $673 billion annually. Current scientific evidence indicates that DM is the consequence of an interaction of environmental, epigenetic, and genetic factors [1]. Among the environmental factors are fundamentally infections and the microbiota involved—of particular importance is the microbiota affecting the oral and intestinal cavities—diet and others. Epigenetics is currently considered as the link between the environment and genetics, altering gene and protein expression. Epigenetic factors—including DNA methylation, histone modification, and microRNAs (e.g., miR-15b, miR-29, or miR-122 [2])—regulate gene expression. These key events are implicated in autoimmunity and in the vulnerability of beta cells of pancreatic islets. Finally, genetic factors promote a special susceptibility to the development of the disease [3]. In this aspect, more than 60 genes, altered chromosomal loci and polymorphisms (e.g., rs12255372 and rs7903146 variants of *TCF7L2* [4]), have been implicated. Type 1 diabetes mellitus (DM1) responds to a multifactorial pathogenesis essentially linked to an autoimmune aggression mediated by autoantibodies that generates a progressive loss of insulin-producing β-cells in the pancreas [5]. On the other hand, the pathogenesis of type 2 diabetes mellitus (DM2) is essentially linked to the development of a state of resistance to the actions of insulin [6].

Oral cavity is found among the organs and systems affected in the course of DM (Table 1). Nevertheless, the information on many of the diabetic related oral diseases—with regard to diagnosis, treatment, and prevention—is limited among health care providers in diabetic patients, especially endocrinologists and family doctors. Likewise, the knowledge that dentists have on the relationships between oral health and DM, and the information on the implications of the dentist in the control of diabetic patients seem limited. Furthermore, knowledge about the aforementioned aspects is frequently based on scant scientific evidence. Undoubtedly, the prevention and control of oral pathology in diabetic patients improves their quality of life and most likely facilitates the long-term control of DM and consequently improves their prognosis. The health care providers for the treatment and follow-up of diabetic patients should be well informed of oral pathologies frequently associated with DM in order to be able to prevent, diagnose, and treat them, or if necessary, refer patients to specialized centers for their management. This most likely requires the implementation of educational programs that convey evidence-based information. In this critical review, the existing knowledge and its degree of evidence, the preventive, clinical, diagnosis, prognosis, and therapeutic aspects of oral diseases occurring with a significant higher frequency in the diabetic population are developed in extension, attending to both type 1 and type 2 DM.

Table 1. Oral manifestations that may be present in patients with Diabetes Mellitus.

Oral Manifestations	Description	References
Periodontitis	The concept of periodontitis refers to a chronic inflammatory process characterized by microbially-associated, host-mediated inflammation that results in loss of periodontal attachment (i.e., by loss of marginal periodontal ligament fibers, apical migration of the junctional epithelium, and apical spread of the bacterial biofilm along the root surface of teeth). Initially, bacterial biofilm formation begins gingival inflammation (i.e., dental-biofilm induced gingivitis) with periodontitis initiation and progression. Furthermore, a multifactorial origin influenced by additional risk factors, such as smoking, is now supported on the immunoinflammatory bases of periodontitis. The relationship between periodontitis and DM (i.e., high prevalence and magnitude of association) is based on a solid evidence level.	[7,8]
Oral candidiasis	Fungal infections, particularly by species of the genus *Candida* sp. Common clinical manifestations are the presence of extensive reddened areas (erythematous candidiasis) along the oral mucosa, generally associated with patchy lingual depapillation and commissural cheilitis. DM patients may present whitish lumps, similar to milk or yogurt clots (speudomembranous candidiasis). Oral candidiasis is usually symptomatic, causing discomfort, burning, or frank pain.	[9,10]
Oral cancer	Oral cancer is the malignant neoplasm affecting lips, oral cavity, or oropharynx. Oral squamous cell carcinoma represents around 90% cases and has a 5-year mortality rate of 50%. The reasons for the increased development of oral cancer in diabetics are not well known, although clinical, biochemical, and molecular reasons have been proposed.	[11,12]
Oral potentially malignant disorders (OPMD)	OPMDs are a significant group of mucosal disorders that may have an increased susceptibility to develop oral cancer, which are essentially oral leukoplakia, oral lichen planus (OLP), proliferative verrucous leukoplakia, erythroplakia and actinic cheilitis. Leukoplakia and OLP—both prevalent OPMDs, associated with considerable malignant transformation rates—have a higher prevalence in subjects with DM than in general population.	[12,13]
Dental caries	Dental caries also known as tooth decays are caused by a breakdown of the tooth tissues. This breakdown is the result of dental plaque's bacterias on teeth that produce acid destroying tooth tissues (e.g., enamel) and results in tooth decay. Diabetic patients, as a consequence of a series of associated oral conditions—xerostomia, high levels of dental plaque, etc.—would be more predisposed to the development of dental caries.	[14,15]

Table 1. *Cont.*

Oral Manifestations	Description	References
Burning mouth syndrome (BMS)	BMS is an atypical chronic pain essentially characterized by the presence of a burning sensation, stinging, or frank pain that is located mainly on the tongue, lips, and palate, although it can spread to any other location, without that there are recognizable mucosal lesions that may justify this condition. BMS seems to present an increased prevalence in patients with DM compared to healthy subjects. It could be associated with the peripheral neuropathy frequently reported in diabetic patients.	[16,17]
Salivary secretion alterations	Alterations in salivary secretion are generically known by the term "dry mouth", which however refers to two different processes, the first related to an objective reduction of salivary flow due to salivary hypofunction (i.e., unstimulated whole saliva flow rate of <0.1 mL/min); and the second, the subjective sensation of lack of saliva in the absence of flow disorders. Dry mouth is one of the most common complaints in diabetic patients, with a partially unknown pathophysiology, which could be related to diabetic neuropathy of parotid gland, pathologic alterations in the salivary glands structure (e.g., vacuolization or acinar atrophy), or hyperglycemia and poorly controlled DM.	[18,19]
Taste perception alterations	Taste perception alterations, mainly hypogeusia (i.e., a partial loss of taste) have been reported in patients with DM. The reasons for the increased development of taste perception alterations in diabetics are not well known, although it has been proposed that it could be associated with the peripheral neuropathy frequently reported in diabetic patients.	[20,21]
Halitosis	Halitosis is a symptom where a person has bad breath. It can be caused by bad oral health, singularly dental care, caries, or periodontitis. Patients with DM are predisposed to halitosis, probably related to the frequent prevalence of these diseases in diabetic patients.	[22,23]
Delayed wound healing	Delayed wound healing is a complication in diabetics after oral surgery, especially in patients with poorly controlled DM. The probable cause of delayed wound healing is damaged small terminal vessels, responsible of reduced blood flow, with an insufficient supply of cellular nutrients through the blood circulation, decreased inflammatory and immune response.	[24–26]

2. Scientific Framework

We chose the critical narrative review design as the scientific framework of this paper on the basis that this type of design covers a wide range of aspects in a given topic. Furthermore, this study design offer the reader global information on a health problem with different facets (not easily achievable through other designs such as systematic reviews and meta-analyses). In this paper, we follow the concept of critical review used by Grant and Booth [27]. A critical review aims to demonstrate that the writer has extensively researched the literature and critically assessed its quality. It goes beyond merely describing the articles identified and includes some degree of analysis and conceptual innovation. An effective critical review presents, analyzes, and synthesizes material from a variety of sources. This concept is widely accepted in the international literature as evidenced by the high number of citations their work has received (5198 citations to date). The main strength of a critical review is based on offering an opportunity to "take stock" and evaluate what is the previous body of a health problem while at the same time making it possible to contribute the authors' own opinions and experiences.

We searched MEDLINE through PubMed (as main electronic database) and Web of Science (for bibliometric analysis purposes) for studies published before the year 2021 (upper limit), with no lower date limit. Search strategy was conducted by combining thesaurus terms used by the databases (i.e., MeSH) with free terms, constructed to maximize sensitivity. In a first line general search, the root keywords and synonyms combined were "diabetes mellitus", "oral health", "periodontal diseases", "oral candidiasis", "oral cancer", "oral potentially malignant disorders", "caries", "burning mouth syndrome", and "salivary secretion alterations". In addition, several more specific searches were conducted by combining relevant aspects of the goals to be reviewed (i.e., relationships between oral diseases and diabetes mellitus, prevention, diagnosis, prognosis, and therapeutic implications). We also manually screened the reference lists of the handled studies for additional relevant studies. Most of the revised studies were included or excluded according to an exhaustive analysis of the title, abstract, year of publication, impact of the journal, and number of citations received. Although these last two criteria may introduce a potential selection bias, its application is necessary when handling a large number of records (e.g., in the first line general search context, simply using the following syntax: ("Diabetes Mellitus"[mh] OR "type 1 diabetes"[all] OR "T1DM"[all] OR "type 2 diabetes"[all] OR "T2DM"[all] OR "diabetes"[all]) AND ("Oral Health"[mh] OR "oral health"[all] OR "mouth diseases"[all] OR "Periodontitis"[mh] OR "periodontitis"[all] OR "periodontal diseases"[all] OR "Mouth Neoplasms"[mh] OR "Mouth Neoplasms"[all] OR "oral squamous cell carcinoma"[all] OR "oral cancer"[all] OR "oral potentially malignant disorders"[all] OR "OPMD"[all] OR ("oral"[all] AND precancer*[all]) OR "Leukoplakia, Oral"[mh] OR "leukoplakia"[all] OR "erythroplakia"[all] OR "Lichen Planus, Oral"[mh] OR "oral lichen planus"[all] OR "Oral Submucous Fibrosis"[mh] OR "oral submucous fibrosis"[all] OR "Dental Caries"[mh] OR "caries"[all] OR "carious"[all] OR "dental decay"[all] OR "Burning Mouth Syndrome"[mh] OR "Burning Mouth Syndrome"[all] OR "BMS"[all] OR "Salivary Gland Diseases"[mh] OR "xerostomia"[mh] OR "xerostomia"[all] OR "dry mouth"[all] OR "hyposalivation"[all]), more than 7000 registers were retrieved). We would also like to clarify that a potential selection bias would only affect to the identification of primary-level studies. Given our effort to develop this review from an evidence-based scientific context, we applied optimal search filters designed for retrieving systematic reviews and meta-analyses (i.e., *Centre for Reviews and Dissemination-CRD* filter; sensitivity = 99.5%, 95%CI = 97.3–99.9 [28,29]). This approach should overcome the potential selection bias, decreasing the rate of missing systematic reviews.

3. Periodontitis

The concept of periodontitis (PD)—according to the new classification scheme for periodontal and peri-implant diseases and conditions [7]—is characterized by microbially-associated, host-mediated inflammation that results in loss of periodontal attachment [8]. PD disease drives the activation of host-derived proteinases with loss of marginal periodontal ligament fibers, apical migration of the junctional epithelium, and apical spread of the bacterial biofilm along the root surface of teeth [8]. Initially, bacterial biofilm formation begins gingival inflammation (i.e., dental-biofilm induced gingivitis [7]); nevertheless, PD initiation and progression is dependent on dysbiotic ecological changes in the microbiome. It occurs in response to nutrients from gingival inflammation and tissue breakdown products with the enrichment of some species and anti-bacterial mechanisms that attempt to contain the microorganisms within the gingival sulcus area once inflammation has initiated [8]. Furthermore, a multifactorial origin influenced by additional risk factors, such as smoking, is now supported on the immunoinflammatory response that trigger the dysbiotic microbiome changes, and also likely influence severity of PD for such individuals [8]. PD is an important health problem because of its prevalence and the systemic repercussions that it entails. Epidemiological studies have reported that 10–15% of the worldwide population suffers from advanced PD [30]. Likewise, the association between PD and some systemic disorders including cardiovascular and metabolic diseases is well known [31–33].

DM is the most prevalent systemic disease in which it has been shown, after extensive research, that it predisposes to the development of PD [34–37]. A recent meta-analysis [38] that collected information from 27 studies (3092 diabetic patients and 23,494 controls) has reported a prevalence of PD of 67.8% in patients with DM and 35.5% in controls (odds ratio [OR] = 1.85; 95%CI = 1.61–2.11), results that in an unappealable way give an idea of the magnitude of the problem. Furthermore, cohorts that include patients with DM1 and DM2 report a higher prevalence of PD in DM1 (78.8% compared to DM2 (70.5%); OR = 2.60 vs. OR = 1.71). A recent systematic review and meta-analysis [39] has also confirmed that DM1 is a relevant risk factor for the development of PD, with a proportion of patients affected more than double for DM1 compared to non-diabetic individuals. In addition, another recent systematic review [40] has also reported an evident bidirectional epidemiological relationship between DM2 and PD, such that the prevalence of DM2 was significantly higher in patients with PD (OR = 4.04, $p < 0.001$), and vice versa (OR = 1.58, $p < 0.001$). The association of DM and PD has recently been considered a comorbidity [41,42].

3.1. Mechanisms Linking DM and PD

Poorly controlled DM generates sustained hyperglycemia, which in turn induces an increase in the inflammatory response in the periodontal tissue; this stimulates the receptor activator of nuclear factor κB (RANK)/RANK-Ligand (RANKL) axis with an increase in osteoclastogenesis and destruction of the alveolar bone, which will conclude with the clinical attachment loss, one of the PD hallmarks. The existing scientific evidence on the biological mechanisms linking DM and PD is detailed below (Figure 1).

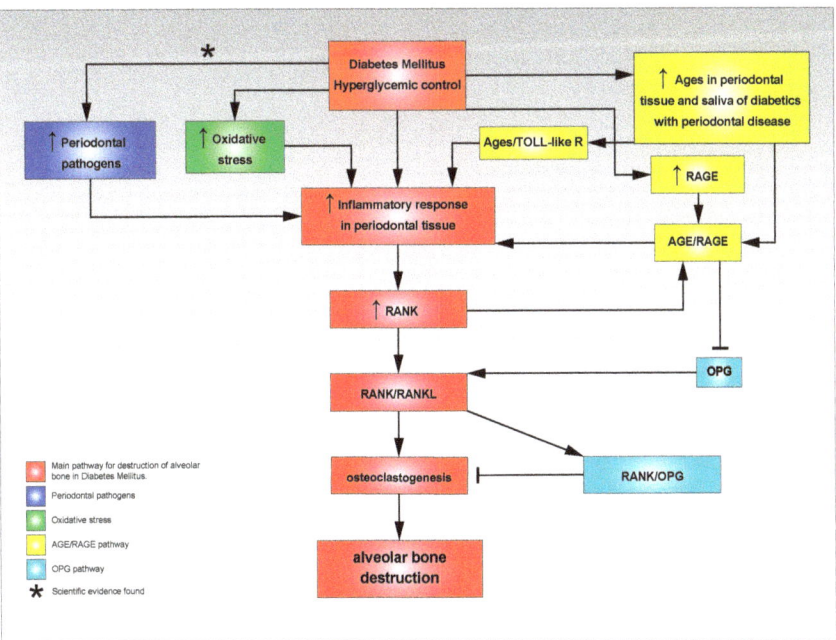

Figure 1. Diabetes Mellitus with a poor control generates sustained hyperglycemia, which in turn induces an increase in the inflammatory response in the periodontal tissue; this in turn stimulates the RANK/RANKL axis with an increase in osteoclastogenesis and destruction of the alveolar bone, which will conclude with the loss of teeth—one of the hallmarks in periodontitis. The increase in the number of periodontal pathogens, the increase in reactive oxygen species (ROS), and the increase in the expression of role of advanced glycation end products (AGE) and its receptor (RAGE) also activate the inflammatory response in the periodontal tissue. The receptor activator of nuclear factor κB (RANK)/RANK-Ligand (RANKL)-RANK/osteoprotegerin (OPG) balance will be important in maintaining periodontal bone homeostasis.

3.1.1. Impact of DM on the Oral Microbiota

It should be recognized that there is very limited and contradictory scientific evidence on the possible impact that DM may exert on the oral microbiota [41,43]. A narrative review [44] has reported that DM1 and DM2 do not have a significant effect on the composition of the periodontal microbiota and that glycemic control level does not seem to significantly influence the composition of the subgingival biofilm. On the contrary, some studies [45–48] indicate that in patients with DM, poor glycemic control could translate into a high number of periodontal pathogens. Currently, we know that these periodontal pathogens are related to the onset and exacerbation of PD [49]. However, the main limitation presented by the evidence on this subject is related to most of these studies are cross-sectional. This study design makes difficult to determine if the more than frequent concomitance of PD and DM responds to a causal relationship or is the result of the presence of common risk factors [41].

3.1.2. Pro-Inflammatory Mediators in Patients with PD and DM

It is currently known that the penetration of periodontal pathogens into the periodontal connective tissue triggers an inflammatory response linked to the development and progression of PD [50]. Evidence from clinical studies supports that DM with poor glycemic control is associated with significantly high levels of pro-inflammatory mediators in gingival tissue [43]. The pathway that best documents the comorbidity between DM with poor glycemic control and PD is inflammation, having shown that an evident local and systemic inflammatory process underlies both conditions that determines its evolution and severity [41]. In vitro and in vivo studies in humans strongly indicate that DM is associated, in a proportional way to glycemic control, with a higher expression of pro-inflammatory mediators in periodontal tissue (TNF-α, IL-6, -8, -10, -12, $\alpha 1\beta$, substance P, eotaxin, macrophage inflammatory protein 1a, GM-CSF, MMP-1, ICAM1, RANKL, PGE2, Toll-like receptor-2, -4, and -9, caspase 3) and with the activation of the Th-17 pathway [44,51–67]. These observations have also been reported in animal models that have evidenced a significantly greater inflammatory response in diabetic vs. non-diabetic, having suggested that periodontal bacteria induce the upregulation of several pro-inflammatory and pro-apoptotic genes in diabetes [68,69].

It has also been pointed out that hyperglycemia and the conditions associated with DM can promote oxidative stress [70] through different pathways with the consequent influence on the inflammatory response. Reactive oxygen species (ROS) has been reported to stimulate the production of pro-inflammatory cytokines through the activation of MAPK, NF-Kβ, Wnt, NALP3 inflammosome pathways, and the activation of the transcription factor FoxO [71–74].

3.1.3. Role of Advanced Glycation End Products (AGE) and Its Receptor (RAGE) in the Development of PD in Diabetes

An important effect of chronic hyperglycemia in uncontrolled DM is related to the non-enzymatic glycation of proteins and lipids, which results in the formation of AGEs. Higher levels of AGEs have been reported in the serum of patients with DM2 in relation to the extent of their PD [75]. The accumulation of AGEs can lead to cellular stress exerting pro-inflammatory and oxidative effects directly or through their interaction with RAGEs. RAGE is a multiligand receptor belonging to the immunoglobulin superfamily of cell-surface molecules [76] that is overexpressed in DM and has been shown to play a role in the development and progression of some complications of diabetes [77] and also in PD in these patients. In this sense, in diabetic mice it has been shown that the loss of bone linked to the infection by *Porphyromonas gingivalis* was mediated by the overexpression of AGE and RAGE [44]. It has also been reported that RAGE contributes to impaired tissue repair in surgical wounds in a diabetic mouse model, and that inhibition of RAGE-mediated signaling increased the rate of tissue healing and repair [78]. Likewise, it has been shown that the AGE-RAGE interaction delays bone healing in the absence of infection, both in osteoblast cultures and in craniotomies in animal models [79]. Finally, AGE could also bind to Toll-like receptors [44]. A significant increase in the expression of these receptors has been observed in the gingival tissue of patients with DM and PD [80], having reported that their activation exerts a pro-inflammatory effect in diabetics similar to that displayed by RAGE, which is especially significant for the Toll-like receptor 4 [81]. Through this pathway, the AGE-Toll-like receptors interaction can increase inflammation and tissue destruction in diabetic PD.

3.1.4. Role of Hyperglycemia in Bone Destruction in PD

The final biological event with the greatest clinical implications in PD is tissue destruction, including destruction of the alveolar bone with consequent tooth loss. The destruction of the alveolar bone is essentially due to the stimulus of the RANK for its ligand (RANKL). RANK is mainly expressed in the membrane of osteoclasts and preosteoclasts and binds to RANKL which is secreted by T cells, indicating that the inflammation inherent in PD induces destruction of the alveolar bone through the stimulation of osteoclastogenesis related to the pathway RANK/RANKL [41]. The natural antagonist of RANKL is osteoprotegerin (OPG), in such a way that the RANK/OPG binding induces the inhibition of osteoclastogenesis. The RANK/OPG ratio is therefore a determining factor in the metabolism and homeostasis of the alveolar bone [41]. Several studies have indicated that DM with poor glycemic control favors the destruction of the alveolar bone in patients with PD mediated by the activation of the RANK/RANKL axis [82–85]. Increased levels of RANKL have been reported in periodontal tissue and crevicular fluid from diabetic patients with poor glycemic control [44,86,87], as well as increased levels of soluble RANKL [82,88] and an increase in the RANK/OPG ratio in poorly controlled DM [82,83]. Studies on animal experimentation also indicate an increase in osteoclastic activity linked to an increase in RANKL levels [89–92]. Finally, it has been interestingly pointed out that the AGE/RAGE axis can also contribute to osteoclastogenesis via increased expression of RANKL and downregulation of OPG in various cell types [93,94]. In an animal model, an increase in osteoclastic activity linked to overexpression of AGEs has been reported, while animals lacking RAGEs exhibited an increase in bone mass and a decrease in the number of osteoclasts [94,95].

3.2. DM Increases the Severity of PD

The existing evidence in this regard indicates that patients with DM are at greater risk of developing more severe PD [96–102]. The parameters most commonly used to measure the severity of PD are the probing depth or pocket depth, the bacterial plaque index, the level of clinical anchorage, which constitutes an important indicator of tissue damage, the number of missing teeth, and the rate of bleeding on probing. A systematic review and meta-analysis [38] has indicated that all these severity indicators are significantly more altered in DM compared to controls. Probing depth was significantly deeper in diabetics compared with controls (mean difference [MD] = 0.23 mm, 95% CI = 0.17–0.29, $p < 0.001$) [38]; plaque index was significantly elevated in the diabetic group (MD = 0.20 mm, 95% CI = 0.18–0.23, $p < 0.001$) [38]; clinical attachment level also reflected higher degree of damage to periodontal tissue in diabetics (MD = 0.39 mm; 95% CI = 0.28–0.50, $p < 0.001$) [38]; diabetics with periodontitis had on average less teeth than the non-diabetic group with periodontitis (MD = −2.14 teeth, 95% CI= −2.87 to −1.40, $p < 0.001$) [38]; bleeding on probing was found affecting more teeth in the diabetic group compared with the control group (MD = 7.90 teeth; 95% CI, 4.24–1.56, $p < 0.001$) [38]. In summary, this systematic review shows with the higher quality of evidence to date that severity of periodontitis is greater in patients with diabetes than in non-diabetic populations. This is relevant for clinical practice and confirms that oral cavity assessment should form a routine part in the clinical evaluation of patients with DM [38].

3.3. PD Worsens the Control and Prognosis of DM

Several studies provide evidence on the negative effect that PD has on the prognosis of diabetes both in terms of mortality and the appearance of DM typical complications [103–108]. A study carried out in Pima Indians—an ethnic group that lives in the state of Arizona (USA) and in the states of Sonora and Chihuahua (Mexico) that shows a high prevalence of DM—reported a significant increase in mortality adjusted for sex and age directly related to the control of their PD. Thus, in diabetic patients without PD or with PD with good control, mortality was 3.7 deaths/1000 inhabitants/year, while in diabetic patients with poor control of PD, mortality amounted to 28.4 deaths/1000 inhabitants/year [103]. Likewise, a large study [104] has reported an increase in cardiovascular mortality in diabetic patients with PD and chronic kidney disease.

Diabetic patients with PD also have a higher risk of complications typical of DM [105,106]; it was published after a joint consensus meeting between the International Diabetes Federation and the European Federation of Periodontology [43], derived from the analysis of 14 studies that included 31,988 patients, so diabetic retinopathy is significantly associated with PD (OR = 1.2–2.8) and the severity of PD is correlated with the severity of retinopathy. Likewise, in patients with DM1 and DM2 with PD there is a higher frequency of kidney complications. Furthermore, a significant association was also reported between DM with PD and the risk of neuropathic foot ulcers development (OR = 6.6); finally, the risk of cardiovascular complications (coronary heart disease, cerebrovascular events and subclinical heart disease) is also significantly increased in diabetic patients with PD.

There is sufficient evidence to support that adequate periodontal treatment generates an improvement in glycemic control in type 2 diabetic patients, evidenced by a reduction in glycated hemoglobin (HbA1c) levels between 0.29% and 0.48% that remains for at least three months after treatment. Although there is insufficient evidence on whether this reduction is maintained after six months of periodontal treatment [14,43,109–111]. This result has also been corroborated by other studies with a moderate quality of evidence [112–118] and by a Cochrane review [117]. The beneficial effect of periodontal treatment in diabetics also seems to translate into a reduction in inflammatory mediators evidenced through a reduction in serum levels of TNF-α and CRP [119,120]. However, it does not seem that the different types of periodontal treatment (surgical, non-surgical, accompanied or not by antibiotics, antiseptics, or with oral hygiene instructions) exert different effects on glycemic control in patients with DM.

Finally, there is reasonable evidence that indicates that PD could increase the risk of developing diabetes, since HbA1c levels have been increased in people with PD without diabetes [107,108]. The joint consensus meeting between the International Diabetes Federation and the European Federation of Periodontology [43] analyzed six representative studies from USA, Japan, and Taiwan populations, (n = 77,716 patients) showing a greater probability of developing prediabetes and diabetes (hazard ratio [HR] = 1.19–1.33) in patients with PDs.

3.4. Dental Implants, Peri-Implantitis, and DM

As mentioned, one of the fundamental consequences of PD in patients with DM is the loss of teeth, which occurs more markedly in elderly patients [69], and thus, one of the more subtle effects of the DM, especially DM2, could be the decrease in quality of life associated with tooth loss and compromised mastication function [121]. Modern dentistry restores lost teeth essentially through dental implants, which has been a real revolution in this field. However, questions have arisen regarding the feasibility and safety of dental implants in the diabetic population. On this issue there is scant and sometimes confusing evidence on how poorly controlled DM affects the prevalence of peri-implant disease, a process equivalent to PD [122,123], which implies bone loss around the implant [124]. In addition, there is also no consistent evidence about whether in patients with DM there is a significantly greater loss of dental implants after their placement [125–127], although apparently there is a delay in osseointegration of the implants related to the poor glycemic control [50,124,128]. A recent systematic review and meta-analysis [129] has indicated that there were statistically significant differences between the groups of DM and non-DM with regard to marginal bone loss ($p < 0.001$), probing depth ($p < 0.001$), and bleeding around dental implants ($p < 0.001$), obtaining the non-DM group the lower complication rates. Finally, in some studies it has been suggested that poorly controlled DM constitutes a relative contraindication for implant therapy [69], although on the contrary, numerous studies support the use of dental implant therapy in diabetic patients even with poor control of the glycaemia [130–133].

4. Oral Candidiasis

The relationship between fungal infections, and in particular infection by species of the genus *Candida* sp., with DM has been widely studied [10,134–136]. It has been clearly established that diabetic patients have an increased susceptibility to fungal infections compared to non-diabetics [137,138]. These susceptibility requires predisposing factors that decisively alter the balance between the host and the yeasts, allowing the passage of *Candida* sp. from its usual commensal state to pathogen, causing infection.

Among the different types of fungal infections that can occur in diabetic patients, oral candidiasis [6] stands out due to its higher frequency and clinical consequences. Significantly higher rates of colonization of the oral mucosa by *Candida* sp. have been described in patients with DM1 (85%) and DM2 (68%) compared with non-diabetics (27%) [138]. One study revealed that 66% of the yeasts isolated from DM patients were *C. albicans* [139]. However, fungal colonization of the oral mucosa is not equivalent to infection, requiring some pathophysiological conditions and associated factors for the infection to finally occur [9,140–144]. These factors are firmly established in diabetic patients and are as follows: (a) Maintained hyperglycemia with increased levels of HbA1c and high levels of glucose in saliva favors the multiplication of *Candida* sp., the increase in the number of receptors available for *Candida* sp., decreased neutrophil activity and increased adherence of *Candida* sp. to the epithelial cells of the oral mucosa [145–151]; (b) the decrease in salivary pH favors the growth of *Candida* sp., the increase in phospholipase and extracellular acid protease levels and the increase in the levels of yeast adhesion to epithelial cells [152–154]; (c) in DM there is a diminished response of the tissue to the injury favoring the colonization of the oral mucosa by *Candida* sp. even in the absence of clinical manifestations [155,156]; (d) and finally, poor oral hygiene, advanced age, female gender and xerostomia are also factors that can appear in DM and have been shown to be associated with a greater tendency to develop fungal infections in diabetics [157–160].

The common clinical manifestations of oral candidiasis are the presence of extensive reddened areas (erythematous candidiasis) along the oral mucosa, which are generally associated with patchy lingual depapilation and commissural cheilitis. Diabetic patients may present also speudomembranous candidiasis characterized by the presence of whitish lumps, similar to milk or yogurt clots, on an erythematous mucosa. These lumps are easily dislodged when scraped off with gauze leaving an erythematous mucosa. Oral candidiasis is usually symptomatic, causing discomfort, burning, or frank pain. Examination of the oral mucosa usually reveals, together with the events described, an absence of salivation or thick and pasty saliva. Diabetic patients may also develop a type of candidiasis associated with the use of removable dental prostheses called prosthetic stomatitis. It is characterized by the appearance of a reddened area under the prosthesis resin, being the mucosa not covered by the prosthesis respected. This form of candidiasis is usually asymptomatic, although a degree of discomfort may also occasionally occur.

5. Oral Cancer and Oral Potentially Malignant Disorders

Oral cancer is a global oral health problem. The most recent data published by prestigious entities (Global cancer incidence, mortality and prevalence [GLOBOCAN] project, International Agency for Research on Cancer [IARC], World Health Organization [WHO]) indicate the appearance of 354,864 new cases and 177,384 patients death per year [161], and a five-year-mortality rate of 50% directly related to this tumor [11]. A fact of great concern is that mortality from oral cancer has not decreased substantially in recent years, despite the fact that the oral cavity is explored by multiple specialists (otolaryngologists, maxillofacial surgeons, dermatologists, dentists, and family doctors). A systematic review and meta-analysis recently published by our research group indicates that diabetic patients have a significantly higher prevalence and risk of developing oral cancer compared to the general population [12]. Worldwide studies on oral cancer incidence and prevalence [162] indicate a strong geographical predisposition for the development of oral cancer, with India and Southeast Asian countries showing the highest figures. This geographical distribution seems to depend on the high levels of tobacco consumption in these countries as this habit is the most relevant etiological factor for the development of oral cancer. However, in our meta-analysis, the subgroup analysis showed the increased risk of development of oral cancer in the diabetic population not dependent on the geographical area studied. In our opinion, and based on these results, the predisposition to the development of cancer in the diabetic population depends directly from conditions associated with DM.

The reasons for the increased development of oral cancer in diabetics are not well known, although clinical, biochemical, and molecular reasons have been proposed. Furthermore, oral cancer and DM share some epidemiological facts and etiological factors, among which are obesity, sedentary lifestyle, advanced age, and diet [163]. On the other hand, hyperinsulinemia due to insulin resistance, through the activation of EGF1R, gives rise to the upregulation of some pro-proliferative and antiapoptotic pathways that have also been documented activated in oral cancer in non-diabetics (PI3K-akt-mTor, MAPK [Ras-Raf-MEK-Erk], and Bcl-2) [164]. Upregulation of these pathways conclusively concludes with the upregulation the *CCND1* gene [165,166]. Our research group has recently pointed out that the upregulation of *CCND1* and the overexpression of its product (cyclin D1) play a determining role in the cascade of molecular events that occur in the malignant transformation of the oral epithelium [167,168]. Therefore, it could be hypothesized that the link between DM and the development of oral cancer is hyperinsulinemia and insulin resistance [12]. Furthermore, as previously mentioned in this paper, hyperglycemia by generating oxidative stress with the release of ROS could cause DNA damage [169]. Hyperglycemia could also be accompanied by an increase in glucose consumption by tumor cells, also known as Warburg effect. This is a well-known hallmark of cancer proposed by Hanahan and Weinberg [170], which seems to induce an increase in cell proliferation associated with an activation of GLUT-1 and GLUT-3, and EGF, EGFR, and PKC-α [171–173].

We have also documented in our research line an increase in oral cancer-related mortality 2.09 times higher in the diabetic population compared to the non-diabetic (95%CI = 1.36–3.22, p = 0.001). This fact, which has also been observed in other types of cancers (liver, pancreas, ovarian, colon, lung, bladder, and breast carcinomas [174,175]) could be due to the phenotype more aggressive—proliferative and invasive—that develops cancer in diabetics as well as the deterioration of the general health of the diabetic related with complications (kidney disease, ischemic disease, etc. [176]) as well as the limitations for surgical treatment linked to postoperative risks, together with higher postoperative mortality [177].

Our research group has also reported the increased risk of development of oral potentially malignant disorders (OPMD) experienced by diabetic patients compared to the general population [12]. OPMDs are a significant group of mucosal disorders that may precede the diagnosis of oral squamous cell carcinoma (OSCC) [13,178], among which are essentially oral leukoplakia [179,180], oral lichen planus (OLP) [181–183], proliferative verrucous leukoplakia [184–186], erythroplakia, and actinic cheilitis [187,188]. Patients diagnosed with OPMDs may have an increased susceptibility to develop cancer anywhere in their mouth during their lifetime [13]. Our previous meta-analysis has shown that oral leukoplakia occurs with a prevalence of 2.49% in the diabetic population (2490 per 100,000 patients with DM) being the risk of developing oral leukoplakia in a diabetic 4.34 times higher compared to the general population. (95%CI = 1.14–16.55, p = 0.03; 10 studies, 7440 patients). A recent study by the WHO collaborative group for the study of cancer and OPMD [179] has reported a risk of oral cancer in oral leukoplakia close to 9%, which indicates the concern of the diagnosis of leukoplakia in a diabetic patient. The risk of developing oral leukoplakia in diabetics does not depend on the geographical area, nor does it depend on tobacco consumption, which indicates that it is probably related to factors exclusively associated with diabetes.

Our results are also strong for OLP, another important and highly prevalent OPMD [189] and associated with considerable malignant transformation rates [181–183]. Patients with DM present a prevalence of OLP of 2.72% (2720 per 100,000) with a chance of developing OLP 1.87 times higher than in the non-diabetic (95%CI = 1.37–2.57, p < 0.001; 22 studies, 5830 patients) [12,190]. Nowadays, the premalignant character of OLP and its progression to cancer high rate have been clearly documented [181], so it is reasonable to hypothesize that in a considerable number of patients diabetics, the appearance of oral cancer may come from the malignant evolution of a previous OLP.

6. Other Oral Conditions Associated with DM

6.1. Dental Caries

The analyses on the prevalence of dental caries in the diabetic population present contradictory and conflicting results [14]. It would seem logical to think that diabetic population, as a consequence of a series of associated oral conditions (xerostomia, high levels of dental plaque, etc.) would be more predisposed to the development of dental caries [191]. A recent systematic review and meta-analysis [15] has reported DM1 patients having significantly higher caries prevalence compared to controls. Although no significant differences were found between DM2 and controls and between well-controlled and poorly controlled diabetics. On the contrary, a study [192] with a large sample (300 diabetics vs. 300 controls) reported a higher prevalence of dental caries in non-diabetics, which the authors attribute to the fact that perhaps the diet of patients with DM generally contains less fermentable carbohydrates and more protein [193]. Another analysis did not find differences in the prevalence of crown caries, although significant differences were found for the prevalence of root caries [194].

6.2. Burning Mouth Syndrome (BMS)

It is an atypical chronic pain essentially characterized by the presence of a burning sensation, stinging or frank pain that is located mainly on the tongue, lips and palate, although it can spread to any other location, without that there are recognizable mucosal lesions that may justify this condition. BMS usually appears in women over 30 years of age and is frequently associated with a history of various emotional disorders [195]. It is a common disease, with an estimated prevalence ranging from 0.7% to 4.6% of the general population [16]. BMS is a process with an impact on the patients quality life, although, despite its frequency and relevance, the pathogenesis is unknown to a large extent [196]. In general, there is an absence of epidemiological primary-level studies focused on the association between BMS and DM. Increased prevalence of BMS in patients with DM compared to healthy subjects has been reported [197,198], while others did not find any differences in prevalence of BMS [199]. A significant association between BMS and peripheral neuropathy has been reported in diabetic patients [17]. It could indicate that BMS in diabetic patients constitutes another manifestation of diabetic neuropathy, although this is an unconfirmed theory.

6.3. Salivary Secretion Alterations

Alterations in salivary secretion are generically called by the term "dry mouth", which however refers to two different processes, the first related to an objective reduction of salivary flow due to salivary hypofunction, defined by an unstimulated whole saliva flow rate of <0.1 mL/min, collected for 5 to 15 min, or chewing-stimulated whole saliva flow rate of <0.7 mL/min, collected for 5 min [200]; and secondly, "dry mouth" can also refer to the subjective sensation of lack of saliva in the absence of flow disorders [18]. The prevalence of salivary hypofunction with decreased salivary flow is estimated to range widely from 1% to 65% of the general population [201].

Dry mouth is one of the most common complaints in diabetic patients. Numerous cross-sectional studies have reported decreased salivary flow from both DM1 [19,202–207] as in DM2 [19,205,208–218]. The pathophysiology of the lack of salivary flow in DM is partly unknown. It has been hypothesized that the parotid innervation involvement in the context of diabetic neuropathy could somehow be involved in the decrease of salivary flow in these patients, although the studies present contradictory results [19,202,219–221]. It should also be noted that the tricyclic antidepressant, frequently used in the treatment of this disorder associated with diabetic neuropathy, produce dry mouth [222]. Some studies have reported alterations in the structure of the salivary glands in patients with DM, including vacuolization or acinar atrophy [223,224]. Likewise, in patients with DM it is common to find asymptomatic parotid enlargement that has been interpreted as a compensatory mechanism for salivary hypofunction [225].

Hyperglycemia seems to be another of the mechanisms responsible for the lack of saliva in diabetics. Significant decreases in salivary flow have been shown in poorly controlled DM compared to those with good glycemic control [19,202,211,212]. In this sense, the overexpression of AGE and RAGE, secondary to hyperglycemia, has been increased in the lacrimal gland tissue in diabetic animal models and associated with dry eyes [226]. Although something equivalent has not been investigated in lacrimal glands, at least theoretically this mechanism could also be operating to salivary hypofunction. RAGE overexpression has been observed in the submaxillary gland of diabetic rats [227]. It is also known that polyuria and osmotic diuresis secondary to hyperglycemia frequently appear in DM, which can trigger dehydration and compensatory hyposalivation [228,229].

6.4. Taste Perception Alterations

Taste perception alterations, mainly hypogeusia, have been reported both in patients with DM1 and DM2, in a significantly higher proportion than in controls [192]. These alterations have also been related to the development of obesity [21] secondary to hyperphagia [20]. Although the alterations in taste perception at the moment are of unknown cause, it has been hypothesized that the disorders of diabetic neuropathy and salivary hypofunction could be in the background of these alterations [192].

6.5. Halitosis

Patients with diabetes are predisposed to halitosis [22], having been reported that approximately 25% of patients with diabetes mellitus suffer from halitosis [230]. The pathogenesis of this disorder is probably related to the frequent presentation of gingivitis, periodontitis, dental caries and xerostomia, which prevents adequate self-cleaning of the oral mucosa. In addition, some of the bacteria that are frequently isolated in the infections of diabetic patients are anaerobes that contribute to the production of volatile products that increase halitosis [23]. In this sense, under the background of periodontitis, bacterial putrefaction and the generation of volatile sulfur compounds could lead to sulfide compound odor [22,231]. On the other hand, under the background of xerostomia, Koshimune et al. [232] found higher concentrations of methyl mercaptan and hydrogen sulfide in patients with salivary secretion alterations. Another study found an association between halitosis and increased HbA1c levels among type 2 diabetic subjects [233]. It was hypothesized that this relationship could be related to the phenomenon of ketoacidosis associated with poorly controlled diabetes [233]. Further studies are needed to explain the nature of this association.

6.6. Delayed Wound Healing

A tendency towards delayed wound healing has been described, especially in patients with poor control of their diabetes in whom long-term complications occur [24]. Probably these long-term complications affect the small terminal vessels, damaging them [25], which produces an insufficient supply of cellular nutrients through the blood circulation, decreasing the inflammatory and antibacterial response [26]. Elevated HbA1c levels $\geq$ 6.5% significantly increase the risk of developing infections after dental interventions and complications of surgical wound healing. For this reason, it is advisable to obtain better control of glycosylated hemoglobin figures [234]. However, those pathological processes in which it is suspected that their presence is contributing to poor diabetes control, and in which surgical treatment is required, should not be delayed in order to achieve a better metabolic control of the disease [234]. In these cases, post-surgical wound care should be maximized and clinical considerations should be made on the convenience of using antibiotics in each specific case [234]. Regarding the type of antibiotic to be used in diabetic patients, the basic rules of antibiotherapy should be respected, i.e., cultures should be performed in these patients in order to select the most effective antibiotic [235]. If necessary, the administration of a broad-spectrum antibiotic should be initiated pending the results of the sensitivity study, and this should be maintained if the study demonstrates its efficacy [235].

Finally, DM is frequently related to other pathological processes, such as hypertension, that require drugs that could also cause decreased salivary flow [19].

7. Need for an Interdisciplinary Team in the Care of Diabetic Patients in Relation to Their Oral Health. Information to the Diabetic Patients about Their Oral Health

From the foregoing it is deduced the importance of oral health in diabetic patients and the reciprocal relationships that exist between good metabolic control of DM and oral health. From this derives the need to establish interdisciplinary teams in the management of diabetic patients, among which dentists should necessarily be. The information available in this regard indicates, however, that at least half of primary care physicians and diabetes specialists do not have adequate knowledge about the importance of oral health in general and about PD in particular in diabetic patients. Furthermore, those clinicians who claim to have knowledge on the subject do not transfer it to their clinical practice and only a third of the professionals refer their patients for a dental consultation [236]. In fact, some studies conclude that active collaboration between dentists, primary care physicians and diabetes specialists does not exist, and the referral of patients to share their care according to competencies is absent. In this way, diabetic patients in many cases are receiving neither the information nor the adequate treatment in relation to their oral health problems [237].

7.1. Attitude of Primary Care Physicians and Specialists Involved in the Management of Diabetic Patients in Relation to Their Oral Health Care

- Clinicians should discuss with diabetic patients the importance of oral health in their disease in relation to the influence it exerts on the metabolic control of the disease and on the reduction of the risk of developing some of the potential complications of DM. Likewise, diabetic patient should be advised to periodically go to the dental clinic for review their oral status [69];
- Clinicians should screen for the main oral conditions that occur in diabetes. This screening should include the evaluation of the periodontal status through simple questions about the existence of spontaneous gingival bleeding or during mastication and brushing, the appearance of mobility or displacement of teeth, the loss of teeth, the presence of halitosis, and the existence of suppuration or periodontal abscesses. Likewise, the presence of erythematous or pseudomembranous candidiasis should be evaluated both through the presence of its symptoms (itching or oral pain) and its signs (oral mucosa affected by extensive red areas and imprecise limits or white areas in the form of lumps that come off easily when scraped with gauze);
- Clinicians should screen the main OPMDs that appear in diabetic patients with a higher prevalence than in the general population (essentially oral leukoplakia and OLP), as well as oral cancer (delimited red areas, ulcers or overgrowths of the oral mucosa older than 15 days) [13,178];
- Clinicians should perform a scrutiny of salivary flow alterations, essentially questioning the patient about the presence of dry mouth symptoms and examining the oral mucosa (obvious absence of saliva or thick saliva, with a parchment-like appearance of the oral mucosa);
- Clinicians should refer diabetic patients to the dental office in the event of any oral health problem detected during control and follow-up visits;
- Clinicians should seek basic training in oral health that allows them to detect the presence of oral disorders that appear in diabetes.

7.2. Attitude of Dentists in the Management of Diabetic Patients in Relation to Their Oral Health Care

- Dentists should discuss with their patients the mutual influences between oral health and diabetes by seeking information on how diabetes can affect oral health [238–243];

- Dentists should promote lifestyle changes on the habits of diabetic patients in order to exert a favorable impact on their oral and general health;
- Dentists must promote attitudes aimed at obtaining the maximum efficiency of oral care in diabetics [43,244]:
    - The medical history should be meticulous and detailed;
    - Communication with primary care physicians and other specialists involved in the care of diabetics should be fluid;
    - The intraoral examination should be meticulous looking for the frequent oral alterations in diabetics, with special reference to the signs and symptoms of PD, oral candidiasis, dry mouth and the presence of OPMD and oral cancer.
- The dental treatment of diabetics should focus on the control of acute infection, offering a therapy plan that is as less complex as possible. Likewise, emergencies in the dental clinic (hyperglycemia, hypoglycemia) must be recognized early and adequately managed. Considerations should be given to which are the most appropriate times to perform dental treatments and what should be the optimal duration of appointments, planning the treatment according to difficulties. Deep anesthesia and good pain and stress control should be provided during treatment;
- Dentists should advise and promote the replacement of missing teeth, the restoration of decayed teeth, and the implementation of preventive oral health habits;
- The dentist must be aware of the existence of the growing number of diabetics in the world [245], many of whom are undiagnosed [246,247]. Dental clinics could act as linkers involved in diabetes screening. In this sense, the suspicion of diabetes in a dental patient should prompt the dentist to request a check of glucose levels in venous blood and in case of alteration, the referral of the patient to his primary care physician for study and treatment if necessary [248];
- Dentists should seek basic training on DM and its complications.

7.3. Information Diabetic Patients Should Receive about Their Oral Health

- Diabetic patients should be given information about their oral health and its relationship to diabetes;
- Diabetic patients should receive information from dentists on the higher prevalence of PD in DM and on the negative consequences this has for the metabolic control of diabetes and on the presentation of complications of diabetes;
- Diabetic patients should receive information from dentists on habits and lifestyle that prevent the development of oral complications of diabetes;
- Diabetic patients should know that they are at risk of developing oral candidiasis;
- Diabetic patients should know that they are at risk of developing oral cancer and OPMD, through accurate, evidence-based information;
- Diabetic patients should know that they could develop alterations in salivary flow with dryness related to their disease;
- Diabetic patients should know the importance of making regular visits to the dental clinic;
- Diabetic patients must make commitments to their oral care.

7.4. Practical Measures and Recommendations to Follow in a Routine Dental Care Session

- Prior to dental treatment, a comprehensive medical history should be performed, singularly recording the type of diabetes, complications, treatment, and control status [249];
- International consensus guidelines state HbA1c levels <6.5% as the main parameter to measure and confirm an appropriate metabolic control [250];
- Pre-prandial blood glucose levels ranging between 70 and 130 mg/dL and post-prandial blood glucose levels < 180 mg/dL also should be confirmed to ensure an adequate metabolic control [250];
- Although well-controlled DM patients could be treated similarly to non-diabetics, short appointments in the morning are preferably to reduce stress of patients [248,251];

- At the beginning of each appointment, the dentist should make sure that the diabetic patient has eaten (fasting must be imperatively avoided) and taken their medications as usual, to avoid a hypoglycemic episode [248,251].

8. Conclusions

Diabetic patients present a notable predisposition to the development of oral pathologies, among which PD stands out, which reaches a prevalence of 67.8%. DM patients have a special predisposition to the development of fungal infections, especially of the *Candida* sp. genus, with significantly higher rates of oral mucosa colonization by *Candida* sp. both in patients with DM1 (85%) and DM2 (68%) compared to non-diabetics (27%). A higher prevalence of oral cancer and OPMD in diabetics has been reported, including oral leukoplakia, with a prevalence of 2.49% in patients, and oral lichen planus with a prevalence of 2.72%. Dental caries, burning mouth syndrome, alterations in saliva secretion, altered taste perception, halitosis, and delayed wound healing are also conditions associated with DM. All these disorders generate important complications that notably worsen the already deteriorated health status of diabetic patients. The frequent involvement of the oral cavity in these patients requires an interdisciplinary approach to its management and adequate guidelines for informing patients about these aspects. It is also essential to increase the training of diabetes care providers as well as patients in relation to their oral health.

Author Contributions: Conceptualization, M.Á.G.-M. and P.R.-G.; methodology, M.Á.G.-M. and P.R.-G.; software, M.Á.G.-M. and P.R.-G.; validation, M.Á.G.-M. and P.R.-G.; formal analysis, M.Á.G.-M. and P.R.-G.; investigation, M.Á.G.-M. and P.R.-G.; resources, M.Á.G.-M.; data curation, M.Á.G.-M. and P.R.-G.; writing—original draft preparation, M.Á.G.-M.; writing—review and editing, M.Á.G.-M. and P.R.-G.; visualization, M.Á.G.-M. and P.R.-G.; supervision, M.Á.G.-M. and P.R.-G.; project administration, M.Á.G.-M.; funding acquisition, M.Á.G.-M. All authors have read and agreed to the published version of the manuscript.

Funding: This research received no external funding.

Institutional Review Board Statement: Not applicable.

Informed Consent Statement: Not applicable.

Conflicts of Interest: The authors declare no conflict of interest.

References

1. Diedisheim, M.; Carcarino, E.; Vandiedonck, C.; Roussel, R.; Gautier, J.-F.; Venteclef, N. Regulation of inflammation in diabetes: From genetics to epigenomics evidence. *Mol. Metab.* **2020**, *41*, 101041. [CrossRef] [PubMed]
2. Karolina, D.S.; Armugam, A.; Sepramaniam, S.; Jeyaseelan, K. miRNAs and diabetes mellitus. *Expert Rev. Endocrinol. Metab.* **2012**, *7*, 281–300. [CrossRef] [PubMed]
3. Xie, Z.; Chang, C.; Huang, G.; Zhou, Z. The Role of Epigenetics in Type 1 Diabetes. *Epigenet. Allergy Autoimmun.* **2020**, *1253*, 223–257. [CrossRef]
4. Florez, J.C.; Jablonski, K.A.; Bayley, N.; Pollin, T.I.; de Bakker, P.I.W.; Shuldiner, A.R.; Knowler, W.C.; Nathan, D.M.; Altshuler, D. TCF7L2 Polymorphisms and progression to diabetes in the diabetes prevention program. *N. Engl. J. Med.* **2006**, *355*, 241–250. [CrossRef] [PubMed]
5. Blake, R.; Trounce, I.A. Mitochondrial dysfunction and complications associated with diabetes. *Biochim. Biophys. Acta-Gen. Subj.* **2014**, *1840*, 1404–1412. [CrossRef] [PubMed]
6. Rodrigues, C.; Rodrigues, M.; Henriques, M. *Candida* sp. Infections in patients with diabetes mellitus. *J. Clin. Med.* **2019**, *8*, 76. [CrossRef] [PubMed]
7. Caton, J.G.; Armitage, G.; Berglundh, T.; Chapple, I.L.C.; Jepsen, S.; Kornman, K.S.; Mealey, B.L.; Papapanou, P.N.; Sanz, M.; Tonetti, M.S. A new classification scheme for periodontal and peri-implant diseases and conditions—Introduction and key changes from the 1999 classification. *J. Periodontol.* **2018**, *89*, S1–S8. [CrossRef]
8. Tonetti, M.S.; Greenwell, H.; Kornman, K.S. Staging and grading of periodontitis: Framework and proposal of a new classification and case definition. *J. Periodontol.* **2018**, *89*, S159–S172. [CrossRef] [PubMed]
9. Lamey, P.-J.; Darwaza, A.; Fisher, B.M.; Samaranayake, L.P.; Macfarlane, T.W.; Frier, B.M. Secretor status, candidal carriage and candidal infection in patients with diabetes mellitus. *J. Oral Pathol. Med.* **1988**, *17*, 354–357. [CrossRef] [PubMed]
10. Belazi, M.; Velegraki, A.; Fleva, A.; Gidarakou, I.; Papanaum, L.; Baka, D.; Daniilidou, N.; Karamitsos, D. Candidal overgrowth in diabetic patients: Potential predisposing factors. *Mycoses* **2005**, *48*, 192–196. [CrossRef]

11. Chi, A.C.; Day, T.A.; Neville, B.W. Oral cavity and oropharyngeal squamous cell carcinoma-an update. *CA Cancer J. Clin.* **2015**, *65*, 401–421. [CrossRef] [PubMed]
12. Ramos-Garcia, P.; Roca-Rodriguez, M.D.M.; Aguilar-Diosdado, M.; Gonzalez-Moles, M.A. Diabetes mellitus and oral cancer/oral potentially malignant disorders: A systematic review and meta-analysis. *Oral Dis.* **2021**, *27*, 404–421. [CrossRef] [PubMed]
13. Warnakulasuriya, S.; Kujan, O.; Aguirre-Urizar, J.M.; Bagan, J.V.; González-Moles, M.Á.; Kerr, A.R.; Lodi, G.; Mello, F.W.; Monteiro, L.; Ogden, G.R.; et al. Oral potentially malignant disorders: A consensus report from an international seminar on nomenclature and classification, convened by the WHO collaborating centre for oral cancer. *Oral Dis.* **2021**, *27*, 1862–1880. [CrossRef]
14. D'Aiuto, F.; Gable, D.; Syed, Z.; Allen, Y.; Wanyonyi, K.L.; White, S.; Gallagher, J.E. Evidence summary: The relationship between oral diseases and diabetes. *Br. Dent. J.* **2017**, *222*, 944–948. [CrossRef] [PubMed]
15. Coelho, A.S.; Amaro, I.F.; Caramelo, F.; Paula, A.; Marto, C.M.; Ferreira, M.M.; Botelho, M.F.; Carrilho, E.V. Dental caries, diabetes mellitus, metabolic control and diabetes duration: A systematic review and meta-analysis. *J. Esthet. Restor. Dent.* **2020**, *32*, 291–309. [CrossRef]
16. Scala, A.; Checchi, L.; Montevecchi, M.; Marini, I.; Giamberardino, M.A. Update on burning mouth syndrome: Overview and patient management. *Crit. Rev. Oral Biol. Med.* **2003**, *14*, 275–291. [CrossRef] [PubMed]
17. Moore, P.A.; Guggenheimer, J.; Orchard, T. Burning mouth syndrome and peripheral neuropathy in patients with type 1 diabetes mellitus. *J. Diabetes Complicat.* **2007**, *21*, 397–402. [CrossRef] [PubMed]
18. Guggenheimer, J.; Moore, P. Xerostomia. *J. Am. Dent. Assoc.* **2003**, *134*, 61–69. [CrossRef]
19. Sreebny, L.M.; Yu, A.; Green, A.; Valdini, A. Xerostomia in diabetes mellitus. *Diabetes Care* **1992**, *15*, 900–904. [CrossRef] [PubMed]
20. Stolbová, K.; Hahn, A.; Benes, B.; Andel, M.; Treslová, L. Gustometry of diabetes mellitus patients and obese patients. *Int. Tinnitus J.* **1999**, *5*, 135–140.
21. Leite, R.S.; Marlow, N.M.; Fernandes, J.K.; Hermayer, K. Oral health and type 2 diabetes. *Am. J. Med. Sci.* **2013**, *345*, 271–273. [CrossRef] [PubMed]
22. Ahmad, R.; Haque, M. Oral health messiers: Diabetes mellitus relevance. *Diabetes Metab. Syndr. Obes. Targets Ther.* **2021**, *14*, 3001–3015. [CrossRef]
23. Mohanty, S.; Mohanty, N.; Rath, S. Analysis of oral health complications in diabetic patients—A diagnostic perspective. *J. Oral Res.* **2018**, *7*, 278–281. [CrossRef]
24. Jha, R.; Kalyani, P.; Bavishi, R. Oral manifestations of diabetes. *J. Res. Med. Dent. Sci.* **2014**, *2*, 6. [CrossRef]
25. Sasaki, H.; Hirai, K.; M Martins, C.; Furusho, H.; Battaglino, R.; Hashimoto, K. Interrelationship between periapical lesion and systemic metabolic disorders. *Curr. Pharm. Des.* **2016**, *22*, 2204–2215. [CrossRef] [PubMed]
26. Buranasin, P.; Mizutani, K.; Iwasaki, K.; Pawaputanon Na Mahasarakham, C.; Kido, D.; Takeda, K.; Izumi, Y. High glucose-induced oxidative stress impairs proliferation and migration of human gingival fibroblasts. *PLoS ONE* **2018**, *13*, e0201855. [CrossRef] [PubMed]
27. Grant, M.J.; Booth, A. A typology of reviews: An analysis of 14 review types and associated methodologies. *Health Inf. Libr. J.* **2009**, *26*, 91–108. [CrossRef] [PubMed]
28. Centre for Reviews and Disseminatio. CRD's Guidance for Undertaking Reviews in Health Care. In *Systematic Reviews*; York Publishing Services Ltd.: Layerthorpe, UK, 2009.
29. Lee, E.; Dobbins, M.; Decorby, K.; McRae, L.; Tirilis, D.; Husson, H. An optimal search filter for retrieving systematic reviews and meta-analyses. *BMC Med. Res. Methodol.* **2012**, *12*, 1–11. [CrossRef] [PubMed]
30. Papapanou, P.N.; Lindhe, J. Epidemiology of periodontal diseases. In *Clinical Periodontology and Implant Dentistry*; Lang, N.P., Lindhe, J., Eds.; John Wiley Sons: Chichester, UK, 2015; pp. 125–168.
31. Gotsman, I.; Lotan, C.; Soskolne, W.A.; Rassovsky, S.; Pugatsch, T.; Lapidus, L.; Novikov, Y.; Masrawa, S.; Stabholz, A. Periodontal destruction is associated with coronary artery disease and periodontal infection with acute coronary syndrome. *J. Periodontol.* **2007**, *78*, 849–858. [CrossRef]
32. Jeffcoat, M.K.; Hauth, J.C.; Geurs, N.C.; Reddy, M.S.; Cliver, S.P.; Hodgkins, P.M.; Goldenberg, R.L. Periodontal disease and preterm birth: Results of a pilot intervention study. *J. Periodontol.* **2003**, *74*, 1214–1218. [CrossRef]
33. Khader, Y.S.; Dauod, A.S.; El-Qaderi, S.S.; Alkafajei, A.; Batayha, W.Q. Periodontal status of diabetics compared with nondiabetics: A meta-analysis. *J. Diabetes Complicat.* **2006**, *20*, 59–68. [CrossRef]
34. Kinane, D.F.; Stathopoulou, P.G.; Papapanou, P.N. Periodontal diseases. *Nat. Rev. Dis. Prim.* **2017**, *3*, 17038. [CrossRef] [PubMed]
35. Nascimento, G.G.; Leite, F.R.M.; Vestergaard, P.; Scheutz, F.; López, R. Does diabetes increase the risk of periodontitis? A systematic review and meta-regression analysis of longitudinal prospective studies. *Acta Diabetol.* **2018**, *55*, 653–667. [CrossRef]
36. Shlossman, M.; Knowler, W.C.; Pettitt, D.J.; Genco, R.J. Type 2 diabetes mellitus and periodontal disease. *J. Am. Dent. Assoc.* **1990**, *121*, 532–536. [CrossRef] [PubMed]
37. Nelson, R.G.; Shlossman, M.; Budding, L.M.; Pettitt, D.J.; Saad, M.F.; Genco, R.J.; Knowler, W.C. Periodontal disease and NIDDM in Pima Indians. *Diabetes Care* **1990**, *13*, 836–840. [CrossRef]
38. Zheng, M.; Wang, C.; Ali, A.; Shih, Y.A.; Xie, Q.; Guo, C. Prevalence of periodontitis in people clinically diagnosed with diabetes mellitus: A meta-analysis of epidemiologic studies. *Acta Diabetol.* **2021**, *58*, 1307–1327. [CrossRef] [PubMed]
39. Dicembrini, I.; Serni, L.; Monami, M.; Caliri, M.; Barbato, L.; Cairo, F.; Mannucci, E. Type 1 diabetes and periodontitis: Prevalence and periodontal destruction—A systematic review. *Acta Diabetol.* **2020**, *57*, 1405–1412. [CrossRef] [PubMed]

40. Wu, C.; Yuan, Y.; Liu, H.; Li, S.; Zhang, B.; Chen, W.; An, Z.; Chen, S.; Wu, Y.; Han, B.; et al. Epidemiologic relationship between periodontitis and type 2 diabetes mellitus. *BMC Oral Health* **2020**, *20*, 204. [CrossRef] [PubMed]
41. Polak, D.; Sanui, T.; Nishimura, F.; Shapira, L. Diabetes as a risk factor for periodontal disease—plausible mechanisms. *Periodontology 2000* **2020**, *83*, 46–58. [CrossRef] [PubMed]
42. Comprehensive medical evaluation and assessment of comorbidities: Standards of medical care in diabetes—2018. *Diabetes Care* **2018**, *44*, S28–S37.
43. Sanz, M.; Ceriello, A.; Buysschaert, M.; Chapple, I.; Demmer, R.T.; Graziani, F.; Herrera, D.; Jepsen, S.; Lione, L.; Madianos, P.; et al. Scientific evidence on the links between periodontal diseases and diabetes: Consensus report and guidelines of the joint workshop on periodontal diseases and diabetes by the International diabetes Federation and the European Federation of Periodontology. *Diabetes Res. Clin. Pract.* **2018**, *137*, 231–241. [CrossRef]
44. Taylor, J.J.; Preshaw, P.M.; Lalla, E. A review of the evidence for pathogenic mechanisms that may link periodontitis and diabetes. *J. Clin. Periodontol.* **2013**, *40*, S113–S134. [CrossRef]
45. Casarin, R.; Barbagallo, A.; Meulman, T.; Santos, V.; Sallum, E.; Nociti, F.; Duarte, P.; Casati, M.; Goncalves, R. Subgingival biodiversity in subjects with uncontrolled type-2 diabetes and chronic periodontitis. *J. Periodontal Res.* **2013**, *48*, 30–36. [CrossRef]
46. Aemaimanan, P.; Amimanan, P.; Taweechaisupapong, S. Quantification of key periodontal pathogens in insulin-dependent type 2 diabetic and non-diabetic patients with generalized chronic periodontitis. *Anaerobe* **2013**, *22*, 64–68. [CrossRef] [PubMed]
47. Merchant, A.T.; Shrestha, D.; Chaisson, C.; Choi, Y.H.; Hazlett, L.J.; Zhang, J. Association between serum antibodies to oral microorganisms and hyperglycemia in adults. *J. Dent. Res.* **2014**, *93*, 752–759. [CrossRef] [PubMed]
48. Demmer, R.T.; Jacobs, D.R., Jr.; Singh, R.; Zuk, A.; Rosenbaum, M.; Papapanou, P.N.; Desvarieux, M. Periodontal bacteria and prediabetes prevalence in ORIGINS: The oral infections, glucose intolerance, and insulin resistance study. *J. Dent. Res.* **2015**, *94*, 201s–211s. [CrossRef] [PubMed]
49. Kumar, V.; Abbas, A.K.; Fausto, N.; Aster, J.C. *Cotran Robbins and Cotran Pathologic Basis of Disease*; Elsevier: Amsterdam, The Netherlands, 2009; ISBN 1-4377-2015-3.
50. Monje, A.; Catena, A.; Borgnakke, W.S. Association between diabetes mellitus/hyperglycaemia and peri-implant diseases: Systematic review and meta-analysis. *J. Clin. Periodontol.* **2017**, *44*, 636–648. [CrossRef]
51. Duarte, P.M.; Bezerra, J.P.; Miranda, T.S.; Feres, M.; Chambrone, L.; Shaddox, L.M. Local levels of inflammatory mediators in uncontrolled type 2 diabetic subjects with chronic periodontitis. *J. Clin. Periodontol.* **2014**, *41*, 11–18. [CrossRef] [PubMed]
52. Shikama, Y.; Kudo, Y.; Ishimaru, N.; Funaki, M. Possible involvement of palmitate in pathogenesis of periodontitis. *J. Cell. Physiol.* **2015**, *230*, 2981–2989. [CrossRef] [PubMed]
53. Hung, S.-L.; Lee, N.-G.; Chang, L.-Y.; Chen, Y.-T.; Lai, Y.-L. Stimulatory effects of glucose and porphyromonas gingivalis lipopolysaccharide on the secretion of inflammatory mediators from human macrophages. *J. Periodontol.* **2014**, *85*, 140–149. [CrossRef] [PubMed]
54. Liu, J.; Wu, Y.; Wang, Y.; Yuan, X.; Fang, B. High levels of glucose induced the Caspase-3/PARP signaling pathway, leading to apoptosis in human periodontal ligament fibroblasts. *Cell Biochem. Biophys.* **2013**, *66*, 229–237. [CrossRef] [PubMed]
55. Chang, L.C.; Kuo, H.C.; Chang, S.F.; Chen, H.J.; Lee, K.F.; Lin, T.H.; Huang, T.Y.; Choe, C.S.; Lin, L.T.; Chen, C.N. Regulation of ICAM-1 expression in gingival fibroblasts infected with high-glucose-treated *P. gingivalis*. *Cell. Microbiol.* **2013**, *15*, 1722–1734. [CrossRef]
56. Xu, J.; Xiong, M.; Huang, B.; Chen, H. Advanced glycation end products upregulate the endoplasmic reticulum stress in human periodontal ligament cells. *J. Periodontol.* **2015**, *86*, 440–447. [CrossRef]
57. Catalfamo, D.L.; Calderon, N.L.; Harden, S.W.; Sorenson, H.L.; Neiva, K.G.; Wallet, S.M. Augmented LPS responsiveness in type 1 diabetes-derived osteoclasts. *J. Cell. Physiol.* **2013**, *228*, 349–361. [CrossRef]
58. Chang, P.C.; Chien, L.Y.; Chong, L.Y.; Kuo, Y.P.; Hsiao, J.K. Glycated matrix up-regulates inflammatory signaling similarly to Porphyromonas gingivalis lipopolysaccharide. *J. Periodontal Res.* **2013**, *48*, 184–193. [CrossRef]
59. Kim, J.H.; Lee, D.E.; Choi, S.H.; Cha, J.H.; Bak, E.J.; Yoo, Y.J. Diabetic characteristics and alveolar bone loss in streptozotocin- and streptozotocin-nicotinamide-treated rats with periodontitis. *J. Periodontal Res.* **2014**, *49*, 792–800. [CrossRef] [PubMed]
60. Ozlurk, A.; Bilgici, B.; Odyakmaz, S.; Konas, E. The relationship of periodontal disease severity to serum and GCF substance p levels in diabetics. *Quintessence Int.* **2012**, *43*, 587–58796.
61. Jiang, S.Y.; Wei, C.C.; Shang, T.T.; Lian, Q.; Wu, C.X.; Deng, J.Y. High glucose induces inflammatory cytokine through protein kinase C-induced toll-like receptor 2 pathway in gingival fibroblasts. *Biochem. Biophys. Res. Commun.* **2012**, *427*, 666–670. [CrossRef] [PubMed]
62. Bastos, A.S.; Graves, D.T.; Loureiro, A.P.D.M.; Júnior, C.R.; Abdalla, D.S.P.; Faulin, T.D.E.S.; Câmara, N.O.; Andriankaja, O.M.; Orrico, S.R.P. Lipid peroxidation is associated with the severity of periodontal disease and local inflammatory markers in patients with type 2 diabetes. *J. Clin. Endocrinol. Metab.* **2012**, *97*, E1353–E1362. [CrossRef] [PubMed]
63. Lamster, I.B.; Novak, M.J. Host mediators in gingival crevicular fluid: Implications for the pathogenesis of periodontal disease. *Crit. Rev. Oral Biol. Med.* **1992**, *3*, 31–60. [CrossRef]
64. Wu, Y.; Liu, F.; Zhang, X.; Shu, L. Insulin modulates cytokines expression in human periodontal ligament cells. *Arch. Oral Biol.* **2014**, *59*, 1301–1306. [CrossRef] [PubMed]
65. Chang, P.-C.; Tsai, S.-C.; Chong, L.Y.; Kao, M.-J. N-Phenacylthiazolium Bromide Inhibits the Advanced Glycation End Product (AGE)–AGE receptor axis to modulate experimental periodontitis in Rats. *J. Periodontol.* **2014**, *85*, e268–e276. [CrossRef] [PubMed]

66. Yang, X.; Zhang, J.; Ni, J.; Ouyang, B.; Wang, D.; Luo, S.; Xie, B.; Xuan, D. Toll-Like Receptor 4–Mediated hyper-responsiveness of gingival epithelial cells to lipopolysaccharide in high-glucose environments. *J. Periodontol.* **2014**, *85*, 1620–1628. [CrossRef]
67. Javed, F.; Al-Daghri, N.M.; Wang, H.L.; Wang, C.Y.; Al-Hezaimi, K. Short-term effects of non-surgical periodontal treatment on the gingival crevicular fluid cytokine profiles in sites with induced periodontal defects: A study on dogs with and without streptozotocin-induced diabetes. *J. Periodontol.* **2014**, *85*, 1589–1595. [CrossRef] [PubMed]
68. Graves, D.T.; Li, J.; Cochran, D.L. Inflammation and uncoupling as mechanisms of periodontal bone loss. *J. Dent. Res.* **2011**, *90*, 143–153. [CrossRef] [PubMed]
69. Albert, D.A.; Ward, A.; Allweiss, P.; Graves, D.T.; Knowler, W.C.; Kunzel, C.; Leibel, R.L.; Novak, K.F.; Oates, T.W.; Papapanou, P.N.; et al. Diabetes and oral disease: Implications for health professionals. *Ann. N. Y. Acad. Sci.* **2012**, *1255*, 1–15. [CrossRef]
70. Bullon, P.; Morillo, J.M.; Ramirez-Tortosa, M.C.; Quiles, J.L.; Newman, H.N.; Battino, M. Metabolic syndrome and periodontitis: Is oxidative stress a common link? *J. Dent. Res.* **2009**, *88*, 503–518. [CrossRef] [PubMed]
71. Graves, D.T.; Naguib, G.; Lu, H.; Leone, C.; Hsue, H.; Krall, E. Inflammation is more persistent in type 1 diabetic mice. *J. Dent. Res.* **2005**, *84*, 324–328. [CrossRef]
72. Martinon, F. Signaling by ROS drives inflammasome activation. *Eur. J. Immunol.* **2010**, *40*, 616–619. [CrossRef] [PubMed]
73. Almeida, M.; Han, L.; Ambrogini, E.; Weinstein, R.S.; Manolagas, S.C. Glucocorticoids and tumor necrosis factor α increase oxidative stress and suppress Wnt protein signaling in osteoblasts. *J. Biol. Chem.* **2011**, *286*, 44326–44335. [CrossRef]
74. Galli, C.; Passeri, G.; Macaluso, G.M. FoxOs, Wnts and oxidative stress-induced bone loss: New players in the periodontitis arena? *J. Periodontal Res.* **2011**, *46*, 397–406. [CrossRef] [PubMed]
75. Takeda, M.; Ojima, M.; Yoshioka, H.; Inaba, H.; Kogo, M.; Shizukuishi, S.; Nomura, M.; Amano, A. Relationship of serum advanced glycation end products with deterioration of periodontitis in type 2 diabetes patients. *J. Periodontol.* **2006**, *77*, 15–20. [CrossRef] [PubMed]
76. Schmidt, A.M.; Weidman, E.; Lalla, E.; Yan, S.D.; Hori, O.; Cao, R.; Brett, J.G.; Lamster, I.B. Advanced glycation endproducts (AGEs) induce oxidant stress in the gingiva: A potential mechanism underlying accelerated periodontal disease associated with diabetes. *J. Periodontal Res.* **1996**, *31*, 508–515. [CrossRef]
77. Yuan, K.; Chang, C.J.; Hsu, P.C.; Sun, H.S.; Tseng, C.C.; Wang, J.R. Detection of putative periodontal pathogens in non-insulin-dependent diabetes mellitus and non-diabetes mellitus by polymerase chain reaction. *J. Periodontal Res.* **2001**, *36*, 18–24. [CrossRef] [PubMed]
78. Goova, M.T.; Li, J.; Kislinger, T.; Qu, W.; Lu, Y.; Bucciarelli, L.G.; Nowygrod, S.; Wolf, B.M.; Caliste, X.; Yan, S.F.; et al. Blockade of receptor for advanced glycation end-products restores effective wound healing in diabetic mice. *Am. J. Pathol.* **2001**, *159*, 513–525. [CrossRef]
79. Santana, R.B.; Xu, L.; Chase, H.B.; Amar, S.; Graves, D.T.; Trackman, P.C. A role for advanced glycation end products in diminished bone healing in type 1 diabetes. *Diabetes* **2003**, *52*, 1502–1510. [CrossRef] [PubMed]
80. Rojo-Botello, N.R.; García-Hernández, A.L.; Moreno-Fierros, L. Expression of toll-like receptors 2, 4 and 9 is increased in gingival tissue from patients with type 2 diabetes and chronic periodontitis. *J. Periodontal Res.* **2012**, *47*, 62–73. [CrossRef]
81. Veloso, C.A.; Fernandes, J.S.; Volpe, C.M.O.; Fagundes-Netto, F.S.; Reis, J.S.; Chaves, M.M.; Nogueira-Machado, J.A. TLR4 and RAGE: Similar routes leading to inflammation in type 2 diabetic patients. *Diabetes Metab.* **2011**, *37*, 336–342. [CrossRef] [PubMed]
82. Vieira Ribeiro, F.; de Mendonça, A.C.; Santos, V.R.; Bastos, M.F.; Figueiredo, L.C.; Duarte, P.M. Duarte Cytokines and bone-related factors in systemically healthy patients with chronic periodontitis and patients with type 2 diabetes and chronic periodontitis. *J. Periodontol.* **2011**, *82*, 1187–1196. [CrossRef] [PubMed]
83. Santos, V.R.; Lima, J.A.; Gonçalves, T.E.D.; Bastos, M.F.; Figueiredo, L.C.; Shibli, J.A.; Duarte, P.M. Receptor activator of nuclear factor-kappa B ligand/osteoprotegerin ratio in sites of chronic periodontitis of subjects with poorly and well-controlled type 2 diabetes. *J. Periodontol.* **2010**, *81*, 1455–1465. [CrossRef] [PubMed]
84. Shetty, B.; Divakar, D.D.; Al-Kheraif, A.A.; Alharbi, A.O.; Almutairi, M.S.T.; Alanazi, M.M. Role of PDT as an adjunct to SRP on whole salivary RANKL and OPG ratio in type-2 diabetic and normoglycemic individuals with chronic periodontitis. *Photodiagn. Photodyn. Ther.* **2021**, *34*. [CrossRef] [PubMed]
85. Xu, J.L.; Meng, H.X.; He, L.; Wang, X.E.; Zhang, L. The effects of initial periodontal therapy on the serum receptor activator of nuclear factor-κβ ligand/osteoprotegerin system in patients with type 2 diabetes mellitus and periodontitis. *J. Periodontol.* **2016**, *87*, 303–311. [CrossRef] [PubMed]
86. Mahamed, D.A.; Marleau, A.; Alnaeeli, M.; Singh, B.; Zhang, X.; Penninger, J.M.; Teng, Y.T.A. G(-) anaerobes-reactive CD4+ T-cells trigger RANKL-mediated enhanced alveolar bone loss in diabetic NOD mice. *Diabetes* **2005**, *54*, 1477–1486. [CrossRef] [PubMed]
87. Duarte, P.M.; De Oliveira, M.C.G.; Tambeli, C.H.; Parada, C.A.; Casati, M.Z.; Nociti Jr, F.H. Overexpression of interleukin-1beta and interleukin-6 may play an important role in periodontal breakdown in type 2 diabetic patients. *J. Periodontal Res.* **2007**, *42*, 377–381. [CrossRef]
88. Drosatos-Tampakaki, Z.; Drosatos, K.; Siegelin, Y.; Gong, S.; Khan, S.; Van Dyke, T.; Goldberg, I.J.; Schulze, P.C.; Schulze-Späte, U. Palmitic acid and DGAT1 deficiency enhance osteoclastogenesis, while oleic acid-induced triglyceride formation prevents it. *J. Bone Miner. Res.* **2014**, *29*, 1183–1195. [CrossRef]
89. Kayal, R.A.; Tsatsas, D.; Bauer, M.A.; Allen, B.; Al-Sebaei, M.O.; Kakar, S.; Leone, C.W.; Morgan, E.F.; Gerstenfeld, L.C.; Einhorn, T.A.; et al. Diminished bone formation during diabetic fracture healing is related to the premature resorption of cartilage associated with increased osteoclast activity. *J. Bone Miner. Res.* **2007**, *22*, 560–568. [CrossRef] [PubMed]

90. Childs, L.M.; Paschalis, E.P.; Xing, L.; Dougall, W.C.; Anderson, D.; Boskey, A.L.; Puzas, J.E.; Rosier, R.N.; O'Keefe, R.J.; Boyce, B.F.; et al. In vivo RANK signaling blockade using the receptor activator of NF-κB:Fc effectively prevents and ameliorates wear debris-induced osteolysis via osteoclast depletion without inhibiting osteogenesis. *J. Bone Miner. Res.* **2002**, *17*, 192–199. [CrossRef]
91. Cappellen, D.; Luong-Nguyen, N.H.; Bongiovanni, S.; Grenet, O.; Wanke, C.; Mira Šuša, M. Transcriptional program of mouse osteoclast differentiation governed by the macrophage colony-stimulating factor and the ligand for the receptor activator of NFκB. *J. Biol. Chem.* **2002**, *277*, 21971–21982. [CrossRef] [PubMed]
92. Graves, D.T.; Alshabab, A.; Albiero, M.L.; Mattos, M.; Corrêa, J.D.; Chen, S.; Yang, Y. Osteocytes play an important role in experimental periodontitis in healthy and diabetic mice through expression of RANKL. *J. Clin. Periodontol.* **2018**, *45*, 285–292. [CrossRef]
93. Yoshida, T.; Flegler, A.; Kozlov, A.; Stern, P.H. Direct inhibitory and indirect stimulatory effects of RAGE ligand S100 on sRANKL-induced osteoclastogenesis. *J. Cell. Biochem.* **2009**, *107*, 917–925. [CrossRef]
94. Ding, K.H.; Wang, Z.Z.; Hamrick, M.W.; Deng, Z.B.; Zhou, L.; Kang, B.; Yan, S.L.; She, J.X.; Stern, D.M.; Isales, C.M.; et al. Disordered osteoclast formation in RAGE-deficient mouse establishes an essential role for RAGE in diabetes related bone loss. *Biochem. Biophys. Res. Commun.* **2006**, *340*, 1091–1097. [CrossRef]
95. Miyata, T.; Kawai, R.; Taketomi, S.; Sprague, S.M. Possible involvement of advanced glycation end-products in bone resorption. *Nephrol. Dial. Transplant.* **1996**, *11*, 54–57. [CrossRef]
96. Battancs, E.; Gheorghita, D.; Nyiraty, S.; Lengyel, C.; Eördegh, G.; Baráth, Z.; Várkonyi, T.; Antal, M. Periodontal disease in diabetes mellitus: A case–control study in smokers and non-smokers. *Diabetes Ther.* **2020**, *11*, 2715–2728. [CrossRef] [PubMed]
97. Torrungruang, K.; Ongphiphadhanakul, B.; Jitpakdeebordin, S.; Sarujikumjornwatana, S. Mediation analysis of systemic inflammation on the association between periodontitis and glycaemic status. *J. Clin. Periodontol.* **2018**, *45*, 548–556. [CrossRef] [PubMed]
98. Noack, B.; Aslanhan, Z.; Boué, J.; Petig, C.; Teige, M.; Schaper, F.; Hoffmann, T.; Hannig, C. Potential association of paraoxonase-1, type 2 diabetes mellitus, and periodontitis. *J. Periodontol.* **2013**, *84*, 614–623. [CrossRef] [PubMed]
99. Winning, L.; Patterson, C.C.; Neville, C.E.; Kee, F.; Linden, G.J. Periodontitis and incident type 2 diabetes: A prospective cohort study. *J. Clin. Periodontol.* **2017**, *44*, 266–274. [CrossRef]
100. Chokwiriyachit, A.; Dasanayake, A.P.; Suwannarong, W.; Hormdee, D.; Sumanonta, G.; Prasertchareonsuk, W.; Wara-Aswapati, N.; Combellick, J.; Pitiphat, W. Periodontitis and gestational diabetes mellitus in non-smoking females. *J. Periodontol.* **2013**, *84*, 857–862. [CrossRef]
101. Hodge, P.J.; Robertson, D.; Paterson, K.; Smith, G.L.F.; Creanor, S.; Sherriff, A. Periodontitis in non-smoking type 1 diabetic adults: A cross-sectional study. *J. Clin. Periodontol.* **2012**, *39*, 20–29. [CrossRef] [PubMed]
102. Hintao, J.; Teanpaisan, R.; Chongsuvivatwong, V.; Dahlen, G.; Rattarasarn, C. Root surface and coronal caries in adults with type 2 diabetes mellitus. *Community Dent. Oral Epidemiol.* **2007**, *35*, 302–309. [CrossRef]
103. Saremi, A.; Nelson, R.G.; Tulloch-Reid, M.; Hanson, R.L.; Sievers, M.L.; Taylor, G.W.; Knowler, W.C. Periodontal disease and mortality in type 2 diabetes. *Diabetes Care* **2005**, *28*, 27–32. [CrossRef] [PubMed]
104. Sharma, P.; Dietrich, T.; Ferro, C.J.; Cockwell, P.; Chapple, I.L.C. Association between periodontitis and mortality in stages 3-5 chronic kidney disease: NHANES III and linked mortality study. *J. Clin. Periodontol.* **2016**, *43*, 104–113. [CrossRef]
105. Thorstensson, H. Medical status and complications in relation to periodontal disease experience in insulin-dependent diabetics. *J. Clin. Periodontol.* **1996**, *23*, 194–202. [CrossRef] [PubMed]
106. Shultis, W.A.; Weil, E.J.; Looker, H.C.; Curtis, J.M.; Shlossman, M.; Genco, R.J.; Knowler, W.C.; Nelson, R.G. Effect of periodontitis on overt nephropathy and end-stage renal disease in type 2 diabetes. *Diabetes Care* **2007**, *30*, 306–311. [CrossRef] [PubMed]
107. Demmer, R.T.; Jacobs, D.R.; Desvarieux, M. Periodontal disease and incident type 2 diabetes: Results from the first national health and nutrition examination survey and its epidemiologic follow-up study. *Diabetes Care* **2008**, *31*, 1373–1379. [CrossRef] [PubMed]
108. Graziani, F.; Gennai, S.; Solini, A.; Petrini, M. A systematic review and meta-analysis of epidemiologic observational evidence on the effect of periodontitis on diabetes An update of the EFP-AAP review. *J. Clin. Periodontol.* **2018**, *45*, 167–187. [CrossRef]
109. Simpson, T.C.; Weldon, J.C.; Worthington, H.V.; Needleman, I.; Wild, S.H.; Moles, D.R.; Stevenson, B.; Furness, S.; Iheozor-Ejiofor, Z. Treatment of periodontal disease for glycaemic control in people with diabetes mellitus. *Cochrane Database Syst. Rev.* **2015**, 1–138. [CrossRef] [PubMed]
110. Madianos, P.N.; Koromantzos, P.A. An update of the evidence on the potential impact of periodontal therapy on diabetes outcomes. *J. Clin. Periodontol.* **2018**, *45*, 188–195. [CrossRef] [PubMed]
111. Hsu, Y.; Nair, M.; Angelov, N.; Lalla, E.; Lee, C. Impact of diabetes on clinical periodontal outcomes following non-surgical periodontal therapy. *J. Clin. Periodontol.* **2019**, *46*, 206–217. [CrossRef]
112. Borgnakke, W.S.; Yelostalo, P.V.; Taylor, G.W.; Genco, R.J. Effect of periodontal disease on diabetes: Systematic review of epidemiologic observational evidence. *J. Periodontol.* **2013**, *84*, S135–S152. [CrossRef]
113. Engebretson, S.; Kocher, T. Evidence that periodontal treatment improves diabetes outcomes: A systematic review and meta-analysis. *J. Clin. Periodontol.* **2013**, *40*, S153–S163. [CrossRef]
114. Li, Q.; Hao, S.; Fang, J.; Xie, J.; Kong, X.H.; Yang, J.X. Effect of non-surgical periodontal treatment on glycemic control of patients with diabetes: A meta-analysis of randomized controlled trials. *Trials* **2015**, *16*, 1–8. [CrossRef] [PubMed]

115. Sgolastra, F.; Severino, M.; Pietropaoli, D.; Gatto, R.; Monaco, A. Effectiveness of periodontal treatment to improve metabolic control in patients with chronic periodontitis and type 2 diabetes: A meta-analysis of randomized clinical trials. *J. Periodontol.* **2013**, *84*, 958–973. [CrossRef]
116. Corbella, S.; Francetti, L.; Taschieri, S.; De Siena, F.; Fabbro, M. Del Effect of periodontal treatment on glycemic control of patients with diabetes: A systematic review and meta-analysis. *J. Diabetes Investig.* **2013**, *4*, 502–509. [CrossRef] [PubMed]
117. Wang, T.F.; Jen, I.A.; Chou, C.; Lei, Y.P. Effects of periodontal therapy on metabolic control in patients with type 2 diabetes mellitus and periodontal disease: A meta-analysis. *Medicine* **2014**, *93*, e292. [CrossRef] [PubMed]
118. Sun, Q.; Feng, M.; Zhang, M.; Zhang, Y.; Cao, M.; Bian, L.; Guan, Q.; Song, K. Effects of periodontal treatment on glycemic control in type 2 diabetic patients: A meta-analysis of randomized controlled trials. *Chin. J. Physiol.* **2014**, *57*, 305–314. [CrossRef]
119. Artese, H.P.C.; Foz, A.M.; Rabelo, M.D.S.; Gomes, G.H.; Orlandi, M.; Suvan, J.; D'Aiuto, F.; Romito, G.A. Periodontal therapy and systemic inflammation in type 2 diabetes mellitus: A meta-analysis. *PLoS ONE* **2015**, *10*, e0128344. [CrossRef]
120. Baeza, M.; Morales, A.; Cisterna, C.; Cavalla, F.; Jara, G.; Isamitt, Y.; Pino, P.; Gamonal, J. Effect of periodontal treatment in patients with periodontitis and diabetes: Systematic review and meta-analysis. *J. Appl. Oral Sci.* **2020**, *28*, e20190248. [CrossRef]
121. McGrath, C.; Bedi, R. Can dentures improve the quality of life of those who have experienced considerable tooth loss? *J. Dent.* **2001**, *29*, 243–246. [CrossRef]
122. Chrcanovic, B.R.; Albrektsson, T.; Wennerberg, A. Diabetes and oral implant failure: A systematic review. *J. Dent. Res.* **2014**, *93*, 859–867. [CrossRef] [PubMed]
123. Javed, F.; Romanos, G.E. Impact of diabetes mellitus and glycemic control on the osseointegration of dental implants: A systematic literature review. *J. Periodontol.* **2009**, *80*, 1719–1730. [CrossRef] [PubMed]
124. Oates, T.W.; Huynh-Ba, G.; Vargas, A.; Alexander, P.; Feine, J. A critical review of diabetes, glycemic control, and dental implant therapy. *Clin. Oral Implants Res.* **2013**, *24*, 117–127. [CrossRef] [PubMed]
125. Bornstein, M.M.; Cionca, N.; Mombelli, A. Systemic conditions and treatments as risks for implant therapy. *Int. J. Oral Maxillofac. Implant.* **2009**, *24*, 12–27.
126. Mombelli, A.; Cionca, N. Systemic diseases affecting osseointegration therapy. *Clin. Oral Implant. Res.* **2006**, *17*, 97–103. [CrossRef]
127. Chen, H.; Liu, N.; Xu, X.; Qu, X.; Lu, E. Smoking, radiotherapy, diabetes and osteoporosis as risk factors for dental implant failure: A meta-analysis. *PLoS ONE* **2013**, *8*, e71955. [CrossRef] [PubMed]
128. Graves, D.T.; Ding, Z.; Yang, Y. The impact of diabetes on periodontal diseases. *Periodontol. 2000* **2020**, *82*, 214–224. [CrossRef]
129. Jiang, X.; Zhu, Y.; Liu, Z.; Tian, Z.; Zhu, S. Association between diabetes and dental implant complications: A systematic review and meta-analysis. *Acta Odontol. Scand.* **2021**, *79*, 9–18. [CrossRef]
130. Dowell, S.; Oates, T.W.; Robinson, M. Implant success in people with type 2 diabetes mellitus with varying glycemic control: A pilot study. *J. Am. Dent. Assoc.* **2007**, *138*, 355–361. [CrossRef] [PubMed]
131. Tawil, G.; Younan, R.; Azar, P.; Sleilati, G. Conventional and advanced implant treatment in the type II diabetic patient: Surgical protocol and long-term clinical results. *Int. J. Oral Maxillofac. Implant.* **2008**, *23*, 744–752.
132. Oates, T.W.; Dowell, S.; Robinson, M.; McMahan, C.A. Glycemic control and implant stabilization in type 2 diabetes mellitus. *J. Dent. Res.* **2009**, *88*, 367–371. [CrossRef] [PubMed]
133. Turkyilmaz, I. One-year clinical outcome of dental implants placed in patients with type 2 diabetes mellitus: A case series. *Implant Dent.* **2010**, *19*, 323–329. [CrossRef] [PubMed]
134. Tang, H.-J.; Liu, W.-L.; Lin, H.-L.; Lai, C.-C. Epidemiology and prognostic factors of candidemia in elderly patients. *Geriatr. Gerontol. Int.* **2015**, *15*, 688–693. [CrossRef]
135. Darwazeh, A.M.G.; Lamey, P.-J.; Samaranayake, L.P.; Macfarlane, T.W.; Flisher, B.M.; Macrury, S.M.; Maccuish, A.C. The relationship between colonisation, secretor status and in-vitro adhesion of Candida albicans to buccal epithelial cells from diabetics. *J. Med. Microbiol.* **1990**, *33*, 43–49. [CrossRef]
136. Gonçalves, R.H.P.; Miranda, E.T.; Zaia, J.E.; Giannini, M.J.S.M. Species diversity of yeast in oral colonization of insulin-treated diabetes mellitus patients. *Mycopathologia* **2006**, *162*, 83–89. [CrossRef] [PubMed]
137. Gudlaugsson, O.; Gillespie, S.; Lee, K.; Berg, J.V.; Hu, J.; Messer, S.; Herwaldt, L.; Pfaller, M.; Diekema, D. Attributable Mortality of Nosocomial Candidemia, Revisited. *Clin. Infect. Dis.* **2003**, *37*, 1172–1177. [CrossRef] [PubMed]
138. Kumar, B.V.; Padshetty, N.S.; Bai, K.Y.; Rao, M.S. Prevalence of Candida in the oral cavity of diabetic subjects. *J. Assoc. Physicians India* **2005**, *53*, 599–602. [PubMed]
139. Aitken-Saavedra, J.; Lund, R.G.; González, J.; Huenchunao, R.; Perez-Vallespir, I.; Morales-Bozo, I.; Urzúa, B.; Tarquinio, S.C.; Maturana-Ramírez, A.; Martos, J.; et al. Diversity, frequency and antifungal resistance of Candida species in patients with type 2 diabetes mellitus. *Acta Odontol. Scand.* **2018**, *76*, 580–586. [CrossRef] [PubMed]
140. Javed, F.; Klingspor, L.; Sundin, U.; Altamash, M.; Klinge, B.; Engström, P.-E. Periodontal conditions, oral Candida albicans and salivary proteins in type 2 diabetic subjects with emphasis on gender. *BMC Oral Health* **2009**, *9*, 12. [CrossRef] [PubMed]
141. Mulu, A.; Kassu, A.; Anagaw, B.; Moges, B.; Gelaw, A.; Alemayehu, M.; Belyhun, Y.; Biadglegne, F.; Hurissa, Z.; Moges, F.; et al. Frequent detection of 'azole' resistant Candida species among late presenting AIDS patients in northwest Ethiopia. *BMC Infect. Dis.* **2013**, *13*, 82. [CrossRef] [PubMed]
142. Goregen, M.; Miloglu, O.; Buyukkurt, M.C.; Caglayan, F.; Aktas, A.E. Median rhomboid glossitis: A clinical and microbiological study. *Eur. J. Dent.* **2011**, *5*, 367–372. [CrossRef] [PubMed]

143. Arendorf, T.M.; Walker, D.M. Tobacco smoking and denture wearing as local aetiological factors in median rhomboid glossitis. *Int. J. Oral Surg.* **1984**, *13*, 411–415. [CrossRef]
144. Flaitz, C.M.; Nichols, C.M.; Hicks, M.J. An overview of the oral manifestations of AIDS-related Kaposi's sarcoma. *Compend. Contin. Educ. Dent.* **1995**, *16*, 136–138. [PubMed]
145. Darwazeh, A.M.G.; MacFarlane, T.W.; McCuish, A.; Lamey, P.-J. Mixed salivary glucose levels and candidal carriage in patients with diabetes mellitus. *J. Oral Pathol. Med.* **1991**, *20*, 280–283. [CrossRef] [PubMed]
146. Reinhart, H.; Muller, G.; Sobel, J.D. Specificity and mechanism of in vitro adherence of Candida albicans. *Ann. Clin. Lab. Sci.* **1985**, *15*, 406–413. [PubMed]
147. Naik, R.; Ahmed Mujib, B.R.; Raaju, U.R.; Telagi, N. Assesing oral candidal carriage with mixed salivary glucose levels as non-invasive diagnostic tool in type-2 Diabetics of Davangere, Karnataka, India. *J. Clin. Diagn. Res.* **2014**, *8*, ZC69. [CrossRef] [PubMed]
148. Sashikumar, R.; Kannan, R. Salivary glucose levels and oral candidal carriage in type II diabetics. *Oral Surg. Oral Med. Oral Pathol. Oral Radiol. Endodont.* **2010**, *109*, 706–711. [CrossRef]
149. Geerlings, S.E.; Hoepelman, A.I. Immune dysfunction in patients with diabetes mellitus (DM). *FEMS Immunol. Med. Microbiol.* **1999**, *26*, 259–265. [CrossRef]
150. Ferguson, D. The physiology and biology of saliva. In *Color Atlas and Text of Salivary Gland: Disease, Disorders and Surgery*; Wolfe Pub Ltd.: London, UK, 1995; pp. 40–48.
151. Dorocka-Bobkowska, B.; Budtz-Jorgensen, E.; WlSoch, S. Non-insulin-dependent diabetes mellitus as a risk factor for denture stomatitis. *J. Oral Pathol. Med.* **1996**, *25*, 411–415. [CrossRef] [PubMed]
152. Balan, P.; B Gogineni, S.; Kumari N, S.; Shetty, V.; Lakshman Rangare, A.; L Castelino, R.; Areekat K, F. Candida carriage rate and growth characteristics of saliva in diabetes mellitus patients: A case-control study. *J. Dent. Res. Dent. Clin. Dent. Prospects* **2015**, *9*, 274–279. [CrossRef] [PubMed]
153. Samaranayake, L.P.; Hughes, A.; Weetman, D.A.; MacFarlane, T.W. Growth and acid production of Candida species in human saliva supplemented with glucose. *J. Oral Pathol. Med.* **1986**, *15*, 251–254. [CrossRef]
154. Samaranayake, L.P.; MacFarlane, T.W. Factors affecting the in-vitro adherence of the fungal oral pathogen Candida albicans to epithelial cells of human origin. *Arch. Oral Biol.* **1982**, *27*, 869–873. [CrossRef]
155. Pallavan, B.; Ramesh, V.; Dhanasekaran, B.P.; Oza, N.; Indu, S.; Govindarajan, V. Comparison and correlation of candidal colonization in diabetic patients and normal individuals. *J. Diabetes Metab. Disord.* **2014**, *13*, 66. [CrossRef] [PubMed]
156. Mantri, S.S.; Parkhedkar, R.D.; Mantri, S.P. Candida colonisation and the efficacy of chlorhexidine gluconate on soft silicone-lined dentures of diabetic and non-diabetic patients. *Gerodontology* **2013**, *30*, 288–295. [CrossRef]
157. Malic, S.; Hill, K.E.; Ralphs, J.R.; Hayes, A.; Thomas, D.W.; Potts, A.J.; Williams, D.W. Characterization of Candida albicans infection of an in vitro oral epithelial model using confocal laser scanning microscopy. *Oral Microbiol. Immunol.* **2007**, *22*, 188–194. [CrossRef]
158. Wang, J.; Ohshima, T.; Yasunari, U.; Namikoshi, S.; Yoshihara, A.; Miyazaki, H.; Maeda, N. The carriage of Candida species on the dorsal surface of the tongue: The correlation with the dental, periodontal and prosthetic status in elderly subjects. *Gerodontology* **2006**, *23*, 157–163. [CrossRef] [PubMed]
159. de Carvalho Bianchi, C.M.P.; Bianchi, H.A.; Tadano, T.; de Paula, C.R.; Hoffmann-Santos, H.D.; Leite, D.P., Jr.; Hahn, R.C. Factors related to oral candidiasis in elderly users and non-users of removable dental prostheses. *Rev. Inst. Med. Trop. Sao Paulo* **2016**, *58*, 17. [CrossRef]
160. Cardoso, M.B.R.; Lago, E.C. Oral changes in elderly from an association center. *Rev. Para. Med. V* **2010**, *24*, 35–41.
161. Bray, F.; Ferlay, J.; Soerjomataram, I.; Siegel, R.L.; Torre, L.A.; Jemal, A. Global cancer statistics 2018: GLOBOCAN estimates of incidence and mortality worldwide for 36 cancers in 185 countries. *CA. Cancer J. Clin.* **2018**, *68*, 394–424. [CrossRef] [PubMed]
162. Warnakulasuriya, S. Global epidemiology of oral and oropharyngeal cancer. *Oral Oncol.* **2009**, *45*, 309–316. [CrossRef] [PubMed]
163. Giovannucci, E.; Harlan, D.M.; Archer, M.C.; Bergenstal, R.M.; Gapstur, S.M.; Habel, L.A.; Pollak, M.; Regensteiner, J.G.; Yee, D. Diabetes and cancer: A consensus report. *CA. Cancer J. Clin.* **2010**, *60*, 207–221. [CrossRef]
164. Pollak, M.N. Insulin-like growth factors and neoplasia. *Biol. IGF-1 Its Interact. Insul. Health Malig. States* **2008**, *262*, 84–98. [CrossRef]
165. Ramos-García, P.; Gil-Montoya, J.A.; Scully, C.; Ayén, A.; González-Ruiz, L.; Navarro-Triviño, F.J.; González-Moles, M.A. An update on the implications of cyclin D1 in oral carcinogenesis. *Oral Dis.* **2017**, *23*, 897–912. [CrossRef] [PubMed]
166. Lee, Y.; Dominy, J.E.; Choi, Y.J.; Jurczak, M.; Tolliday, N.; Camporez, J.P.; Chim, H.; Lim, J.-H.; Ruan, H.-B.; Yang, X.; et al. Cyclin D1–Cdk4 controls glucose metabolism independently of cell cycle progression. *Nature* **2014**, *510*, 547–551. [CrossRef] [PubMed]
167. Ramos-García, P.; González-Moles, M.Á.; Ayén, Á.; González-Ruiz, L.; Ruiz-Ávila, I.; Lenouvel, D.; Gil-Montoya, J.A.; Bravo, M. Asymmetrical proliferative pattern loss linked to cyclin D1 overexpression in adjacent non-tumour epithelium in oral squamous cell carcinoma. *Arch. Oral Biol.* **2019**, *97*, 12–17. [CrossRef] [PubMed]
168. Ramos-García, P.; González-Moles, M.Á.; González-Ruiz, L.; Ayén, Á.; Ruiz-Ávila, I.; Bravo, M.; Gil-Montoya, J.A. Clinicopathological significance of tumor cyclin D1 expression in oral cancer. *Arch. Oral Biol.* **2019**, *99*, 177–182. [CrossRef] [PubMed]
169. Asmat, U.; Abad, K.; Ismail, K. Diabetes mellitus and oxidative stress—A concise review. *Saudi Pharm. J.* **2016**, *24*, 547–553. [CrossRef] [PubMed]
170. Hanahan, D.; Weinberg, R.A. Hallmarks of cancer: The next generation. *Cell* **2011**, *144*, 646–674. [CrossRef]

171. Hahn, T.; Barth, S.; Hofmann, W.; Reich, O.; Lang, I.; Desoye, G. Hyperglycemia regulates the glucose-transport system of clonal choriocarcinoma cells in vitro. A potential molecular mechanism contributing to the adjunct effect of glucose in tumor therapy. *Int. J. Cancer* **1998**, *78*, 353–360. [CrossRef]
172. Han, L.; Ma, Q.; Li, J.; Liu, H.; Li, W.; Ma, G.; Xu, Q.; Zhou, S.; Wu, E. High glucose promotes pancreatic cancer cell proliferation via the induction of EGF expression and transactivation of EGFR. *PLoS ONE* **2011**, *6*, e27074. [CrossRef]
173. Okumura, M.; Yamamoto, M.; Sakuma, H.; Kojima, T.; Maruyama, T.; Jamali, M.; Cooper, D.R.; Yasuda, K. Leptin and high glucose stimulate cell proliferation in MCF-7 human breast cancer cells: Reciprocal involvement of PKC-α and PPAR expression. *Biochim. Biophys. Acta-Mol. Cell Res.* **2002**, *1592*, 107–116. [CrossRef]
174. Barone, B.B.; Yeh, H.C.; Snyder, C.F.; Peairs, K.S.; Stein, K.B.; Derr, R.L.; Wolff, A.C.; Brancati, F.L. Long-term all-cause mortality in cancer patients with preexisting diabetes mellitus: A systematic review and meta-analysis. *JAMA* **2008**, *300*, 2754–2764. [CrossRef] [PubMed]
175. Seshasai, S.R.K.; Kaptoge, S.; Thompson, A.; Di Angelantonio, E.; Gao, P.; Sarwar, N.; Whincup, P.H.; Mukamal, K.J.; Gillum, R.F.; Holme, I.; et al. Diabetes mellitus, fasting glucose, and risk of cause-specific death. *N. Engl. J. Med.* **2011**, *364*, 829–841. [CrossRef]
176. Van De Poll-Franse, L.V.; Houterman, S.; Janssen-Heijnen, M.L.G.; Dercksen, M.W.; Coebergh, J.W.W.; Haak, H.R. Less aggressive treatment and worse overall survival in cancer patients with diabetes: A large population based analysis. *Int. J. Cancer* **2007**, *120*, 1986–1992. [CrossRef] [PubMed]
177. Lee, D.H.; Kim, S.Y.; Nam, S.Y.; Choi, S.-H.; Choi, J.W.; Roh, J.-L. Risk factors of surgical site infection in patients undergoing major oncological surgery for head and neck cancer. *Oral Oncol.* **2011**, *47*, 528–531. [CrossRef] [PubMed]
178. Warnakulasuriya, S.; Johnson, N.W.; van der Waal, I. Nomenclature and classification of potentially malignant disorders of the oral mucosa. *J. Oral Pathol. Med.* **2007**, *36*, 575–580. [CrossRef] [PubMed]
179. Aguirre-Urizar, J.M.; Lafuente-Ibáñez de Mendoza, I.; Warnakulasuriya, S. Malignant transformation of oral leukoplakia: Systematic review and meta-analysis of the last 5 years. *Oral Dis.* **2021**, *27*, 1881–1895. [CrossRef]
180. Warnakulasuriya, S.; Ariyawardana, A. Malignant transformation of oral leukoplakia: A systematic review of observational studies. *J. Oral Pathol. Med.* **2016**, *45*, 155–166. [CrossRef] [PubMed]
181. González-Moles, M.Á.; Ruiz-Ávila, I.; González-Ruiz, L.; Ayén, Á.; Gil-Montoya, J.A.; Ramos-García, P. Malignant transformation risk of oral lichen planus: A systematic review and comprehensive meta-analysis. *Oral Oncol.* **2019**, *96*, 121–130. [CrossRef] [PubMed]
182. González-Moles, M.Á.; Ramos-García, P.; Warnakulasuriya, S. An appraisal of highest quality studies reporting malignant transformation of oral lichen planus based on a systematic review. *Oral Dis.* **2020**. [CrossRef]
183. Ramos-García, P.; Gonzalez-Moles, M.A.; Warnakulasuriya, S. Oral cancer development in lichen planus and related conditions-3.0 evidence level-: A systematic review of systematic reviews. *Oral Dis.* **2021**, *27*, 1908–1918. [CrossRef] [PubMed]
184. Ramos-García, P.; González-Moles, M.Á.; Mello, F.W.; Bagan, J.V.; Warnakulasuriya, S. Malignant transformation of oral proliferative verrucous leukoplakia: A systematic review and meta-analysis. *Oral Dis.* **2021**, *27*, 1896–1907. [CrossRef] [PubMed]
185. González-Moles, M.Á.; Ramos-García, P.; Warnakulasuriya, S. A scoping review on gaps in the diagnostic criteria for proliferative verrucous leukoplakia: A conceptual proposal and diagnostic evidence-based criteria. *Cancers* **2021**, *13*, 3669. [CrossRef]
186. González-Moles, M.Á.; Warnakulasuriya, S.; Ramos-García, P. Prognosis parameters of oral carcinomas developed in proliferative verrucous leukoplakia: A systematic review and meta-analysis. *Cancers* **2021**, *13*, 4843. [CrossRef]
187. Iocca, O.; Sollecito, T.P.; Alawi, F.; Weinstein, G.S.; Newman, J.G.; De Virgilio, A.; Di Maio, P.; Spriano, G.; Pardiñas López, S.; Shanti, R.M. Potentially malignant disorders of the oral cavity and oral dysplasia: A systematic review and meta-analysis of malignant transformation rate by subtype. *Head Neck* **2019**, *42*, 539–555. [CrossRef]
188. Dancyger, A.; Heard, V.; Huang, B.; Suley, C.; Tang, D.; Ariyawardana, A. Malignant transformation of actinic cheilitis: A systematic review of observational studies. *J. Investig. Clin. Dent.* **2018**, *9*, e12343. [CrossRef] [PubMed]
189. González-Moles, M.Á.; Warnakulasuriya, S.; González-Ruiz, I.; González-Ruiz, L.; Ayén, Á.; Lenouvel, D.; Ruiz-Ávila, I.; Ramos-García, P. Worldwide prevalence of oral lichen planus: A systematic review and meta-analysis. *Oral Dis.* **2020**, *27*, 813–828. [CrossRef] [PubMed]
190. Otero Rey, E.M.; Yáñez-Busto, A.; Rosa Henriques, I.F.; López-López, J.; Blanco-Carrión, A. Lichen planus and diabetes mellitus: Systematic review and meta-analysis. *Oral Dis.* **2019**, *25*, 1253–1264. [CrossRef]
191. Ismail, A.F.; McGrath, C.P.; Yiu, C.K.Y. Oral health of children with type 1 diabetes mellitus: A systematic review. *Diabetes Res. Clin. Pract.* **2015**, *108*, 369–381. [CrossRef]
192. Mauri-Obradors, E.; Estrugo-Devesa, A.; Jane-Salas, E.; Vinas, M.; Lopez-Lopez, J. Oral manifestations of diabetes mellitus. A systematic review. *Med. Oral Patol. Oral Cir. Bucal.* **2017**, *22*, e586. [CrossRef]
193. Bharateesh, J.V.; Ahmed, M.; Kokila, G. Diabetes and oral health: A case-control study. *Int. J. Prev. Med.* **2012**, *3*, 806–809. [PubMed]
194. Meurman, J.H.; Collin, H.L.; Niskanen, L.; Töyry, J.; Alakuijala, P.; Keinänen, S.; Uusitupa, M. Saliva in non-insulin-dependent diabetic patients and control subjects: The role of the autonomic nervous system. *Oral Surg. Oral Med. Oral Pathol. Oral Radiol. Endodontol.* **1998**, *86*, 69–76. [CrossRef]
195. Bookout, G.P.; Ladd, M.; Short, R.E. *Burning Mouth Syndrome.*; StatPearls Publishing: Treasure Island, FL, USA, 2021.
196. Verhulst, M.J.L.; Loos, B.G.; Gerdes, V.E.A.; Teeuw, W.J. Evaluating all potential oral complications of diabetes mellitus. *Front. Endocrinol. (Lausanne)* **2019**, *10*, 56. [CrossRef] [PubMed]

197. Collin, H.-L.; Niskanen, L.; Uusitupa, M.; Töyry, J.; Collin, P.; Koivisto, A.-M.; Viinamäki, H.; Meurman, J.H. Oral symptoms and signs in elderly patients with type 2 diabetes mellitus. *Oral Surg. Oral Med. Oral Pathol. Oral Radiol. Endodontol.* **2000**, *90*, 299–305. [CrossRef] [PubMed]
198. Eltas, A.; Tozoğlu, Ü.; Keleş, M.; Canakci, V. Assessment of oral health in peritoneal dialysis patients with and without diabetes mellitus. *Perit. Dial. Int. J. Int. Soc. Perit. Dial.* **2012**, *32*, 81–85. [CrossRef] [PubMed]
199. Vesterinen, M.; Ruokonen, H.; Furuholm, J.; Honkanen, E.; Meurman, J.H. Clinical questionnaire study of oral health care and symptoms in diabetic vs. non-diabetic predialysis chronic kidney disease patients. *Clin. Oral Investig.* **2012**, *16*, 559–563. [CrossRef] [PubMed]
200. Bültzingslöwen, V.I.; Sollecito, T.P.; Fox, P.C.; Daniels, T.; Jonsson, R.; Lockhart, P.B.; Wray, D.; Brennan, M.T.; Carrozzo, M.; Gandera, B.; et al. Salivary dysfunction associated with systemic diseases: Systematic review and clinical management recommendations. *Oral Surg. Oral Med. Oral Pathol. Oral Radiol. Endodontol.* **2007**, *103*, S57.e1–S57.e15. [CrossRef]
201. Orellana, M.F.; Lagravère, M.O.; Boychuk, D.G.; Major, P.W.; Flores-Mir, C.; Ortho, C. Prevalence of xerostomia in population-based samples: A systematic review. *J. Public Health Dent.* **2006**, *66*, 152–158. [CrossRef] [PubMed]
202. Moore, P.A.; Guggenheimer, J.; Etzel, K.R.; Weyant, R.J.; Orchard, T. Type 1 diabetes mellitus, xerostomia, and salivary flow rates. *Oral Surg. Oral Med. Oral Pathol. Oral Radiol. Endodontol.* **2001**, *92*, 281–291. [CrossRef]
203. Ben-Aryeh, H.; Cohen, M.; Kanter, Y.; Szargel, R.; Laufer, D. Salivary composition in diabetic patients. *J. Diabet. Complicat.* **1988**, *2*, 96–99. [CrossRef]
204. López, M.E.; Colloca, M.E.; Páez, R.G.; Schallmach, J.N.; Koss, M.A.; Chervonagura, A. Salivary characteristics of diabetic children. *Braz. Dent. J.* **2003**, *14*, 26–31. [CrossRef]
205. Mata, A.D.; Marques, D.; Rocha, S.; Francisco, H.; Santos, C.; Mesquita, M.F.; Singh, J. Effects of diabetes mellitus on salivary secretion and its composition in the human. *Mol. Cell. Biochem.* **2004**, *261*, 137–142. [CrossRef] [PubMed]
206. Karjalainen, K.M. Salivary factors in children and adolescents with insulin-dependent diabetes mellitus. *Pediatr. Dent.* **1996**, *18*, 306–307.
207. Malicka, B.; Kaczmarek, U.; Skośkiewicz-Malinowska, K. Prevalence of xerostomia and the salivary flow rate in diabetic patients. *Adv. Clin. Exp. Med.* **2014**, *23*, 225–233. [CrossRef] [PubMed]
208. Vasconcelos, A.C.U.; Soares, M.S.M.; Almeida, P.C.; Soares, T.C. Comparative study of the concentration of salivary and blood glucose in type 2 diabetic patients. *J. Oral Sci.* **2010**, *52*, 293–298. [CrossRef] [PubMed]
209. Montaldo, L.; Montaldo, P.; Papa, A.; Caramico, N.; Toro, G. Effects of saliva substitutes on oral status in patients with Type 2 diabetes. *Diabet. Med.* **2010**, *27*, 1280–1283. [CrossRef] [PubMed]
210. Lasisi, T.J.; Fasanmade, A.A. Salivary flow and composition in diabetic and non-diabetic subjects. *Niger. J. Physiol. Sci.* **2012**, *27*, 79–82. [PubMed]
211. Chávez, E.M.; Borrell, L.N.; Taylor, G.W.; Ship, J.A. A longitudinal analysis of salivary flow in control subjects and older adults with type 2 diabetes. *Oral Surgery Oral Med. Oral Pathol. Oral Radiol. Endodontol.* **2001**, *91*, 166–173. [CrossRef]
212. Chavez, E.M.; Taylor, G.W.; Borrell, L.N.; Ship, J.A. Salivary function and glycemic control in older persons with diabetes. *Oral Surg. Oral Med. Oral Pathol. Oral Radiol. Endodontol.* **2000**, *89*, 305–311. [CrossRef]
213. Jawed, M.; Khan, R.N.; Shahid, S.M.; Azhar, A. protective effects of salivary factors in dental caries in diabetic patients of Pakistan. *Exp. Diabetes Res.* **2012**, *2012*, 1–5. [CrossRef] [PubMed]
214. Sandberg, G.E.; Sundberg, H.E.; Fjellstrom, C.A.; Wikblad, K.F. Type 2 diabetes and oral health. *Diabetes Res. Clin. Pract.* **2000**, *50*, 27–34. [CrossRef]
215. Kao, C.-H.; Tsai, S.-C.; Sun, S.-S. Scintigraphic evidence of poor salivary function in type 2 diabetes. *Diabetes Care* **2001**, *24*, 952–953. [CrossRef] [PubMed]
216. Khovidhunkit, S.O.P.; Suwantuntula, T.; Thaweboon, S.; Mitrirattanakul, S.; Chomkhakhai, U.; Khovidhunkit, W. Xerostomia, hyposalivation, and oral microbiota in type 2 diabetic patients: A preliminary study. *J. Med. Assoc. Thail.* **2009**, *92*, 1220–1228.
217. Lin, C.-C.; Sun, S.-S.; Kao, A.; Lee, C.-C. Impaired salivary function in patients with noninsulin-dependent diabetes mellitus with xerostomia. *J. Diabetes Complicat.* **2002**, *16*, 176–179. [CrossRef]
218. Quirino, M.R.; Birman, E.G.; Paula, C.R. Oral manifestations of diabetes mellitus in controlled and uncontrolled patients. *Braz. Dent. J.* **1995**, *6*, 131–136. [PubMed]
219. Newrick, P.G.; Bowman, C.; Green, D.; O'Brien, I.A.D.; Porter, S.R.; Scully, C.; Corrall, R.J.M. Parotid salivary secretion in diabetic autonomic neuropathy. *J. Diabet. Complicat.* **1991**, *5*, 35–37. [CrossRef]
220. Sandberg, G.E.; Wikblad, K.F. Oral dryness and peripheral neuropathy in subjects with type 2 diabetes. *J. Diabetes Complicat.* **2003**, *17*, 192–198. [CrossRef]
221. Lamey, P. -J.; Fisher, B.M.; Frier, B.M. The effects of diabetes and autonomic neuropathy on parotid salivary flow in man. *Diabet. Med.* **1986**, *3*, 537–540. [CrossRef]
222. Scully Cbe, C. Drug effects on salivary glands: Dry mouth. *Oral Dis.* **2003**, *9*, 165–176. [CrossRef] [PubMed]
223. Monteiro, M.M.; D'Epiro, T.T.S.; Bernardi, L.; Fossati, A.C.M.; dos Santos, M.F.; Lamers, M.L. Long-and short-term diabetes mellitus type 1 modify young and elder rat salivary glands morphology. *Arch. Oral Biol.* **2017**, *73*, 40–47. [CrossRef] [PubMed]
224. Carda, C.; Carranza, M.; Arriaga, A.; Díaz, A.; Peydró, A.; Gomez De Ferraris, M.E. Structural differences between alcoholic and diabetic parotid sialosis. *Med. Oral Patol. Oral Cir. Bucal* **2005**, *10*, 309–314.

225. Russotto, S.B. Asymptomatic parotid gland enlargement in diabetes mellitus. *Oral Surg. Oral Med. Oral Pathol.* **1981**, *52*, 594–598. [CrossRef]
226. Alves, M.; Calegari, V.C.; Cunha, D.A.; Saad, M.J.A.; Velloso, L.A.; Rocha, E.M. Increased expression of advanced glycation end-products and their receptor, and activation of nuclear factor kappa-B in lacrimal glands of diabetic rats. *Diabetologia* **2005**, *48*, 2675–2681. [CrossRef]
227. Fukuoka, C.Y.; Simões, A.; Uchiyama, T.; Arana-Chavez, V.E.; Abiko, Y.; Kuboyama, N.; Bhawal, U.K. The effects of low-power laser irradiation on inflammation and apoptosis in submandibular glands of diabetes-induced rats. *PLoS ONE* **2017**, *12*, e0169443. [CrossRef] [PubMed]
228. Ship, J.A.; Fischer, D.J. The relationship between dehydration and parotid salivary gland function in young and older healthy adults. *J. Gerontol. Ser. A: Biol. Sci. Med. Sci.* **1997**, *52*, M310–M319. [CrossRef]
229. Sreebny, L.M.; Schwartz, S.S. A reference guide to drugs and dry mouth. *Gerodontology* **1986**, *5*, 75–99. [CrossRef] [PubMed]
230. Ravindran, R.; Deepa, M.G.; Sruthi, A.K.; Kuruvila, C.; Priya, S.; Sunil, S.; Roopesh, G. Roopesh evaluation of oral health in type II diabetes mellitus patients. *Oral Maxillofac. Pathol. J.* **2015**, *6*, 525–531.
231. Kamaraj, D.R.; Bhushan, K.S.; Laxman, V.K.; Mathew, J. Detection of odoriferous subgingival and tongue microbiota in diabetic and nondiabetic patients with oral malodor using polymerase chain reaction. *Indian J. Dent. Res.* **2011**, *22*, 260–265. [CrossRef]
232. Koshimune, S.; Awano, S.; Gohara, K.; Kurihara, E.; Ansai, T.; Takehara, T. Low salivary flow and volatile sulfur compounds in mouth air. *Oral Surg. Oral Med. Oral Pathol. Oral Radiol. Endod.* **2003**, *96*, 38–41. [CrossRef]
233. Al-Zahrani, M.S.; Zawawi, K.H.; Austah, O.N.; Al-Ghamdi, H.S. Self reported halitosis in relation to glycated hemoglobin level in diabetic patients. *Open Dent. J.* **2011**, *5*, 154–157. [CrossRef] [PubMed]
234. Wray, L. The diabetic patient and dental treatment: An update. *Br. Dent. J.* **2011**, *211*, 209–215. [CrossRef] [PubMed]
235. Ship, J. Diabetes and oral health. *J. Am. Dent. Assoc.* **2003**, *134*, 4S–10S. [CrossRef]
236. Siddiqi, A.; Zafar, S.; Sharma, A.; Quaranta, A. Diabetes mellitus and periodontal disease: The call for interprofessional education and interprofessional collaborative care—A systematic review of the literature. *J. Interprof. Care* **2020**, 1–9. [CrossRef] [PubMed]
237. Siddiqi, A.; Zafar, S.; Sharma, A.; Quaranta, A. Diabetic patients' knowledge of the bidirectional link: Are dental health care professionals effectively conveying the message? *Aust. Dent. J.* **2019**, *64*, 312–326. [CrossRef] [PubMed]
238. Allen, E.M.; Ziada, H.M.; O'Halloran, D.; Clerehugh, V.; Allen, P.F. Attitudes, awareness and oral health-related quality of life in patients with diabetes. *J. Oral Rehabil.* **2008**, *35*, 218–223. [CrossRef] [PubMed]
239. Tomar, S.L.; Lester, A. Dental and other health care visits among U.S. adults with diabetes. *Diabetes Care* **2000**, *23*, 1505–1510. [CrossRef] [PubMed]
240. Sandberg, G.E.; Sundberg, H.E.; Wikblad, K.F. A controlled study of oral self-care and self-perceived oral health in type 2 diabetic patients. *Acta Odontol. Scand.* **2001**, *59*, 28–33. [CrossRef]
241. Moore, P.A.; Orchard, T.; Guggenheimer, J.; Weyant, R.J. Diabetes and oral health promotion: A survey of disease prevention behaviors. *J. Am. Dent. Assoc.* **2000**, *131*, 1333–1341. [CrossRef] [PubMed]
242. Jansson, H.; Lindholm, E.; Lindh, C.; Groop, L.; Bratthall, G. Type 2 diabetes and risk for periodontal disease: A role for dental health awareness. *J. Clin. Periodontol.* **2006**, *33*, 408–414. [PubMed]
243. Al Habashneh, R.; Khader, Y.; Hammad, M.M.; Almuradi, M. Knowledge and awareness about diabetes and periodontal health among Jordanians. *J. Diabetes Complicat.* **2010**, *24*, 409–414. [CrossRef] [PubMed]
244. Chapple, I.L.C.; Genco, R. Diabetes and periodontal diseases: Consensus report of the Joint EFP/AAP workshop on periodontitis and systemic diseases. *J. Periodontol.* **2013**, *84*, S106–S112. [CrossRef]
245. Ogurtsova, K.; da Rocha Fernandes, J.D.; Huang, Y.; Linnenkamp, U.; Guariguata, L.; Cho, N.H.; Cavan, D.; Shaw, J.E.; Makaroff, L.E. IDF Diabetes Atlas: Global estimates for the prevalence of diabetes for 2015 and 2040. *Diabetes Res. Clin. Pract.* **2017**, *128*, 40–50. [CrossRef]
246. Estrich, C.G.; Araujo, M.W.B.; Lipman, R.D. Prediabetes and diabetes screening in dental care settings: NHANES 2013 to 2016. *JDR Clin. Transl. Res.* **2019**, *4*, 76–85. [CrossRef]
247. Beagley, J.; Guariguata, L.; Weil, C.; Motala, A.A. Global estimates of undiagnosed diabetes in adults. *Diabetes Res. Clin. Pract.* **2014**, *103*, 150–160. [CrossRef] [PubMed]
248. Miller, A.; Ouanounou, A. Diagnosis, management, and dental considerations for the diabetic patient. *J. Can. Dent. Assoc.* **2020**, *86*, k8. [PubMed]
249. Marti Alamo, S.; Jimenez Soriano, Y.; Sarrion Perez, M. Dental considerations for the patient with diabetes. *J. Clin. Exp. Dent.* **2011**, *3*, e25–e30. [CrossRef]
250. Nathan, D.M.; Buse, J.B.; Davidson, M.B.; Ferrannini, E.; Holman, R.R.; Sherwin, R.; Zinman, B.; American Diabetes Association. European association for study of diabetes medical management of hyperglycemia in type 2 diabetes: A consensus algorithm for the initiation and adjustment of therapy: A consensus statement of the American diabetes association and the European association for the study of diabetes. *Diabetes Care* **2009**, *32*, 193–203. [CrossRef]
251. Bergman, S.A. Perioperative management of the diabetic patient. *Oral Surg. Oral Med. Oral Pathol. Oral Radiol. Endodontol.* **2007**, *103*, 731–737. [CrossRef] [PubMed]

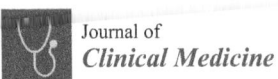

Article

Good Metabolic Control in Children with Type 1 Diabetes Mellitus: Does Glycated Hemoglobin Correlate with Interstitial Glucose Monitoring Using FreeStyle Libre?

Rocio Porcel-Chacón [1], Cristina Antúnez-Fernández [2], Maria Mora Loro [3], Ana-Belen Ariza-Jimenez [4,*], Leopoldo Tapia Ceballos [5], Jose Manuel Jimenez Hinojosa [5], Juan Pedro Lopez-Siguero [5] and Isabel Leiva Gea [5]

[1] Pediatrics, Hospital Costa del Sol, 29603 Marbella, Spain; rocio.porcel.86@gmail.com
[2] Endocrinology and Diabetes, Hospital de Algeciras, 11207 Cadiz, Spain; cristinaantunez1991@gmail.com
[3] Pediatrics, Hospital Regional de Malaga, 29010 Malaga, Spain; maria.mora.sspa@juntadeandalucia.es
[4] Pediatric Endocrinology, Hospital Universitario Reina Sofia, 14004 Cordoba, Spain
[5] Pediatric Endocrinology, Hospital Regional Materno-Infantil de Malaga, 29011 Malaga, Spain; leotapiaceb@hotmail.com (L.T.C.); jmjhinojosa@hotmail.com (J.M.J.H.); lopez.siguero@gmail.com (J.P.L.-S.); isabeleiva@hotmail.com (I.L.G.)
* Correspondence: micodemas@hotmail.com

Abstract: Background: Good metabolic control of Type 1 diabetes (T1D) leads to a reduction in complications. The only validated parameter for establishing the degree of control is glycated hemoglobin (HbA1c). We examined the relationship between HbA1c and a continuous glucose monitoring (CGM) system. Materials and methods: A cohort prospective study with 191 pediatric patients with T1D was conducted. Time in range (TIR), time below range (TBR), coefficient of variation (CV), number of capillary blood glucose tests, and HbA1c before sensor insertion and at one year of use were collected. Results: Patients were classified into five groups according to HbA1c at one year of using CGM. They performed fewer capillary blood glucose test at one year using CGM ($-6 +/- 2$, $p < 0.0001$). We found statistically significant differences in TIR between categories. Although groups with HbA1c < 6.5% and HbA1c 6.5–7% had the highest TIR (62.214 and 50.462%), their values were highly below optimal control according to CGM consensus. Groups with TBR < 5% were those with HbA1c between 6.5% and 8%. Conclusions: In our study, groups classified as well-controlled by guidelines were not consistent with good control according to the CGM consensus criteria. HbA1c should not be considered as the only parameter for metabolic control. CGM parameters allow individualized targets.

Keywords: type 1 diabetes mellitus; pediatric diabetes; continuous glucose monitoring; time in range; HbA1c; capillary blood glucose test

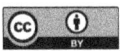

1. Introduction

Type 1 diabetes mellitus (T1D) is one of the most common chronic diseases in children. Due to its onset early in life and the lack of a definitive treatment, those affected live with the disease for a long time and, therefore, have a high burden of morbidity and mortality, since complications can arise both in the short and long term [1].

It has been shown that good metabolic control of the disease leads to a reduction in these complications [2,3]. The only currently validated parameter for establishing the degree of control of the disease is glycated hemoglobin (HbA1c), which, although providing very useful information, has a number of important limitations. It is an analytical parameter that reflects the average blood glucose values in the preceding two to three months. The main limitations are that it does not consider acute hypoglycemic and hyperglycemic events or the frequency and magnitude of intraday and interday blood glucose variability. Similarly, HbA1c values may be affected in situations such as anemia, hemoglobinopathies, or transfusions, among others [4,5].

In the 1980s, the Diabetes Control and Complications Trial (DCCT) demonstrated that those patients with T1D who were able to maintain HbA1c levels closer to those without diabetes had a lower incidence of microvascular and cardiovascular complications, both avoiding or delaying their onset (primary prevention) and slowing their progression (secondary prevention). In addition, it was found that initial metabolic control had a long-term influence on the subsequent clinical course, which was termed "metabolic memory". These data have been validated 30 years after the initial study with the Diabetes Control and Complications Trial/Epidemiology of Diabetes Interventions and Complications Study at 30 years (DCCT-EDIC) [6].

Targets for good disease control based on HbA1c levels vary depending on the consensus used [1,7]. All these guidelines agree that targets should be individualized for each patient (Table 1).

Table 1. Reference values for blood glucose and HbA1c according to different societies.

	NICE	ISPAD	ADA
Preprandial blood glucose (mg/dL)	70–126	70–130	90–130
Postprandial blood glucose (mg/dL)	90–162	90–180	
Bedtime glucose (mg/dL)	70–126	80–140	90–150
HbA1C (%)	≤6.5	<7	<7.5

NICE: The National Institute for Health and Care Excellence. ISPAD: International Society for Pediatric and Adolescent Diabetes. ADA: American Diabetes Association. HbA1c: glycated hemoglobin.

Since the advent of continuous glucose monitoring (CGM) systems, we have gained more information on the variability of blood glucose and on acute hypoglycemic and hyperglycemic events, all while decreasing the number of capillary blood glucose tests required.

From the data obtained from the CGM system downloads, efforts were made to identify a set of data that would serve as criteria for good or poor control of the disease. Accordingly, the ATTD (Advanced Technologies and Treatments for Diabetes) congress, reached a new consensus in which 10 parameters were defined [4,8] (Table 2).

Table 2. Standardized CGM parameters in the ATTD 2019 consensus and target values for T1D.

Variable	Target
1. Number of days of CGM	14 days
2. Percentage of time CGM was active	>70%
3. Mean glucose/standard deviation	<154 mg/dL/<29%
4. Glucose management indicator/estimated HbA1C	<7%
5. Glucose variability (coefficient of variation) (%)	<36%
6. Time in range from 70 to 180 mg/dL (% of time)	>70%/>16 h 48 min
7. Time above range >180 mg/dL (% of time) Hyperglycemia level 1	<25%
8. Duration hyperglycemia level 1	<6 h
9. Time above range >250 mg/dL (% of time) Hyperglycemia level 2	<5%
10. Duration hyperglycemia level 2	<1h 12 min
11. Time below range <70 mg/dL (% of time) Hypoglycemia level 1	<4%
12. Duration hypoglycemia level 1	<1 h
13. Time below range <54 mg/dL (% of time) Hypoglycemia level 2	<1%
14. Duration hypoglycemia level 2	<15 min

CGM: continuous glucose monitoring. ATTD: Advanced Technologies and Treatments for Diabetes. HbA1c: glycated hemoglobin. T1D: type 1 diabetes.

The FreeStyle Libre flash glucose monitoring system 1 (Abbott Diabetes Care, Witney, UK) is an established technology that measures interstitial fluid glucose levels. A sensor worn on the back of the upper arm takes a reading every minute that can be scanned using a hand-held reader or smartphone to receive a current glucose result along with historic results with a 15-min frequency. The FreeStyle Libre sensors are calibrated in the factory and have a wear time of up to 14 days without the need for the user to perform daily calibration using finger-prick tests [9].

The IMPACT and REPLACE studies [10,11] conducted with the FreeStyle Libre 1 sensor in adults with T1D or type 2 diabetes (T2D) on insulin therapy showed no decrease in HbA1c compared to SMBG. The SELFY study [12], performed in children and adolescents with T1D, reported a decrease in HbA1c from 7.9% to 7.4% after 8 weeks of sensor use compared to SMBG ($p < 0.001$). A meta-analysis [13] performed in 2019 analyzing results from 271 studies found a 0.55% (95% CI -0.70, -0.39) decrease in HbA1c 2–4 months after initiation of FreeStyle Libre 1 use in patients with T1D and T2D. In the 447 children and adolescents included, the mean decrease in HbA1c was 0.54% (95% CI -0.84, -0.23), and this improvement was maintained at 12 months. It was concluded that initiation of sensor use as part of diabetes management resulted in a decrease in HbA1c in adults and children with T1D and in adults with T2D.

The objective of our study is the evaluation of pediatric patients with T1D after one year of use of the Free Style Libre system, categorizing them by their HbA1c, in order to be able to know the differences in the number of capillary blood glucose controls before and after implantation, as well as CGM parameters that presents each category of HbA1c.

2. Material and Methods

2.1. Study Design and Participants

The funding of this study was in accordance with the regulations of the Official Gazette of the Andalusian Government (BOJA), resolution of 17 April 2018, regarding the organization of the Andalusian Health Service (SAS) to include CGM systems among the benefits provided by the Andalusian Public Health Service and a research project funded by the Andalusian Ministry of Health and Family (PIGE 0533-219).

This study was carried out from June of 2018 to September of 2019, following approval by the Ethics Committee of the Regional Hospital of Malaga. This prospective study was undertaken following insertion of the FreeStyle Libre 1 sensor in 191 pediatric patients with T1D. The inclusion criteria were presence of T1D with disease duration of more than one year, age between 4 and 18 years at the start of the study, and no previous experience using the FreeStyle Libre 1. Furthermore, only those patients who had more than 80% use of the sensor were included.

The exclusion criteria were having previously used interstitial blood glucose monitoring or having anemia or hemoglobinopathy that could constitute a bias.

Finally, we subdivided all patients in different groups according to cut-off points of HbA1c:

Group 1 HbA1c $\leq 6.5\%$
Group 2 HbA1c 6.5–7% (more than 6.5 and less than or equal to 7)
Group 3 HbA1c 7–7.5% (more than 7 and less than or equal to 7.5)
Group 4 HbA1c 7.5–8% (more than 7 and less than or equal to 8)
Group 5 HbA1c $\geq 8\%$

2.2. Variables

The data were extracted using the LibreView® platform (Abbott Diabetes Care, Witney, UK) one year after insertion of the FreeStyle Libre 1 sensor (Abbott Diabetes Care, Witney, UK), taking into account the last 14 days of use prior to the office visit. The parameters collected were those accepted in the consensus guidelines on the interpretation of CGM [4,5,7]: time in range (TIR), percentage of time below range (TBR), and coefficient of variation (CV), as well as average number of scans per day. In addition to these variables, we also analyzed sex, age, and the number of capillary blood glucose tests performed before sensor insertion and one year later. HbA1c values were also obtained before sensor insertion and at one year of use. The determination was made through a capillary blood sample using the DCA Vantage analyzer system (immunoassay technique) in the laboratory of the Regional Hospital of Malaga.

Capillary blood glucose measurements were collected after downloading the last 14 days of the glucometer in use prior to sensor insertion. Collection of capillary blood glucose readings at one year was performed by downloading the glucometer in use. For all patients, this could be done through the LibreView® platform, as they were using the reader with a glucometer function with FreeStyle Optium® capillary blood glucose strips.

Clinical data were collected through a written questionnaire completed by the primary caregiver and supervised by the healthcare team.

3. Statistical Analysis

All analyses were performed with R (R Core Team, 2020, University of Auckland, CAL, USA). Normality and homoscedasticity were tested using the Anderson–Darling and Fligner–Killeen tests, respectively. For quantitative variables, the statistics (mean and standard deviation) were reported, and for categorical variables, the absolute and relative frequencies were reported. To study the relationship between each of the quantitative variables of two groups or samples, the p-value associated with the Student's t-test or nonparametric test such as Wilcoxon test, when normality was not proven were conducted. To study the relationship between each of the quantitative variables of several groups or samples, the p-value associated with the Kruskall–Wallis test was used. In the case of two categorical variables, Fisher's test or the chi-square test was used.

4. Results

4.1. Difference in the Number of Capillary Blood Glucose Tests Performed per Day

The patients were classified into five groups according to their HbA1c at one year of using the FreeStyle Libre 1 sensor. The differences in the effect of the sensor were explored between the different groups and within the same group, before using the sensor and at one year of use (Table 3).

In most of the groups, the patients performed fewer capillary blood glucose tests one year after insertion of the sensor (mean: −6.0, standard deviation: 2.0). For statistical analysis, the Wilcoxon signed-rank test for paired samples was used. Statistically significant differences were found between the number of capillary blood glucose tests before and after the use of the sensor within each group (V = 23, p-value < 0.0001).

To assess the difference in the number of capillary blood glucose tests between the different groups, we used the Kruskal–Wallis nonparametric test. There were no significant differences between the groups (Kruskal–Wallis, chi-squared = 4.5977, standard deviation = 4.0, p-value 0.3311) (Figure 1).

4.2. Monitoring Parameters

TIR is defined as the time during which blood glucose levels are between two points, usually in the range 70–180 mg/dL or 70–140 mg/dL. Statistically significant differences were found in both TIRs 70–180 mg/dL and 70–140 mg/dL between the different groups (Table 3).

According to the aim of TIR ≥ 70%, 33.33% of group 1 achieved time in range, while 12% of group 2 and 9.37% of group 3 achieved time in range.

TBR is defined as the percentage of time in which blood glucose is ≤70 mg/dL. We found no statistically significant differences between the different HbA1c categories (Table 3).

CV is a measure of glucose variability derived from the standard deviation and the interquartile range. No statistical significance was observed between the different HbA1c categories (p-value 0.054) (Table 3).

Table 3. Patients categorized by level of glycated hemoglobin one year after sensor use with results of different variables.

		HbA1c ≤ 6.5% (n = 58)	HbA1c 6.5–7% (n = 49)	HbA1c 7–7.5% (n = 38)	HbA1C 7.5–8% (n = 28)	HbA1c ≥ 8% (n = 18)	p-Value (Kruskal–Wallis)
Sex	Boys	28 (48.3%)	28 (57.1%)	18 (47.4%)	15 (53.6%)	10 (55.6%)	NS
	Girls	30 (51.7%)	21 (42.9%)	20 (42.9%)	13 (46.4%)	8 (44.4%)	
Age (years) Mean (SD)		10.8 (3.3)	11.7 (3)	10.8 (3.4)	10.6 (2.5)	12.2 (2.3)	NS
No. capillary blood glucose/day baseline Mean (SD)		7.0 (1.4)	7.2 (1.4)	6.7 (1.1)	7.3 (1.6)	6.4 (1.1)	NS
Miss		9	5	9	1	2	
No. capillary blood glucose/day after a year Mean (SD)		1.3 (1.9)	0.9 (1.5)	0.7 (1.2)	1 (1.6)	1.4 (2.2)	NS
Miss		5	2	0	1	0	
% TIR (Glucose 70–180 ng/mL) Mean (SD)		62.214 (11.584)	50.462 (10.856)	47.625 (13.995)	39.385 (6.104)	32.636 (7.953)	<0.001
Miss		2	0	0	0	0	
% TIR (Glucose 70–140 ng/mL) Mean (SD)		40.923 (12.114)	30.885 (9.253)	26.781 (9.797)	22.538 (3.843)	17.636 (5.143)	<0.001
Miss		3	0	0	0	0	
% TBR Mean (SD)		5.397 (5.474)	4.271 (4.321)	3.789 (3.699)	3.667 (4.010)	5.167 (4.890)	NS
Miss		0	1	0	1	0	
CV Mean (SD)		38.562 (10.315)	38.983 (8.899)	40.170 (7.359)	37.544 (6.224)	44.078 (8.917)	0.054
Miss		0	1	0	1	0	
Scanning frequency (SD)		9.857 (3.035)	9.120 (3.113)	10.875 (7.129)	11.538 (4.612)	7.545 (3.830)	0.238
Miss		2	1	0	0	0	

TIR: time in range measured in percentage. TBR: percentage of time below 70 mg/dL. CV: coefficient of variation measured in percentage. SD: standard deviation. NS: Not significant. HbA1c: glycated hemoglobin.

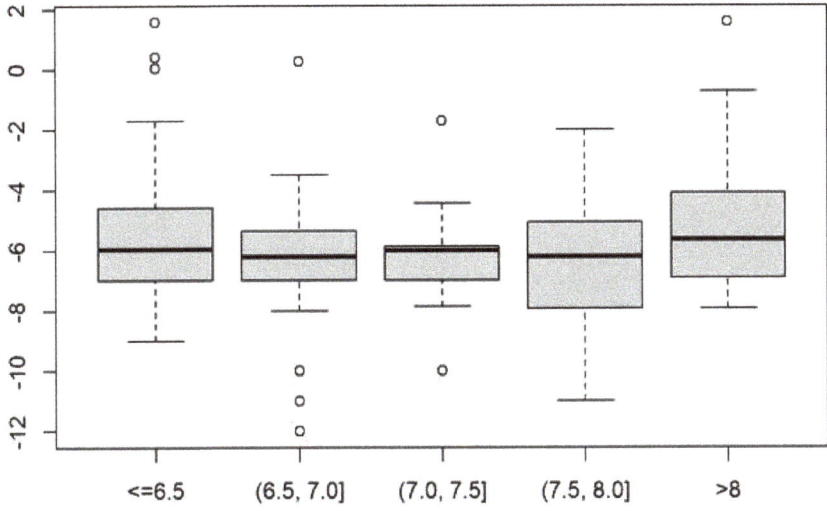

Figure 1. Difference in the lowest number of capillary blood glucose readings per day between the different capillary glycated hemoglobin groups one year after sensor insertion.

Table 3 reports TBR, which allowed us to observe that the lower TIR was not due to the higher TBR, since in most categories it was close to the recommended one (less than 5%); thus, it is the highest time above range which would explain the shortest time in range that we observed in the data.

5. Discussion

According to the data extracted from the latest ISPAD consensus, good metabolic control based solely on HbA1c is considered to have a value less than 7% [1,7]. However, although group 1 (HbA1c ≤ 6.5%) had the highest TIR between 70 and 180 mg/dL, the mean of this percentage was 62.214%, below the value accepted by the CGM Consensus [4,8] for optimal control, which is set at TIR ≥ 70%. Group 2 (HbA1c 6.5–7%) (which would also be within the good control group per the ISPAD) had a mean TIR of 50.462%. Thus, we can conclude that the HbA1c accepted as optimal for good metabolic control (≤7%) does not correspond to an adequate TIR value (≥70%). The data obtained from our study indicate that the groups classified as well-controlled by the NICE (The National Institute for Health and Care Excellence, UK), ISPAD (International Society for Pediatric and Adolescent Diabetes, Berlin, Germany), and ADA (American Diabetes Association, Virginia, USA) guidelines (≤6.5%, ≤7%, and ≤7.5%, respectively) [1,7] are not consistent with good control according to the CGM consensus criteria. With these results, data are presented that support a new paradigm for metabolic control of T1D, in which the validity of HbA1c is not considered as the only parameter for metabolic control of the disease. The incorporation of CGM parameters allows for clear and individualized metabolic control targets in terms of hyperglycemia, hypoglycemia, and variability, underscoring the need for scalability of therapies that allow these targets to be achieved. Longer studies to correlate the recommended monitoring parameters with long-term macrovascular and microvascular complications are needed.

Several studies to date have attempted to correlate HbA1c with TIR in T1D patients. In 2019, two meta-analyses [14,15] were performed that sought evidence of this association. The first of these [14] studied 545 adult patients with T1D and compared HbA1c with different CGM parameters. It was concluded that CGM measures relevant to hyperglycemia (including TIR and mean glucose) were highly correlated with each other but moderately correlated with HbA1c, meaning that a particular TIR or change in a patient's TIR could be associated with a wide range of HbA1c values. The second [15] included a total of 1137 adult patients with T1D in whom data correlating percentage of TIR and HbA1c were analyzed. It was concluded that there was a strong relationship between the two, with every 10% change in TIR resulting in a 0.8% change in HbA1c.

The percentage of TBR considered optimal is ≤5%. We found that the groups meeting this parameter were those with HbA1c 6.5–7%, 7–7.5%, and 7.5–8%, while the groups with HbA1c ≤ 6.5% and over 8% had higher values than those recommended.

We also noted a sharp decrease in the number of daily capillary glucose tests in all groups with the use of the FreeStyle Libre system 1, which is associated with greater convenience for the patient. Pediatric patients with T1D had a mean of 7–8 capillary blood glucose tests per day for metabolic control, with physical deterioration (skin of the hands) and the social stigmatization associated with the continuous handling of blood.

6. Conclusions

Harmonization of the recommendations for glycated hemoglobin and for time-in-range is lacking, as patients with glycated hemoglobin considered to be adequately controlled have lower time-in-range averages than those recommended for the pediatric population. Long-term studies correlating monitoring parameters with long-term complications are needed to identify monitoring targets that reduce macrovascular and microvascular complications.

Author Contributions: Writing-original draft, R.P.-C.; Investigation, C.A.-F.; Formal analysis, M.M.L.; Writing-review, A.-B.A.-J.; Data curation, L.T.C.; Resources and project administration, J.M.J.H.; Supervision and validation, J.P.L.-S.; Methodology and conceptualization, I.L.G. All authors have read and agreed to the published version of the manuscript.

Funding: The funding of this study was in accordance with the regulations of the Official Gazette of the Andalusian Government (BOJA), resolution of 17 April 2018, regarding the organization of the Andalusian Health Service (SAS) to include CGM systems among the benefits provided by the Andalusian Public Health Service and a research project funded by the Andalusian Ministry of Health and Family (PIGE 0533-219).

Institutional Review Board Statement: The study was conducted according to the guidelines of Declaration of Helsinki, and approved by Ethics Committee of the Regional Hospital of Malaga.

Informed Consent Statement: Informed consent was obtained from all subjects involved in the study.

Conflicts of Interest: The authors declare no conflict of interest.

References

1. American Diabetes Association. 13. Children and Adolescents: *Standards of Medical Care in Diabetes—2019*. Diabetes Care **2019**, *42* (Suppl. 1), S148–S164. [CrossRef] [PubMed]
2. Maahs, D.M.; Hermann, J.M.; DuBose, S.N.; Miller, K.M.; Heidtmann, B.; Di Meglio, L.A.; Rami-Merhar, B.; Beck, R.W.; Schober, E.; Tamborlane, W.V.; et al. Contrasting the clinical care and outcomes of 2622 children with type 1 diabetes less than 6 years of age in the United States T1D Exchange and German/Austrian DPV registries. *Diabetologia* **2014**, *57*, 1578–1585. [CrossRef] [PubMed]
3. Swift, P.G.; Skinner, T.C.; de Beaufort, C.E.; Cameron, F.J.; Aman, J.; Aanstoot, H.J.; Castaño, L.; Chiarelli, F.; Daneman, D.; Hvidoere Study Group on Childhood Diabetes. Target setting in intensive insulin management is associated with metabolic control: The Hvidoere childhood diabetes study group centre differences study 2005. *Pediatr. Diabetes* **2010**, *11*, 271–278. [CrossRef] [PubMed]
4. Danne, T.; Nimri, R.; Battelino, T.; Bergenstal, R.M.; Close, K.L.; DeVries, J.H.; Garg, S.; Heinemann, L.; Hirsch, I.; Amiel, S.A.; et al. International Consensus on Use of Continuous Glucose Monitoring. *Diabetes Care* **2017**, *40*, 1631–1640. [CrossRef] [PubMed]
5. American Diabetes Association. 6. Glycemic Targets: *Standards of Medical Care in Diabetes—2019*. Diabetes Care **2019**, *42* (Suppl. 1), S61–S70.
6. Nathan, D.M.; DCCT/EDIC Research Group. The diabetes control and complications trial/epidemiology of diabetes interventions and complications study at 30 years: Overview. *Diabetes Care* **2014**, *37*, 9–16. [CrossRef] [PubMed]
7. DiMeglio, L.A.; Acerini, C.L.; Codner, E.; Craig, M.E.; Hofer, S.E.; Pillay, K.; Maahs, D.M. ISPAD Clinical Practice Consensus Guidelines 2018: Glycemic control targets and glucose monitoring for children, adolescents, and young adults with diabetes. *Pediatr. Diabetes* **2018**, *19* (Suppl. 27), 105–114. [CrossRef] [PubMed]
8. Battelino, T.; Danne, T.; Bergenstal, R.M.; Amiel, S.A.; Beck, R.; Biester, T.; Bosi, E.; Buckingham, B.A.; Cefalu, W.T.; Close, K.L.; et al. Clinical Targets for Continuous Glucose Monitoring Data Interpretation: Recommendations from the International Consensus on Time in Range. *Diabetes Care* **2019**, *42*, 1593–1603. [CrossRef] [PubMed]
9. Bailey, T.; Bode, B.W.; Christiansen, M.P.; Klaff, L.J.; Alva, S. The Performance and Usability of a Factory-Calibrated Flash Glucose Monitoring System. *Diabetes Technol. Ther.* **2015**, *17*, 787–794. [CrossRef] [PubMed]
10. Bolinder, J.; Antuna, R.; Geelhoed-Duijvestijn, P.; Kröger, J.; Weitgasser, R. Novel glucose-sensing technology and hypoglycaemia in type 1 diabetes: A multicentre, non-masked, randomised controlled trial. *Lancet* **2016**, *388*, 2254–2263. [CrossRef]
11. Haak, T.; Hanaire, H.; Ajjan, R.; Hermanns, N.; Riveline, J.P.; Rayman, G. Flash Glucose-Sensing Technology as a Replacement for Blood Glucose Monitoring for the Management of Insulin-Treated Type 2 Diabetes: A Multicenter, Open-Label Randomized Controlled Trial. *Diabetes Ther.* **2017**, *8*, 55–73. [CrossRef] [PubMed]
12. Campbell, F.M.; Murphy, N.P.; Stewart, C.; Biester, T.; Kordonouri, O. Outcomes of using flash glucose monitoring technology by children and young people with type 1 diabetes in a single arm study. *Pediatr. Diabetes* **2018**, *19*, 1294–1301. [CrossRef] [PubMed]
13. Evans, M.; Welsh, Z.; Ells, S.; Seibold, A. The Impact of Flash Glucose Monitoring on Glycaemic Control as Measured by HbA1c: A Meta-analysis of Clinical Trials and Real-World Observational Studies. *Diabetes Ther.* **2020**, *11*, 83–95. [CrossRef] [PubMed]
14. Beck, R.W.; Bergenstal, R.M.; Cheng, P.; Kollman, C.; Carlson, A.L.; Johnson, M.L.; Rodbard, D. The Relationships Between Time in Range, Hyperglycemia Metrics, and HbA1c. *J. Diabetes Sci. Technol.* **2019**, *13*, 614–626. [CrossRef] [PubMed]
15. Vigersky, R.A.; McMahon, C. The Relationship of Hemoglobin A1C to Time-in-Range in Patients with Diabetes. *Diabetes Technol. Ther.* **2019**, *21*, 81–85. [CrossRef] [PubMed]

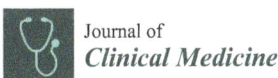

Review

Heart Failure in Type 1 Diabetes: A Complication of Concern? A Narrative Review

Ana María Gómez-Perez [1,2,3], **Miguel Damas-Fuentes** [1,2], **Isabel Cornejo-Pareja** [1,2,3],* and **Francisco J. Tinahones** [1,2,3]

1. Department of Endocrinology and Nutrition, Virgen de la Victoria University Hospital, 29010 Málaga, Spain; anamgp86@gmail.com (A.M.G.-P.); migueldamasf@hotmail.com (M.D.-F.); fjtinahones@hotmail.com (F.J.T.)
2. Instituto de Investigación Biomédica de Málaga (IBIMA), Cellular and Molecular Endocrinology, Virgen de la Victoria University Hospital, 29010 Málaga, Spain
3. Spanish Biomedical Research Center in Physiopathology of Obesity and Nutrition (CIBERObn), Instituto de Salud Carlos III, 28029 Madrid, Spain
* Correspondence: isabelmaria_cornejo@hotmail.com; Tel.: +34-95-103-4044

Abstract: Heart failure (HF) has been a hot topic in diabetology in the last few years, mainly due to the central role of sodium-glucose cotransporter 2 inhibitors (iSGLT2) in the prevention and treatment of cardiovascular disease and heart failure. It is well known that HF is a common complication in diabetes. However, most of the knowledge about it and the evidence of cardiovascular safety trials with antidiabetic drugs refer to type 2 diabetes (T2D). The epidemiology, etiology, and pathophysiology of HF in type 1 diabetes (T1D) is still not well studied, though there are emerging data about it since life expectancy for T1D has increased in the last decades and there are more elderly patients with T1D. The association of T1D and HF confers a worse prognosis than in T2D, thus it is important to investigate the characteristics, risk factors, and pathophysiology of this disease in order to effectively design prevention strategies and therapeutic tools.

Keywords: type 1 diabetes; heart failure; cardiovascular disease; diabetic myocardiopathy

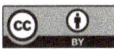

1. Introduction

Heart failure (HF) is one of the most frequent causes of hospital admission and has a poor prognosis in most cases, despite great pharmacological advances developed in recent decades for heart failure with reduced ejection fraction (HFrEF; left ventricular ejection fraction < 40%) [1]. In addition, there is a group of patients with an ejection fraction > 50% (heart failure with preserved ejection fraction or HFpEF), who also have a poor prognosis, but for whom there are still no proven effective therapies [2]. In the field of diabetes, thanks to the role of several pharmacological groups in the prevention of cardiovascular events, among which is hospitalization for HF, this condition has acquired a central role as one of the most frequent complications of type 2 diabetes (T2D) [3]. However, it is also gaining more interest in patients with type 1 diabetes (T1D), especially due to the longer life expectancy that makes it easier to find older patients with long-standing T1D. In fact, epidemiological evidence shows us that diabetes increases the risk of HF twice in men and up to five times in women [4]. Among patients with diabetes, an estimated 40% have HF, with higher mortality and risk of hospitalization than patients without diabetes [5].

Although due to the development of sodium-glucose cotransporter 2 inhibitors (iSGLT2) and glucagon-like peptide 1 analogues (aGLP1), the evidence on heart failure in T2D is growing and extensive, in T1D there is a paucity of data. In this review, we will focus on the evidence about HF in T1D with a special interest in the epidemiology, risk factors, and pathophysiology of this complication.

2. Epidemiology and Risk Factors

2.1. Epidemiology

Until a few years ago, most epidemiological and long-term follow-up studies on diabetes were focused on classic cardiovascular complications with an atherosclerotic profile. However, thanks to the data from the cardiovascular safety studies of new antidiabetic drugs, more and more studies with epidemiological data are being published also on T1D, though its incidence and prevalence are not well established. In a 10-year retrospective study performed by McAllister et al. of over 3.25 million people without DM and with T2D and T1D, there were 1313 events of HF among patients with T1D. The crude incidence rate of hospitalization for HF in the T1D group was 5.6 per 1000 person-years compared to 2.4 in patients without diabetes and 12.4 in patients with T2D. However, the case-fatality rate was higher in patients with T1D than people without diabetes mellitus; the difference was larger for men (OR, 1.91; 95% CI, 1.68–2.18) than for women (OR, 1.31; 95% CI, 1.05–1.65) [6].

In a recent observational study, Kristófi et al. analyzed a population of 59,331 patients with T1D and 484,241 patients with T2D in Sweden and Norway, looking for the prevalence and event rates of myocardial infarction, HF, stroke, chronic kidney disease, all-cause death, and cardiovascular death. They observed that patients with T1D had a higher risk of HF and renal disease in different age groups than patients with T2D. The age-adjusted risk for patients 65–79 years showed that the risk of heart failure was 1.3 to 1.4 times higher in patients with T1D than with T2D. They also found greater cardiovascular mortality in T1D in patients above 55 years [7]. Similarly, in a recent meta-analysis carried out by Cai et al. that included 10 observational studies with 166,027 patients, a relative risk of heart failure of 4.29 (95% CI 3.42–4.86) was observed in patients with T1D compared with healthy controls. This meta-analysis suggests that T1D is associated with an increased risk of several cardiovascular diseases, among them HF [8].

In another recent paper, Chadalavada et al. investigated the effect of diabetes in mortality and incident HF with the entire population of the UK Biobank. They included a total population of 493,167 participants, of which 22,685 had diabetes (4.6%). They found a hazard ratio (HR) for HF of 1.9 (CI 95% 1.7–2) among patients with diabetes compared to healthy controls. Interestingly, they found that women with T1D had an 88% increased risk of HF compared to men (HR 4.7 (CI 95% 3.6-6.2) vs 2.5 (CI 95% 2.0–3.0), respectively) and this association was independent of confounding factors. In T2D, the risk of HF was also greater in women but to a lesser extent [9]. On the incidence of HF in T1D, Avogaro et al. performed a systematic review and meta-analysis, including 6 studies published between 1990 and 2018. In their age-adjusted model, the incidence rate of HF in patients with T1D was 3.18 ($p < 0.001$) compared to the general population [10]. Finally, in a nationwide retrospective study performed in Korea, Lee et al. explored HR for cardiovascular disease and early death in people with T1D compared with people with T2D and healthy controls. During more than 93,300,000 person-years of follow-up, they found an HR of hospitalization for HF of 2.105 (CI 95% 1.901–2.330) in T1D compared to T2D and an HR of 3.024 (CI 95% 2.730–3.350) compared to the non-diabetes group. This greater risk for HF in T1D remained after adjustment for fasting plasma glucose and some cardiovascular risk factors, such as smoking, dyslipidemia, hypertension, physical activity, or body mass index, among others [11].

2.2. Risk Factors

Cardiovascular risk factors are well established and data from the Diabetes Control and Complications Trial (DCCT) and its observational follow-up Epidemiology of Diabetes Interventions and Complications (EDIC) demonstrated that an early period of 6–7 years of intensive glycemic control significantly reduced the risk for cardiovascular disease. Although the effect tends to decrease over the years, it remains highly significant 30 years later (a reduction of 30% compared to conventional treatment; $p = 0.016$) [12,13]. However, the presence of diastolic dysfunction has been demonstrated even in adolescent and young adult patients with T1D, as potential early markers of heart failure [14,15]. Moreover, some studies suggest that multiple risk factor control reduces the risk for myocardial infarction or stroke but has little association with the risk for HF in T1D [16]. Therefore, the study and identification of risk factors for HF in people with T1D are key points to improve the detection, management, and prognosis of this complication.

Regarding glycemic control, the data from DCCT/EDIC studies showed that glycemic control represented as HbA1c was the strongest modifiable risk factor for congestive heart failure after 29 years of follow-up in 1441 patients with T1D. Each 1% increase in HbA1c produced an incidence ratio of 3.15 ($p < 0.01$) for congestive heart failure [12]. Therefore, early intensive therapy seems to have an effect in reducing HF risk in the long-term (five-fold difference among intensive therapy group and conventional treatment), though in the analysis at 30 years, the number of events related to HF were too small to establish a definitive conclusion [13]. In line with these results, Rawshani et al. assessed the relative prognostic importance of 17 risk factors on cardiovascular outcomes in a nationwide register of patients with diabetes in Sweden. For HF, they found that the most important predictors were albuminuria (β-coefficient 3.63 (3.05–4.31)), HbA1c (β-coefficient 1.025 (1.020–1.030)), and systolic blood pressure ((β-coefficient 1.35 (1.25–1.44)) [17]. Kristófi et al. [7], in line with previously published data that identified albuminuria and chronic kidney disease (CKD) as risk factors for cardiovascular disease in T1D [18,19], found that prevalent and incident CKD are more common in T1D than in T2D. These higher levels of kidney impairment may play a role in higher rates of cardiovascular disease, reinforcing the importance of cardiorenal syndrome.

A possible explanation for this greater risk of renal and cardiovascular disease, and among them HF, is that the disease duration is often longer in T1D than T2D. Therefore, the probability of microvascular complications and the effects of hyperglycemia in cardiovascular outcomes are greater in T1D [7]. In fact, in the meta-regression analysis performed by Avogaro et al., age was significantly associated with the incidence ratio of HF [10]. Another study by McAllister and colleagues of over 3.25 million people among which there were 18,240 subjects with T1D, found that by the age of 20 years the prevalence of HF is similar among patients with T1D and T2D, but by the age of 80 years the prevalence of HF is higher in T1D and the same occurs with case-fatality rate, suggesting that the accumulation of risk factors and more prevalent microvascular complications in this group may contribute to higher incident and prevalent HF. Another hypothesis suggested in this study was that lower rates of prescription drugs known to reduce the risk of HF, such as antihypertensives, drugs acting on the renin-angiotensin system, or lipid lowering drugs, may also contribute to higher incident and prevalent HF. However, differences remained despite the older mean age of patients with T2D and after adjusting for individual risk of HF according to baseline characteristics. Though these are data from a retrospective study and some information was taken from clinical recordings with a risk of missing information, it is a very interesting hypothesis to consider [6].

Another emerging field of investigation in HF in T1D that may be intimately linked to glycemic control is cardiac autoimmunity. In an analysis derived from DCCT/EDIC, Sousa et al. measured the prevalence and profiles of cardiac autoantibodies in samples from DCCT and divided them in two groups, patients with HbA1c > 9% (n = 83) and patients with HbA1c < 7% (n = 83) at 26 years of follow-up. The same analysis was performed in similar groups of patients with T2D. They found that the DCCT HbA1c > 9% group had significantly higher levels of cardiac autoantibodies than the DCCT HbA1 < 7% group, while glycemic control was not related to cardiac autoimmunity in T2D. Moreover, positivity for two or more autoantibodies during DCCT was associated with a greater risk of cardiovascular disease (HR 16.1 [95% CI 3.0–88.2]) and coronary artery calcification (OR 60.1 [95% CI 8.4–410.0]) [20]. The same authors recently published a study showing that cardiac autoimmunity is related to subclinical myocardial dysfunction, independent of classical cardiovascular disease risk factors. They observed in a sample from DCCT that patients with two or more cardiac autoantibodies had greater left ventricular end-diastolic volume, end-systolic volume, left ventricular mass, and lower left ventricular ejection fraction [21]. These observations suggest that there are different mechanisms for cardiovascular disease and thus for HF in T1D and T2D and those mechanisms may be tightly related to long exposure to hyperglycemia in T1D.

Finally, regarding risk factors, there is an interesting study carried out by Khedr et al. on 78 adolescents with T1D of at least 6 years of duration, in whom they analyzed some lipid biomarkers as predictors of diastolic dysfunction. They found diastolic failure to occur in 50% of the females and 66.6% of the males, and described that lower high-density lipoproteins (HDL) (OR 0.93, 95% CI 0.88–0.99) and a higher total cholesterol/HDL ratio (OR 2.55, 95% CI 1.9–5.45) and triglycerides/HDL ratio (OR 2.74, 95% CI 1.12–6.71) were associated with diastolic failure [22].

Considering that classical risk factors seem to be important, but it also seems that HF in T1D has differential characteristics, it is necessary to continue investigating the most important risk factors for the development of this complication (Figure 1).

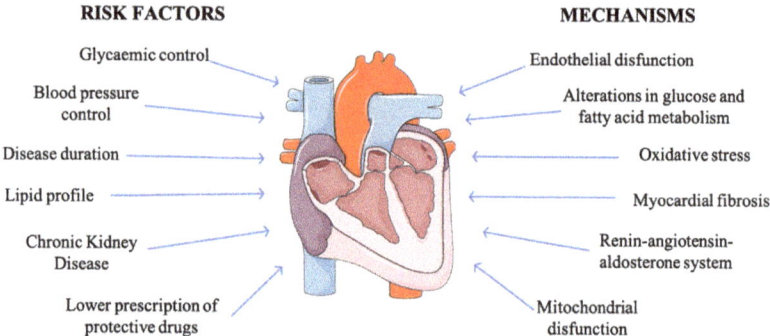

Figure 1. Risk factors and pathophysiology of heart failure in diabetes.

3. Pathophysiology

The mechanisms responsible for the association between diabetes and heart failure are not entirely clear, although a great variety of them have been proposed, such as endothelial dysfunction, alterations in glucose and fatty acid metabolism at the myocardial level, myocardial fibrosis, the increase in oxidative stress, or the activation of local neurohormonal systems, such as the renin-angiotensin-aldosterone system, endothelin, or the sympathetic nervous system [23] (Figure 1). It has also been proposed that some of these mechanisms can cause systolic or diastolic ventricular dysfunction even in the absence of coronary artery disease or structural disease [5]. There is a multitude of preclinical data, but they are still to be clarified.

Diabetic cardiomyopathy pathophysiology is widely studied in T2D, while its mechanisms in T1D are less clear. Hyperglycemia and chronic inflammation present in both types, promoting cardiac hypertrophy and fibrosis, increasing myocardial stiffness, and resulting in diastolic and systolic dysfunction. Increased levels of glucose lead to a higher production of advanced glycation end products (AGEs), which have been suggested to trigger deleterious effects on ventricular function through the formation of crosslinks between collagen molecules in the extracellular matrix, impairing its degradation and leading to myocardial stiffness and diastolic dysfunction [24]. Activated endothelial cells also contribute by promoting the uncoupling of endothelial nitric oxide synthase (NOS) resulting in diminished nitric oxide (NO) levels. This decreases soluble guanylate cyclase (sGC) activity and cyclic guanosine monophosphate (cGMP) content in the myocardium, which impairs the protective effects of protein kinase G (PKG) [25].

Due to the insulinopenia in T1DM, fatty acid β-oxidation is increased to maintain adenosine triphosphate (ATP) producti; however, this process becomes ineffective during diabetes evolution, resulting in intracellular lipid accumulation and lipotoxicity [26]. Increased intracellular fatty acid concentration and mitochondrial dysfunction lead to an increased production of reactive oxygen species (ROS). Excess ROS production causes the activation of cellular and mitochondrial nitrogen oxides (NOX), which leads to the generation of superoxide and hydrogen peroxide [27]. These effects result in cardiomyocyte loss, cardiac hypertrophy, and inflammation with fibrosis of the extracellular matrix [28]. N-acetylcysteine (NAC) has been used as an antioxidant in mouse models of T1D to normalize oxidative stress and therefore prevent the development of cardiomyopathy [29].

Mitochondrial dysfunction is usually found in cardiac tissue in T1D patients. Decreased mitochondrial oxidative capacity is caused by altered mitochondrial ultrastructure, proteomic remodeling, and oxidative damage to proteins and mitochondrial DNA [30].

Concerning cardiac inflammation, the infiltration of macrophages and lymphocytes is usual in DM. These inflammatory cells secrete cytokines, such as tumor necrosis factor (TNF), interleukin 6 (IL-6), interleukin 1β (IL-1β), interferon-γ, and transforming growth factor β (TGFβ) that can produce profibrotic responses, leading to further adverse remodeling. Studies in mice have detected higher T-cell infiltration in the myocardium in T1D [31] and some attempts to reduce cardiac fibrosis by decreasing T-cell trafficking have been successful [32]. Regarding the immune system, as we mention before, Sousa et al. observed higher levels of cardiac autoantibodies in patients with T1D and poor glycemic control, and patients positive for ≥2 cardiac autoantibodies were more likely to have subclinical myocardial dysfunction as well as a higher cardiovascular disease risk. Chronic hyperglycemia may cause subclinical myocardial injury favoring the exposure of heart muscle proteins as α-myosin to the immune system. In patients with T1D and poor glycemic control, the immune system is dysregulated and may overreact to these proteins, producing an expansion of proinflammatory CD4 T-cells specific to α-myosin and the development of autoantibodies [20,21].

Another mechanism implicated in the pathophysiology in T1D mouse models is increased cardiomyocyte intracellular Ca^{2+} due to lower sarcoplasmic reticulum Ca^{2+} pump activity because of the decreased glucose transporter type 4 (GLUT 4) recruitment to the plasma membrane, mediating this disturbance in contractile dysfunction and arrhythmia [33].

Renin-Angiotensin-Aldosterone activity is increased under diabetic conditions. Angiotensin-II receptor type 1 (AT1R) density and synthesis are increased in T1D hearts, and the increase in fibrosis is partially inhibited following treatment with ACE inhibitors and AT receptor blockers [34]. Moreover, a frequent complication related to sustained hyperglycemia is cardiac autonomic neuropathy which includes abnormalities in heart rate control, vascular hemodynamics, and cardiac structure and function. An early characteristic of cardiac autonomic neuropathy is the reduction of parasympathetic activity with an imbalance toward higher sympathetic activity [35].

Among the new fields that are opening in the pathophysiology of heart failure, the intestinal microbiota and some of its metabolites stand out [36]. In some models, *Akkermansia, Prevotella 9, Paraprevoltella,* and *Phascolarctobaterium* have been associated with changes in cardiac structure and function [37]. The "intestinal hypothesis" of heart failure postulates that the reduction in cardiac output causes damage to the intestinal barrier that generates dysbiosis, favoring the proliferation of pathogenic species such as *Candida* and the reduction of anti-inflammatory bacteria such as *Faecalibacterium prausnitzii*. Similarly, the microbiota can promote heart failure through the modulation of intestinal immunity. Segmented filamentous bacteria favor the production of IL-6 and interleukin 23 [38] and *Bacteroides Fragilis* favors the production of anti-inflammatory cytokines that, in murine models, have been shown to reduce ventricular remodeling after myocardial infarction [39]. Bacterial metabolites also seem to have a role; for example, the reduction of short-chain fatty acids can favor the damage of the intestinal barrier and promote dysbiosis and the translocation of endotoxins to the bloodstream [40]. Trimethylamine N-oxide (TMAO) also seems to act as a risk factor for heart failure, since it has been observed in animal models to facilitate the release of calcium in the heart muscle by altering contractility and may also increase myocardial fibrosis [41,42]. It has also been observed that higher levels of TMAO in blood appear to be associated with a worse prognosis [43].

4. Diagnosis

The pathophysiological timeline of diabetic cardiomyopathy seems to follow the trend observed in other non-structural heart diseases, with the initial development of left ventricular diastolic dysfunction followed by subclinical systolic dysfunction with preserved ejection fraction and finally progressing to HFrEF [44,45]. In advanced stages, the diagnosis of HF is based on a combination of clinical data of the patient—compatible signs and symptoms based on the classic Framingham criteria—supported by diagnostic tests. Diagnostic confirmation is necessary in all cases, given its prognostic implication and the need to carry out an adequate therapeutic adjustment [46].

However, in the population with T1D, it is important to diagnose diastolic dysfunction and subclinical systolic dysfunction, to do an early diagnosis of the disease using sensitive cardiac markers that are easy to incorporate in routine clinical practice. Type B natriuretic peptides (BNP, NT-ProBNP) are plasmatic biomarkers, which are released in response to ventricular stretching and volume overload within the cardiac chambers, and can be affected by parameters such as age, sex, BMI, or renal function. These markers are a useful tool to guide the diagnosis of HF in the acute setting, in either diabetic or non-diabetic patients. Data from the multinational Breathing Not Properly trial suggest that diabetes is not a confounding variable in the interpretation of BNP levels in this situation [47]. A recent study [48] determined that higher NT-ProBNP levels were independently associated with HF in 664 subjects with T1D [HR 1.7 (95% CI: 1.1–2.4), $p = 0.01$]. The latest guidelines for the diagnosis and treatment of HF recommend the use of these natriuretic peptides both in acute and non-acute settings to rule out HF, given its high negative predictive value, but not to establish its diagnosis. Thus, the diagnosis in diabetic patients in the non-acute setting should follow the diagnostic algorithm that emphasizes that patients with a high probability of HF may have an echocardiogram to confirm or rule out the diagnosis [49]. Echocardiography is postulated as a central tool in the diagnosis of HF, given its safety, easy access, and highly informative character (cardiac chamber volumes, ventricular and valve function, and myocardial wall thickness, among other aspects) [50].

For the study of diastolic dysfunction in young people with T1D [51], it is recommended to follow the general indications of the American Society of Echocardiography and the European Association of Cardiovascular Imaging, through indices that include involving pulse Doppler transmitral inflow velocities (E and A waves) and tissue Doppler early and late mitral annular diastolic velocities (e' and a'), atrial size measurements, and pulmonary venous flow evaluation [52]. Thus, in recent years, more sensitive ultrasound techniques have been incorporated to detect the more subtle abnormalities of cardiac function that would go unnoticed with conventional techniques and measurements (such as ventricular deformation and desynchrony indices). Although left ventricular diastolic dysfunction is the earliest manifestation of HF in the diabetic population [53], recently, the role of left atrial dysfunction as an active contributor to the initial diastolic dysfunction suffered by these patients has been revealed [54]. Ifuku M et al. [14] observed left atrial dysfunction (such as left Atrial phasic strain) in adolescents and young people with T1D ($n = 53$) compared to non-diabetic controls ($n = 53$) and assert that it could constitute an early and sensitive marker of diastolic dysfunction in T1D. The E/e' ratio is frequently used as a marker of diastolic dysfunction (Yoldaş T, 2018). Bradley TJ et al. [55] observed an E/e' ratio (7.3 ± 1.2 vs. 6.7 ± 1.3; $p = 0.0003$) increased in patients with T1D ($n = 199$) compared to non-diabetic subjects ($n = 178$). However, not all the findings are consistent in this regard [56].

Kaushik A et al. [57], in a recent study, found the presence of preclinical ventricular dysfunction echocardiographic alterations in the population with T1D. Specifically, they found lower left ventricular strain indices [basal lateral LV (21.39 ± 4.12 vs. 23.78 ± 2.02; $p = 0.001$), mid-lateral LV (21.43 ± 4.27 vs. 23.17 ± 1.92 $p = 0.02$), basal septum (20.59 ± 5.28 vs. 22.91 ± 2.00; $p = 0.01$), and mid septum (22.06 ± 4.75 vs. 24.10 ± 1.99; $p = 0.01$] in children and adolescents with T1D ($n = 50$) compared to non-diabetic controls ($n = 25$), despite the absence of manifest heart failure and normal ejection fraction. In addition, greater endothelial dysfunction was detected by flow-mediated dilatation (FMD) in subjects with T1D compared to non-diabetic patients (8.36 ± 4.27 vs. 10.57 ± 4.12, $p = 0.04$). These myocardial alteration parameters correlated with HbA1c levels ($r = -0.327, p = 0.017$). These findings reinforce the hypothesis of the possible early effect of the diabetic metabolic environment on myocardial function.

Some studies that evaluate systolic function in T1D with HFrEF expose a parallel reduction in ultrasound parameters such as longitudinal tension and global ventricular circumference, as well as a reduction in the systolic strain rate using speckle-tracking echocardiography [58], although not all studies have reported changes in this regard [59,60]. Different studies have also reported subclinical cardiac dysfunction in young subjects with T1D [61–63] although other studies have not reached this conclusion [60,61]. This controversy could probably be due to differences in the characteristics of the subjects with T1D -glycemic control, time of evolution of the disease [64], and the use of different ultrasound protocols for the determination of ultrasound parameters in the comprehensive evaluation of cardiac dysfunction, which calls for standardized approaches to facilitate their interpretation.

These basic and central examinations based on clinical, analytical, and mainly ultrasound parameters can be completed with other modalities such as cardiac magnetic resonance imaging. Cardiac MRI allows for calculating improved rates of myocardial deformation of diastolic incoordination, including biventricular desynchrony and incoordination. The EMERALD study, carried out in a young population with T1D, reports alterations in the diastolic pressure of the ventricular septum and the diastolic relaxation fraction, which reflects an uncoordinated and energetically less favorable myocardial relaxation compared to non-diabetic subjects [65].

Although the identification of this underlying heart problem in T1D can be very important to delay or prevent the development of manifest HF, it is necessary follow-up with these patients, through longitudinal studies, to accurately determine the clinical importance of the preclinical myocardial changes detected in this population.

5. Treatment

According to the latest European guidelines for the treatment and diagnosis of HF [49], in patients with HFrEF, interventions that reduce morbidity and mortality confer a similar benefit in the presence or absence of diabetes. In addition to the control of classic cardiovascular risk factors, the use of beta-blockers, angiotensin-converting enzyme inhibitors (ACEIs), spironolactone, or eplerenone is proposed. Meanwhile, other drugs are recommended only in selected patients with symptomatic HFrEF, both diabetics and non-diabetics, as is the case with the use of diuretics, sacubitril/valsartan, ivabradine, hydralazine, isosorbide dinitrate, or angiotensin II type I receptor blockers.

The identification of asymptomatic T1D patients with cardiac dysfunction may favor the development of useful therapeutic strategies in diabetic cardiomyopathy, to optimize the treatment of these patients and improve the prognosis of the disease. As we mentioned before, McAllister et al. [6] and Kristófi et al. [7] found that the total age-adjusted CVRD burden and risks were greater among patients with T1D compared with those with T2D and HF rates were significantly higher in T1D patients depending on the age group. They also highlighted that the use of antihypertensive, antiplatelet, and statin drugs was much higher in T2D than in T1D, although these differences could be explained by differences in age and comorbidities. These findings highlight the need to improve preventive strategies beyond glycemic control in the T1D population from an early age.

The gold-standard treatment in T1D is the use of basal-bolus insulin therapy and the early intensive therapy is a fundamental aspect to reduce HF risk in the long-term [13]. Currently, new strategies to measure glucose levels, including the detection of interstitial glucose through Continuous Glucose Monitoring (iCGM) or Flash Glucose Monitoring (FGM), allow the adjustment of insulin therapy to improve metabolic control and achieve optimal control, as well as a more accurate assessment of glycemic variability and its reduction [66,67]. Besides, because glycemic variability is an independent risk factor for developing long-term complications in diabetic patients, continuous glucose monitoring might be a valuable tool in this context [67].

Certain drugs approved for the treatment of T2D such as metformin, aGLP1, and iSGLT2 are being evaluated as potential complementary drugs to insulin therapy in T1D [68]. Reflections in this regard underline the importance of the proper selection of patients with T1D and a close follow-up of them, in the case of the use of iSGLT2 due to the associated risk of developing "normoglycemic" diabetic ketoacidosis (DKA) [69]. Based on recent positive results from the DEPICT study [70], dapagliflozin 5 mg was the first iSGLT2 to have its marketing authorization in Europe in March 2019 as an additional drug to insulin therapy in patients with T1D with a body mass index (BMI) ≥ 27 kg/m^2 [71]. It also recently received Scottish Medicines Consortium (SMC) approval [72] as well as National Institute for Health and Care Excellence (NICE) approval following health economic analysis, in which dapagliflozin was found to be a highly cost-effective treatment option in people with T1D inadequately controlled by insulin alone [73]. However, its non-authorization in other places such as the U.S., and the BMI restrictions reflect safety concerns regarding the "normoglycemic" DKA risk. Since the available data are unclear, it is important to proceed on an individual basis for people that fall into these categories. Selecting appropriate people with T1D for iSGLT2 treatment is critical for minimizing the DKA risk and maximizing the potential benefits associated with this treatment. Those most likely to benefit from dapagliflozin treatment include overweight/obese people, established on stable optimized insulin therapy (i.e., not recently diagnosed), with high insulin needs (i.e., > 0.5 units/kg of body weight/day), and a low DKA risk profile, who have demonstrated adherence to their insulin regimen and the ability to understand and utilize relevant education relating to DKA risk [74].

In recent years, the development of these hypoglycemic molecules such as aGLP1 or iSGLT2 and the performance of cardiovascular safety studies for their commercialization have shown that they are not only beneficial in glycemic control, but also have cardioprotective effects in both T2D and non-diabetic patients. This opens the door to a clinical entity with important clinical repercussions, highly prevalent as we have seen in the general diabetic population and T1D. Furthermore, in certain stages, the lack of therapeutic options stands out, and although the studies show promising results, there are no specific data on the use of these drugs in the T1D population.

Metformin is the first-line treatment in T2D. In recent years, cohort studies and systematic reviews have analyzed its role in cardiovascular disease, finding that metformin seems to be associated with a reduction in mortality from all causes in T2D patients with HF, as well as with a reduction in readmissions by HF [75,76], so it is recommended in the current guidelines of the European Society of Cardiology [49] as a first-line drug in patients with T2D and HF. In T1D, REMOVAL a placebo-controlled trial to Metformin, data suggest that it might have a wider role in cardiovascular risk management, but do not support the use of metformin to improve glycemic control in adults with long-standing T1D [77].

Relative to iSGLT2, in the DECLARE-TIMI 58 trial, dapagliflozin treatment was associated with a lower rate of HF-related death and hospitalization than the placebo [78]. Likewise, dapagliflozin treatment has also been associated with a reduction in HF-related hospitalization rates in patients with or without HFrEF and a reduction in cardiovascular mortality and all-cause mortality compared to the placebo in patients with T2D and HFrEF [79], as well as in patients with T2D and previous myocardial infarction [80]. These benefits are the same in patients without diabetes with HFrEF [81], so its cardiovascular benefit would be independent of the hypoglycemic effect. The cardioprotective effects of empagliflozin are very similar [82]. These data are reinforced by later trials such as EMPRISE, where empagliflozin showed greater efficacy in the incidence of HF compared to sitagliptin, in reducing hospitalization for HF in T2D patients with and without cardiovascular disease [83]. Moreover, in the EMPEROR-Reduced trial, the use of empagliflozin reduced the risk of hospitalization for HF and cardiovascular mortality, regardless of the presence or absence of diabetes [84].

In this line, the EMPA-TROPISM (ATRU-4) study supports the benefit of empagliflozin in the treatment of HF regardless of its glycemic status, by demonstrating significant improvement in the key parameters of cardiac dysfunction, such as left ventricular (LV) volume, LV mass, LV systolic function, functional capacity, and quality of life of non-diabetic HFrEF patients [85]. Finally, results from the EMPEROR-preserve trial have been recently published, showing a reduction of the combined risk of cardiovascular death or hospitalization for HF with 10 mg empagliflozin in patients with HFpEF, regardless of the presence or absence of diabetes [86]. Other molecules of this pharmacological group have also shown benefits concerning cardiovascular mortality and hospitalization for HF (canagliflozin, CANVAS) [87], (sotagliflozin, SOLOIST-WHF) [88] or (ertugliflozin, VERTIS) [89]. In the case of sotagliflozin, they found benefits in HFpEF as well.

Regarding aGLP1, trials have shown heterogeneous information with favorable results in the reduction of cardiovascular mortality events for some molecules (Table 1): LEADER (liraglutide) [90], SUSTAIN-6 (semaglutide) [91], REWIND (dulaglutide) [92]; and neutral effects for other: ELIXA (lisixenatide) [93] and EXSCEL (long-acting exenatide) [94], without finding favorable specific results on HF. Subsequently, more specific trials have been conducted with liraglutide in patients with or without diabetes and HFrEF, which have further increased the uncertainty about the use of this molecule in subjects with established HF. The FIGHT trial, carried out in 300 patients recently hospitalized for HF, found that the use of liraglutide did not lead to greater clinical stability after hospitalization. Likewise, in the LIVE study ($n = 241$), it was found that the use of liraglutide did not affect left ventricular systolic function (LVEF) compared to the placebo in patients with stable HF, although it was associated with an increase in heart rate and serious adverse cardiac events, such as sustained ventricular tachycardia, atrial fibrillation, or worsening ischemic heart disease (10% vs 3%, $p = 0.04$). A meta-analysis published in recent years showed encouraging results regarding cardiovascular safety with the use of aGLP1, suggesting that they can reduce major adverse cardiovascular events, cardiovascular mortality, and all-cause mortality risk; no significant effect was identified in relation to hospitalization for HF [95] or even with reduced risk of hospitalization for HF [96]. A double-blind clinical trial [97] performed on T2D patients ($n = 49$) showed that treatment for 26 weeks with liraglutide versus a placebo reduced early diastolic LV filling and LV filling pressure to normal levels, pathogenic characteristics of HFpEF. However, future studies are needed to investigate these potential effects of aGLP1 in HF in its early stages and its benefits in other populations such as non-diabetic, obese, or T1D subjects.

Table 1. Evidence on hospitalization for heart failure and cardiovascular mortality with glucagon-like peptides 1 agonist (aGLP1) and sodium-glucose cotransporter 2 inhibitor (i-SGLT2) from randomized controlled trials.

		Study	Hospitalization for HF	CV Mortality
GLP1 receptor agonists	Liraglutide	LEADER [90]		↓
	Semaglutide	SUSTAIN-6 [91]		↓
	Dulaglutide	REWIND [92]		↓
SGLT2 inhibitors	Dapagliflozin	DECLARE-TIMI 58 [78]	↓	
	Empagliflozin	EMPRISE [83]	↓	
		EMPEROR-Reduced [84]	↓	↓
		EMPEROR-Preserve [86]	↓	↓
	Canagliflozin	CANVAS [87]	↓	↓
	Ertugliflozin	VERTIS [89]	↓	

GLP1: glucagon-like peptide 1; SGLT-2: sodium-glucose cotransporter 2; HF: heart failure; CV: cardiovascular.

Regarding the position of the different international cardiology and endocrinology societies in the use of iSGLT-2 and aGLP1, both are the recommended therapies in cases of T2D with cardiovascular disease, preferably leaning towards the use of the former in HF cases without ruling out the use of aGLP1 [68,98–101]. However, the American Heart Failure Society specifies the precaution of its use in situations of acute decompensation [102].

6. Conclusions

HF is a complication of increasing concern in diabetes, and given the high incidence of HF and the risk of hospitalization for HF in the population with T1D, more studies should be developed in this regard to clarify pathophysiological aspects, determine specific risk factors to control, and develop standardized protocols to establish specific precision biomarkers for the diagnosis of this entity in T1D patients from early stages.

The relationship between classic cardiovascular risk factors—such as hyperglycemia, hypertension, or dyslipidemia—and the cardiac and vascular abnormalities seen in people with T1D is not fully understood, so further research is required to identify potential treatment targets allowing for the development of therapeutic agents in this field. Some therapeutic groups, such as iSLGT2 and aGLP1, have shown a clear benefit in preventing cardiovascular complications in T2D. In particular, iSGLT2 have shown to be very effective in reducing HF-related deaths and hospitalization for HF in both T2D and non-diabetic patients. However, it remains to be determined if they are useful and safe in patients with HF and T1D.

Author Contributions: Conceptualization, F.J.T. and I.C.-P.; investigation, I.C-P., A.M.G.-P. and I.C-P.; resources, M.D.-F. and A.M.G.-P.; writing—original draft preparation, I.C.-P., M.D.-F. and A.M.G.-P.; writing—review and editing, I.C.-P., M.D.-F. and A.M.G.-P.; visualization, M.D.-F.; supervision, F.J.T. All authors have read and agreed to the published version of the manuscript.

Funding: ICP was supported by Rio Hortega and now for Juan Rodes from the Spanish Ministry of Economy and Competitiveness (ISCIII) and cofounded by Fondo Europeo de Desarrollo Regional-FEDER (CM 17/00169, JR 19/00054). AMGP was supported by a research contract from Servicio Andaluz de Salud (B-0033-2014). MDF was supported by Rio Hortega from the Spanish Ministry of Economy and Competitiveness (ISCIII) and cofounded by Fondo Europeo de Desarrollo Regional-FEDER (CM20/00183). This study was supported by the "Centros de Investigación Biomédica en Red" (CIBER) of the Institute of Health Carlos III (ISCIII) (CB06/03/0018), and research grants from the ISCIII (PI18/01160), and co-financed by the European Regional Development Fund (ERDF).The funders had no role in the manuscript.

Acknowledgments: We thank smart.servier.com for providing the image that illustrates this review.

Conflicts of Interest: The authors declare no conflict of interest.

References

1. Bress, A.P.; King, J.B.; Brixner, D.; Kielhorn, A.; Patel, H.K.; Maya, J.; Lee, V.C.; Biskupiak, J.; Munger, M. Pharmacotherapy Treatment Patterns, Outcomes, and Health Resource Utilization Among Patients with Heart Failure with Reduced Ejection Fraction at a U.S. Academic Medical Center. *Pharmacotherapy* **2016**, *36*, 174–186. [CrossRef]
2. Dunlay, S.M.; Roger, V.L.; Redfield, M.M. Epidemiology of Heart Failure with Preserved Ejection Fraction. *Nat. Rev. Cardiol.* **2017**, *14*, 591–602. [CrossRef]
3. Butler, J.; Januzzi, J.L.; Rosenstock, J. Management of Heart Failure and Type 2 Diabetes Mellitus: Maximizing Complementary Drug Therapy. *Diabetes Obes. Metab.* **2020**, *22*, 1243–1262. [CrossRef]
4. Dauriz, M.; Mantovani, A.; Bonapace, S.; Verlato, G.; Zoppini, G.; Bonora, E.; Targher, G. Prognostic Impact of Diabetes on Long-Term Survival Outcomes in Patients with Heart Failure: A Meta-Analysis. *Diabetes Care* **2017**, *40*, 1597–1605. [CrossRef]
5. Shaw, J.A.; Cooper, M.E. Contemporary Management of Heart Failure in Patients with Diabetes. *Diabetes Care* **2020**, *43*, 2895–2903. [CrossRef] [PubMed]
6. McAllister, D.A.; Read, S.H.; Kerssens, J.; Livingstone, S.; McGurnaghan, S.; Jhund, P.; Petrie, J.; Sattar, N.; Fischbacher, C.; Kristensen, S.L.; et al. Incidence of Hospitalization for Heart Failure and Case-Fatality Among 3.25 Million People With and Without Diabetes Mellitus. *Circulation* **2018**, *138*, 2774–2786. [CrossRef]

7. Kristófi, R.; Bodegard, J.; Norhammar, A.; Thuresson, M.; Nathanson, D.; Nyström, T.; Birkeland, K.I.; Eriksson, J.W. Cardiovascular and Renal Disease Burden in Type 1 Compared With Type 2 Diabetes: A Two-Country Nationwide Observational Study. *Diabetes Care* **2021**, *44*, 1211–1218. [CrossRef]
8. Cai, X.; Li, J.; Cai, W.; Chen, C.; Ma, J.; Xie, Z.; Dong, Y.; Liu, C.; Xue, R.; Zhao, J. Meta-Analysis of Type 1 Diabetes Mellitus and Risk of Cardiovascular Disease. *J. Diabetes Complicat.* **2021**, *35*, 107833. [CrossRef] [PubMed]
9. Chadalavada, S.; Jensen, M.T.; Aung, N.; Cooper, J.; Lekadir, K.; Munroe, P.B.; Petersen, S.E. Women with Diabetes Are at Increased Relative Risk of Heart Failure Compared to Men: Insights From UK Biobank. *Front. Cardiovasc. Med.* **2021**, *8*. [CrossRef] [PubMed]
10. Avogaro, A.; Azzolina, D.; Fadini, G.P.; Baldi, I. Incidence of Heart Failure in Patients with Type 1 Diabetes: A Systematic Review of Observational Studies. *J. Endocrinol. Investig.* **2021**, *44*, 745–753. [CrossRef]
11. Lee, Y.-B. Risk of Early Mortality and Cardiovascular Disease in Type 1 Diabetes: A Comparison with Type 2 Diabetes, a Nationwide Study. *Cardiovasc Diabetol.* **2019**, *18*, 157. [CrossRef] [PubMed]
12. Risk Factors for First and Subsequent CVD Events in Type 1 Diabetes: The DCCT/EDIC Study l Cochrane Library. Available online: https://www.cochranelibrary.com/central/doi/10.1002/central/CN-02208916/full (accessed on 9 July 2021).
13. Diabetes Control and Complications Trial (DCCT)/Epidemiology of Diabetes Interventions and Complications (EDIC) Study Research Group Intensive Diabetes Treatment and Cardiovascular Outcomes in Type 1 Diabetes: The DCCT/EDIC Study 30-Year Follow-Up. *Diabetes Care* **2016**, *39*, 686–693. [CrossRef] [PubMed]
14. Ifuku, M.; Takahashi, K.; Hosono, Y.; Iso, T.; Ishikawa, A.; Haruna, H.; Takubo, N.; Komiya, K.; Kurita, M.; Ikeda, F.; et al. Left Atrial Dysfunction and Stiffness in Pediatric and Adult Patients with Type 1 Diabetes Mellitus Assessed with Speckle Tracking Echocardiography. *Pediatr. Diabetes* **2021**, *22*, 303–319. [CrossRef] [PubMed]
15. Iso, T.; Takahashi, K.; Yazaki, K.; Ifuku, M.; Nii, M.; Fukae, T.; Yazawa, R.; Ishikawa, A.; Haruna, H.; Takubo, N.; et al. In-Depth Insight into the Mechanisms of Cardiac Dysfunction in Patients with Type 1 Diabetes Mellitus Using Layer-Specific Strain Analysis. *Circ. J.* **2019**, *83*, 1330–1337. [CrossRef]
16. Rawshani, A.; Rawshani, A.; Franzén, S.; Eliasson, B.; Svensson, A.-M.; Miftaraj, M.; McGuire, D.K.; Sattar, N.; Rosengren, A.; Gudbjörnsdottir, S. Range of Risk Factor Levels: Control, Mortality, and Cardiovascular Outcomes in Type 1 Diabetes Mellitus. *Circulation* **2017**, *135*, 1522–1531. [CrossRef]
17. Rawshani, A.; Rawshani, A.; Sattar, N.; Franzén, S.; McGuire, D.K.; Eliasson, B.; Svensson, A.-M.; Zethelius, B.; Miftaraj, M.; Rosengren, A.; et al. Relative Prognostic Importance and Optimal Levels of Risk Factors for Mortality and Cardiovascular Outcomes in Type 1 Diabetes Mellitus. *Circulation* **2019**, *139*, 1900–1912. [CrossRef]
18. Miller, R.G.; Costacou, T.; Orchard, T.J. Risk Factor Modeling for Cardiovascular Disease in Type 1 Diabetes in the Pittsburgh Epidemiology of Diabetes Complications (EDC) Study: A Comparison with the Diabetes Control and Complications Trial/Epidemiology of Diabetes Interventions and Complications Study (DCCT/EDIC). *Diabetes* **2019**, *68*, 409–419. [CrossRef]
19. Groop, P.-H.; Thomas, M.C.; Moran, J.L.; Wadèn, J.; Thorn, L.M.; Mäkinen, V.-P.; Rosengård-Bärlund, M.; Saraheimo, M.; Hietala, K.; Heikkilä, O.; et al. The Presence and Severity of Chronic Kidney Disease Predicts All-Cause Mortality in Type 1 Diabetes. *Diabetes* **2009**, *58*, 1651–1658. [CrossRef]
20. Sousa, G.R.; Pober, D.; Galderisi, A.; Lv, H.; Yu, L.; Pereira, A.C.; Doria, A.; Kosiborod, M.; Lipes, M.A. Glycemic Control, Cardiac Autoimmunity, and Long-Term Risk of Cardiovascular Disease in Type 1 Diabetes Mellitus. *Circulation* **2019**, *139*, 730–743. [CrossRef]
21. Sousa, G.R.; Kosiborod, M.; Bluemke, D.A.; Lipes, M.A. Cardiac Autoimmunity Is Associated With Subclinical Myocardial Dysfunction in Patients With Type 1 Diabetes Mellitus. *Circulation* **2020**, *141*, 1107–1109. [CrossRef]
22. Khedr, D.; Hafez, M.; Lumpuy-Castillo, J.; Emam, S.; Abdel-Massih, A.; Elmougy, F.; Elkaffas, R.; Mahillo-Fernández, I.; Lorenzo, O.; Musa, N. Lipid Biomarkers as Predictors of Diastolic Dysfunction in Diabetes with Poor Glycemic Control. *Int. J. Mol. Sci.* **2020**, *21*, 5079. [CrossRef]
23. Tan, Y.; Zhang, Z.; Zheng, C.; Wintergerst, K.A.; Keller, B.B.; Cai, L. Mechanisms of Diabetic Cardiomyopathy and Potential Therapeutic Strategies: Preclinical and Clinical Evidence. *Nat. Rev. Cardiol.* **2020**, *17*, 585–607. [CrossRef]
24. Singh, V.P.; Bali, A.; Singh, N.; Jaggi, A.S. Advanced Glycation End Products and Diabetic Complications. *Korean J. Physiol. Pharm.* **2014**, *18*, 1–14. [CrossRef] [PubMed]
25. Cruz, L.; Ryan, J.J. Nitric Oxide Signaling in Heart Failure with Preserved Ejection Fraction. *JACC Basic Transl. Sci.* **2017**, *2*, 341–343. [CrossRef] [PubMed]
26. Herrero, P.; Peterson, L.R.; McGill, J.B.; Matthew, S.; Lesniak, D.; Dence, C.; Gropler, R.J. Increased Myocardial Fatty Acid Metabolism in Patients with Type 1 Diabetes Mellitus. *J. Am. Coll Cardiol.* **2006**, *47*, 598–604. [CrossRef]
27. Cai, L.; Kang, Y.J. Oxidative Stress and Diabetic Cardiomyopathy: A Brief Review. *Cardiovasc Toxicol.* **2001**, *1*, 181–193. [CrossRef] [PubMed]
28. Hölscher, M.E.; Bode, C.; Bugger, H. Diabetic Cardiomyopathy: Does the Type of Diabetes Matter? *Int. J. Mol. Sci.* **2016**, *17*, 2136. [CrossRef] [PubMed]
29. Xia, Z.; Kuo, K.-H.; Nagareddy, P.R.; Wang, F.; Guo, Z.; Guo, T.; Jiang, J.; McNeill, J.H. N-Acetylcysteine Attenuates PKCβ2 Overexpression and Myocardial Hypertrophy in Streptozotocin-Induced Diabetic Rats. *Cardiovasc. Res.* **2007**, *73*, 770–782. [CrossRef]

30. How, O.-J.; Aasum, E.; Severson, D.L.; Chan, W.Y.A.; Essop, M.F.; Larsen, T.S. Increased Myocardial Oxygen Consumption Reduces Cardiac Efficiency in Diabetic Mice. *Diabetes* **2006**, *55*, 466–473. [CrossRef]
31. Lin, Y.; Tang, Y.; Wang, F. The Protective Effect of HIF-1α in T Lymphocytes on Cardiac Damage in Diabetic Mice. *Ann. Clin. Lab. Sci.* **2016**, *46*, 32–43.
32. Abdullah, C.S.; Li, Z.; Wang, X.; Jin, Z.-Q. Depletion of T Lymphocytes Ameliorates Cardiac Fibrosis in Streptozotocin-Induced Diabetic Cardiomyopathy. *Int. Immunopharmacol.* **2016**, *39*, 251–264. [CrossRef]
33. Zhao, X.-Y.; Hu, S.-J.; Li, J.; Mou, Y.; Chen, B.-P.; Xia, Q. Decreased Cardiac Sarcoplasmic Reticulum Ca2+ -ATPase Activity Contributes to Cardiac Dysfunction in Streptozotocin-Induced Diabetic Rats. *J. Physiol. Biochem.* **2006**, *62*, 1–8. [CrossRef]
34. Singh, V.P.; Le, B.; Khode, R.; Baker, K.M.; Kumar, R. Intracellular Angiotensin II Production in Diabetic Rats Is Correlated with Cardiomyocyte Apoptosis, Oxidative Stress, and Cardiac Fibrosis. *Diabetes* **2008**, *57*, 3297–3306. [CrossRef] [PubMed]
35. Olshansky, B.; Sabbah, H.N.; Hauptman, P.J.; Colucci, W.S. Parasympathetic Nervous System and Heart Failure: Pathophysiology and Potential Implications for Therapy. *Circulation* **2008**, *118*, 863–871. [CrossRef]
36. Tang, W.H.W.; Kitai, T.; Hazen, S.L. Gut Microbiota in Cardiovascular Health and Disease. *Circ. Res.* **2017**, *120*, 1183–1196. [CrossRef]
37. Gutiérrez-Calabrés, E.; Ortega-Hernández, A.; Modrego, J.; Gómez-Gordo, R.; Caro-Vadillo, A.; Rodríguez-Bobada, C.; González, P.; Gómez-Garre, D. Gut Microbiota Profile Identifies Transition from Compensated Cardiac Hypertrophy to Heart Failure in Hypertensive Rats. *Hypertension* **2020**, *76*, 1545–1554. [CrossRef]
38. Tang, W.H.W.; Li, D.Y.; Hazen, S.L. Dietary Metabolism, the Gut Microbiome, and Heart Failure. *Nat. Rev. Cardiol.* **2019**, *16*, 137–154. [CrossRef] [PubMed]
39. Jia, Q.; Li, H.; Zhou, H.; Zhang, X.; Zhang, A.; Xie, Y.; Li, Y.; Lv, S.; Zhang, J. Role and Effective Therapeutic Target of Gut Microbiota in Heart Failure. *Cardiovasc Ther.* **2019**, *2019*, 5164298. [CrossRef] [PubMed]
40. Nagatomo, Y.; Wilson Tang, W.H. Intersections between Microbiome and Heart Failure: Revisiting the Gut Hypothesis. *J. Card. Fail.* **2015**, *21*, 973–980. [CrossRef] [PubMed]
41. Savi, M.; Bocchi, L.; Bresciani, L.; Falco, A.; Quaini, F.; Mena, P.; Brighenti, F.; Crozier, A.; Stilli, D.; Del Rio, D. Trimethylamine-N-Oxide (TMAO)-Induced Impairment of Cardiomyocyte Function and the Protective Role of Urolithin B-Glucuronide. *Molecules* **2018**, *23*, 549. [CrossRef]
42. Organ, C.L.; Otsuka, H.; Bhushan, S.; Wang, Z.; Bradley, J.; Trivedi, R.; Polhemus, D.J.; Tang, W.H.W.; Wu, Y.; Hazen, S.L.; et al. Choline Diet and Its Gut Microbe-Derived Metabolite, Trimethylamine N-Oxide, Exacerbate Pressure Overload-Induced Heart Failure. *Circ. Heart Fail.* **2016**, *9*, e002314. [CrossRef] [PubMed]
43. Li, W.; Huang, A.; Zhu, H.; Liu, X.; Huang, X.; Huang, Y.; Cai, X.; Lu, J.; Huang, Y. Gut Microbiota-Derived Trimethylamine N-Oxide Is Associated with Poor Prognosis in Patients with Heart Failure. *Med. J. Aust.* **2020**, *213*, 374–379. [CrossRef] [PubMed]
44. From, A.M.; Scott, C.G.; Chen, H.H. The Development of Heart Failure in Patients with Diabetes Mellitus and Pre-Clinical Diastolic Dysfunction a Population-Based Study. *J. Am. Coll Cardiol.* **2010**, *55*, 300–305. [CrossRef] [PubMed]
45. Seferović, P.M.; Paulus, W.J. Clinical Diabetic Cardiomyopathy: A Two-Faced Disease with Restrictive and Dilated Phenotypes. *Eur. Heart J.* **2015**, *36*, 1718–1727. [CrossRef] [PubMed]
46. Maestre, A.; Gil, V.; Gallego, J.; Aznar, J.; Mora, A.; Martín-Hidalgo, A. Diagnostic Accuracy of Clinical Criteria for Identifying Systolic and Diastolic Heart Failure: Cross-Sectional Study. *J. Eval. Clin. Pract.* **2009**, *15*, 55–61. [CrossRef] [PubMed]
47. Wu, A.H.B.; Omland, T.; Duc, P.; McCord, J.; Nowak, R.M.; Hollander, J.E.; Herrmann, H.C.; Steg, P.G.; Wold Knudsen, C.; Storrow, A.B.; et al. The Effect of Diabetes on B-Type Natriuretic Peptide Concentrations in Patients with Acute Dyspnea: An Analysis from the Breathing Not Properly Multinational Study. *Diabetes Care* **2004**, *27*, 2398–2404. [CrossRef] [PubMed]
48. Tofte, N.; Theilade, S.; Winther, S.A.; Birkelund, S.; Goetze, J.P.; Hansen, T.W.; Rossing, P. Comparison of Natriuretic Peptides as Risk Markers for All-Cause Mortality and Cardiovascular and Renal Complications in Individuals with Type 1 Diabetes. *Diabetes Care* **2021**, *44*, 595–603. [CrossRef]
49. Ponikowski, P.; Voors, A.A.; Anker, S.D.; Bueno, H.; Cleland, J.G.F.; Coats, A.J.S.; Falk, V.; González-Juanatey, J.R.; Harjola, V.-P.; Jankowska, E.A.; et al. 2016 ESC Guidelines for the Diagnosis and Treatment of Acute and Chronic Heart Failure: The Task Force for the Diagnosis and Treatment of Acute and Chronic Heart Failure of the European Society of Cardiology (ESC)Developed with the Special Contribution of the Heart Failure Association (HFA) of the ESC. *Eur. Heart J.* **2016**, *37*, 2129–2200. [CrossRef]
50. Caballero, L.; Kou, S.; Dulgheru, R.; Gonjilashvili, N.; Athanassopoulos, G.D.; Barone, D.; Baroni, M.; Cardim, N.; Gomez de Diego, J.J.; Oliva, M.J.; et al. Echocardiographic Reference Ranges for Normal Cardiac Doppler Data: Results from the NORRE Study. *Eur. Heart J. Cardiovasc. Imaging* **2015**, *16*, 1031–1041. [CrossRef]
51. Schäfer, M.; Nadeau, K.J.; Reusch, J.E.B. Cardiovascular Disease in Young People with Type 1 Diabetes: Search for Cardiovascular Biomarkers. *J. Diabetes Complicat.* **2020**, *34*, 107651. [CrossRef]
52. Nagueh, S.F.; Smiseth, O.A.; Appleton, C.P.; Byrd, B.F.; Dokainish, H.; Edvardsen, T.; Flachskampf, F.A.; Gillebert, T.C.; Klein, A.L.; Lancellotti, P.; et al. Recommendations for the Evaluation of Left Ventricular Diastolic Function by Echocardiography: An Update from the American Society of Echocardiography and the European Association of Cardiovascular Imaging. *J. Am. Soc. Echocardiogr.* **2016**, *29*, 277–314. [CrossRef] [PubMed]
53. Schilling, J.D.; Mann, D.L. Diabetic Cardiomyopathy: Bench to Bedside. *Heart Fail. Clin.* **2012**, *8*, 619–631. [CrossRef] [PubMed]

54. Sanchis, L.; Gabrielli, L.; Andrea, R.; Falces, C.; Duchateau, N.; Perez-Villa, F.; Bijnens, B.; Sitges, M. Left Atrial Dysfunction Relates to Symptom Onset in Patients with Heart Failure and Preserved Left Ventricular Ejection Fraction. *Eur. Heart J. Cardiovasc. Imaging* **2015**, *16*, 62–67. [CrossRef]
55. Bradley, T.J.; Slorach, C.; Mahmud, F.H.; Dunger, D.B.; Deanfield, J.; Deda, L.; Elia, Y.; Har, R.L.H.; Hui, W.; Moineddin, R.; et al. Early Changes in Cardiovascular Structure and Function in Adolescents with Type 1 Diabetes. *Cardiovasc. Diabetol.* **2016**, *15*, 31. [CrossRef]
56. Flachskampf, F.A.; Biering-Sørensen, T.; Solomon, S.D.; Duvernoy, O.; Bjerner, T.; Smiseth, O.A. Cardiac Imaging to Evaluate Left Ventricular Diastolic Function. *JACC Cardiovasc. Imaging* **2015**, *8*, 1071–1093. [CrossRef]
57. Kaushik, A.; Kapoor, A.; Dabadghao, P.; Khanna, R.; Kumar, S.; Garg, N.; Tewari, S.; Goel, P.K.; Sinha, A. Use of Strain, Strain Rate, Tissue Velocity Imaging, and Endothelial Function for Early Detection of Cardiovascular Involvement in Young Diabetics. *Ann. Pediatr. Cardiol.* **2021**, *14*, 1–9. [CrossRef] [PubMed]
58. Yoldaş, T.; Örün, U.A.; Sagsak, E.; Aycan, Z.; Kaya, Ö.; Özgür, S.; Karademir, S. Subclinical Left Ventricular Systolic and Diastolic Dysfunction in Type 1 Diabetic Children and Adolescents with Good Metabolic Control. *Echocardiography* **2018**, *35*, 227–233. [CrossRef]
59. Hensel, K.O.; Grimmer, F.; Jenke, A.C.; Wirth, S.; Heusch, A. The Influence of Real-Time Blood Glucose Levels on Left Ventricular Myocardial Strain and Strain Rate in Pediatric Patients with Type 1 Diabetes Mellitus—A Speckle Tracking Echocardiography Study. *BMC Cardiovasc. Disord.* **2015**, *15*, 175. [CrossRef]
60. Palmieri, V.; Capaldo, B.; Russo, C.; Iaccarino, M.; Pezzullo, S.; Quintavalle, G.; Di Minno, G.; Riccardi, G.; Celentano, A. Uncomplicated Type 1 Diabetes and Preclinical Left Ventricular Myocardial Dysfunction: Insights from Echocardiography and Exercise Cardiac Performance Evaluation. *Diabetes Res. Clin. Pr.* **2008**, *79*, 262–268. [CrossRef] [PubMed]
61. Hodzic, A.; Ribault, V.; Maragnes, P.; Milliez, P.; Saloux, E.; Labombarda, F. Decreased Regional Left Ventricular Myocardial Strain in Type 1 Diabetic Children: A First Sign of Diabetic Cardiomyopathy? *J. Transl. Int. Med.* **2016**, *4*, 81–87. [CrossRef]
62. Labombarda, F.; Leport, M.; Morello, R.; Ribault, V.; Kauffman, D.; Brouard, J.; Pellissier, A.; Maragnes, P.; Manrique, A.; Milliez, P.; et al. Longitudinal Left Ventricular Strain Impairment in Type 1 Diabetes Children and Adolescents: A 2D Speckle Strain Imaging Study. *Diabetes Metab.* **2014**, *40*, 292–298. [CrossRef]
63. Cori, A.D.; Bello, V.D.; Miccoli, R.; Talini, E.; Palagi, C.; Donne, M.G.D.; Penno, G.; Nardi, C.; Bianchi, C.; Mariani, M.; et al. Left Ventricular Function in Normotensive Young Adults with Well-Controlled Type 1 Diabetes Mellitus. *Am. J. Cardiol.* **2007**, *99*, 84–90. [CrossRef]
64. Altun, G.; Babaoğlu, K.; Binnetoğlu, K.; Özsu, E.; Yeşiltepe Mutlu, R.G.; Hatun, Ş. Subclinical Left Ventricular Longitudinal and Radial Systolic Dysfunction in Children and Adolescents with Type 1 Diabetes Mellitus. *Echocardiography* **2016**, *33*, 1032–1039. [CrossRef]
65. Schäfer, M.; Bjornstad, P.; Frank, B.S.; Baumgartner, A.; Truong, U.; Enge, D.; von Alvensleben, J.C.; Mitchell, M.B.; Ivy, D.D.; Barker, A.J.; et al. Frequency of Reduced Left Ventricular Contractile Efficiency and Discoordinated Myocardial Relaxation in Patients Aged 16 to 21 Years with Type 1 Diabetes Mellitus (from the Emerald Study). *Am. J. Cardiol.* **2020**, *128*, 45–53. [CrossRef]
66. Mancini, G.; Berioli, M.G.; Santi, E.; Rogari, F.; Toni, G.; Tascini, G.; Crispoldi, R.; Ceccarini, G.; Esposito, S. Flash Glucose Monitoring: A Review of the Literature with a Special Focus on Type 1 Diabetes. *Nutrients* **2018**, *10*, 992. [CrossRef] [PubMed]
67. Siegelaar, S.E.; Holleman, F.; Hoekstra, J.B.L.; DeVries, J.H. Glucose Variability; Does It Matter? *Endocr. Rev.* **2010**, *31*, 171–182. [CrossRef] [PubMed]
68. Association, A.D. 9. Pharmacologic Approaches to Glycemic Treatment: Standards of Medical Care in Diabetes—2019. *Diabetes Care* **2019**, *42*, S90–S102. [CrossRef] [PubMed]
69. Danne, T.; Garg, S.; Peters, A.L.; Buse, J.B.; Mathieu, C.; Pettus, J.H.; Alexander, C.M.; Battelino, T.; Ampudia-Blasco, F.J.; Bode, B.W.; et al. International Consensus on Risk Management of Diabetic Ketoacidosis in Patients with Type 1 Diabetes Treated With Sodium-Glucose Cotransporter (SGLT) Inhibitors. *Diabetes Care* **2019**, *42*, 1147–1154. [CrossRef]
70. Dandona, P.; Mathieu, C.; Phillip, M.; Hansen, L.; Tschöpe, D.; Thorén, F.; Xu, J.; Langkilde, A.M. DEPICT-1 Investigators Efficacy and Safety of Dapagliflozin in Patients with Inadequately Controlled Type 1 Diabetes: The DEPICT-1 52-Week Study. *Diabetes Care* **2018**, *41*, 2552–2559. [CrossRef]
71. EMA. Accepts Marketing Authorisation for Forxiga in Type-1 Diabetes. *Eur. Pharm. Rev.* **2021**, *38*, e14458.
72. Dapagliflozin (Forxiga). Available online: https://www.scottishmedicines.org.uk/medicines-advice/dapagliflozin-forxiga-full-smc2185/ (accessed on 16 September 2021).
73. National Institute for Health and Clinical Excellence. Technology Appraisal Guidance [TA597]: Dapagliflozin with Insulin for Treating Type 1 Diabetes 2019. 2020. Available online: https://www.nice.org.uk/guidance/TA597 (accessed on 14 September 2021).
74. Evans, M.; Hicks, D.; Patel, D.; Patel, V.; McEwan, P.; Dashora, U. Optimising the Benefits of SGLT2 Inhibitors for Type 1 Diabetes. *Diabetes* **2020**, *11*, 37–52. [CrossRef]
75. Eurich, D.T.; Weir, D.L.; Majumdar, S.R.; Tsuyuki, R.T.; Johnson, J.A.; Tjosvold, L.; Vanderloo, S.E.; McAlister, F.A. Comparative Safety and Effectiveness of Metformin in Patients with Diabetes Mellitus and Heart Failure: Systematic Review of Observational Studies Involving 34,000 Patients. *Circ. Heart Fail.* **2013**, *6*, 395–402. [CrossRef]

76. Crowley, M.J.; Diamantidis, C.J.; McDuffie, J.R.; Cameron, C.B.; Stanifer, J.W.; Mock, C.K.; Wang, X.; Tang, S.; Nagi, A.; Kosinski, A.S.; et al. Clinical Outcomes of Metformin Use in Populations with Chronic Kidney Disease, Congestive Heart Failure, or Chronic Liver Disease: A Systematic Review. *Ann. Intern. Med.* **2017**, *166*, 191–200. [CrossRef] [PubMed]
77. Petrie, J.R.; Chaturvedi, N.; Ford, I.; Brouwers, M.C.G.J.; Greenlaw, N.; Tillin, T.; Hramiak, I.; Hughes, A.D.; Jenkins, A.J.; Klein, B.E.K.; et al. Cardiovascular and Metabolic Effects of Metformin in Patients with Type 1 Diabetes (REMOVAL): A Double-Blind, Randomised, Placebo-Controlled Trial. *Lancet Diabetes Endocrinol.* **2017**, *5*, 597–609. [CrossRef]
78. Wiviott, S.D.; Raz, I.; Bonaca, M.P.; Mosenzon, O.; Kato, E.T.; Cahn, A.; Silverman, M.G.; Zelniker, T.A.; Kuder, J.F.; Murphy, S.A.; et al. Dapagliflozin and Cardiovascular Outcomes in Type 2 Diabetes. *N. Engl. J. Med.* **2019**, *380*, 347–357. [CrossRef] [PubMed]
79. Kato, E.T.; Silverman, M.G.; Mosenzon, O.; Zelniker, T.A.; Cahn, A.; Furtado, R.H.M.; Kuder, J.; Murphy, S.A.; Bhatt, D.L.; Leiter, L.A.; et al. Effect of Dapagliflozin on Heart Failure and Mortality in Type 2 Diabetes Mellitus. *Circulation* **2019**, *139*, 2528–2536. [CrossRef] [PubMed]
80. Furtado, R.H.M.; Bonaca, M.P.; Raz, I.; Zelniker, T.A.; Mosenzon, O.; Cahn, A.; Kuder, J.; Murphy, S.A.; Bhatt, D.L.; Leiter, L.A.; et al. Dapagliflozin and Cardiovascular Outcomes in Patients with Type 2 Diabetes Mellitus and Previous Myocardial Infarction. *Circulation* **2019**, *139*, 2516–2527. [CrossRef] [PubMed]
81. McMurray, J.J.V.; Solomon, S.D.; Inzucchi, S.E.; Køber, L.; Kosiborod, M.N.; Martinez, F.A.; Ponikowski, P.; Sabatine, M.S.; Anand, I.S.; Bělohlávek, J.; et al. Dapagliflozin in Patients with Heart Failure and Reduced Ejection Fraction. *N. Engl. J. Med.* **2019**, *381*, 1995–2008. [CrossRef]
82. Fitchett, D.; Zinman, B.; Wanner, C.; Lachin, J.M.; Hantel, S.; Salsali, A.; Johansen, O.E.; Woerle, H.J.; Broedl, U.C.; Inzucchi, S.E.; et al. Heart Failure Outcomes with Empagliflozin in Patients with Type 2 Diabetes at High Cardiovascular Risk: Results of the EMPA-REG OUTCOME® Trial. *Eur. Heart J.* **2016**, *37*, 1526–1534. [CrossRef]
83. Patorno, E.; Pawar, A.; Franklin, J.M.; Najafzadeh, M.; Déruaz-Luyet, A.; Brodovicz, K.G.; Sambevski, S.; Bessette, L.G.; Santiago Ortiz, A.J.; Kulldorff, M.; et al. Empagliflozin and the Risk of Heart Failure Hospitalization in Routine Clinical Care. *Circulation* **2019**, *139*, 2822–2830. [CrossRef]
84. Packer, M.; Anker, S.D.; Butler, J.; Filippatos, G.; Pocock, S.J.; Carson, P.; Januzzi, J.; Verma, S.; Tsutsui, H.; Brueckmann, M.; et al. Cardiovascular and Renal Outcomes with Empagliflozin in Heart Failure. *N. Engl. J. Med.* **2020**, *383*, 1413–1424. [CrossRef] [PubMed]
85. Santos-Gallego, C.G.; Vargas-Delgado, A.P.; Requena-Ibanez, J.A.; Garcia-Ropero, A.; Mancini, D.; Pinney, S.; Macaluso, F.; Sartori, S.; Roque, M.; Sabatel-Perez, F.; et al. Randomized Trial of Empagliflozin in Nondiabetic Patients With Heart Failure and Reduced Ejection Fraction. *J. Am. Coll. Cardiol.* **2020**, *77*, 243–255. [CrossRef] [PubMed]
86. Anker, S.D.; Butler, J.; Filippatos, G.; Ferreira, J.P.; Bocchi, E.; Böhm, M.; Brunner–La Rocca, H.-P.; Choi, D.-J.; Chopra, V.; Chuquiure-Valenzuela, E.; et al. Empagliflozin in Heart Failure with a Preserved Ejection Fraction. *N. Engl. J. Med.* **2021**, NEJMoa2107038. [CrossRef] [PubMed]
87. Neal, B.; Perkovic, V.; Mahaffey, K.W.; de Zeeuw, D.; Fulcher, G.; Erondu, N.; Shaw, W.; Law, G.; Desai, M.; Matthews, D.R. Canagliflozin and Cardiovascular and Renal Events in Type 2 Diabetes. *N. Engl. J. Med.* **2017**, *377*, 644–657. [CrossRef] [PubMed]
88. Bhatt, D.L.; Szarek, M.; Steg, P.G.; Cannon, C.P.; Leiter, L.A.; McGuire, D.K.; Lewis, J.B.; Riddle, M.C.; Voors, A.A.; Metra, M.; et al. Sotagliflozin in Patients with Diabetes and Recent Worsening Heart Failure. *N. Engl. J. Med.* **2021**, *384*, 117–128. [CrossRef] [PubMed]
89. Cannon, C.P.; Pratley, R.; Dagogo-Jack, S.; Mancuso, J.; Huyck, S.; Masiukiewicz, U.; Charbonnel, B.; Frederich, R.; Gallo, S.; Cosentino, F.; et al. Cardiovascular Outcomes with Ertugliflozin in Type 2 Diabetes. *N. Engl. J. Med.* **2020**, *383*, 1425–1435. [CrossRef]
90. Marso, S.P.; Daniels, G.H.; Brown-Frandsen, K.; Kristensen, P.; Mann, J.F.E.; Nauck, M.A.; Nissen, S.E.; Pocock, S.; Poulter, N.R.; Ravn, L.S.; et al. Liraglutide and Cardiovascular Outcomes in Type 2 Diabetes. *N. Engl. J. Med.* **2016**, *375*, 311–322. [CrossRef]
91. Marso, S.P.; Bain, S.C.; Consoli, A.; Eliaschewitz, F.G.; Jódar, E.; Leiter, L.A.; Lingvay, I.; Rosenstock, J.; Seufert, J.; Warren, M.L.; et al. Semaglutide and Cardiovascular Outcomes in Patients with Type 2 Diabetes. *N. Engl. J. Med.* **2016**, *375*, 1834–1844. [CrossRef]
92. Gerstein, H.C.; Colhoun, H.M.; Dagenais, G.R.; Diaz, R.; Lakshmanan, M.; Pais, P.; Probstfield, J.; Riesmeyer, J.S.; Riddle, M.C.; Rydén, L.; et al. Dulaglutide and Cardiovascular Outcomes in Type 2 Diabetes (REWIND): A Double-Blind, Randomised Placebo-Controlled Trial. *Lancet* **2019**, *394*, 121–130. [CrossRef]
93. Pfeffer, M.A.; Claggett, B.; Diaz, R.; Dickstein, K.; Gerstein, H.C.; Køber, L.V.; Lawson, F.C.; Ping, L.; Wei, X.; Lewis, E.F.; et al. Lixisenatide in Patients with Type 2 Diabetes and Acute Coronary Syndrome. *N. Engl. J. Med.* **2015**, *373*, 2247–2257. [CrossRef]
94. Holman, R.R.; Bethel, M.A.; Mentz, R.J.; Thompson, V.P.; Lokhnygina, Y.; Buse, J.B.; Chan, J.C.; Choi, J.; Gustavson, S.M.; Iqbal, N.; et al. Effects of Once-Weekly Exenatide on Cardiovascular Outcomes in Type 2 Diabetes. *N. Engl. J. Med.* **2017**, *377*, 1228–1239. [CrossRef] [PubMed]
95. Bethel, M.A.; Patel, R.A.; Merrill, P.; Lokhnygina, Y.; Buse, J.B.; Mentz, R.J.; Pagidipati, N.J.; Chan, J.C.; Gustavson, S.M.; Iqbal, N.; et al. Cardiovascular Outcomes with Glucagon-like Peptide-1 Receptor Agonists in Patients with Type 2 Diabetes: A Meta-Analysis. *Lancet Diabetes Endocrinol.* **2018**, *6*, 105–113. [CrossRef]
96. Kristensen, S.L.; Rørth, R.; Jhund, P.S.; Docherty, K.F.; Sattar, N.; Preiss, D.; Køber, L.; Petrie, M.C.; McMurray, J.J.V. Cardiovascular, Mortality, and Kidney Outcomes with GLP-1 Receptor Agonists in Patients with Type 2 Diabetes: A Systematic Review and Meta-Analysis of Cardiovascular Outcome Trials. *Lancet Diabetes Endocrinol.* **2019**, *7*, 776–785. [CrossRef]

97. Bizino, M.B.; Jazet, I.M.; Westenberg, J.J.M.; van Eyk, H.J.; Paiman, E.H.M.; Smit, J.W.A.; Lamb, H.J. Effect of Liraglutide on Cardiac Function in Patients with Type 2 Diabetes Mellitus: Randomized Placebo-Controlled Trial. *Cardiovasc. Diabetol.* **2019**, *18*, 55. [CrossRef] [PubMed]
98. Das, S.R.; Everett, B.M.; Birtcher, K.K.; Brown, J.M.; Cefalu, W.T.; Januzzi, J.L.; Kalyani, R.R.; Kosiborod, M.; Magwire, M.L.; Morris, P.B.; et al. 2018 ACC Expert Consensus Decision Pathway on Novel Therapies for Cardiovascular Risk Reduction in Patients With Type 2 Diabetes and Atherosclerotic Cardiovascular Disease: A Report of the American College of Cardiology Task Force on Expert Consensus Decision Pathways. *J. Am. Coll Cardiol.* **2018**, *72*, 3200–3223. [CrossRef] [PubMed]
99. Buse, J.B.; Wexler, D.J.; Tsapas, A.; Rossing, P.; Mingrone, G.; Mathieu, C.; D'Alessio, D.A.; Davies, M.J. 2019 Update to: Management of Hyperglycaemia in Type 2 Diabetes, 2018. A Consensus Report by the American Diabetes Association (ADA) and the European Association for the Study of Diabetes (EASD). *Diabetologia* **2020**, *63*, 221–228. [CrossRef]
100. Arnett, D.K.; Blumenthal, R.S.; Albert, M.A.; Buroker, A.B.; Goldberger, Z.D.; Hahn, E.J.; Himmelfarb, C.D.; Khera, A.; Lloyd-Jones, D.; McEvoy, J.W.; et al. 2019 ACC/AHA Guideline on the Primary Prevention of Cardiovascular Disease: A Report of the American College of Cardiology/American Heart Association Task Force on Clinical Practice Guidelines. *J. Am. Coll Cardiol.* **2019**, *74*, e177–e232. [CrossRef] [PubMed]
101. Garber, A.J.; Handelsman, Y.; Grunberger, G.; Einhorn, D.; Abrahamson, M.J.; Barzilay, J.I.; Blonde, L.; Bush, M.A.; DeFronzo, R.A.; Garber, J.R.; et al. Consensus statement by the American association of clinical endocrinologists and american college of endocrinology on the comprehensive type 2 diabetes management algorithm—2020 executive summary. *Endocr. Pract.* **2020**, *26*, 107–139. [CrossRef]
102. Dunlay, S.M.; Givertz, M.M.; Aguilar, D.; Allen, L.A.; Chan, M.; Desai, A.S.; Deswal, A.; Dickson, V.V.; Kosiborod, M.N.; Lekavich, C.L.; et al. Type 2 Diabetes Mellitus and Heart Failure: A Scientific Statement from the American Heart Association and the Heart Failure Society of America: This Statement Does Not Represent an Update of the 2017 ACC/AHA/HFSA Heart Failure Guideline Update. *Circulation* **2019**, *140*, e294–e324. [CrossRef]

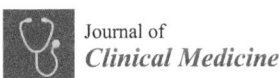

Article

Effects of Weight Gain after 20 Years of Age and Incidence of Hyper-Low-Density Lipoprotein Cholesterolemia: The Iki Epidemiological Study of Atherosclerosis and Chronic Kidney Disease (ISSA-CKD)

Shota Okutsu [1,2], Yoshifumi Kato [1], Shunsuke Funakoshi [2], Toshiki Maeda [2], Chikara Yoshimura [2], Miki Kawazoe [2], Atsushi Satoh [2], Soichiro Yokota [3], Kazuhiro Tada [3], Koji Takahashi [3], Kenji Ito [3], Tetsuhiko Yasuno [3], Hideyuki Fujii [4], Shigeaki Mukoubara [5], Hitoshi Nakashima [3], Daiji Kawanami [4], Kosuke Masutani [3], Hisatomi Arima [2,*] and Shigeki Nabeshima [1]

1. General Medicine, Fukuoka University Hospital, Fukuoka 814-0180, Japan; shota.o.19870528@gmail.com (S.O.); ykato@fukuoka-u.ac.jp (Y.K.); snabeshi@fukuoka-u.ac.jp (S.N.)
2. Department of Preventive Medicine and Public Health, Fukuoka University, Fukuoka 814-0180, Japan; shunsuke.funakoshi@gmail.com (S.F.); tmaeda@fukuoka-u.ac.jp (T.M.); ychikara@fukuoka-u.ac.jp (C.Y.); miki1024@fukuoka-u.ac.jp (M.K.); atsushis@fukuoka-u.ac.jp (A.S.)
3. Division of Nephrology and Rheumatology, Department of Internal Medicine, Fukuoka University, Fukuoka 814-0180, Japan; syokota@fukuoka-u.ac.jp (S.Y.); ktada@fukuoka-u.ac.jp (K.T.); reply_09030728174@yahoo.co.jp (K.T.); kito@fukuoka-u.ac.jp (K.I.); yasuno9584@fukuoka-u.ac.jp (T.Y.); hitscenenakashima@gmail.com (H.N.); kmasutani@fukuoka-u.ac.jp (K.M.)
4. Department of Endocrinology and Diabetes Mellitus, Fukuoka University School of Medicine, Fukuoka 814-0180, Japan; joeten1cho@yahoo.co.jp (H.F.); kawanami@fukuoka-u.ac.jp (D.K.)
5. Nagasaki Prefecture Iki Hospital, Nagasaki 811-5365, Japan; s-mukoubara@ikihp.jp
* Correspondence: harima@fukuoka-u.ac.jp; Tel.: +81-92-801-1011; Fax: +81-92-862-8200

Abstract: The aim of this study was to investigate the effects of long-term weight gain from the age of 20 on incidence of hyper-low-density-lipoprotein (LDL) cholesterolemia in the general population of Japanese people. Methods: We conducted a population-based retrospective cohort study using annual health checkup data for residents of Iki City, Nagasaki Prefecture, Japan. A total of 3179 adult ($\geq$30 years old) men and women without hyper-LDL cholesterolemia at baseline, who underwent two or more health checkups were included in the analysis. Information on weight gain ($\geq$10 kg) after 20 years of age was obtained using questionnaire. The outcome of this study was development of hyper-LDL cholesterolemia defined as LDL-cholesterol level $\geq$3.62 mmol/L and/or initiation of lipid-lowering medications. Results: During a mean follow-up period of 4.53 years, 665 of the 3179 participants developed hyper-LDL cholesterolemia (46.5/1000 person-years). The incidence of hyper-LDL cholesterolemia was higher in participants with a weight gain of $\geq$10 kg (55.3/1000 person-years) than among those with a weight gain of <10 kg (41.8/1000 person-years). This association remained statistically significant even after adjustment for age, sex, smoking, daily drinking, exercise, obesity, hypertension, and diabetes (multivariable hazard ratio 1.31, 95% confidence interval 1.08–1.58, p = 0.006). Conclusion: A weight gain of $\geq$10 after 20 years of age affected the development of hyper-LDL cholesterol regardless of age, sex, and obesity in a general population of Japanese.

Keywords: weight gain; LDL cholesterol; hyper-LDL cholesterolemia; longitudinal study; general population

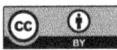

1. Introduction

Cardiovascular disease is one of the leading causes of death in Japan as well as worldwide, with 18 million fatalities accounting for 32% of total deaths worldwide [1]. The risks of cardiovascular disease are associated with lifestyle factors such as smoking, diet, and exercise habits, and metabolic factors such as obesity, serum lipid levels, hypertension, and diabetes [2,3]. Of these, elevated low-density lipoprotein (LDL) cholesterol levels are among the most important [4]. Randomized controlled trials have demonstrated the short-term effects of interventions to reduce body weight on LDL cholesterol levels [5]. However, the effects of long-term weight changes on LDL cholesterol levels are not clear. The objective of this study was to investigate the effects of long-term weight gain from the age of 20 on incidence of hyper-low-density-lipoprotein (LDL) cholesterolemia in the general population of Japanese.

2. Materials and Methods

2.1. Study Design and Participants

The Iki Epidemiological Study of Atherosclerosis and Chronic Kidney Disease (ISSA-CKD) project was a retrospective open cohort study of the general population of Iki City, Nagasaki Prefecture, Japan. The details of the study methods have been previously reported [6–11]. In brief, Iki Island is in the north of Nagasaki Prefecture and the population is approximately 27,000. In Iki City, medical examinations are conducted annually for residents over 30 years of age. A total of 7895 people who participated in these medical examinations at least once during study period between 2008 and 2017. We excluded 1879 individuals who underwent a health checkup only once, 2289 individuals who had previously been diagnosed with hyper-LDL cholesterolemia (LDL-C levels ≥3.62 mmol/L and/or use of lipid-lowering medications), and 548 individuals with missing information on weight gain after 20 years of age. Therefore, this study enrolled 3179 individuals. The study was approved by the Fukuoka University Clinical Research Ethics Center (approval number: 2017M010).

2.2. Data Collection

Information on weight change after 20 years of age was collected using a standardized yes/no questionnaire ("has your weight increased by 10 kg or more since 20 years of age?"). The cut-off point of 10 kg was defined based on recommendation from the Ministry of Health, Labour and Welfare to detect people who gained weight by 10 kg or more after 20 years of age because they are at high risk of diabetes and hypertension [12]. We also used a standardized questionnaire regarding smoking, daily alcohol intake, and regular exercise habits, as well as the use of blood pressure, lipid-lowering, and glucose-lowering drugs. A current smoker was defined as a participant who smoked ≥100 cigarettes or had smoked continuously for ≥6 months. A current alcohol drinker was defined as a participant who drank daily. A regular exercise habit was defined as exercise performed for ≥30 min at least twice weekly. Height and weight were measured without shoes and body mass index (BMI; kg/m^2) was calculated. Obesity was defined as a BMI ≥ 25 kg/m^2 [13]. Blood pressure (BP) was measured by trained staff using a mercury, automatic, or aneroid sphygmomanometer with an appropriately sized cuff, measured with the right upper arm according to standard guidelines after at least 5 min of rest in a sitting position [14]. Hypertension was defined as BP ≥ 140/90 mmHg, or use of BP-lowering medications [15]. Casual blood samples were also collected. LDL cholesterol levels were determined using a direct enzymatic method. High-density lipoprotein (HDL) cholesterol and triglyceride levels were also measured using the enzymatic method. Blood glucose and HbA1c levels were measured enzymatically, and diabetes was defined as a fasting blood glucose level ≥7.0 mmol/L, non-fasting blood glucose ≥11.1 mmol/L, HbA1c (National Glycohemoglobin Standardization Program) ≥6.5%, or use of glucose-lowering drugs [16].

2.3. Outcome

During the follow-up period from 2008 to 2017, we defined the first time when each participant received a medical examination as the baseline and followed the patients up to 2017. The outcome of this study was incidence of hyper-LDL cholesterolemia. The onset of hyper-LDL cholesterolemia was defined as an LDL-C level of ≥3.62 mmol/L or the initiation of lipid-lowering drugs during the follow-up period [17], which was confirmed at the end of follow-up.

2.4. Statistical Analysis

We applied Wilcoxon test for continuous variables and Chi-square tests for categorical variables to compare baseline characteristics between the two groups: those whose weight had increased by ≥10 kg after 20 years of age and those who did not. The incidence of hyper-LDL cholesterolemia was calculated in person-years. The effect of weight gain of ≥10 kg after 20 years of age on the development of hyper-LDL cholesterolemia was estimated using univariable and multivariable Cox proportional hazard models. The multivariable analysis was adjusted for age, sex, smoking, drinking, exercise, obesity, hypertension, and diabetes. We conducted a subgroup analysis to stratify the effect of weight gain on the development of hyper-LDL cholesterolemia by subgroup (under 65 years or over 65 years of age, male or female sex, non-obese or obese). The differences between subgroups were tested by adding an interaction term to the statistical model. Statistical Analysis System (SAS) version 9.4 (SAS Institute Inc., Cary, NC, USA) was used to perform the statistical analyses. All p-values reported were two-sided, and the significance level was set at $p < 0.05$.

3. Results

Table 1 shows the baseline characteristics according to weight gain after 20 years of age. Participants with a weight gain of ≥10 kg were more likely to be men, obese, hypertensive, and diabetic, as well as higher levels of BMI, blood pressure, HbA1c, HDL-C, LDL-C, and triglycerides. During a mean follow-up period of 4.53 years, 665 of the 3179 participants developed hyper-LDL cholesterolemia (46.5/1000 person-years).

Table 1. Participant baseline characteristics according to weight gain after 20 years of age.

	Weight Change after 20 Years of Age		p Value
	<10 kg (N = 2146)	≥10 kg (N = 1033)	
Age	58.9 ± 11.7	58.9 ± 10.4	0.977
Female	1111 (51.8%)	413 (40.0%)	<0.0001
Current smoker	474 (22.1%)	232 (22.4%)	0.810
Daily drinking	574 (26.9%)	331 (32.3%)	0.0018
Exercise	1549 (73.3)	769 (75.2%)	0.250
Body mass index	22.0 ± 2.63	26.1 ± 3.18	<0.0001
Obesity	256 (11.9%)	635 (61.5%)	<0.0001
Systolic blood pressure, mmHg	127 ± 18.9	132 ± 18.4	<0.0001
Diastolic blood pressure, mmHg	73.7 ± 11.0	77.0 ± 11.3	<0.0001
Hypertension	787 (36.7%)	534 (51.7%)	<0.0001
LDL-cholesterol, mmol/L (mg/dL)	2.74 ± 0.54 (106 ± 21.0)	2.90 ± 0.50 (112 ± 19.5)	<0.0001
HDL-cholesterol, mmol/L (mg/dL)	1.67 ± 0.44 (64.6 ± 16.9)	1.46 ± 0.39 (56.5 ± 15.0)	<0.0001
Triglyceride, mmol/L (mg/dL)	1.15 ± 0.87 (102 ± 76.9)	1.56 ± 1.21 (138 ± 107)	<0.0001
HbA1c, %	5.30 ± 0.63	5.50 ± 0.80	<0.0001
Diabetes	133 (6.2%)	106 (10.7%)	<0.0001

LDL, low-density lipoprotein; HDL, high-density lipoprotein; HbA1c, glycated hemoglobin.

Table 2 shows the risks of hyper-LDL cholesterolemia according to weight gain after 20 years of age. The incidence of hyper-LDL cholesterolemia was higher in participants with a weight gain of ≥10 kg (55.3/1000 person-years) than among those with a weight gain of <10 kg (41.8/1000 person-years). This association remained statistically significant even after adjustment for age, sex, smoking, daily drinking, exercise, obesity, hypertension, and diabetes (multivariable-adjusted hazard ratio 1.31, 95% confidence interval 1.08–1.58,

$p = 0.006$). Similar results were obtained after adjustment for more detailed categories for alcohol intake (no drinkers, occasional drinkers or daily drinkers [<22 g/day, 22–43 g/day or ≥44 g/day]): multivariable hazard ratio 1.31, 95% confidence interval 1.08–1.58, $p = 0.005$. Sensitivity analysis with adjustment of BMI instead of obesity demonstrated that the hazard ratio of weight gain ≥10 kg after 20 years of age for development of hyper-LDL cholesterolemia was 1.18 (95% confidence interval 0.97–1.43) but the association was not statistically significant (p value = 0.100). Likewise, sensitivity analysis with adjustment of waist circumference instead of obesity demonstrated that the hazard ratio of weight gain ≥10 kg after 20 years of age for development of hyper-LDL cholesterolemia was 1.16 (95% confidence interval 0.96–1.41) but the association was not statistically significant (p value = 0.122).

Table 2. Risks of hyper-LDL cholesterolemia according to weight gain after 20 years of age.

	Weight Change after 20 Years of Age		p Value
	<10 kg (N = 2146)	≥10 kg (N = 1033)	
Number of events	406	259	
Person-years	9721.38	4679.49	
Incidence/1000 person-years	41.8	55.3	
Crude hazard ratio (95%CI)	Reference	1.33 (1.14–1.55)	<0.001
Multivariable-adjusted * hazard ratio (95%CI)	Reference	1.31 (1.08–1.58)	0.006

* Adjusted for age, sex, smoking, daily drinking, exercise, obesity, hypertension, and diabetes. CI, confidence interval.

Table 3 shows the results of subgroup analyses. There were no clear differences in the effects of weight gain of ≥10 kg after 20 years of age for the development of hyper-LDL cholesterolemia between subgroups defined by age (<65 vs. ≥65 years), sex, and obesity (all $p > 0.1$ for interaction).

Table 3. Subgroup analyses.

	Adjusted * Hazard Ratio	p for Interaction
Age (years)		
<65	1.40 (1.10–1.77)	
>65	1.12 (0.82–1.54)	0.13
Sex		
Male	1.26 (0.96–1.65)	
Female	1.33 (1.02–1.72)	0.90
Obesity		
Absent	1.26 (0.99–1.59)	
Present	1.38 (1.00–1.91)	0.63

* Adjusted for age (except for subgroup analysis by age), sex (except for subgroup analysis by sex), smoking, daily drinking, exercise, obesity (except for subgroup analysis by obesity), hypertension, and diabetes.

4. Discussion

The results of this large-scale longitudinal study of the general Japanese population showed that a weight gain of ≥10 kg after 20 years of age was significantly associated with the incidence of hyper-LDL cholesterolemia. This outcome remained significant even after adjusting for age, sex, smoking, daily drinking, exercise, obesity, hypertension, and diabetes. A similar association was observed between subgroups defined by age, sex, and obesity.

Previous studies have investigated the effects of body weight changes on serum LDL cholesterol levels. A meta-analysis of 73 randomized trials including 32,496 participants (mean age 48 years, weight 102 kg, BMI 36.3 kg/m^2) reported that short-term body weight reduction due to lifestyle-related interventions was associated with decreased LDL cholesterol levels in both men and women [4]. A prospective observational study of

3388 overweight Polish individuals aged 45–64 years reported was no significant association between a two-year change in body weight and serum LDL cholesterol levels [18]. Regarding the effects of long-term body weight change, a cross-sectional study investigating the association between body weight gain after 20 years of age and the prevalence of hyper-LDL cholesterolemia in 1715 Chinese participants in the general population aged 45–60 years reported that women with a weight gain of ≥ 10 kg after 20 years of age had a higher prevalence of hyper-LDL cholesterolemia than those without; however, this association was not observed in men [19]. In the present large-scale, longitudinal study of the general Japanese population, long-term body weight change age 20 years of age was associated with increased risks of the future development of hyper-LDL cholesterolemia. The effects of long-term body weight change on hyper-LDL cholesterolemia were comparable between sexes. Based on these findings, long-term weight gain is likely to affect the future development of hyper-LDL cholesterolemia.

The mechanisms underlying the association between long-term weight gain and hyper-LDL cholesterolemia have not been fully elucidated. Weight gain from the age of 20 years appears to mainly reflect an increase in visceral fat volume owing to decreased muscle mass volume and basal metabolic rate after this age [20–22]. Increased visceral fat volume causes insulin resistance [23–25], which is associated with an increased pool of LDL precursors including very-low-density lipoprotein (VLDL) [26,27]. Insulin resistance is also associated with a reduction in the number of LDL receptors, a decrease in the LDL-binding affinity of these receptors, and a subsequent reduction in the clearance of LDL particles [26–28]. Increased pooled LDL precursors and decreased clearance of LDL particles, which are associated with visceral fat, might be attributable to the development of hyper-LDL cholesterolemia.

This is the first longitudinal study of the association between a weight gain of ≥ 10 kg after 20 years of age and hyper-LDL cholesterolemia in the general population including adult Japanese men and women. The limitations of this study were its retrospective design, the use of a recall-based questionnaire, and the analysis of data from medical examinations of the general public, which may have resulted in a bias toward health-conscious participants.

5. Conclusions

In conclusion, in adult Japanese men and women, a weight gain of ≥ 10 kg after 20 years of age affected the development of hyper-LDL cholesterol regardless of age, sex, and obesity. A population strategy with interventions to maintain a proper weight is important to prevent the subsequent occurrence of cardiovascular events, increased risk of death, and medical costs.

Author Contributions: Conceptualization, H.A.and S.O.; data curation, H.A.; formal analysis, T.M. and H.A.; investigation, H.F., S.F., A.S., M.K., S.Y., C.Y., S.N., K.T. (Kazuhiro Tada), K.T. (Koji Takahashi),Y.K. and S.O.; methodology, H.A.; project administration, H.A.; software, H.A.; supervision, H.A.; writing—original draft, S.O. and H.A.; writing—review and editing, D.K., H.A., S.N., Y.K., H.N., K.I., T.Y., S.M., K.M. and S.O. All authors were informed about each step of manuscript processing including the submission, revision, revision reminder, etc. via emails from our system or assigned assistant editor. All authors have read and agreed to the published version of the manuscript.

Funding: This research received grants from Iki City.

Institutional Review Board Statement: The study was conducted according to the guidelines of the Declaration of Helsinki of 1975, revised in 2013, and approved by Fukuoka University Clinical Research and Ethics Centre (No.2017M010).

Informed Consent Statement: Consent of participants was obtained using opt-out approach.

Data Availability Statement: The data are not publicly available in order to preserve the anonymity of the subjects involved in the study.

Conflicts of Interest: H.A. received research grants from Daiichi Sankyo and Takeda, lecture fees from Bayer, Daiichi Sankyo, Fukuda Denshi, MSD, Takeda, Teijin and fees for consultancy from Kyowa Kirin. D.K. received research support from Böehringer Ingelheim, Sumitomo Dainippon Pharma, Takeda Pharmaceutical.

References

1. Roth, G.A.; Johnson, C.; Abajobir, A.; Abd-Allah, F.; Abera, S.F.; Abyu, G.; Ahmed, M.; Aksut, B.; Alam, T.; Alam, K.; et al. Global, Regional, and National Burden of Cardiovascular Diseases for 10 Causes, 1990 to 2015. *J. Am. Coll. Cardiol.* **2017**, *70*, 1–25. [CrossRef]
2. Zmysłowski, A.; Szterk, A. Current knowledge on the mechanism of atherosclerosis and pro-atherosclerotic properties of oxysterols. *Lipids Health Dis.* **2017**, *16*, 188. [CrossRef]
3. Catapano, A.L.; Graham, I.; De Backer, G.; Wiklund, O.; Chapman, M.J.; Drexel, H.; Hoes, A.W.; Jennings, C.S.; Landmesser, U.; Pedersen, T.R.; et al. 2016 ESC/EAS Guidelines for the Management of Dyslipidaemias: The Task Force for the Management of Dyslipidaemias of the European Society of Cardiology (ESC) and European Atherosclerosis Society (EAS). *Eur. Heart J.* **2016**, *37*, 2999–3058. [CrossRef]
4. Nabel, E.G.; Braunwald, E. A tale of coronary artery disease and myocardial infarction. *N. Engl. J. Med.* **2012**, *366*, 54–63, Erratum in **2012**, *366*, 970. [CrossRef]
5. Hasan, B.; Nayfeh, T.; Alzuabi, M.; Wang, Z.; Kuchkuntla, A.R.; Prokop, L.J.; Newman, C.B.; Murad, M.H.; Rajjo, T.I. Weight loss and serum lipids in overweight and obese adults: A systematic review and meta-analysis. *J. Clin. Endocrinol. Metab.* **2020**, *105*, 3695–3703. [CrossRef] [PubMed]
6. Ishida, S.; Kondo, S.; Funakoshi, S.; Satoh, A.; Maeda, T.; Kawazoe, M.; Yoshimura, C.; Tada, K.; Takahashi, K.; Ito, K.; et al. White blood cell count and incidence of hypertension in the general Japanese population: ISSA-CKD study. *PLoS ONE* **2021**, *16*, e0246304. [CrossRef]
7. Miyabayashi, I.; Mori, S.; Satoh, A.; Kawazoe, M.; Funakoshi, S.; Ishida, S.; Maeda, T.; Yoshimura, C.; Tada, K.; Takahashi, K.; et al. Uric acid and prevalence of hypertension in a general population of Japanese: ISSA-CKD Study. *J. Clin. Med. Res.* **2020**, *12*, 431–435. [CrossRef]
8. Yasuno, T.; Maeda, T.; Tada, K.; Takahashi, K.; Ito, K.; Abe, Y.; Mukoubara, S.; Masutani, K.; Arima, H.; Nakashima, H. Effects of HbA1c on the development and progression of chronic kidney disease in elderly and middle-aged Japanese: Iki Epidemiological Study of Atherosclerosis and Chronic Kidney Disease (ISSA-CKD). *Intern. Med.* **2020**, *59*, 175–180. [CrossRef]
9. Ito, K.; Maeda, T.; Tada, K.; Takahashi, K.; Yasuno, T.; Masutani, K.; Mukoubara, S.; Arima, H.; Nakashima, H. The role of cigarette smoking on new-onset of chronic kidney disease in a Japanese population without prior chronic kidney disease: Iki epidemiological study of atherosclerosis and chronic kidney disease (ISSA-CKD). *Clin. Exp. Nephrol.* **2020**, *24*, 919–926. [CrossRef] [PubMed]
10. Maeda, T.; Yoshimura, C.; Takahashi, K.; Ito, K.; Yasuno, T.; Abe, Y.; Masutani, K.; Nakashima, H.; Mukoubara, S.; Arima, H. Usefulness of the blood pressure classification in the new 2017 ACC/AHA hypertension guidelines for the prediction of new-onset chronic kidney disease. *J. Hum. Hypertens.* **2019**, *33*, 873–878. [CrossRef]
11. Fujii, H.; Funakoshi, S.; Maeda, T.; Satoh, A.; Kawazoe, M.; Ishida, S.; Yoshimura, C.; Yokota, S.; Tada, K.; Takahashi, K.; et al. Eating Speed and Incidence of Diabetes in a Japanese General Population: ISSA-CKD. *J. Clin. Med.* **2021**, *10*, 1949. [CrossRef]
12. *Standard Program of Health Check-Up and Health Guidance*; Ministry of Health, Labor and Welfare: Tokyo, Japan, 2007.
13. Examination Committee of Criteria for 'Obesity Disease' in Japan: Japan Society for the Study of Obesity New Criteria for "Obesity Disease" in Japan. *Circ. J.* **2002**, *66*, 987–992.
14. The Japanese Society of Cardiovascular Disease Prevention. *Handbook for Cardiovascular Prevention*; Hokendojinsha: Tokyo, Japan, 2014.
15. Umemura, S.; Arima, H.; Arima, S.; Asayama, K.; Dohi, Y.; Hirooka, Y.; Horio, T.; Hoshide, S.; Ikeda, S.; Ishimitsu, T.; et al. The Japanese Society of Hypertension Guidelines for the Management of Hypertension (JSH 2019). *Hypertens. Res.* **2019**, *42*, 1235–1481. [CrossRef]
16. Shurraw, S.; Hemmelgarn, B.; Lin, M.; Majumdar, S.R.; Klarenbach, S.; Manns, B.; Bello, A.; James, M.; Turin, T.C.; Tonelli, M. Alberta Kidney Disease Network: Association between glycemic control and adverse outcomes in people with diabetes mellitus and chronic kidney disease: A population-based cohort study. *Arch. Intern. Med.* **2011**, *171*, 1920–1927. [CrossRef]
17. Kinoshita, M.; Yokote, K.; Arai, H.; Iida, M.; Ishigaki, Y.; Ishibashi, S.; Umemoto, S.; Egusa, G.; Ohmura, H.; Okamura, T.; et al. Japan Atherosclerosis Society (JAS) Guidelines for Prevention of Atherosclerotic Cardiovascular Diseases 2017. *J. Atheroscler. Thromb.* **2018**, *25*, 846–984. [CrossRef]
18. Macek, P.; Terek-Derszniak, M.; Biskup, M.; Krol, H.; Smok-Kalwat, J.; Gozdz, S.; Zak, M. A two-year follow-up cohort study-improved clinical control over CVD risk factors through weight loss in middle-aged and older adults. *J. Clin. Med.* **2020**, *9*, 2904. [CrossRef]
19. Zhou, Y.; Xuan, Y.J.; Yang, L.S.; Rutayisire, E.; Zhang, L.J.; Xuan, P.; Tao, X.Y.; Sheng, J.; Tao, F.B.; Wang, S.F. Weight changes since age 20 and cardiovascular risk factors in a middle-aged Chinese population. *J. Public Health* **2018**, *40*, 253–261. [CrossRef]
20. Kitazoe, Y.; Kishino, H.; Tanisawa, K.; Udaka, K.; Tanaka, M. Renormalized basal metabolic rate describes the human aging process and longevity. *Aging Cell* **2019**, *18*, e12968. [CrossRef] [PubMed]
21. Hunter, G.R.; Gower, B.A.; Kane, B.L. Age related shift in visceral fat. *Int. J. Body Compos. Res.* **2010**, *8*, 103–108. [PubMed]

22. Jensen, M.D.; Ryan, D.H.; Apovian, C.M.; Ard, J.D.; Comuzzie, A.G.; Donato, K.A.; Hu, F.B.; Hubbard, V.S.; Jakicic, J.M.; Kushner, R.F.; et al. American College of Cardiology/American Heart Association Task Force on Practice Guidelines; Obesity Society: 2013 AHA/ACC/TOS guideline for the management of overweight and obesity in adults: A report of the American College of Cardiology/American Heart Association Task Force on Practice Guidelines and The Obesity Society. *Circulation* **2014**, *129* (Suppl. 2), S102–S138.
23. Jung, U.J.; Choi, M.S. Obesity and its metabolic complications: The role of adipokines and the relationship between obesity, inflammation, insulin resistance, dyslipidemia and nonalcoholic fatty liver disease. *Int. J. Mol. Sci.* **2014**, *15*, 6184–6223. [CrossRef] [PubMed]
24. Pennings, N.; Jaber, J.; Ahiawodzi, P. Ten-year weight gain is associated with elevated fasting insulin levels and precedes glucose elevation. *Diabetes Metab. Res. Rev.* **2018**, *34*, e2986. [CrossRef] [PubMed]
25. Chang, Y.; Sung, E.; Yun, K.E.; Jung, H.S.; Kim, C.W.; Kwon, M.J.; Cho, S.I.; Ryu, S. Weight change as a predictor of incidence and remission of insulin resistance. *PLoS ONE* **2013**, *8*, e63690. [CrossRef]
26. Kawanami, D.; Matoba, K.; Utsunomiy, K. Dyslipidemia in diabetic nephropathy. *Ren. Replace Ther.* **2016**, *2*, 16. [CrossRef]
27. Bjornstad, P.; Eckel, R.H. Pathogenesis of lipid disorders in insulin resistance: A brief review. *Curr. Diabetes Rep.* **2018**, *18*, 127. [CrossRef]
28. Vergès, B. Pathophysiology of diabetic dyslipidaemia: Where are we? *Diabetologia* **2015**, *58*, 886–899. [CrossRef]

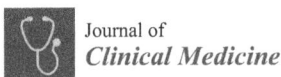

Review

A Practical Guide for the Management of Steroid Induced Hyperglycaemia in the Hospital

Felix Aberer [1,2], Daniel A. Hochfellner [1], Harald Sourij [1,2,*] and Julia K. Mader [1]

[1] Division of Endocrinology and Diabetology, Medical University of Graz, 8036 Graz, Austria; felix.aberer@medunigraz.at (F.A.); daniel.hochfellner@medunigraz.at (D.A.H.); julia.mader@medunigraz.at (J.K.M.)

[2] Interdisciplinary Metabolic Medicine Trials Unit, Medical University of Graz, 8036 Graz, Austria

* Correspondence: ha.sourij@medunigraz.at; Tel.: +43-316-385-81310

Abstract: Glucocorticoids represent frequently recommended and often indispensable immunosuppressant and anti-inflammatory agents prescribed in various medical conditions. Despite their proven efficacy, glucocorticoids bear a wide variety of side effects among which steroid induced hyperglycaemia (SIHG) is among the most important ones. SIHG, potentially causes new-onset hyperglycaemia or exacerbation of glucose control in patients with previously known diabetes. Retrospective data showed that similar to general hyperglycaemia in diabetes, SIHG in the hospital and in outpatient settings detrimentally impacts patient outcomes, including mortality. However, recommendations for treatment targets and guidelines for in-hospital as well as outpatient therapeutic management are lacking, partially due to missing evidence from clinical studies. Still, SIHG caused by various types of glucocorticoids is a common challenge in daily routine and clinical guidance is needed. In this review, we aimed to summarize clinical evidence of SIHG in inpatient care impacting clinical outcome, establishment of diagnosis, diagnostic procedures and therapeutic recommendations.

Keywords: steroid induced hyperglycaemia; hospital; practical guide

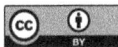

1. Introduction

Steroidal therapies in particular glucocorticoids (GC), represent therapeutic agents of great importance in the treatment and prophylaxis of various acute and chronic inflammatory as well as autoimmune disorders [1]. Despite their efficacy, the use of steroids is associated with a variety of side effects that can be pragmatically divided into three categories: (1) Immediate side effects include the occurrence of fluid retention with oedema, blurriness of vision, impairments of mood, immune response modulation and the development of steroid induced hyperglycaemia (SIHG). (2) Idiosyncratic side effects summarize the development of avascular necrosis, cataract formation, glaucoma and psychosis. (3) More gradual side effects affecting the endocrine system and inducing the development of bone disease, dyslipidaemia, obesity and adrenal suppression [2]. As GCs decrease peripheral insulin sensitivity, increase hepatic gluconeogenesis, trigger insulin resistance on the level of the lipid metabolism and adipose tissue, as well as inhibit pancreatic insulin production and secretion, they represent a drug class with the highest risk of provoking the development of hyperglycaemia and overt diabetes mellitus (DM) [3–5].

2. Prevalence of Steroid Induced Hyperglycaemia in the Hospital

The prevalence of SIHG is dependent on the dose, indication and setting of use. Individual conditions such as age, baseline body mass index (BMI) and family history of diabetes are known to impact the risk of SIHG development. Older observational data indicate that 2% of incident diabetes cases in a primary care population are associated with GC therapy and the odds ratios for presenting with new-onset diabetes after introduction of GCs in various studies has been described to range from 1.36–2.31 [6]. Patients without history of diabetes developed in-hospital hyperglycaemia (≥10 mmol/L; ≥180 mg/dL) in 70% when relevant doses of GCs were administered [7]. A meta-analysis summarized studies in which patients without pre-existing diabetes who received systemic GCs and showed a rate of SIHG development in 32.3% and in further 18.6% diabetes was sustainable during the follow up [8]. In patients who received solid organ transplantation and GC therapy the prevalence was described to be between 17% and 32% [9,10] and in a high-risk population of people who received high dose systemic therapy for acute Graft-versus-Host disease, two thirds of the cohort showed median glucose readings in the hyperglycaemic range (defined as fasting glucose ≥7 mmol/L or ≥126 mg/dL) [11]. As SIHG is suggested to be a transient problem resolving after the discontinuation of GCs, data indicate that diabetes can persist and GCs just unmasked a pre-existing glucose metabolism disorder [12,13]. While mainly systemic steroids were identified to expose the patient to an increased risk for hyperglycaemia, recently, topically used GCs were also shown to be associated with an elevated risk of diabetes [14].

3. Impact of Steroid Induced Hyperglycaemia

It has been shown that acute and chronic hyperglycaemia that are present in many cases in the hospital setting are important risk factors for prolonged hospital stays, infectious complications, poorer surgical outcomes and increased mortality [15–17]. Data of people with SIHG without previously known DM are scarce. Some studies reported an association of reduced response to chemotherapeutics and increased mortality in patients with haematological disorders as well as in patients with solid cancer [11,18–21]. Similar outcome with inferior prognosis is reported for patients who underwent kidney transplantation [22] or in case of being hospitalized for acute exacerbated chronic obstructive pulmonary disease [23]. However, the question whether elevated blood glucose is just a surrogate parameter for severe illness and adverse outcome [24] or if blood glucose might be a modifiable risk factor has not been answered yet. Given the fact that most of the studies yet performed employed observational designs and data derived from randomized controlled clinical studies are still substantially lacking, uncertainties whether asymptomatic and transient inpatient hyperglycaemia should be treated, remain [25].

4. Definition of Steroid Induced Hyperglycaemia

SIHG is defined as abnormally elevated blood glucose associated with the use of GCs in patients with or without pre-existing DM. The diagnostic criteria for SIHG do not differ from other types of diabetes and include a confirmed fasting blood glucose ≥7 mmol/L (≥126 mg/dL), a glucose level of ≥11.1 mmol/L (≥200 mg/dL) at 2 h following ingestion of 75 g glucose in an oral glucose tolerance test (OGTT), an HbA1c ≥6.5% (≥48 mmol/mol) or a random blood glucose ≥11.1 mmol/L (≥200 mg/dL) [26]. However, in patients with SIHG, diagnosis can be more challenging: fasting blood glucose might be normal especially when short- or intermediate-acting GCs are administered in single morning doses. Apart from its difficulties in implementation of oGTT in hospitalized patients, hyperglycaemia might be absent after glucose exposure in an oGTT, especially when it is performed in the morning when the diabetogenic effect of the GCs is not yet present. HbA1c might be inconspicuous especially in those with new-onset GC therapy as it reflects the glycaemic situation in the weeks prior to the time point of measurement. In addition, several conditions such as chronic kidney disease or hemoglobinopathies, that are frequently present in people requiring steroids, affect the reliability of HbA1c measurements. Nevertheless, determination of HbA1c can be useful to evaluate glycaemic control in patients who are on long-term GC therapy or to distinguish between new-onset diabetes and pre-existing DM in a situation of hyperglycaemia after GC initiation. Due to the mentioned limitations of the usual diagnostic approach to detect SIHG, it is recommended to perform frequent (capillary) glucose monitoring in those who receive high doses of GCs (defined as >20 mg prednisolone or equivalent). This approach is particularly recommended in people with a high risk to develop SIHG (e.g., advanced age, higher BMI, previously present impaired glucose tolerance, prediabetes or family history of diabetes). Then, a random glucose value ≥11.1 mmol/L (≥200 mg/dL) can be utilized to establish the diagnosis of SIHG [27].

5. Treatment Targets

No clear evidence is available for the establishment of therapeutic goals for patients with SIHG [28]. According to the American Diabetes Association (ADA) glucose targets for patients with SIHG do not differ from those with any other type of diabetes and should be individualized according to specific factors such as life expectancy, comorbidities, patient compliance and risk of hypoglycaemia [29]. In hospitalized patients a target glucose range of 7.8–10.0 mmol/L (140–180 mg/dL) is recommended for the majority of critically and non-critically ill patients. More stringent goals such as 6.1–7.8 mmol/L (110–140 mg/dL) may be appropriate for selected patients, if this goal can be achieved without relevant hypoglycaemia [30]. However, when aiming to achieve lower target glucose levels it has to be considered that people with SIHG often suffer from severe underlying disease (e.g., cancer), are in the perioperative care setting (e.g., recently transplanted patients or those requiring steroids as supportive therapy [31]), receive concomitant complex therapies (chemotherapy, immunosuppressants, antimicrobial therapy, etc.) and thus, might be prone to larger glucose fluctuations. In the course of treatment, GCs need frequent dose adaptions that result in altered requirements of glucose lowering therapies. As a consequence, the risk for hypoglycaemia is increased when stringent glucose targets were chosen. Therefore, in specific patient populations (incurable disease with short life expectancy, advanced age and comorbidities, susceptibility for hypoglycaemia and impaired awareness of hypoglycaemia) the major aim will be the avoidance of hypoglycaemia and hyperglycaemic symptoms [29,32,33].

6. Admission to the Hospital

HbA1c should be assessed in all people with previous DM in order to evaluate glycaemic control prior to GC initiation. In people who were not previously diagnosed with DM and who require relevant amounts of GCs (>20 mg prednisolone or equivalent) or who are at high risk to develop diabetes or SIHG (criteria see Figure 2), HbA1c should be assessed at admission [34]. This helps to distinguish whether a pre-existing unrecognized DM is present which would result in a more pronounced glycaemic excursion following GC therapy initiation. It can also be assumed that hyperglycaemia is self-limiting after cessation of GC treatment and glucose levels return to normal, given that HbA1c levels were inconspicuous prior to GC treatment [35]. A position statement released by the Joint British Diabetes Societies (JBDS) has defined an algorithm for glucose monitoring in hospitalized patients requiring GC treatment. They postulate that determinations of glucose should be performed at least once daily, preferably prior to lunch or 1–2 h post lunch or before the evening meal in people without diabetes in whom GC therapy was initiated. Once daily glucose measurements should be continued and if glucose readings exceed 11.1 mmol/L (200 mg/dL) repeatedly, frequency of testing should be increased to 4 times daily (before each meal and at bedtime) which is mandatory in patients with pre-existing diabetes treated with GC [33]. In the course of hospitalization and scheduling of GC initiation, patients should be well informed about potential side effects of GCs including SIHG and its therapeutic consequences.

7. Initiation of Glucose Lowering Therapy

A practical approach when the implementation of glucose lowering therapy should be initiated was published by Suh et al. who recommend initiating therapy when pre- or post-prandial glucose repeatedly exceed 7.8 (140 mg/dL) or 11.1 mmol/L (200 mg/dL), respectively [28,33]. Similar to the management strategies to lower glucose in patients with type 2 diabetes (T2DM), stepwise intensification of antihyperglycaemic therapy and frequent re-evaluation should be performed in SIHG. The glucose lowering agents of choice should match daily glucose profiles and the mechanism of action should fit to the corresponding GC agent.

8. Treatment of Steroid Induced Hyperglycaemia in the Hospital
8.1. Oral Antihyperglycaemic Agents

In the outpatient setting some oral hypoglycaemic agents (OHA) might have the potential to improve glycaemic control and prevent or delay the development of SIHG [36,37]. There is only very little evidence available showing clinical efficacy of using OHA for in-hospital hyperglycaemia caused by GCs. Insulin sensitizers such as metformin and pioglitazone might be used to enhance insulin sensitivity and reduce insulin resistance [38–41] and can be continued in preexisting T2DM unless contraindications exist. However, in hospitalized patients, specifically in those who are acutely ill, susceptibility to hypoxia or acute kidney injury as well as fluid retention can limit the use of these agents. In addition, in particular pioglitazone, needs an expanded time to exert full action which disqualifies it to be applied for acute SIHG. Insulin secretagogues, stimulating endogenous insulin production might be suitable to tackle mild SIHG in the inpatient setting, specifically in inpatients who are non-severely ill and who receive short-acting steroids once daily in the morning [33]. However, insulin secretagogues should be used with caution as there is an increased risk of hypoglycaemia especially when steroid doses are tapered or meals are skipped. The safe side effect profile of incretin mimetics such as DPP4 inhibitors might support their application in hospitalized patients with SIHG, their acute glucose lowering effect is of moderate extent and mostly they are mostly used as an adjunct to insulin therapy. The use of GLP1-receptor agonists bears the risk of gastrointestinal adverse effects in particular during the initiation phase which limits their broad usage for acutely ill, hospitalized patients with SIHG [28]. The use of the sodium-glucose co transporter-2 (SGLT2) inhibitor dapagliflozin has shown to be safe in patients hospitalized for chronic obstructive pulmonary disease (COPD) developing SIHG, but did not improve glycaemic control or clinical outcomes [42].

OHAs might be an adequate choice in inpatients with stable and non-critical disease and mild hyperglycaemic excursions. In those with significant hyperglycaemia and severe illness, insulin remains the treatment of choice in the hospital setting as also suggested by the current guidelines for inpatient diabetes management [30].

8.2. GC Dependent Glucose Increase and the Choice of Insulin Therapy

The hyperglycaemic effect of different GCs can be pragmatically transferred to the pharmacokinetic profiles of different GCs. Thus, the insulin therapy chosen for SIHG has to take the used agent, the current dose, the time point and interval of the GC administration into account. Table 1 summarizes the pharmacokinetics of available GCs adapted from the literature [43,44], Table 2 indicates potential glucose profiles according to the administered GC agent.

Table 1. Different corticosteroids and their equivalent doses, steroidal kinetics and potential to trigger hyperglycaemia.

Glucocorticoids		Approximate Equivalent Dose (mg)	Plasma Peak Concentration (minutes)	Elimination Half-Life (hours)	Duration of Action (hours)	Hyperglycaemic Effects (hours)		
						Onset	Peak	Resolution
Short-acting	Hydrocortisone	20	10	2	8–12	1	3	6
Intermediate-acting	Predniso(lo)ne	5	60–180	2.5	12–36	4	8	12–16
	Methylprednisolone	4	60	2.5	12–36	4	8	12–16
Long-acting	Dexamethasone	0.75	60–120	4	36–72	8	variable	24–36

Table 2. Schematic illustration of different glucocorticoids and their potential effect on glycaemia. Long-acting agents are usually administered only once daily. These examples are presuming people with normal glucose homeostasis prior to start of glucocorticoid therapy. X-axis: time of the day; y-axis: potential influence on glucose.

Glucocorticoids		Hyperglycaemic Effects (hours)			Glucose Profiles (GC Given Once Daily [8 a.m.])	Glucose Profiles (GC Given Twice Daily [8 a.m. and 20 p.m.])
		Onset	Peak	Resolution		
Short-acting	Hydrocortisone	1	3	6		
Intermediate-acting	Predniso(lo)ne	4	8	12–16		
	Methylprednisolone	4	8	12–16		
Long-acting	Dexamethasone	8	variable	24–36		n.a.

The upcoming paragraphs describe different scenarios of patients with normal glucose homeostasis under regular conditions as well as patients with T2DM well-controlled under dietary recommendations or treated with OHA in whom relevant hyperglycaemia is a consequence of GC administration who subsequently require insulin therapy. The paragraphs contain recently available recommendations which were given for people with new-onset hyperglycaemia or previously known T2DM.

8.2.1. Scenario 1: Short-Acting Glucocorticoids (Hydrocortisone)

Short-acting hydrocortisone has a considerably high mineralocorticoid activity and is therefore suitable as first-line agent in the therapy of adrenal insufficiency. In its usual application as hormone replacement therapy, hydrocortisone should not cause relevant hyperglycaemia if the substance is administered in physiological doses. For these reasons, no data of SIHG induced by short-acting GCs are available and the recommendations arise from speculations. However, the required physiological doses are often overestimated and exogenous Cushing syndrome including SIHG can occur [45]. In addition, in specific conditions such as acute illness, stress or during surgery substantial dose increases can be required that might induce SIHG. Hydrocortisone is characterized by a fast onset and short duration of the intended effect. Simultaneously, the expectable glucose profile in selected patients will show to have a fast and strong increase but only of short duration. Hence, these commonly transient and mostly self-limiting glucose peaks remain often unrecognized. Whether these short-term hyperglycaemic episodes require glucose lowering therapy has to be decided on an individual basis. In patients with significant hyperglycaemia or impaired health status, the agent of choice is short-acting insulin (rapid-acting insulin analogues or regular insulin) which should be injected at the time or shortly after GC administration. As hydrocortisone is usually administered twice or thrice daily, multiple rapid-acting insulin doses might be suitable to improve glycaemic control. However, it has to be taken into account that morning doses during replacement therapy are usually higher than doses throughout the day and insulin requirements thus might be lowered subsequently. Initiation of the dose can be recommended with 0.1 IU/kilogram (kg) bodyweight (BW) [46]. In addition, insulin therapy can be intensified by including insulin corrections in case of higher subsequent glucose values or persisting post-prandial hyperglycaemia assuming that the intensification requires pre/post-prandial glucose assessments. In these cases, schematic increments of 0.04 IU/kg for pre-prandial values from 11.1–16.7 mmol/L (200–300 mg/dL) or 0.08 IU/kg for values $\geq$ 16.7 mmol/L ($\geq$300 mg/dL) can be added to the scheduled insulin dose. It is important to mention that insulin requirements are GC dose-dependent; hence, reduction of GC is usually related to an improvement of glycaemia. Reduction of rapid-acting insulin should be performed proportionally to the reduction in GC dose, vice versa rapid-acting insulin dose can be increased when doses of GCs are recommended to be increased [2,46].

8.2.2. Scenario 2: Intermediate-Acting Glucocorticoids (Predniso(lo)ne and Methylprednisolone)

Intermediate-acting glucocorticoids represent the most commonly prescribed steroid agents. Their high glucocorticoid activity makes them useful for long-term anti-inflammatory and immunosuppressant treatment especially in solid-organ transplant patients and those with COPD. Considering a single dose administration in the morning, which corresponds to the typical prescription, hyperglycaemia develops slowly, but continuously, mostly lasts until the evening and gradually recovers until the next morning simultaneously following the peak and duration of action of the steroid agent. To best fit this glucose pattern short- or intermediate-acting basal insulins such as insulin detemir or NPH (neutral protamine Hagedorn) insulin is recommended. A clinical recommendation to initiate insulin was issued by Clore et al. who suggest initiating a weight-dependent scheme with 0.4 IU/kg of NPH insulin [47]. Another study described clinical efficacy when lower doses of NPH (0.2–0.3 IU/kg) dependent of the GC dose were administered and whether patients were fasting or not [48]. While the kinetics of intermediate-acting glucocorticoids appear to fit best to the glucose lowering property of NPH insulin, two randomized studies with insulin glargine U100 at a fixed starting dose of 0.5 IU/kg [49] or initiated according to admission glucose (0.3 or 0.4 IU/kg) [50] demonstrated non-inferiority compared to NPH insulin in regards of efficacy and safety, including nocturnal hypoglycaemia. A sufficient performance was also confirmed in a study which used insulin glargine U100 incorporated in a clinical decision support system for the treatment of in hospital SIHG [51]. Probably a reasonable and simple approach is to initiate basal insulin in a GC dose-dependent dose, starting with 0.1 IU/kg BW if patients receive 10 mg of prednisone or equivalent and 0.2 IU/kg BW in case GC dose is 20 mg, 0.3 IU/kg BW when dose was set at 30 mg and so on [47,52]. Insulin dose finding based on patient age and kidney function has been proposed, indicating that initial doses should be lower in those with impaired kidney function (eGFR < 30 mL/min/1.73 m^2) or older than 70 years [17,33]. Subsequent dose adjustments should be based on achievement of glycaemic targets assessed by glucose measurements performed the next morning given that the GC is taken in the morning. Multiple daily administrations of intermediate-acting GCs are more complex as hyperglycaemia might overlap and persistent hyperglycaemia can occur (see glucose profile in Table 2). In this case, NPH insulin once daily will not be sufficient and NPH twice daily or a switch to longer-acting insulin (e.g., glargine) is required. If necessary, additional rapid-acting insulin boluses might be added. This can be established by either correctional bolus insulin (correction factor see scenario 1) or by switching to premixed insulin with a mixture of 70% rapid-acting and 30% basal insulin administered simulously to the GC intake [46].

8.2.3. Scenario 3: Long-Acting Glucocorticoids (Dexamethasone)

Dexamethasone, as the most potent GC agent, is characterized by a prolonged duration of action lasting for more than 24 h. It is clinically used in various scenarios such as in inflammatory diseases, as an analgesic or for the reduction of brain pressure in cerebral cancer or cerebral edema. In the recent severe acute respiratory syndrome coronavirus type 2 (COVID-19) pandemic, dexamethasone has been recommended for those with impairments in gas exchange due to viral pneumonia [53], irrespective of diabetes status. This approach needs to be further investigated in people with diabetes as deterioration of glycaemic control and new-onset hyperglycaemia were associated with inferior outcome in people with COVID-19 [54–57]. For hyperglycaemia during dexamethasone treatment for COVID-19, Rayman et al. have recently published a guidance article. In insulin naïve patients, they recommend to start NPH insulin when glucose exceeds a threshold of 12 mmol/L (~216 mg/dL) in a dose of 0.3 IU/kg/day while 2/3 should be administered in the morning and the remaining third in the evening. They also propose a dose reduction to 0.15 IU/kg in case of age >70 years or eGFR below 30 mL/min. Insulin doses are recommended to be titrated according to morning or evening glucose vales in a manner of a reduction of 20% if glucose falls below 4.1 mmol/L (~70 mg/dL) or decreased by 10% in case of glucose between 4.1–6.0 mmol/L (~70–110 mg/dL). Vice versa, insulin dose should be up-titrated by 20% if glucose values exceed 18 mmol/L (~320 mg/dL) and by 10% if glucose values are between 12.1 and 18 mmol/L (~220–320 mg/dL) [58]. In general, hyperglycaemia in association with long-acting GCs, which are usually administered in the morning, develops slowly, peaks during the day (varying time point) and is sustained for 24 h after intake. Thus, intermediate-acting basal insulins (NPH insulin, insulin detemir) should be prescribed twice daily (initial dose 0.3 IU/kg BW). Alternatively, long- or ultralong-acting basal insulin analogues (insulin glargine U100/U300 or insulin degludec) might be the most appropriate insulin to control hyperglycaemia in this situation (initial dose 0.2 IU/kg BW). Insulin dose should be adjusted according to glucose 24 h after GC intake and onset of hyperglycaemia. To date, to the best of our knowledge, not a single study has been conducted to test new generation ultra-long-acting basal insulin analogues for the treatment of SIHG.

8.3. Insulin Intensification and Adjustments

Especially in those without pre-existing diabetes prior to GC treatment, it is of utmost importance for insulin titration to know current GC dose and GC dose changes (tapering or increase). In a pragmatic approach, insulin dose can be adjusted by half the percentage of the GC dose change. For example, when GCs are increased or tapered by 50%, insulin dose is suggested to be increased or reduced by 25%, respectively. In patients with pre-existing DM a deterioration of glycaemic control secondary to GC therapy can be expected. In this regard, type of GC agent as well as time point and interval of GC application have to be taken into account.

8.3.1. Adjustment of Basal Insulin Therapy

When basal insulin therapy was already initiated, up-titration by 10–20% should be performed in case of sustained hyperglycaemia (fasting glucose exceeding 11.1 mmol/L [200 mg/dL]) on 2–3 subsequent days [17,33]. Alternatively, adjustments can be performed in 2 IU increments (conservative approach) to reach the individual glucose target; however, a steady dose adjustment must be warranted. Persisting hyperglycaemia despite basal insulin titration with predominantly postprandial hyperglycaemia requires additional rapid-acting insulin administrations either as rapid-acting insulin injection or incorporated in premixed insulins.

8.3.2. Adjustment of Rapid-Acting Insulin Therapy

Rapid-acting insulins should be primarily administered at the time point of GC administration and can be initiated with 0.1 IU/kg BW. In addition, rapid-acting insulin should be used to correct pre-prandial and spontaneous hyperglycaemia. In such cases add-on of 0.04 IU/kg for pre-prandial values from 11.1–16.7 mmol/L (200–300 mg/dL) or 0.08 IU/kg for values $\geq$ 16.7 mmol/L ($\geq$300 mg/dL) can be additionally added to the scheduled insulin dose. It is important to mention that insulin requirements depend on GC dose; hence, reduction of GC is usually accompanied by an improvement of glycaemia. Reduction of rapid-acting insulin should be performed proportionally to the reduction in GC dose, vice versa rapid-acting insulin dose can be increased when GC doses are increased [2,46].

8.3.3. Adjustment of Basal-Bolus Insulin

In patients with pre-existing basal-bolus insulin therapy doses of basal and bolus insulin should be adjusted according to the above recommendations. However, those with endogenous insulin deficiency (as people with type 1 diabetes) are more prone to hypoglycaemia which has to be considered when doses are increased [59]. A specific approach how to adjust insulin in people with preexisting type 1 diabetes is given in Section 8.3.5.

A schematic algorithm for the initiation and intensification of glucose lowering therapy in SIHG is illustrated in Figure 1. This algorithm is not valid for patients with preexisting type 1 diabetes.

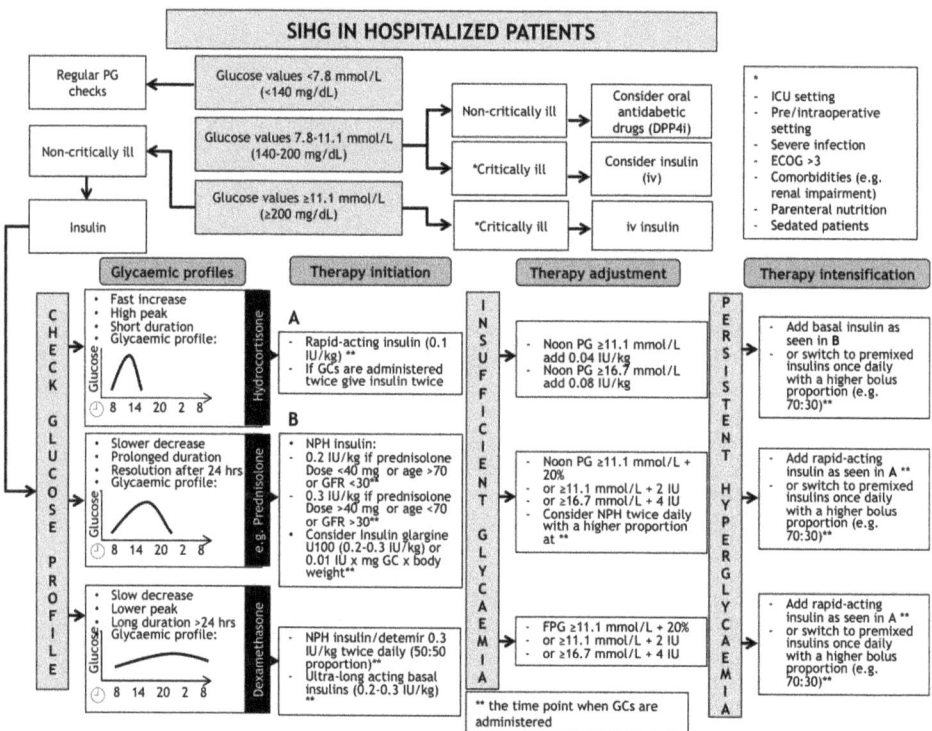

Figure 1. Opinion-based schematic algorithm for initiation, adjustment and intensification of insulin therapy for treatment of SIHG. DPP4i = Dipeptidyl-Peptidase4-inhibitor, ECOG = Karnofsky index, FPG = Fasting plasma glucose, GC = Glucocorticoid, ICU = Intensive Care Unit, IU = International Units, NPH = Neutral Protamine Hagedorn, SIHG = Steroid induced hyperglycaemia. * = definition of critical illness, ** = indicating the time point when glucocorticoids are administered. (**A**) indicates recommendations for initiation of rapid-acting insulin. (**B**) indicates recommendations to initiate basal in-sulin.

8.3.4. Adjustment of Insulin Therapy in Patients with Type 1 Diabetes (T1DM)

It has been shown that relevant doses of transiently administered GCs (in the referenced study 60 mg prednisone/day) lead to an increase in insulin requirements of 70% on average with considerable inter-individual variation to normalize blood glucose levels in patients with previously known well controlled T1DM. This glucose increase was sustained the day after GC therapy was discontinued, indicating a longer lasting hyperglycaemic effect despite the use of an intermediate-acting GC agent. Interestingly, the GC induced additional insulin requirements to achieve reasonable glycaemic control varied considerably and independently from previous insulin dose (30–100% increase) which makes recommendations for adjustments challenging. [60]. Dashora et al. described a 50%

increase in insulin requirements in females with T1DM requiring variable doses of GC therapy for treatment of hyperemesis gravidarum [61].

Due to the heterogeneity of the effect of GC on glucose metabolism in patients with T1DM it is recommended to intensify frequent monitoring of glucose upon initiation of GC therapy, as deterioration of glycaemic control has to be expected. As patients with T1DM are more prone to hypoglycaemia in comparison to patients with T2DM, initial dose adjustments have to be taken very carefully and in an iterative manner [33]. GCs are a well-known trigger for diabetic ketoacidosis in patients with deficiency or absence of endogenous insulin secretion, thus proper insulin dose adjustments to the GC therapy are recommended and transient hyperglycaemia should not be trivialized in these patients. Clinical evidence for insulin dose adjustments for patients with T1DM on GC therapy both, in the inpatient or in the outpatient setting, is largely lacking and not described in detail in any treatment guideline [62]. Moreover, the present article discusses SIHG in the hospital setting where besides GC therapy, numerous other factors such as acute disease and altered daily routine additionally influence glucose control. As there is only very little evidence available we suggest a cautious increase in total daily insulin dose (TDD) according to prednisolone (or prednisolone equivalent [PE]) dose, a suggestion that needs further scrutiny in clinical practice:

- PE of 20 mg → 10% increase in TDD
- PE of 40 mg → 20% increase in TDD
- PE of 60 mg → 30% increase in TDD

Taking these estimations into account the following considerations are important:

- Adjustments of insulin therapy when short-acting steroids (hydrocortisone) are used:
    - If short acting GCs are used, then an increase of rapid-acting insulin at the time point of GC intake might be sufficient. A correctional rapid-acting insulin dose can be administered in case of persistent hyperglycaemia after 3–4 h when the rapid-acting insulin action has tapered off. As a consequence, the ratio of rapid-acting to basal insulin will exceed the usual 50:50 ratio.
- Adjustments of insulin therapy when intermediate-acting steroids (e.g., prednisolone) are used:
    - Approach A: An increased dose of rapid-acting insulin at the time of intermediate-acting prednisolone administration might be appropriate aiming to achieve glucose control at noon.
    - Approach B: In case of pre-existing therapy with intermediate-acting basal-insulins (NPH insulin or insulin detemir) that are usually injected twice daily, a dose increases at the time point of GC intake (usually in the morning) is recommended.
    - Approach C: In patients previously using (ultra-)long acting basal-insulins (insulin glargine U100/U300 or insulin degludec), approach A might be sufficient; in case of an expected long-term GC treatment, these patients might benefit most from a switch to intermediate-acting basal insulins (NPH insulin, insulin detemir. In such case, the basal insulin should be injected twice daily with a proportionally higher dose at the time point when the GC agent is administered.
- Adjustments of insulin therapy when long-acting steroids (e.g., dexamethasone) are used:
    - Long-acting GCs will trigger continuous and long-lasting hyperglycaemia over 24 h, thus it might be suitable to adjust the total daily basal-insulin dose according to the GC dose as outlined above.

Of note, the continuation of using preexisting insulin pump therapy (continuous subcutaneous insulin infusion [CSII]) in the hospital is not recommended in the majority of cases especially in those who are acutely hospitalized and severely ill. In patients without physical or mental disorders, the self-managed continuation of CSII therapy might be justified [63,64]. CSII systems provide adjustable basal rates, programming of different basal rate profiles as well as a temporary % increase/decrease of the current basal rate.

Moreover, bolus dosing can be performed more frequently to administer correctional insulin when required without an additional injection as in pen-based therapy. Thus, in insulin pump users the continuation of insulin pump therapy with according to adjustment of insulin dose might be a considerable option if deemed practicable by the physicians in charge. However, clinical evidence supporting this presumption is not available yet.

In summary, the adjustment of insulin doses in patients with complex previous insulin therapies (i.e. T1DM) can be performed according to the above recommendations, which are quite carefully elaborated, but still require additional individualization, frequent glucose monitoring and close-meshed therapy adjustments.

8.3.5. The Critically Ill Patient

Hyperglycaemic derailments as well as severe and subsequent hypoglycaemia might complicate the clinical course in patients hospitalized on intensive medical care units and might impact on adverse outcomes. During critical illness, factors such as stress, inflammation, failure of kidney function or administered therapeutics, specifically GCs, detrimentally impact on glucose metabolism in people with and without previously known diabetes. In most of patients with critical illness and hyperglycaemia, insulin therapy should be introduced as continuous intravenous application [30]. Intravenous insulin provides the advantage of more rapid insulin adjustments to hyperglycaemic levels. Rapid-acting human insulin or analogues should be prepared by 50 IU rapid-acting insulin mixed with 50 mL sodium chloride (0.9%) with a starting dose of 0.1 IU/kg/h [64]. The switch to subcutaneous insulin is recommended when patient status improves (e.g., uptake of oral nutrition, scheduled transfer to general ward) and metabolic status is balanced. Basal insulin can be started at a dose of 50% of the previous 24 h insulin dose as administered intravenously in an overlapping manner (basal insulin application 2 h prior to cessation of intravenous insulin) in order to prevent rebound hyperglycaemia or acidosis [64]. Of course, also critically ill patients with SIHG should be treated with intravenous insulin, however, no specific recommendations for the treatment with intravenous insulin differing from the recommendation in "usual" critical care hyperglycaemia are available. The used insulin dose of the intravenous insulin application can help to estimate the appropriate dose of subcutaneously administered insulin.

9. Discharge from the Hospital

GCs frequently need to be continued after the inpatient stay and hence, hyperglycaemia also might persist [12]. Of note, hyperglycaemic state remains often also in those where GC therapy was discontinued indicating that people with SIHG are prone to develop T2DM.

Based on recommendations of a guideline published by the Joint British Diabetes Societies [33], it is necessary that all patients should be informed about the nature of SIHG, symptoms of hypo- and hyperglycaemia and its consequences if not properly treated. If applicable, patients should be trained in the use of insulin pens and self-monitoring of blood glucose (SMBG). Patients should be advised in the frequency of necessary SMBG and recommended to document glucose values and if applicable insulin doses. Optimally, all patients, irrespective of diabetes therapy at hospital discharge should have access to adequate glucose monitoring technology at home in order to avoid subsequent relevant hyperglycaemia. Adequate and individualized treatment plans should be made available to patients to avoid consecutive presentations at emergency departments potentially resulting in hospital readmissions. Individual therapy regimens should be prepared which contain recommendations for insulin dosing and which give a chance of self-adjustments especially taking into account possible dose changes in the GC therapy. Patients should be offered the possibility to regularly contact the medical staff of the outpatient clinic in case of concerns or problems regarding current glycaemic control. The general practitioner should be introduced in the case and preferentially take the lead concerning the management of the hyperglycaemic state. In addition, HbA1c should be measured every three months [65]. A possible admission and discharge algorithm is illustrated in Figure 2.

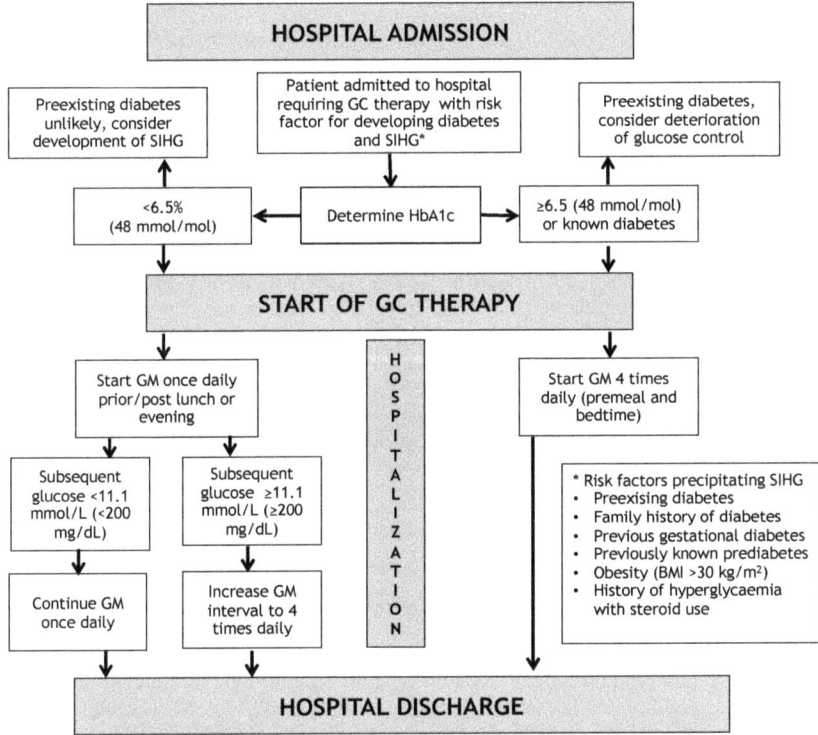

Figure 2. Opinion based admission and discharge algorithm for hospitalized patients with SIHG modified from [33]. BMI = Body mass index, GC = Glucocorticoids, GM = Glucose Monitoring, GP = General practitioner, SIHG = Steroid induced hyperglycaemia, SMBG = self-monitored blood glucose. * = risk factors for steroid induced hyperglycaemia.

10. Discussion

GCs are frequently prescribed as they have been confirmed to potentially improve outcomes in various autoimmune and inflammatory diseases, as well as recently also in COVID 19 [66]. Relevant doses of GC therapy potentially lead to hyperglycaemia in both hospitalized patients and patients in outpatient care exposing them to a higher risk of acute and chronic complications.

Diagnosis, monitoring and in particular the management of SIHG represents an everyday challenge and often physicians not specifically working in the field of diabetes and endocrinology have to deal with the management. Therefore, this review aims to provide summary figures that can be used by clinicians for the management of SIHG in routine care. There is a large amount of data available which confirmed the potential burden of chronic hyperglycaemia in both type 1 and type 2 diabetes. In contrast, whether mild, asymptomatic and mostly transient hyperglycaemia, specifically in hospitalized patients impacts on outcome, has not been systematically investigated, specifically not in those with SIHG [25]. Observational data identified elevated glucose as potential biomarker for adverse surgical outcomes, longer hospital stays and an increased mortality [67–69]. Vice versa, aggressive glucose lowering therapy in hospitalized patients, in particular using insulin with the risk of causing hypoglycaemia has also shown to negatively impact mortality [70]. For SIHG, which represents a different but important entity, clinical data, both from observational and interventional trials, is largely lacking.

Certainly, there is an increasing need to provide more evidence which, first, identifies the most safe and efficient therapy modalities to treat SIHG, secondly, sets a basis for defining recommended glucose targets and thirdly, allows to answer the question whether improved glycaemia translates to superior outcomes. In addition, novel diabetes technology such as continuous glucose monitors, electronic decision support systems and automated insulin delivery systems might be beneficial to better control SIHG and provide more outcome data in the near future.

Author Contributions: All of the four authors have sufficiently contributed to this work. F.A. drafted the manuscript, D.A.H., J.K.M. and H.S. approved the latest version to be published. All authors have read and agreed to the published version of the manuscript.

Funding: No funding was received for this work.

Institutional Review Board Statement: Not applicable.

Informed Consent Statement: Not applicable.

Data Availability Statement: Not applicable.

Conflicts of Interest: F.A. received speaker honoraria from Eli Lilly, Merck Sharp & Dome, Boehringer Ingelheim, Astra Zeneca and travel grants from Sanofi, Novo Nordisk, Takeda, Merck Sharp & Dome and Amgen. D.A.H. received travel grants from NovoNordisk, Novartis and Eli Lilly. H.S. received research grants from Boehringer Ingelheim, Eli Lilly, MSD, NovoNordisk and Sanofi. H.S. received lecture fees or honoraria for advisory boards from AstraZeneca, BMS, Boehringer Ingelheim, Eli Lilly, MSD, Novartis, NovoNordisk, Sanofi. J.K.M. is a member in the advisory board of Becton-Dickinson, Boehringer Ingelheim, Eli Lilly, Medtronic, Prediktor SA and Sanofi and received speaker honoraria from Abbott Diabetes Care, Astra Zeneca, Eli Lilly, Dexcom, Medtronic, Novo Nordisk, Roche Diabetes Care, Sanofi, Servier and Takeda.

References

1. Coutinho, A.E.; Chapman, K.E. The anti-inflammatory and immunosuppressive effects of glucocorticoids, recent developments and mechanistic insights. *Mol. Cell Endocrinol.* **2011**, *335*, 2–13. [CrossRef] [PubMed]
2. Trence, D.L. Management of patients on chronic glucocorticoid therapy: An endocrine perspective. *Prim. Care* **2003**, *30*, 593–605. [CrossRef]
3. van Raalte, D.H.; Diamant, M. Steroid diabetes: From mechanism to treatment? *Neth. J. Med.* **2014**, *72*, 62–72. [PubMed]
4. Bonaventura, A.; Montecucco, F. Steroid-induced hyperglycemia: An underdiagnosed problem or clinical inertia? A narrative review. *Diabetes Res. Clin. Pract.* **2018**, *139*, 203–220. [CrossRef]
5. Geer, E.B.; Islam, J.; Buettner, C. Mechanisms of glucocorticoid-induced insulin resistance: Focus on adipose tissue function and lipid metabolism. *Endocrinol. Metab. Clin. N. Am.* **2014**, *43*, 75–102. [CrossRef]
6. Gulliford, M.C.; Charlton, J.; Latinovic, R. Risk of diabetes associated with prescribed glucocorticoids in a large population. *Diabetes Care* **2006**, *29*, 2728–2729. [CrossRef]
7. Fong, A.C.; Cheung, N.W. The high incidence of steroid-induced hyperglycaemia in hospital. *Diabetes Res. Clin. Pract.* **2013**, *99*, 277–280. [CrossRef]
8. Liu, X.X.; Zhu, X.M.; Miao, Q.; Ye, H.Y.; Zhang, Z.Y.; Li, Y.M. Hyperglycemia induced by glucocorticoids in nondiabetic patients: A meta-analysis. *Ann. Nutr. Metab.* **2014**, *65*, 324–332. [CrossRef]
9. Kwon, S.; Hermayer, K.L.; Hermayer, K. Glucocorticoid-induced hyperglycemia. *Am. J. Med. Sci.* **2013**, *345*, 274–277. [CrossRef]
10. Tufton, N.; Ahmad, S.; Rolfe, C.; Rajkariar, R.; Byrne, J.; Chowdhury, T.A. New-onset diabetes after renal transplantation. *Diabet. Med.* **2014**, *31*, 1284–1292. [CrossRef]
11. Stauber, M.N.; Aberer, F.; Oulhaj, A.; Mader, J.K.; Zebisch, A.; Pieber, T.R.; Neumeister, P.; Greinix, H.T.; Sill, H.; Sourij, H.; et al. Early Hyperglycemia after Initiation of Glucocorticoid Therapy Predicts Adverse Outcome in Patients with Acute Graft-versus-Host Disease. *Biol. Blood Marrow. Transplant.* **2017**, *23*, 1186–1192. [CrossRef]

12. Simmons, L.R.; Molyneaux, L.; Yue, D.K.; Chua, E.L. Steroid-induced diabetes: Is it just unmasking of type 2 diabetes? *ISRN Endocrinol.* **2012**, *2012*, 910905. [CrossRef]
13. Wu, J.; Mackie, S.L.; Pujades-Rodriguez, M. Glucocorticoid dose-dependent risk of type 2 diabetes in six immune-mediated inflammatory diseases: A population-based cohort analysis. *BMJ Open Diabetes Res. Care* **2020**, *8*. [CrossRef]
14. Andersen, Y.M.F.; Egeberg, A.; Ban, L.; Gran, S.; Williams, H.C.; Francis, N.A.; Knop, F.K.; Gislason, G.H.; Skov, L.; Thyssen, J.P. Association Between Topical Corticosteroid Use and Type 2 Diabetes in Two European Population-Based Adult Cohorts. *Diabetes Care* **2019**, *42*, 1095–1103. [CrossRef]
15. Falciglia, M.; Freyberg, R.W.; Almenoff, P.L.; D'Alessio, D.A.; Render, M.L. Hyperglycemia-related mortality in critically ill patients varies with admission diagnosis. *Crit Care Med.* **2009**, *37*, 3001–3009. [CrossRef]
16. Corsino, L.; Dhatariya, K.; Umpierrez, G. Management of Diabetes and Hyperglycemia in Hospitalized Patients. In *Endotext*; Feingold, K.R., Anawalt, B., Boyce, A., Chrousos, G., Dungan, K., Grossman, A., Hershman, J.M., Kaltsas, G., Koch, C., Kopp, P., et al., Eds.; MDText. com, Inc.: South Dartmouth, MA, USA, 2000.
17. Umpierrez, G.E.; Hellman, R.; Korytkowski, M.T.; Kosiborod, M.; Maynard, G.A.; Montori, V.M.; Seley, J.J.; Van den Berghe, G.; Endocrine, S. Management of hyperglycemia in hospitalized patients in non-critical care setting: An endocrine society clinical practice guideline. *J. Clin. Endocrinol. Metab.* **2012**, *97*, 16–38. [CrossRef]
18. Aberer, F.; Kremser, S.; Mader, J.K.; Zinke-Cerwenka, W.; Greinix, H.; Tripolt, N.J.; Pieber, T.R.; Zebisch, A.; Sill, H.; Oulhaj, A.; et al. Hyperglycaemia within the first month after allogeneic haematopoietic stem-cell transplantation is an independent risk factor for overall survival in patients with acute myeloid leukaemia. *Diabetes Metab.* **2017**, *43*, 560–562. [CrossRef]
19. Ali, N.A.; O'Brien, J.M., Jr.; Blum, W.; Byrd, J.C.; Klisovic, R.B.; Marcucci, G.; Phillips, G.; Marsh, C.B.; Lemeshow, S.; Grever, M.R. Hyperglycemia in patients with acute myeloid leukemia is associated with increased hospital mortality. *Cancer* **2007**, *110*, 96–102. [CrossRef]
20. Derr, R.L.; Ye, X.; Islas, M.U.; Desideri, S.; Saudek, C.D.; Grossman, S.A. Association between hyperglycemia and survival in patients with newly diagnosed glioblastoma. *J. Clin. Oncol.* **2009**, *27*, 1082–1086. [CrossRef]
21. Sonabend, R.Y.; McKay, S.V.; Okcu, M.F.; Yan, J.; Haymond, M.W.; Margolin, J.F. Hyperglycemia during induction therapy is associated with poorer survival in children with acute lymphocytic leukemia. *J. Pediatr.* **2009**, *155*, 73–78. [CrossRef]
22. Palepu, S.; Prasad, G.V. New-onset diabetes mellitus after kidney transplantation: Current status and future directions. *World J. Diabetes* **2015**, *6*, 445–455. [CrossRef] [PubMed]
23. Baker, E.H.; Janaway, C.H.; Philips, B.J.; Brennan, A.L.; Baines, D.L.; Wood, D.M.; Jones, P.W. Hyperglycaemia is associated with poor outcomes in patients admitted to hospital with acute exacerbations of chronic obstructive pulmonary disease. *Thorax* **2006**, *61*, 284–289. [CrossRef] [PubMed]
24. Newton, C.A.; Smiley, D.; Bode, B.W.; Kitabchi, A.E.; Davidson, P.C.; Jacobs, S.; Steed, R.D.; Stentz, F.; Peng, L.; Mulligan, P.; et al. A comparison study of continuous insulin infusion protocols in the medical intensive care unit: Computer-guided vs. standard column-based algorithms. *J. Hosp. Med.* **2010**, *5*, 432–437. [CrossRef] [PubMed]
25. Dhatariya, K. Should inpatient hyperglycaemia be treated? *BMJ* **2013**, *346*, f134. [CrossRef]
26. American Diabetes, A. 2. Classification and Diagnosis of Diabetes: Standards of Medical Care in Diabetes-2021. *Diabetes Care* **2021**, *44*, S15–S33. [CrossRef]
27. Perez, A.; Jansen-Chaparro, S.; Saigi, I.; Bernal-Lopez, M.R.; Minambres, I.; Gomez-Huelgas, R. Glucocorticoid-induced hyperglycemia. *J. Diabetes* **2014**, *6*, 9–20. [CrossRef]
28. Suh, S.; Park, M.K. Glucocorticoid-Induced Diabetes Mellitus: An Important but Overlooked Problem. *Endocrinol. Metab.* **2017**, *32*, 180–189. [CrossRef]
29. American Diabetes, A. 6. Glycemic Targets: Standards of Medical Care in Diabetes-2021. *Diabetes Care* **2021**, *44*, S73–S84. [CrossRef]
30. American Diabetes, A. 15. Diabetes Care in the Hospital: Standards of Medical Care in Diabetes-2021. *Diabetes Care* **2021**, *44*, S211–S220. [CrossRef]
31. Dhatariya, K., II. Does dexamethasone-induced hyperglycaemia contribute to postoperative morbidity and mortality? *Br. J. Anaesth.* **2013**, *110*, 674–675. [CrossRef]
32. Sinclair, A.J.; Dashora, U.; George, S.; Dhatariya, K.; Group, J.-I.W. Joint British Diabetes Societies for Inpatient Care (JBDS-IP) Clinical Guideline Inpatient care of the frail older adult with diabetes: An Executive Summary. *Diabet. Med.* **2020**, *37*, 1981–1991. [CrossRef]
33. Roberts, A.; James, J.; Dhatariya, K.; Joint British Diabetes Societies for Inpatient, C. Management of hyperglycaemia and steroid (glucocorticoid) therapy: A guideline from the Joint British Diabetes Societies (JBDS) for Inpatient Care group. *Diabet. Med.* **2018**, *35*, 1011–1017. [CrossRef]
34. Dhatariya, K.E.; James, J.; Kong, M.F.; Berrington, R.; Joint British Diabetes Society (JBDS) for Inpatient Care Group; Guidelines Writing Group. Diabetes at the front door. A guideline for dealing with glucose related emergencies at the time of acute hospital admission from the Joint British Diabetes Society (JBDS) for Inpatient Care Group. *Diabet. Med.* **2020**, *37*, 1578–1589. [CrossRef]
35. Imatoh, T.; Sai, K.; Hori, K.; Segawa, K.; Kawakami, J.; Kimura, M.; Saito, Y. Development of a novel algorithm for detecting glucocorticoid-induced diabetes mellitus using a medical information database. *J. Clin. Pharm. Ther.* **2017**, *42*, 215–220. [CrossRef]

36. van Genugten, R.E.; van Raalte, D.H.; Muskiet, M.H.; Heymans, M.W.; Pouwels, P.J.; Ouwens, D.M.; Mari, A.; Diamant, M. Does dipeptidyl peptidase-4 inhibition prevent the diabetogenic effects of glucocorticoids in men with the metabolic syndrome? A randomized controlled trial. *Eur. J. Endocrinol.* **2014**, *170*, 429–439. [CrossRef]
37. van Raalte, D.H.; van Genugten, R.E.; Linssen, M.M.; Ouwens, D.M.; Diamant, M. Glucagon-like peptide-1 receptor agonist treatment prevents glucocorticoid-induced glucose intolerance and islet-cell dysfunction in humans. *Diabetes Care* **2011**, *34*, 412–417. [CrossRef]
38. Seelig, E.; Meyer, S.; Timper, K.; Nigro, N.; Bally, M.; Pernicova, I.; Schuetz, P.; Muller, B.; Korbonits, M.; Christ-Crain, M. Metformin prevents metabolic side effects during systemic glucocorticoid treatment. *Eur. J. Endocrinol.* **2017**, *176*, 349–358. [CrossRef]
39. Willi, S.M.; Kennedy, A.; Brant, B.P.; Wallace, P.; Rogers, N.L.; Garvey, W.T. Effective use of thiazolidinediones for the treatment of glucocorticoid-induced diabetes. *Diabetes Res. Clin. Pract.* **2002**, *58*, 87–96. [CrossRef]
40. Pernicova, I.; Kelly, S.; Ajodha, S.; Sahdev, A.; Bestwick, J.P.; Gabrovska, P.; Akanle, O.; Ajjan, R.; Kola, B.; Stadler, M.; et al. Metformin to reduce metabolic complications and inflammation in patients on systemic glucocorticoid therapy: A randomised, double-blind, placebo-controlled, proof-of-concept, phase 2 trial. *Lancet Diabetes Endocrinol.* **2020**, *8*, 278–291. [CrossRef]
41. He, J.; Xu, C.; Kuang, J.; Liu, Q.; Jiang, H.; Mo, L.; Geng, B.; Xu, G. Thiazolidinediones attenuate lipolysis and ameliorate dexamethasone-induced insulin resistance. *Metabolism* **2015**, *64*, 826–836. [CrossRef]
42. Gerards, M.C.; Venema, G.E.; Patberg, K.W.; Kross, M.; Potter van Loon, B.J.; Hageman, I.M.G.; Snijders, D.; Brandjes, D.P.M.; Hoekstra, J.B.L.; Vriesendorp, T.M.; et al. Dapagliflozin for prednisone-induced hyperglycaemia in acute exacerbation of chronic obstructive pulmonary disease. *Diabetes Obes. Metab.* **2018**, *20*, 1306–1310. [CrossRef]
43. Wallace, M.D.; Metzger, N.L. Optimizing the Treatment of Steroid-Induced Hyperglycemia. *Ann. Pharmacother.* **2018**, *52*, 86–90. [CrossRef]
44. Liu, D.; Ahmet, A.; Ward, L.; Krishnamoorthy, P.; Mandelcorn, E.D.; Leigh, R.; Brown, J.P.; Cohen, A.; Kim, H. A practical guide to the monitoring and management of the complications of systemic corticosteroid therapy. *Allergy Asthma Clin. Immunol.* **2013**, *9*, 30. [CrossRef]
45. Barbot, M.; Ceccato, F.; Scaroni, C. Diabetes Mellitus Secondary to Cushing's Disease. *Front. Endocrinol.* **2018**, *9*, 284. [CrossRef] [PubMed]
46. Tamez-Perez, H.E.; Quintanilla-Flores, D.L.; Rodriguez-Gutierrez, R.; Gonzalez-Gonzalez, J.G.; Tamez-Pena, A.L. Steroid hyperglycemia: Prevalence, early detection and therapeutic recommendations: A narrative review. *World J. Diabetes* **2015**, *6*, 1073–1081. [CrossRef]
47. Clore, J.N.; Thurby-Hay, L. Glucocorticoid-induced hyperglycemia. *Endocr. Pract.* **2009**, *15*, 469–474. [CrossRef]
48. Khowaja, A.; Alkhaddo, J.B.; Rana, Z.; Fish, L. Glycemic Control in Hospitalized Patients with Diabetes Receiving Corticosteroids Using a Neutral Protamine Hagedorn Insulin Protocol: A Randomized Clinical Trial. *Diabetes Ther.* **2018**, *9*, 1647–1655. [CrossRef] [PubMed]
49. Radhakutty, A.; Stranks, J.L.; Mangelsdorf, B.L.; Drake, S.M.; Roberts, G.W.; Zimmermann, A.T.; Stranks, S.N.; Thompson, C.H.; Burt, M.G. Treatment of prednisolone-induced hyperglycaemia in hospitalized patients: Insights from a randomized, controlled study. *Diabetes Obes. Metab.* **2017**, *19*, 571–578. [CrossRef]
50. Ruiz de Adana, M.S.; Colomo, N.; Maldonado-Araque, C.; Fontalba, M.I.; Linares, F.; Garcia-Torres, F.; Fernandez, R.; Bautista, C.; Olveira, G.; de la Cruz, J.L.; et al. Randomized clinical trial of the efficacy and safety of insulin glargine vs. NPH insulin as basal insulin for the treatment of glucocorticoid induced hyperglycemia using continuous glucose monitoring in hospitalized patients with type 2 diabetes and respiratory disease. *Diabetes Res. Clin. Pract.* **2015**, *110*, 158–165. [CrossRef]
51. Aberer, F.; Mader, J.K.; Holzgruber, J.; Trummer, C.; Schwetz, V.; Pandis, M.; Pferschy, P.N.; Greinix, H.; Tripolt, N.J.; Pieber, T.R.; et al. Feasibility and safety of using an automated decision support system for insulin therapy in the treatment of steroid-induced hyperglycemia in patients with acute graft-versus-host disease: A randomized trial. *J. Diabetes Investig.* **2019**, *10*, 339–342. [CrossRef] [PubMed]
52. Seggelke, S.A.; Gibbs, J.; Draznin, B. Pilot study of using neutral protamine Hagedorn insulin to counteract the effect of methylprednisolone in hospitalized patients with diabetes. *J. Hosp. Med.* **2011**, *6*, 175–176. [CrossRef]
53. Wiersinga, W.J.; Rhodes, A.; Cheng, A.C.; Peacock, S.J.; Prescott, H.C. Pathophysiology, Transmission, Diagnosis, and Treatment of Coronavirus Disease 2019 (COVID-19): A Review. *JAMA* **2020**, *324*, 782–793. [CrossRef]
54. Li, G. Inpatient use of glucocorticoids may mediate the detrimental effect of new-onset hyperglycemia on COVID-19 severity. *Diabetes Res. Clin. Pract.* **2020**, *168*, 108441. [CrossRef]
55. Morieri, M.L.; Fadini, G.P.; Boscari, F.; Fioretto, P.; Maran, A.; Busetto, L.; Crepaldi, M.C.; Vedovato, M.; Bonora, B.M.; Selmin, E.; et al. Hyperglycemia, glucocorticoid therapy, and outcome of COVID-19. *Diabetes Res. Clin. Pract.* **2020**, *168*, 108449. [CrossRef]
56. Holman, N.; Knighton, P.; Kar, P.; O'Keefe, J.; Curley, M.; Weaver, A.; Barron, E.; Bakhai, C.; Khunti, K.; Wareham, N.J.; et al. Risk factors for COVID-19-related mortality in people with type 1 and type 2 diabetes in England: A population-based cohort study. *Lancet Diabetes Endocrinol.* **2020**, *8*, 823–833. [CrossRef]
57. Fadini, G.P.; Morieri, M.L.; Boscari, F.; Fioretto, P.; Maran, A.; Busetto, L.; Bonora, B.M.; Selmin, E.; Arcidiacono, G.; Pinelli, S.; et al. Newly-diagnosed diabetes and admission hyperglycemia predict COVID-19 severity by aggravating respiratory deterioration. *Diabetes Res. Clin. Pract.* **2020**, *168*, 108374. [CrossRef]

58. Rayman, G.; Lumb, A.N.; Kennon, B.; Cottrell, C.; Nagi, D.; Page, E.; Voigt, D.; Courtney, H.C.; Atkins, H.; Higgins, K.; et al. Dexamethasone therapy in COVID-19 patients: Implications and guidance for the management of blood glucose in people with and without diabetes. *Diabet. Med.* **2021**, *38*, e14378. [CrossRef]
59. Zenz, S.; Mader, J.K.; Regittnig, W.; Brunner, M.; Korsatko, S.; Boulgaropoulos, B.; Magnes, C.; Raml, R.; Narath, S.H.; Eller, P.; et al. Impact of C-Peptide Status on the Response of Glucagon and Endogenous Glucose Production to Induced Hypoglycemia in T1DM. *J. Clin. Endocrinol. Metab.* **2018**, *103*, 1408–1417. [CrossRef]
60. Bevier, W.C.; Zisser, H.C.; Jovanovic, L.; Finan, D.A.; Palerm, C.C.; Seborg, D.E.; Doyle, F.J., 3rd. Use of continuous glucose monitoring to estimate insulin requirements in patients with type 1 diabetes mellitus during a short course of prednisone. *J. Diabetes Sci. Technol.* **2008**, *2*, 578–583. [CrossRef]
61. Dashora, U.K.; Taylor, R. Maintaining glycaemic control during high-dose prednisolone administration for hyperemesis gravidarum in Type 1 diabetes. *Diabet. Med.* **2004**, *21*, 298–299. [CrossRef]
62. Best, C.J.; Thosani, S.; Ortiz, M.; Levesque, C.; Varghese, S.S.; Lavis, V.R. Co-Managing Patients with Type 1 Diabetes and Cancer. *Curr. Diab. Rep.* **2016**, *16*, 73. [CrossRef] [PubMed]
63. Umpierrez, G.E.; Klonoff, D.C. Diabetes Technology Update: Use of Insulin Pumps and Continuous Glucose Monitoring in the Hospital. *Diabetes Care* **2018**, *41*, 1579–1589. [CrossRef] [PubMed]
64. Mader, J.K.; Brix, J.; Aberer, F.; Vonbank, A.; Resl, M.; Pieber, T.R.; Stechemesser, L.; Sourij, H. Hospital diabetes management (Update 2019). *Wien. Klin. Wochenschr.* **2019**, *131*, 200–211. [CrossRef] [PubMed]
65. Mills, E.; Devendra, S. Steroid-induced hyperglycaemia in primary care. *Lond. J. Prim. Care* **2015**, *7*, 103–106. [CrossRef]
66. Group, R.C.; Horby, P.; Lim, W.S.; Emberson, J.R.; Mafham, M.; Bell, J.L.; Linsell, L.; Staplin, N.; Brightling, C.; Ustianowski, A.; et al. Dexamethasone in Hospitalized Patients with Covid-19—Preliminary Report. *N. Engl. J. Med.* **2020**. [CrossRef]
67. Gandhi, G.Y.; Murad, M.H.; Flynn, D.N.; Erwin, P.J.; Cavalcante, A.B.; Bay Nielsen, H.; Capes, S.E.; Thorlund, K.; Montori, V.M.; Devereaux, P.J. Effect of perioperative insulin infusion on surgical morbidity and mortality: Systematic review and meta-analysis of randomized trials. *Mayo Clin. Proc.* **2008**, *83*, 418–430. [CrossRef]
68. Sampson, M.J.; Dozio, N.; Ferguson, B.; Dhatariya, K. Total and excess bed occupancy by age, specialty and insulin use for nearly one million diabetes patients discharged from all English Acute Hospitals. *Diabetes Res. Clin. Pract.* **2007**, *77*, 92–98. [CrossRef]
69. Evans, N.R.; Dhatariya, K.K. Assessing the relationship between admission glucose levels, subsequent length of hospital stay, readmission and mortality. *Clin. Med.* **2012**, *12*, 137–139. [CrossRef]
70. Investigators, N.-S.S.; Finfer, S.; Liu, B.; Chittock, D.R.; Norton, R.; Myburgh, J.A.; McArthur, C.; Mitchell, I.; Foster, D.; Dhingra, V.; et al. Hypoglycemia and risk of death in critically ill patients. *N. Engl. J. Med.* **2012**, *367*, 1108–1118. [CrossRef]

Article

Eating Speed and Incidence of Diabetes in a Japanese General Population: ISSA-CKD

Hideyuki Fujii [1], Shunsuke Funakoshi [2], Toshiki Maeda [2], Atsushi Satoh [2], Miki Kawazoe [2], Shintaro Ishida [3], Chikara Yoshimura [2], Soichiro Yokota [4], Kazuhiro Tada [4], Koji Takahashi [4], Kenji Ito [4], Tetsuhiko Yasuno [4], Shota Okutsu [5], Shigeaki Mukoubara [6], Hitoshi Nakashima [4], Shigeki Nabeshima [5], Seiji Kondo [3], Masaki Fujita [7], Kosuke Masutani [4], Hisatomi Arima [2] and Daiji Kawanami [1],*

1. Department of Endocrinology and Diabetes Mellitus, Fukuoka University School of Medicine, Fukuoka 814-0180, Japan; joeten1cho@yahoo.co.jp
2. Department of Preventive Medicine and Public Health, Faculty of Medicine, Fukuoka University, Fukuoka 814-0180, Japan; shunsuke.funakoshi@gmail.com (S.F.); tmaeda@fukuoka-u.ac.jp (T.M.); atsushis@fukuoka-u.ac.jp (A.S.); miki1024@fukuoka-u.ac.jp (M.K.); ychikara@fukuoka-u.ac.jp (C.Y.); harima@fukuoka-u.ac.jp (H.A.)
3. Department of Oral and Maxillofacial Surgery, Faculty of Medicine, Fukuoka University, Fukuoka 814-0180, Japan; shintarou19910118@gmail.com (S.I.); kondo@fukuoka-u.ac.jp (S.K.)
4. Division of Nephrology and Rheumatology, Department of Internal Medicine, Faculty of Medicine, Fukuoka University, Fukuoka 814-0180, Japan; syokota@fukuoka-u.ac.jp (S.Y.); ktada@fukuoka-u.ac.jp (K.T.); reply_09030728174@yahoo.co.jp (K.T.); kito@fukuoka-u.ac.jp (K.I.); yasuno9584@fukuoka-u.ac.jp (T.Y.); hitscenenakashima@gmail.com (H.N.); kmasutani@fukuoka-u.ac.jp (K.M.)
5. Department of General Medicine, Fukuoka University Hospital, Fukuoka 814-0180, Japan; shota.o.19870528@gmail.com (S.O.); snabeshi@fukuoka-u.ac.jp (S.N.)
6. Department of Internal Medicine, Nagasaki Prefecture Iki Hospital, Nagasaki 811-5132, Japan; s-mukoubara@ikihp.jp
7. Department of Respiratory Medicine, Faculty of Medicine, Fukuoka University, Fukuoka 814-0180, Japan; mfujita@fukuoka-u.ac.jp
* Correspondence: kawanami@fukuoka-u.ac.jp; Tel.: +81-92-801-1011; Fax: +81-92-865-5163

Abstract: Background: We investigated whether eating speed was associated with the incidence of diabetes in a Japanese general population. Methods: A total of 4853 Japanese individuals without diabetes at baseline were analyzed. Self-reported eating speed was categorized as slow, medium, and fast on the basis of questionnaire responses. The study outcome was the incidence of diabetes. Results: After an average follow-up period of 5.1 years, 234 individuals developed diabetes. The incidence of diabetes per 1000 person-years was 4.9 in the slow eating speed group, 8.8 in the medium eating speed group, and 12.5 in the fast eating speed group, respectively (*** $p < 0.001$ for trend). The HRs were 1.69 (95%CI 0.94–3.06) for the medium eating speed and 2.08 (95%CI 1.13–3.84) for the fast eating speed, compared to the slow eating speed (* $p = 0.014$ for trend) after adjustment for age, gender, smoking status, drinking, exercise, obesity, hypertension, and dyslipidemia. Conclusion: Faster eating speed increased a risk for the incidence of diabetes in a general Japanese population.

Keywords: diabetes; eating speed; primary prevention; lifestyle

1. Introduction

Diabetes is a life-threatening disease that causes microvascular and macrovascular complications [1–6]. Diabetes is considered as a serious disorder that doubles the risk of premature death [7]. A longitudinal study demonstrated that the incidence rate of coronary artery disease per 1000 person-years in Japanese patients with type 2 diabetes was 9.59, which is approximately three times higher than the general population [8]. In Japan, diabetic kidney disease is the leading cause (43.5%) among new dialysis patients [9]. The number of people with diabetes and impaired glucose tolerance in Japan is estimated at 20 million, and this number has been increasing since 1997 [10]. According to the 2016

National Health and Nutrition Survey by the Japanese Ministry of Health, Labor and Welfare, the prevalence rate of type 2 diabetes in Japan was 12.1%. The effective prevention of type 2 diabetes requires up-to-date knowledge of risk factors for the disease.

It has been shown that interventions seeking to impact lifestyle behaviors, including improving dietary and exercise habits, can prevent the onset of type 2 diabetes [11–13]. Obesity [11–14] and insufficient exercise have been implicated as established modifiable risk factors for type 2 diabetes [15–17], as well as impaired glucose tolerance, smoking [18], alcohol intake [19,20], and inadequate diet (calorie intake and content) [11–13,21–23]. Several studies have shown that fast eating is associated with the increased risk of type 2 diabetes [24–26]. Previous studies have used questionnaires to classify eating speed. For example, the question was "Do you eat faster than people who eat together at the same table?" or "Do you eat faster than people of the same generation?" In one study, the eating speed was classified into five groups (very slow, relatively slow, medium, relatively fast, and very fast) [25]. However, the evidence on this topic is mainly derived from case–control studies or studies conducted among special populations (e.g., worksite populations), and it is unclear to what extent this evidence is generalizable to general populations. The aim of this large-scale population-based study was to examine the effect of eating speed on the development of diabetes in a general population in Japan.

2. Materials and Methods

2.1. Study Design

The Iki City Epidemiological Study of Atherosclerosis and Chronic Kidney Disease (ISSA-CKD) is a population-based retrospective cohort study that uses annual health checkup data for the citizens of Iki City, Nagasaki Prefecture, Japan. ISSA-CKD has been described in the accompanying literatures [27–30]. The present study was conducted according to the guidelines of the Declaration of Helsinki of 1975, revised in 2013, and approved by the Fukuoka University Clinical Research and Ethics Center (No.2017M010).

2.2. Participants

A total of 7895 individuals received annual health checkups from 2008–2017. Of these people, 3042 (38.5%) were excluded: 1881 dropped out from consecutive follow-up annual medical checkups, and 1161 had diabetes at baseline. Thus, 4853 citizens were analyzed in this study.

2.3. Data Collection

At baseline, we collected information on eating speed, using a questionnaire with the following question: "How fast is your eating speed compared with others?" The response categories were slow, medium, and fast. Information on smoking, alcohol drinking, regular exercise, family history of diabetes, and current use of medications for hypertension, dyslipidemia, and diabetes was also collected via questionnaire. We defined obesity as a BMI $\geq$ 25 kg/m^2. Participants who had smoked 100 cigarettes or more, or who had smoked regularly for 6 months and more were defined as currently smoking. Drinking behavior was defined as drinking on 5 days or more per week. Regular exercise was defined as exercising $\geq$30 min/day at least twice a week. Hypertension was defined as a systolic blood pressure of 140/90 mmHg or more or use of blood pressure-lowering medicine. Fasting or casual blood and urine samples were collected. Plasma glucose levels were measured by an enzymatic method, and glycated hemoglobin (HbA1c) levels (National Glycohemoglobin Standardization Program value) were determined by a high-performance liquid chromatography method. The diagnosis of diabetes was determined by a fasting glucose level $\geq$ 6.99 mmol/L, casual blood glucose level $\geq$ 11.10 mmol/L, HbA1c $\geq$ 6.5%, or the use of glucose-lowering therapies. Serum low-density lipoprotein (LDL) cholesterol, high-density lipoprotein (HDL) cholesterol and triglyceride concentrations were measured enzymatically. Dyslipidemia was defined as LDL cholesterol $\geq$ 3.62 mmol/L, HDL cholesterol < 1.03 mmol/L, triglycerides $\geq$ 1.69 mmol/L or the use of lipid-lowering medication.

2.4. Outcome

The incidence of diabetes (fasting glucose level ≥ 6.99 mmol/L, casual blood glucose level ≥ 11.10 mmol/L, HbA1c ≥ 6.5%, or the use of glucose-lowering therapies) at the end of follow-up.

2.5. Statistical Analysis

Continuous variables were expressed as means ± SD. Simple regression models were used to determine trends across tertile groups of eating speed. Categorical variables were expressed as the number (percentage) of participants. Logistic regression models were used to test trends across groups. Incidence rates of diabetes were expressed by person-year. We estimated crude and multivariable-adjusted hazard ratios (HRs) and their 95% confidence intervals (CIs) of the effect of eating speed on the development of diabetes by the use of Cox proportional hazards models. Then, we next adjusted for age, sex, smoking status, alcohol drinking, exercise, obesity, hypertension and dyslipidemia. A two-tailed p value of less than 0.05 was considered statistically significant. Analyses were performed using SAS, Version 9.4.

3. Results

The average age of the participants at baseline was 59.6 years, 55.5% were women, and the average BMI was 23.6 kg/m^2. The mean baseline fasting blood glucose level was 5.1 ± 0.5 mmol/L, and the mean HbA1c level was 5.1 ± 0.4%. A total of 1350 people (27.8%) were classified in the fast eating speed group, 2993 (61.7%) were classified in the medium eating speed group, and 510 (10.5%) were classified in the slow eating speed group. Table 1 shows the baseline characteristics. A self-reported faster eating speed was associated with younger age, higher BMI, higher triglycerides, and lower levels of HDL-cholesterol.

Table 1. Baseline characteristics by self-reported eating speed.

	Self-Reported Eating Speed			p Value for Trend
	Slow (N = 510)	Medium (N = 2993)	Fast (N = 1350)	
Age, mean (SD), years	61.6 (±10.7)	59.8 (±10.5)	58.5 (±10.8)	*** < 0.001
Male, N/total N (%)	180/510 (35.3%)	1271/2993 (42.5%)	709/1350 (52.5%)	*** < 0.001
Smoking status, N/total N (%)				
Never smoker	423/510 (82.9%)	2275/2993 (76.0%)	975/1350 (72.2%)	*** < 0.001
Ex-smoker	19/510 (3.7%)	151/2993 (5.0%)	89/1350 (6.6%)	
Current smoker, <20 cigarettes/day	17/510 (3.3%)	134/2993 (4.5%)	72/1350 (5.3%)	
Current smoker, ≥20 cigarettes/day	22/510 (4.3%)	226/2993 (7.6%)	129/1350 (9.6%)	
Current smoker, missing information on the number of cigarettes/day	29/510 (5.7%)	207/2993 (6.9%)	85/1350 (6.3%)	
Alcohol intake [†], N/total N (%)				
No	305/505 (60.4%)	1609/2970 (54.2%)	649/1342 (48.4%)	** 0.004
Occasional alcohol drinking	100/505 (19.8%)	680/2970 (22.9%)	347/1342 (25.9%)	
Daily current alcohol drinking, <20 g/day	43/505 (8.5%)	221/2970 (7.4%)	97/1342 (7.2%)	
Daily current alcohol drinking, 20–39.9 g/day	39/505 (7.7%)	318/2970 (10.7%)	182/1342 (13.6%)	
Daily current alcohol drinking, ≥40 g/day	18/505 (3.6%)	142/2970 (4.8%)	67/1342 (5.0%)	
Regular exercise [‡], N/total N (%)	120/510 (23.5%)	809/2993 (27.0%)	357/1350 (26.4%)	0.451
Body mass index, mean (SD), kg/m^2	22.7 (±3.3)	23.3 (±3.3)	24.5 (±3.6)	*** < 0.001
Obesity [§], N/total N (%)	101/510 (19.8%)	815/2993 (27.2%)	554/1350 (41.0%)	*** < 0.001
Systolic blood pressure, mean (SD), mmHg	128.7 (±19.6)	129.0 (±18.3)	128.9 (±19.0)	0.987
Diastolic blood pressure, mean (SD), mmHg	73.8 (±10.8)	74.8 (±11.1)	75.6 (±11.3)	** 0.002
High-density lipoprotein cholesterol, mean (SD), mmol/L	1.63 (±0.41)	1.62 (±0.42)	1.55 (±0.41)	*** < 0.001
Low density lipoprotein cholesterol, mean (SD), mmol/L	3.10 (±0.82)	3.18 (±0.81)	3.20 (±0.82)	0.06
Triglyceride, mean (SD), mmol/L	1.29 (±0.93)	1.28 (±0.84)	1.44 (±1.03)	*** < 0.001
Dyslipidemia [¶], N/total N (%)	194/510 (38.0%)	1244/2993 (41.6%)	642/1350 (47.6%)	*** < 0.001
Hypertension [††], N/total N (%)	209/510 (41.0%)	1272/2993 (42.5%)	588/1350 (43.6%)	0.308
HbA1c, mean (SD),%	5.1 (±0.3)	5.1 (±0.4)	5.1 (±0.4)	0.669
Fasting blood glucose (SD), mmol/L [†††]	5.0 (±0.5)	5.0 (±0.5)	5.1 (±0.6)	** 0.0013

[†] Habitually drinking on 5 or more days per week. [‡] Habitually exercising ≥ 30 min per day twice or more per week. [§] Body mass index ≥ 25 kg/m^2. [¶] Low-density lipoprotein cholesterol ≥ 3.62 mmol/L, high-density lipoprotein cholesterol < 1.03 mmol/L, triglycerides ≥ 1.69 mmol/L, or use of lipid-lowering medication. [††] Systolic blood pressure ≥ 140 mmHg, diastolic blood pressure ≥ 90 mmHg, or use of blood pressure-lowering medication. [†††] Available for 381 participants in the slow group, 2230 in the medium group, and 1017 in the fast group. ** $p < 0.05$, *** $p < 0.001$.

During an average follow-up of 5.1 years (24,745 person-years), 234 individuals developed diabetes (incidence rate: 9.4 per 1000 person-years). Table 2 shows the risks of diabetes by reported eating speed. The incidence rates (per 1000 person-years) were 4.9 for the slow eating speed group, 8.8 for the medium eating speed group, and 12.5 for the fast eating speed group ($p < 0.001$ for trend). These associations remained statistically significant even after adjustment for age, gender, smoking status, drinking habits, exercise habits, obesity, hypertension, and dyslipidemia: The multivariable-adjusted HRs (95% CIs) were 1.69 (0.94–3.06) for medium eating speed, and 2.08 (1.13–3.84) for fast eating speed, compared with the reference group of slow eating speed (* $p = 0.014$ for trend). When BMI (instead of obesity), systolic blood pressure (instead of hypertension), HDL-c and triglycerides (instead of dyslipidemia) were included in multivariable analysis as covariates, the hazard ratios were 1.72 (95% CIs 0.95–3.11) for medium eating speed and 1.94 (95% CIs 1.05–3.58) for fast eating speed compared with slow eating speed. When waist circumference (instead of BMI) was included in multivariable analysis as covariate, the hazard ratios were 1.72 (95% CIs 0.94–3.08) for medium eating speed and 2.05 (95% CIs 1.15–3.78) for fast eating speed compared with slow eating speed.

Table 2. Risk of diabetes mellitus by self-reported eating speed.

	Self-Reported Eating Speed			
	Slow	Medium	Fast	p Value for Trend
	(N = 510)	(N = 2993)	(N = 1350)	
N of events/person-years	12/2468	134/15,234	88/7034	
Incidence rate (per 1000 person-years)	4.9	8.8	12.5	
Crude hazard ratio	1	1.82	2.61	*** < 0.001
(95% Confidence interval)	(Reference)	(1.01–3.29)	(1.43–4.77)	
Adjusted hazard ratio †	1	1.69	2.08	** 0.014
(95% Confidence interval)	(Reference)	(0.94–3.06)	(1.13–3.84)	

† Adjusted for age, sex, smoking status, alcohol drinking, exercise, obesity, hypertension and dyslipidemia. ** $p < 0.05$, *** $p < 0.001$.

Table 3 shows the results of the subgroup analysis. The effect of reported eating speed on the development of diabetes was comparable across the subgroups defined by age, gender, obesity, hypertension, dyslipidemia, smoking, drinking habits, and regular exercise (all $p > 0.1$ for the interactions).

Table 3. Subgroup analysis.

	Self-Reported Eating Speed			
	Slow	Medium	Fast	p Value for Interaction
	(N = 510)	(N = 2993)	(N = 1350)	
Age				
<65 years	1 (reference)	1.04 (0.48–2.29)	1.52 (0.68–3.36)	0.105
≥65 years	1 (reference)	2.64 (1.06–6.55)	2.61 (1.01–6.79)	
Sex				
Male	1 (reference)	2.48 (0.91–6.80)	3.03 (1.09–8.42)	0.617
Female	1 (reference)	1.28 (0.61–2.68)	1.57 (0.72–3.43)	
Obesity				
Yes	1 (reference)	1.35 (0.54–3.37)	1.94 (0.77–4.87)	0.462
No	1 (reference)	1.97 (0.91–4.29)	2.02 (0.88–4.61)	
Hypertension				
Yes	1 (reference)	1.91 (0.83–4.40)	2.31 (0.98–5.45)	0.895
No	1 (reference)	1.47 (0.63–3.41)	1.74 (0.73–4.17)	
Dyslipidemia				
Yes	1 (reference)	1.77 (0.71–4.41)	2.39 (0.95–6.02)	0.402
No	1 (reference)	1.76 (0.80–3.84)	1.88 (0.82–4.31)	

Table 3. Cont.

	Self-Reported Eating Speed			p Value for Interaction
	Slow	Medium	Fast	
	(N = 510)	(N = 2993)	(N = 1350)	
Current smoking				
Yes	1 (reference)	1.26 (0.38–4.12)	1.10 (0.31–3.84)	0.349
No	1 (reference)	1.82 (0.92–3.61)	2.48 (1.23–5.00)	
Daily alcohol intake				
Yes	1 (reference)	5.20 (0.71–37.88)	5.33 (0.71–39.81)	0.298
No	1 (reference)	1.33 (0.71–2.49)	1.81 (0.94–3.46)	
Regular exercise				
Yes	1 (reference)	1.63 (0.50–5.31)	2.63 (0.79–8.70)	0.662
No	1 (reference)	1.63 (0.82–3.25)	1.81 (0.89–3.69)	

Values are hazard ratios (95% confidence intervals) adjusted for age (except for the subgroup analysis by age), sex (except for the subgroup analysis by sex), obesity (except for the subgroup analysis by obesity), hypertension (except for the subgroup analysis by hypertension), dyslipidemia (except for the subgroup analysis by dyslipidemia), current smoking (except for the subgroup analysis by current smoking), daily alcohol drinking (except for the subgroup analysis by alcohol drinking) and regular exercise (except for the subgroup analysis by regular exercise). Obesity: body mass index ≥ 25 kg/m^2. Hypertension: systolic blood pressure ≥ 140 mmHg, diastolic blood pressure ≥ 90 mmHg or use of blood pressure-lowering medication. Dyslipidemia: low-density lipoprotein cholesterol ≥ 3.62 mmol/L, high-density lipoprotein cholesterol < 1.03 mmol/L, triglycerides ≥ 1.69 mmol/L, or the use of lipid-lowering medication.

4. Discussion

In this large-scale observational study of a general Japanese population, a self-reported faster eating speed was associated with a higher risk of developing diabetes. This association remained significant in the multivariable analysis, including age, sex, smoking status, drinking, regular exercise, obesity, hypertension and dyslipidemia as covariates. The correlation of eating speed with incidence of diabetes was comparable across subgroups defined by age, sex, obesity, hypertension, dyslipidemia, current smoking and drinking.

Previous evidence on the relationship between eating speed and the risk of type 2 diabetes is mainly derived from case–control studies. A case–control study conducted in Lithuania compared 234 individuals with newly diagnosed type 2 diabetes with 468 controls, demonstrating that the risk of type 2 diabetes was more than doubled for people who ate quickly compared with others [31]. In Japan, Sakurai et al. [25] reported that eating quickly increased the risk of diabetes among 2050 middle-aged Japanese male workers undergoing medical examinations. In a 3-year longitudinal study of 172 people in Japan who underwent medical examinations in a single hospital, Totsuka et al. [32] found that self-reported fast eating speed was associated with the incidence of impaired glucose tolerance, which was confirmed using a 75 g glucose tolerance test. One large-scale population-based study of a Japanese population who underwent annual health checkups reported a 1.12-fold higher risk of diabetes in the group of fast eating speed than in the combined group of medium and slow eating speed during 1-year to 3-year follow-up [26]. The present large-scale population-based longitudinal study with long-term follow-up (average 5.1 years) confirmed the findings of previous studies and clearly demonstrated a strong, linear relationship between self-reported eating quickly and the development of diabetes (multivariable-adjusted HRs 1.69 for medium eating speed and 2.08 for fast eating speed compared with the reference group of slow eating speed, * $p = 0.014$ for trend) among a general Japanese population.

The precise mechanisms by which eating speed increases the incidence of diabetes have not been clearly defined, but one possible explanation for the effect is the development of insulin resistance through weight gain. Fast eating has been shown to lead to weight gain, obesity [25,32–39], and the subsequent development of insulin resistance [24,25,32,39]. Second, fast eating may cause postprandial hyperglycemia. It has been reported that, in healthy subjects, thorough mastication was associated with lower levels of postprandial blood glucose compared with normal mastication [40]. Therefore, fast eating, which is associated with lower mastication, may cause postprandial hyperglycemia. Over time, postprandial hyperglycemia may gradually cause pancreatic β-cell exhaustion, leading to a decrease in insulin secretion [41]. Third, a decrease in mastication may lead to an increase in food intake. An animal study found that, in rats, thorough mastication activated histamine in the hypothalamus and binding of histamine to H1 receptors in the paraventricular nucleus and ventromedial lobe of the hypothalamus resulted in food intake suppression [42]. Thus, fast eating, which is associated with decreased mastication, may increase food consumption. Fourth, decreases in the secretion of peptide YY and glucagon-like peptide 1 (GLP-1) by fast eating may cause postprandial hyperglycemia [43]. Fifth, fast eating may be associated with a delayed feeling of fullness and satiety, which leads to over-eating. A previous study reported that slow eating speed reduced ghrelin secretion in response to carbohydrate load in obese adolescents [44]. Furthermore, Rigamonti et al. reported that slow feeding rates increased peptide YY and GLP-1 secretion [43,45]. Taken together, fast eating may cause these changes in hormone secretion, leading to a delay in the feeling of fullness and satiety, which leads to over-eating.

The strengths of the present study were its relatively large sample size and population-based longitudinal design. In addition, the onset of diabetes was evaluated by blood glucose and HbA1c levels at annual medical examinations. Some previous studies have evaluated the onset of diabetes based only on self-reported information. The present study has several limitations. First, eating speed was self-reported and was not objectively evaluated. The accuracy of evaluating eating speed based on self-report is controversial. Woodland et al. demonstrated that the match rate of self-reported eating speed and the objective measure of eating rate was 47.4% [46]. A future study using a reliable method to assess eating speed will be required to obtain more objectivity. Second, a detailed nutritional survey was not conducted in this study. Third, people who are interested in their own health are more likely to undergo medical examinations than those who are not. Our findings obtained from participants of the ISSA-CKD study do not always apply to the general population. Further study will be interesting to elucidate whether or not similar results can be observed in the general Japanese population. Fourth, no information was available on the etiological type of diabetes, although most onsets after age 40 are type 2 diabetes [47,48]. Fifth, a detailed amount of exercise was not available. However, previous studies have shown that exercise ($\geq$4 METs/h/week) of at least 30 min per week on at least 2 days a week is the minimum required to improve physical fitness and musculo-skeletal function [49]. We created the questionnaire about exercise habits on this basis. A future study using a reliable method to assess exercise habits and physical fitness index will be required.

5. Conclusions

In conclusion, a self-reported faster eating speed was clearly associated with a higher risk of developing diabetes in this large-scale observational study of a general Japanese population. A feasible strategy in the future is to work with physicians and registered dietitians to provide nutrition therapy to improve eating speed during medical examination. The population strategy to reduce eating speed appears to provide further protection against the emerging burden of diabetes.

Author Contributions: Conceptualization, D.K. and H.A.; data curation, H.A.; formal analysis, T.M. and H.A.; investigation, H.F., S.F., A.S., M.K., S.I., C.Y., S.Y., K.T. (Kazuhiro Tada), K.T. (Koji Takahashi) and S.O.; methodology, H.A.; project administration, S.F. and H.A.; software, T.M. and H.A.; supervision, D.K.; writing—original draft, H.F. and H.A.; writing—review and editing, D.K., K.I., T.Y., S.M., H.N., S.N., S.K., M.F. and K.M. All authors were informed about each step of manuscript processing including the submission, revision, revision reminder, etc. via emails from our system or assigned Assistant Editor. All authors have read and agreed to the published version of the manuscript.

Funding: This research received no external funding.

Institutional Review Board Statement: The study was conducted according to the guidelines of the Declaration of Helsinki of 1975, revised in 2013, and approved by Fukuoka University Clinical Research & Ethics Centre (No.2017M010).

Informed Consent Statement: Consent of participants was obtained using opt-out approach.

Data Availability Statement: The data presented in this study are available on request from the corresponding author. The data are not publicly available in order to preserve the anonymity of the subjects involved in the study.

Conflicts of Interest: H.A. received research grants from Daiichi Sankyo and Takeda, lecture fees from Bayer, Daiichi Sankyo, Fukuda Denshi, MSD, Takeda, Teijin and fees for consultancy from Kyowa Kirin. D.K. received research support from Böehringer Ingelheim, Sumitomo Dainippon Pharma, Takeda Pharmaceutical.

References

1. Ruderman, N.B.; Saha, A.K.; Vavvas, D.; Heydrick, S.J.; Kurowski, T.G. Lipid Abnormalities in Muscle of Insulin-resistant Rodents the Malonyl CoA Hypothesisa. *Ann. N. Y. Acad. Sci.* **1997**, *827*, 221–230. [CrossRef]
2. Gougeon, R.; Styhler, K.; Morais, J.A.; Jones, P.J.; Marliss, E.B. Effects of oral hypoglycemic agents and diet on protein metabolism in type 2 diabetes. *Diabetes Care* **2000**, *23*, 1–8. [CrossRef] [PubMed]
3. O'Brien, T.; Nguyen, T.T.; Zimmerman, B.R. Hyperlipidemia and Diabetes Mellitus. *Mayo Clin. Proc.* **1998**, *73*, 969–976. [CrossRef]
4. Howard, B.V.; Robbins, D.C.; Sievers, M.L.; Lee, E.T.; Rhoades, D.; Devereux, R.B.; Cowan, L.D.; Gray, R.S.; Welty, T.K.; Go, O.T.; et al. LDL Cholesterol as a Strong Predictor of Coronary Heart Disease in Diabetic Individuals with Insulin Resistance and Low LDL. *Arterioscler. Thromb. Vasc. Biol.* **2000**, *20*, 830–835. [CrossRef] [PubMed]
5. Nathan, D.M.; Singer, D.E.; Godine, J.E.; Harrington, C.H.; Perlmuter, L.C. Retinopathy in older type II diabetics. Association with glucose control. *Diabetes* **1986**, *35*, 797–801. [CrossRef] [PubMed]
6. Cowie, C.C.; Port, F.K.; Wolfe, R.A.; Savage, P.J.; Moll, P.P.; Hawthorne, V.M. Disparities in Incidence of Diabetic End-Stage Renal Disease According to Race and Type of Diabetes. *N. Engl. J. Med.* **1989**, *321*, 1074–1079. [CrossRef]
7. World Health Organization. Global Health Estimates 2016 Summary Tables: DEATHS by Cause, Age and Sex, by World Bank Income Group, 2000–2015. Available online: http://www.who.int/healthinfo/global_burden_disease/en/ (accessed on 18 September 2020).
8. Sone, H.; Tanaka, S.; Tanaka, S.; Suzuki, S.; Seino, H.; Hanyu, O.; Sato, A.; Toyonaga, T.; Okita, K.; Ishibashi, S.; et al. Leisure-Time physical activity is a significant predictor of stroke and total mortality in Japanese patients with type 2 diabetes: Analysis from the Japan Diabetes Complications Study (JDCS). *Diabetologia* **2013**, *56*, 1021–1030. [CrossRef]
9. The Diabetes Control and Complications Trial Research Group (DCCT). The absence of a glycemic threshold for the development of long-term complications: The perspective of the Diabetes Control and Complications Trial. *Diabetes* **1996**, *45*, 1289–1298. [CrossRef]
10. Office of Nutrition, Health Service Division, Health Service Bureau, Ministry of Health, Labour and Welfare, Japan (2017). The National Health and Nutrition Survey in Japan, 2016. Ministry of Health, Labour and Welfare. Available online: http://www.mhlw.go.jp/bunya/kenkou/eiyou/dl/h28-houkoku.pdf (accessed on 10 October 2020).
11. Kosaka, K.; Noda, M.; Kuzuya, T. Prevention of type 2 diabetes by lifestyle intervention: A Japanese trial in IGT males. *Diabetes Res. Clin. Pract.* **2005**, *67*, 152–162. [CrossRef] [PubMed]
12. Kawahara, T.; Takahashi, K.; Inazu, T.; Arao, T.; Kawahara, C.; Tabata, T.; Moriyama, H.; Okada, Y.; Morita, E.; Tanaka, Y. Reduced progression to type 2 diabetes from impaired glucose tolerance after a 2-day in-hospital diabetes educational program: The Joetsu Diabetes Prevention Trial. *Diabetes Care* **2008**, *31*, 1949–1954. [CrossRef] [PubMed]
13. Saito, T.; Watanabe, M.; Nishida, J.; Izumi, T.; Omura, M.; Takagi, T.; Fukunaga, R.; Bandai, Y.; Tajima, N.; Nakamura, Y.; et al. Lifestyle Modification and Prevention of Type 2 Diabetes in Overweight Japanese With Impaired Fasting Glucose Levels: A Randomized Controlled Trial. *Arch. Intern. Med.* **2011**, *171*, 1352–1360. [CrossRef]
14. Maskarinec, G.; Erber, E.; Grandinetti, A.; Verheus, M.; Oum, R.; Hopping, B.N.; Schmidt, M.M.; Uchida, A.; Juarez, D.T.; Hodges, K.; et al. Diabetes incidence based on linkages with health plans: The multiethnic cohort. *Diabetes* **2009**, *58*, 1732–1738. [CrossRef]
15. Kabeya, Y.; Goto, A.; Kato, M.; Matsushita, Y.; Takahashi, Y.; Isogawa, A.; Inoue, M.; Mizoue, T.; Tsugane, S.; Kadowaki, T.; et al. Time Spent Walking and Risk of Diabetes in Japanese Adults: The Japan Public Health Center-Based Prospective Diabetes Study. *J. Epidemiol.* **2016**, *26*, 224–232. [CrossRef]
16. Aune, D.; Norat, T.; Leitzmann, M.; Tonstad, S.; Vatten, L.J. Physical activity and the risk of type 2 diabetes: A systematic review and dose-response meta-analysis. *Eur. J. Epidemiol.* **2015**, *30*, 529–542. [CrossRef]
17. Smith, A.D.; Crippa, A.; Woodcock, J.; Brage, S. Physical activity and incident type 2 diabetes mellitus: A systematic review and dose-response meta-analysis of prospective cohort studies. *Diabetologia* **2016**, *59*, 2527–2545. [CrossRef] [PubMed]
18. Pan, A.; Wang, Y.; Talaei, M.; Hu, F.B.; Wu, T. Relation of active, passive, and quitting smoking with incident type 2 diabetes: A systematic review and meta-analysis. *Lancet Diabetes Endocrinol.* **2015**, *3*, 958–967. [PubMed]

19. Baliunas, D.O.; Taylor, B.J.; Irving, H.; Roerecke, M.; Patra, J.; Mohapatra, S.; Rehm, J. Alcohol as a risk factor for type 2 diabetes: A systematic review and meta-analysis. *Diabetes Care* **2009**, *32*, 2123–2132. [CrossRef]
20. Knott, C.; Bell, S.; Britton, A. Alcohol Consumption and the Risk of Type 2 Diabetes: A Systematic Review and Dose-Response Meta-analysis of More Than 1.9 Million Individuals From 38 Observational Studies. *Diabetes Care* **2015**, *38*, 1804–1812. [CrossRef]
21. Imai, S.; Matsuda, M.; Hasegawa, G.; Fukui, M.; Obayashi, H.; Ozasa, N.; Kajiyama, S. A simple meal plan of 'eating vegetables before carbohydrate' was more effective for achieving glycemic control than an exchange-based meal plan in Japanese patients with type 2 diabetes. *Asia Pac. J. Clin. Nutr.* **2011**, *20*, 161–168. [PubMed]
22. Shukla, A.P.; Andono, J.; Touhamy, S.H.; Casper, A.; Iliescu, R.G.; Mauer, E.; Shan Zhu, Y.; Ludwig, D.S.; Aronne, L.J. Carbohydrate-last meal pattern lowers postprandial glucose and insulin excursions in type 2 diabetes. *BMJ Open Diabetes Res. Care* **2017**, *5*, e000440.
23. Pan, A.; Schernhammer, E.S.; Sun, Q.; Hu, F.B. Rotating night shift work and risk of type 2 diabetes: Two prospective cohort studies in women. *PLoS Med.* **2011**, *8*, e1001141. [CrossRef] [PubMed]
24. Otsuka, R.; Tamakoshi, K.; Yatsuya, H.; Wada, K.; Matsushita, K.; OuYang, P.; Hotta, Y.; Takefuji, S.; Mitsuhashi, H.; Sugiura, K.; et al. Eating fast leads to insulin resistance: Findings in middle-aged Japanese men and women. *Prev. Med.* **2008**, *46*, 154–159. [CrossRef]
25. Sakurai, M.; Nakamura, K.; Miura, K.; Takamura, T.; Yoshita, K.; Nagasawa, S.Y.; Morikawa, Y.; Ishizaki, M.; Kido, T.; Naruse, Y.; et al. Self-Reported speed of eating and 7-year risk of type 2 diabetes mellitus in middle-aged Japanese men. *Metabolism* **2012**, *61*, 1566–1571. [CrossRef]
26. Kudo, A.; Asahi, K.; Satoh, H.; Iseki, K.; Moriyama, T.; Yamagata, K.; Tsuruya, K.; Fujimoto, S.; Narita, I.; Konta, T.; et al. Fast eating is a strong risk factor for new-onset diabetes among the Japanese general population. *Sci. Rep.* **2019**, *9*, 8210. [CrossRef] [PubMed]
27. Maeda, T.; Yoshimura, C.; Takahashi, K.; Ito, K.; Yasuno, T.; Abe, Y.; Masutani, K.; Nakashima, H.; Mukoubara, S.; Arima, H. Usefulness of the blood pressure classification in the new 2017 ACC/AHA hypertension guidelines for the prediction of new-onset chronic kidney disease. *J. Hum. Hypertens.* **2019**, *33*, 873–878. [CrossRef] [PubMed]
28. Yasuno, T.; Maeda, T.; Tada, K.; Takahashi, K.; Ito, K.; Abe, Y.; Mukoubara, S.; Masutani, K.; Arima, H.; Nakashima, H. Effects of HbA1c on the Development and Progression of Chronic Kidney Disease in Elderly and Middle-Aged Japanese: Iki Epidemiological Study of Atherosclerosis and Chronic Kidney Disease (ISSA-CKD). *Intern. Med.* **2020**, *59*, 175–180. [CrossRef] [PubMed]
29. Miyabayashi, I.; Mori, S.; Satoh, A.; Kawazoe, M.; Funakoshi, S.; Ishida, S.; Maeda, T.; Yoshimura, C.; Tada, K.; Takahashi, K.; et al. Uric Acid and Prevalence of Hypertension in a General Population of Japanese: ISSA-CKD Study. *J. Clin. Med. Res.* **2020**, *12*, 431–435. [CrossRef] [PubMed]
30. Ito, K.; Maeda, T.; Tada, K.; Takahashi, K.; Yasuno, T.; Masutani, K.; Mukoubara, S.; Arima, H.; Nakashima, H. The role of cigarette smoking on new-onset of chronic kidney disease in a Japanese population without prior chronic kidney disease: Iki epidemiological study of atherosclerosis and chronic kidney disease (ISSA-CKD). *Clin. Exp. Nephrol.* **2020**, *24*, 919–926. [CrossRef] [PubMed]
31. Radzeviciene, L.; Ostrauskas, R. Fast eating and the risk of type 2 diabetes mellitus: A case-control study. *Clin. Nutr.* **2013**, *32*, 232–235. [CrossRef]
32. Totsuka, K.; Maeno, T.; Saito, K.; Kodama, S.; Asumi, M.; Yachi, Y.; Hiranuma, Y.; Shimano, H.; Yamada, N.; Ono, Y.; et al. Self-reported fast eating is a potent predictor of development of impaired glucose tolerance in Japanese men and women: Tsukuba Medical Center Study. *Diabetes Res. Clin. Pract.* **2011**, *94*, e72–e74. [CrossRef]
33. Sasaki, S.; Katagiri, A.; Tsuji, T.; Shimoda, T.; Amano, K. Self-Reported rate of eating correlates with body mass index in 18-y-old Japanese women. *Int. J. Obes. Relat. Metab. Disord.* **2003**, *27*, 1405–1410. [CrossRef]
34. Otsuka, R.; Tamakoshi, K.; Yatsuya, H.; Murata, C.; Sekiya, A.; Wada, K.; Zhang, H.M.; Matsushita, K.; Sugiura, K.; Takefuji, S.; et al. Eating Fast Leads to Obesity: Findings Based on Self-administered Questionnaires among Middle-aged Japanese Men and Women. *J. Epidemiol.* **2006**, *16*, 117–124. [CrossRef]
35. Tanihara, S.; Imatoh, T.; Miyazaki, M.; Babazono, A.; Momose, Y.; Baba, M.; Uryu, Y.; Une, H. Retrospective longitudinal study on the relationship between 8-year weight change and current eating speed. *Appetite* **2011**, *57*, 179–183. [CrossRef]
36. Takayama, S.; Akamine, Y.; Okabe, T.; Koya, Y.; Haraguchi, M.; Miyata, Y.; Sakai, T.; Sakura, H.; Sasaki, T. Rate of eating and body weight in patients with type 2 diabetes or hyperlipidaemia. *J. Int. Med. Res.* **2002**, *30*, 442–444. [CrossRef]
37. Zhu, B.; Haruyama, Y.; Muto, T.; Yamazaki, T. Association between eating speed and metabolic syndrome in a three-year population-based cohort study. *J. Epidemiol.* **2015**, *25*, 332–336. [CrossRef] [PubMed]
38. Ashizawa, E.; Katano, S.; Harada, A.; Yanagibori, R.; Kobayashi, Y.; Sato, S.; Eguchi, H. Exploring the link between standard lifestyle questionnaires administered during specific medical check-ups and incidence of metabolic syndrome in Chiba Prefecture. *Nihon Koshu Eisei Zasshi.* **2014**, *61*, 176–185. [PubMed]
39. Shigeta, H.; Shigeta, M.; Nakazawa, A.; Nakamura, N.; Yoshikawa, T. Lifestyle, Obesity, and Insulin Resistance. *Diabetes Care* **2001**, *24*, 608. [CrossRef]
40. Suzuki, H.; Fukushima, M.; Okamoto, S.; Takahashi, O.; Shimbo, T.; Kurose, T.; Yamada, Y.; Inagaki, N.; Seino, Y.; Fukui, T. Effects of thorough mastication on postprandial plasma glucose concentrations in nonobese Japanese subjects. *Metabolism* **2005**, *54*, 1593–1599. [CrossRef]

41. Merovci, A.; Tripathy, D.; Chen, X.; Valdez, I.; Abdul-Ghani, M.; Solis-Herrera, C.; Gastaldelli, A.; DeFronzo, R.A. Effect of Mild Physiologic Hyperglycemia on Insulin Secretion, Insulin Clearance and Insulin Sensitivity in Healthy Glucose Tolerant Subjects. *Diabetes* **2020**, *70*, 204–231, db200039. [CrossRef] [PubMed]
42. Sakata, T.; Yoshimatsu, H.; Kurokawa, M. Hypothalamic neuronal histamine: Implications of its homeostatic control of energy metabolism. *Nutrition* **1997**, *13*, 403–411. [CrossRef]
43. Kokkinos, A.; le Roux, C.W.; Alexiadou, K.; Tentolouris, N.; Vincent, R.P.; Kyriaki, D.; Perrea, D.; Ghatei, M.A.; Bloom, S.R.; Katsilambros, N. Eating slowly increases the postprandial response of the anorexigenic gut hormones, peptide YY and glucagon-like peptide-1. *J. Clin. Endocrinol. Metab.* **2010**, *95*, 333–337. [CrossRef]
44. Galhardo, J.; Hunt, L.P.; Lightman, S.L.; Sabin, M.A.; Bergh, C.; Sodersten, P.; Shield, J.P. Normalizing eating behavior reduces body weight and improves gastrointestinal hormonal secretion in obese adolescents. *J. Clin. Endocrinol. Metab.* **2012**, *97*, E193–E201. [CrossRef]
45. Rigamonti, A.E.; Agosti, F.; Compri, E.; Giunta, M.; Marazzi, N.; Muller, E.E.; Cella, S.G.; Sartorio, A. Anorexigenic postprandial responses of PYY and GLP1 to slow ice cream consumption: Preservation in obese adolescents, but not in obese adults. *Eur. J. Endocrinol.* **2013**, *168*, 429–436. [CrossRef]
46. Woodward, E.; Haszard, J.; Worsfold, A.; Venn, B. Comparison of Self-Reported Speed of Eating with an Objective Measure of Eating Rate. *Nutrients* **2020**, *12*, 599. [CrossRef]
47. Melton, L.J.; Palumbo, P.J.; Chu, C.-P. Incidence of Diabetes Mellitus by Clinical Type. *Diabetes Care* **1983**, *6*, 75–86. [CrossRef] [PubMed]
48. Melton, L.J., 3rd; Palumbo, P.J.; Dwyer, M.S.; Chu, C.P. Impact of recent changes in diagnostic criteria on the apparent natural history of diabetes mellitus. *Am. J. Epidemiol.* **1983**, *117*, 559–565. [CrossRef] [PubMed]
49. Wenger, H.A.; Bell, G.J. The Interactions of Intensity, Frequency and Duration of Exercise Training in Altering Cardiorespiratory Fitness. *Sports Med.* **1986**, *3*, 346–356. [CrossRef] [PubMed]

MDPI
St. Alban-Anlage 66
4052 Basel
Switzerland
www.mdpi.com

Journal of Clinical Medicine Editorial Office
E-mail: jcm@mdpi.com
www.mdpi.com/journal/jcm

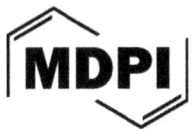

Disclaimer/Publisher's Note: The statements, opinions and data contained in all publications are solely those of the individual author(s) and contributor(s) and not of MDPI and/or the editor(s). MDPI and/or the editor(s) disclaim responsibility for any injury to people or property resulting from any ideas, methods, instructions or products referred to in the content.

www.ingramcontent.com/pod-product-compliance
Lightning Source LLC
LaVergne TN
LVHW070436100526
838202LV00014B/1607

Breast Cancer: A Multi-Disciplinary Approach from Imaging to Therapy

Breast Cancer: A Multi-Disciplinary Approach from Imaging to Therapy

Editor

Daniele Ugo Tari

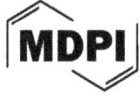 Basel • Beijing • Wuhan • Barcelona • Belgrade • Novi Sad • Cluj • Manchester

Editor
Daniele Ugo Tari
Department of Breast Imaging
Caserta Local Health Authority
Caserta
Italy

Editorial Office
MDPI
St. Alban-Anlage 66
4052 Basel, Switzerland

This is a reprint of articles from the Special Issue published online in the open access journal *Current Oncology* (ISSN 1718-7729) (available at: www.mdpi.com/journal/curroncol/special_issues/breast_cancer_imaging_therapy).

For citation purposes, cite each article independently as indicated on the article page online and as indicated below:

Lastname, A.A.; Lastname, B.B. Article Title. *Journal Name* **Year**, *Volume Number*, Page Range.

ISBN 978-3-7258-0208-1 (Hbk)
ISBN 978-3-7258-0207-4 (PDF)
doi.org/10.3390/books978-3-7258-0207-4

© 2024 by the authors. Articles in this book are Open Access and distributed under the Creative Commons Attribution (CC BY) license. The book as a whole is distributed by MDPI under the terms and conditions of the Creative Commons Attribution-NonCommercial-NoDerivs (CC BY-NC-ND) license.

Contents

About the Editor vii

Daniele Ugo Tari
Breast Cancer: A Multi-Disciplinary Approach from Imaging to Therapy
Reprinted from: *Curr. Oncol.* **2024**, *31*, 598-602, doi:10.3390/curroncol31010043 1

Prarthna V. Bhardwaj, Holly Mason, Seth A. Kaufman, Paul Visintainer and Grace Makari-Judson
Outcomes of a Multidisciplinary Team in the Management of Patients with Early-Stage Breast Cancer Undergoing Neoadjuvant Chemotherapy at a Community Cancer Center
Reprinted from: *Curr. Oncol.* **2023**, *30*, 4861-4870, doi:10.3390/curroncol30050366 6

Derek Muradali, Glenn G. Fletcher, Erin Cordeiro, Samantha Fienberg, Ralph George and Supriya Kulkarni et al.
Preoperative Breast Magnetic Resonance Imaging: An Ontario Health (Cancer Care Ontario) Clinical Practice Guideline
Reprinted from: *Curr. Oncol.* **2023**, *30*, 6255-6270, doi:10.3390/curroncol30070463 16

Anna D'Angelo, Charlotte Marguerite Lucille Trombadori, Flavia Caprini, Stefano Lo Cicero, Valentina Longo and Francesca Ferrara et al.
Efficacy and Accuracy of Using Magnetic Seed for Preoperative Non-Palpable Breast Lesions Localization: Our Experience with Magseed
Reprinted from: *Curr. Oncol.* **2022**, *29*, 8468-8474, doi:10.3390/curroncol29110667 32

Christina Panagiotis Malainou, Nikolina Stachika, Aikaterini Konstantina Damianou, Aristotelis Anastopoulos, Ioanna Ploumaki and Efthymios Triantafyllou et al.
Estrogen-Receptor-Low-Positive Breast Cancer: Pathological and Clinical Perspectives
Reprinted from: *Curr. Oncol.* **2023**, *30*, 9734-9745, doi:10.3390/curroncol30110706 39

Daniela Oliveira, Sofia Fernandes, Isália Miguel, Sofia Fragoso and Fátima Vaz
Is There a Role for Risk-Reducing Bilateral Breast Surgery in *BRCA1/2* Ovarian Cancer Survivors? An Observational Study
Reprinted from: *Curr. Oncol.* **2023**, *30*, 7810-7817, doi:10.3390/curroncol30090567 51

Donato Casella, Daniele Fusario, Dario Cassetti, Anna Lisa Pesce, Alessandro De Luca and Maristella Guerra et al.
Controlateral Symmetrisation in SRM for Breast Cancer: Now or Then? Immediate versus Delayed Symmetrisation in a Two-Stage Breast Reconstruction
Reprinted from: *Curr. Oncol.* **2022**, *29*, 9391-9400, doi:10.3390/curroncol29120737 59

Zeliha Güzelöz, Oğuzhan Ayrancıoğlu, Nesrin Aktürk, Merve Güneş and Zümre Arıcan Alıcıkuş
Dose Volume and Liver Function Test Relationship following Radiotheraphy for Right Breast Cancer: A Multicenter Study
Reprinted from: *Curr. Oncol.* **2023**, *30*, 8763-8773, doi:10.3390/curroncol30100632 69

Katarina Antunac, Ljiljana Mayer, Marija Banovic and Lidija Beketic-Oreskovic
Correlation of High-Sensitivity Cardiac Troponin I Values and Cardiac Radiation Doses in Patients with Left-Sided Breast Cancer Undergoing Hypofractionated Adjuvant Radiotherapy with Concurrent Anti-HER2 Therapy
Reprinted from: *Curr. Oncol.* **2023**, *30*, 9049-9062, doi:10.3390/curroncol30100654 80

Cristina Marinela Oprean, Andrei Dorin Ciocoiu, Nusa Alina Segarceanu, Diana Moldoveanu, Alexandra Stan and Teodora Hoinoiu et al.
Pregnancy in a Young Patient with Metastatic HER2-Positive Breast Cancer—Between Fear of Recurrence and Desire to Procreate
Reprinted from: *Curr. Oncol.* **2023**, *30*, 4833-4843, doi:10.3390/curroncol30050364 . . . . **94**

Anna Isselhard, Zoë Lautz, Kerstin Rhiem and Stephanie Stock
Assessing Psychological Morbidity in Cancer-Unaffected *BRCA1/2* Pathogenic Variant Carriers: A Systematic Review
Reprinted from: *Curr. Oncol.* **2023**, *30*, 3590-3608, doi:10.3390/curroncol30040274 . . . . **105**

Franciéle Marabotti Costa Leite, Andreia Gomes Oliveira, Bruna Lígia Ferreira de Almeida Barbosa, Mariana Zoboli Ambrosim, Neiva Augusta Viegas Vasconcellos and Paulete Maria Ambrósio Maciel et al.
Intimate Partner Violence against Mastectomized Women: Victims' Experiences
Reprinted from: *Curr. Oncol.* **2022**, *29*, 8556-8564, doi:10.3390/curroncol29110674 . . . . **124**

About the Editor

Daniele Ugo Tari

Dr. Daniele Tari, MD, is the Director of the Department of Breast Imaging at Caserta LHA, Italy. After his postgraduate studies in Radiology, he specialized in breast imaging under Prof. GM Giuseppetti's mentorship in Ancona, Italy.

His research focuses on breast imaging and diseases, oncology, and public health. As a member of the Italian College of Senologists and the Italian School of Senology, he contributed to developing Italian breast cancer management guidelines. Dr. Tari emphasizes specialized training in breast imaging and promotes a multimodality approach for comprehensive early diagnoses. With over 80 published papers in national and international journals and more than 470 citations, Dr. Tari's contributions earned recognition at the 2023 EUSOBI Scientific Meeting in Valencia. He serves as an academic editor for Plos One, guest editor for MDPI, and ad hoc reviewer for high-impact journals. Dr. Tari is also affiliated with prestigious organizations like EUSOBI, ESR, and SIRM.

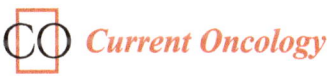

Editorial

Breast Cancer: A Multi-Disciplinary Approach from Imaging to Therapy

Daniele Ugo Tari

Department of Breast Imaging, Caserta Local Health Authority, District 12 "Palazzo della Salute", 81100 Caserta, Italy; daniele.tari@aslcaserta.it

1. Introduction

Breast cancer (BC) is the most prevalent form of cancer among women worldwide, accounting for over 2 million diagnoses annually [1]. The impact of BC extends beyond individual patients, affecting the entire community through its implications in imaging, therapy, and its broader social, economic, and psychological consequences. In the face of ongoing challenges, a comprehensive approach is crucial to ensuring a high standard of care, particularly in the aftermath of the COVID-19 pandemic, which has brought lasting changes to medical practices [2]. The demand for personalized medicine has underscored the importance of a multidisciplinary strategy combining artificial intelligence and human expertise [3].

Early detection of breast cancer has significantly improved survival rates, enabling more effective and targeted treatments. However, a substantial gap persists when early diagnosis is not achieved, particularly among women with dense breasts or those at high risk [4,5]. Additionally, the incidence of male breast cancer has risen by 20–25% in recent decades [6]. Consequently, a multidisciplinary team and enhanced diagnostic-therapeutic pathways (DTCP) are essential for early detection and improved treatments [7].

The primary aim of this Special Issue has been to comprehensively present and discuss all aspects of breast cancer management, from imaging to therapy, addressing knowledge gaps, and exploring the psychological aspects of diagnosis and therapy. Out of nineteen submitted articles, eleven were accepted for publication after the peer-review process, resulting in a 58% acceptance rate. The published articles, briefly described in the following section, cover several topics and aspects significantly influencing breast cancer management.

2. Summary of Published Articles

In the first article of this Special Issue, Bhardwaj et al. (Contribution 1) assessed the efficacy and coordination of a multidisciplinary team (MDT) in the treatment of early-stage breast cancer using neoadjuvant chemotherapy (NAC). The retrospective study covered 94 patients and focused on the timing and outcomes of NAC, surgery, and radiation therapy. The study found significant downstaging of breast tumors in 91.4% of patients and axillary downstaging in 33% of patients. The median time from diagnosis to NAC was 37.5 days, from the end of NAC to surgery was 29 days, and from surgery to radiation therapy was 49.5 days. The study concluded that the MDT provided timely, coordinated, and consistent care, with the time to treatment aligning with national trends. It highlighted the effectiveness of multidisciplinary coordination in managing early-stage breast cancer, suggesting this as a model for other community cancer centers.

Muradali et al. (Contribution 2) synthesized the inconsistencies in the use of preoperative breast magnetic resonance imaging (MRI) following the diagnosis of breast cancer through mammography and/or ultrasound. After conducting a systematic review and meta-analysis, they recommended considering preoperative breast MRI on a case-by-case basis, especially for patients where additional information about disease extent could

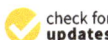

Citation: Tari, D.U. Breast Cancer: A Multi-Disciplinary Approach from Imaging to Therapy. *Curr. Oncol.* 2024, 31, 598–602. https://doi.org/10.3390/curroncol31010043

Received: 15 January 2024
Accepted: 19 January 2024
Published: 22 January 2024

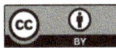

Copyright: © 2024 by the author. Licensee MDPI, Basel, Switzerland. This article is an open access article distributed under the terms and conditions of the Creative Commons Attribution (CC BY) license (https://creativecommons.org/licenses/by/4.0/).

influence treatment decisions. The study substantiated that MRI improves recurrence rates, decreases reoperations, and increases detection of synchronous contralateral breast cancer. It emphasized the need for shared decision-making between care providers and patients, considering the benefits and risks of MRI as well as patient preferences. Specific recommendations are given for using MRI in various clinical scenarios, such as aiding surgical planning, identifying lesions in dense breasts, and determining the presence of muscle or chest wall invasion in certain tumors. The paper underlined the significance of MRI's high sensitivity and specificity in breast cancer diagnosis and staging, advocating for its selective use in enhancing treatment outcomes.

The study proposed by D'Angelo et al. (Contribution 3) is a retrospective investigation into the use of Magseed® (Endomagnetics, Cambridge, UK) for the preoperative localization of non-palpable breast lesions. It involved 45 patients who underwent breast-conserving surgery (BCS) between 2020 and 2022, with Magseed placement primarily under ultrasound guidance. The study boasted a high placement success rate of 97.8%, with only one instance of seed migration, and a 100% retrieval rate post-BCS. Notably, no patients required re-excision due to positive margins. The authors concluded that Magseed is an extremely effective technique for preoperative localization of non-palpable breast lesions, supporting its continued use despite acknowledging certain limitations and rare occurrences of seed migration. The study contributed valuable real-world data to the growing body of literature on Magseed, suggesting it as a viable alternative to traditional wire localization techniques.

Malainou et al. (Contribution 4) delved into the unique challenges and clinical implications of estrogen receptor-low-positive (ER-low-positive) breast cancer. This subtype, characterized by 1–9% ER expression, represents a small but significant portion of breast cancer cases, and its management is less clear-cut due to its nuanced response to standard therapies. The review consolidated various studies that discuss the prevalence, characteristics, and treatment responses of ER-low-positive BC. It highlighted that while these tumors share some similarities with ER-negative and triple-negative breast cancers, they present distinct clinical behaviors and outcomes. The review called for more research, especially randomized clinical trials, to better understand and manage this unique breast cancer subset, emphasizing the need for tailored treatment strategies and the potential of including these patients in clinical trials for more aggressive breast cancer types. This review is a call to action for the medical community to recognize the distinct nature of ER-low-positive BC and to seek more effective management strategies.

Oliveira et al. (Contribution 5) presented an observational analysis of 69 BRCA1/2 ovarian cancer survivors and their subsequent risk of developing breast cancer. The authors found that the median overall survival after ovarian cancer diagnosis was 8 years, with a significantly higher survival rate for BRCA2 patients compared to BRCA1 patients. About 13.2% of the participants developed breast cancer at a median age of 61 years. The study discussed the controversy of risk-reducing bilateral breast surgery in ovarian cancer survivors due to the associated high relapse rates and mortality of ovarian cancer. While the study acknowledged the potential benefits of surgical breast cancer risk management, it emphasized that such decisions should be tailored to individual patient characteristics and preferences, considering the balance between ovarian cancer mortality and breast cancer risk. This study contributes to the ongoing discourse on the management of cancer risks in BRCA1/2 ovarian cancer survivors, suggesting a multidisciplinary approach to decision-making.

Casella et al. (Contribution 6) presented a study exploring the clinical and aesthetic outcomes of immediate versus delayed symmetrization in skin-reducing mastectomy (SRM) for BC. The study involved a randomized observational cohort of 84 patients undergoing SRM, divided into two groups: immediate and delayed symmetrization. The study found that immediate symmetrization provided better aesthetic outcomes and higher patient satisfaction without significantly impacting the second stage of reconstruction. It highlighted immediate symmetrization as a safe and tolerable technique, improving the quality of life for patients. The research underscored the importance of considering immediate symmetrization in reconstructive surgery planning for breast cancer patients to provide better immediate symmetry and overall satisfaction.

The next two papers evaluated the impact of radiotherapy (RT) on right and left BC, respectively. In particular, Guzeloz et al. (Contribution 7) explored the relationship between radiotherapy dose-volume parameters for right breast cancer and subsequent changes in liver function tests (LFTs), specifically alanine aminotransferase (ALT), aspartate aminotransferase (AST), and gamma-glutamyl transferase (GGT). The retrospective analysis included 100 female patients treated across three centers, focusing on liver dosimetry during right breast or chest wall RT and its impact on LFTs pre- and post-RT. The results showed a median increase of up to 15% in AST, ALT, and GGT levels post-radiotherapy, with a significant correlation between higher liver doses and changes in LFTs. The study emphasized the importance of considering liver dose during radiotherapy planning and the necessity of regular LFT monitoring, advocating for a mean liver dose below 208 cGy to minimize potential liver damage. The study contributed to understanding the implications of RT on liver function and underscored the need for careful dose management to prevent liver toxicity, particularly in breast cancer patients with a longer life expectancy.

Antunac K et al. (Contribution 8) investigated the relationship between radiation doses to cardiac structures and the elevation of high-sensitivity cardiac troponin I (hscTnI) as an early marker of cardiotoxicity in patients receiving adjuvant radiotherapy for left-sided breast cancer along with anti-HER2 therapy. Including 61 patients, the study found that patients with an increase in hscTnI values post-radiotherapy had significantly higher mean radiation doses to the heart, left ventricle (LV), and left anterior descending artery (LAD) compared to those without an hscTnI increase. The findings suggested that higher radiation doses to these cardiac structures are associated with subclinical myocardial damage, as indicated by elevated hscTnI levels. The study underscored the importance of optimizing radiation therapy techniques to minimize cardiac exposure and the potential for early cardiac injury in breast cancer treatment.

The last three articles explored the psychological impact that a diagnosis or a potential diagnosis of breast cancer can have on women, assessing its effects on both an individual and familial level.

Oprean C et al. (Contribution 9) proposed a poignant case study of a 31-year-old woman grappling with metastatic HER2-positive breast cancer who chose to pursue pregnancy despite the known risks. The patient initially responded well to first-line treatment but vehemently refused ongoing oncological care due to her strong desire to conceive. This decision led to the cessation of treatment and the subsequent progression of her disease. Unfortunately, her pregnancy and life ended abruptly due to complications from her cancer. This case underscored the complex psychological aspects influencing patient decisions, including cognitive distortion, which led to prioritizing procreation over personal survival. The study emphasized the importance of multidisciplinary care and psychological support in managing such challenging cases, highlighting the urgent need for careful guidance and support for patients making life-altering decisions under the weight of severe illness.

Isselhard et al. (Contribution 10) provided a comprehensive evaluation of the psychological distress experienced by women who carry BRCA1/2 pathogenic variants but are not affected by cancer. This systematic review included 45 studies from 13 countries focusing on measures of distress, depression, and other psychological outcomes. Most studies observed an initial peak in distress following the disclosure of genetic test results, which tended to decline over subsequent months. While depression was frequently investigated, it was generally not found to be clinically significant among carriers. Quality of life appeared largely unaffected, though younger women showed some dissatisfaction with their role functioning. Body image was less frequently assessed, but available evidence suggested a decrease in body image satisfaction, especially after prophylactic mastectomy. The review called for future research to use standardized instruments to enhance comparability and provide more definitive conclusions about the psychological morbidity in this specific population.

Finally, Leite et al. (Contribution 11) delved into the experiences of violence endured by women from their intimate partners following mastectomy. Conducted with 16 Brazilian women who underwent breast cancer treatment, this qualitative study revealed alarming insights into the types of violence—psychological, physical, and sexual—that these women faced during their already vulnerable post-mastectomy period. The results highlighted that 50% of participants encountered psychological violence, 30% physical violence, and 20% sexual violence from their intimate partners. The research underscored the pressing need for healthcare professionals to be vigilant and proactive in identifying and addressing intimate partner violence among mastectomized women, recognizing it as a significant factor affecting their overall treatment and recovery. The study's conclusions advocated for a comprehensive, multidisciplinary approach to supporting these women, including the establishment of a protective and care network to combat the pervasive issue of violence.

3. Conclusions

The interdisciplinary nature of these discussions underscores the need for a holistic understanding and approach to breast cancer, emphasizing the importance of collaborative efforts in advancing knowledge and improving patient outcomes.

In particular, it would be desirable for scientific research to systematically compare practical experiences with extant literature, with the objective of providing empirically grounded guidance for clinical practice and meticulously embodying the principles of evidence-based medicine. Such a rigorous approach holds the potential to substantially contribute to the establishment of uniformity across diverse socio-economic contexts.

In conclusion, the imperative for further in-depth research and development remains crucial. It is vital to thoroughly understand and address the management of breast cancer diagnosis and treatment, facing new challenges with steadfast commitment and dedication.

Funding: This article received no external funding.

Acknowledgments: This Special Issue would not have been possible without the contributions of various talented authors, hardworking and professional reviewers, and dedicated editorial team members of the journal. Congratulations to all authors who submitted articles—no matter what the final decisions of the editors were. Feedback, comments, and suggestions have been offered by peer reviewers and editors to help the authors improve their articles. Finally, I would like to express my gratitude to the Assistant Editor of this Special Issue.

Conflicts of Interest: The author declares no conflicts of interest.

List of Contributions

1. Bhardwaj, P.V.; Mason, H.; Kaufman, S.A.; Visintainer, P.; Makari-Judson, G. Outcomes of a Multidisciplinary Team in the Management of Patients with Early-Stage Breast Cancer Undergoing Neoadjuvant Chemotherapy at a Community Cancer Center. *Curr. Oncol.* **2023**, *30*, 4861–4870. https://doi.org/10.3390/curroncol30050366.
2. Muradali, D.; Fletcher, G.G.; Cordeiro, E.; Fienberg, S.; George, R.; Kulkarni, S.; Seely, J.M.; Shaheen, R.; Eisen, A. Preoperative Breast Magnetic Resonance Imaging: An Ontario Health (Cancer Care Ontario) Clinical Practice Guideline. *Curr. Oncol.* **2023**, *30*, 6255–6270. https://doi.org/10.3390/curroncol30070463.
3. D'Angelo, A.; Trombadori, C.M.L.; Caprini, F.; Lo Cicero, S.; Longo, V.; Ferrara, F.; Palma, S.; Conti, M.; Franco, A.; Scardina, L.; et al. Efficacy and Accuracy of Using Magnetic Seed for Preoperative Non-Palpable Breast Lesions Localization: Our Experience with Magseed. *Curr. Oncol.* **2022**, *29*, 8468–8474. https://doi.org/10.3390/curroncol29110667.
4. Malainou, C.P.; Stachika, N.; Damianou, A.K.; Anastopoulos, A.; Ploumaki, I.; Triantafyllou, E.; Drougkas, K.; Gomatou, G.; Kotteas, E. Estrogen-Receptor-Low-Positive Breast Cancer: Pathological and Clinical Perspectives. *Curr. Oncol.* **2023**, *30*, 9734–9745. https://doi.org/10.3390/curroncol30110706.

5. Oliveira, D.; Fernandes, S.; Miguel, I.; Fragoso, S.; Vaz, F. Is There a Role for Risk-Reducing Bilateral Breast Surgery in *BRCA1/2* Ovarian Cancer Survivors? An Observational Study. *Curr. Oncol.* **2023**, *30*, 7810–7817. https://doi.org/10.3390/curroncol30090567.
6. Casella, D.; Fusario, D.; Cassetti, D.; Pesce, A.L.; De Luca, A.; Guerra, M.; Cuomo, R.; Ribuffo, D.; Neri, A.; Marcasciano, M. Controlateral Symmetrisation in SRM for Breast Cancer: Now or Then? Immediate versus Delayed Symmetrisation in a Two-Stage Breast Reconstruction. *Curr. Oncol.* **2022**, *29*, 9391–9400. https://doi.org/10.3390/curroncol29120737.
7. Güzelöz, Z.; Ayrancıoğlu, O.; Aktürk, N.; Güneş, M.; Alıcıkuş, Z.A. Dose Volume and Liver Function Test Relationship following Radiotheraphy for Right Breast Cancer: A Multicenter Study. *Curr. Oncol.* **2023**, *30*, 8763–8773. https://doi.org/10.3390/curroncol30100632.
8. Antunac, K.; Mayer, L.; Banovic, M.; Beketic-Oreskovic, L. Correlation of High-Sensitivity Cardiac Troponin I Values and Cardiac Radiation Doses in Patients with Left-Sided Breast Cancer Undergoing Hypofractionated Adjuvant Radiotherapy with Concurrent Anti-HER2 Therapy. *Curr. Oncol.* **2023**, *30*, 9049–9062. https://doi.org/10.3390/curroncol30100654.
9. Oprean, C.M.; Ciocoiu, A.D.; Segarceanu, N.A.; Moldoveanu, D.; Stan, A.; Hoinoiu, T.; Chiorean-Cojocaru, I.; Grujic, D.; Stefanut, A.; Pit, D.; et al. Pregnancy in a Young Patient with Metastatic HER2-Positive Breast Cancer-Between Fear of Recurrence and Desire to Procreate. *Curr. Oncol.* **2023**, *30*, 4833–4843. https://doi.org/10.3390/curroncol30050364.
10. Isselhard, A.; Lautz, Z.; Rhiem, K.; Stock, S. Assessing Psychological Morbidity in Cancer-Unaffected *BRCA1/2* Pathogenic Variant Carriers: A Systematic Review. *Curr. Oncol.* **2023**, *30*, 3590–3608. https://doi.org/10.3390/curroncol30040274.
11. Leite, F.M.C.; Oliveira, A.G.; Barbosa, B.L.F.A.; Ambrosim, M.Z.; Vasconcellos, N.A.V.; Maciel, P.M.A.; Amorim, M.H.C.; Furieri, L.B.; Lopes-Júnior, L.C. Intimate Partner Violence against Mastectomized Women: Victims' Experiences. *Curr. Oncol.* **2022**, *29*, 8556–8564. https://doi.org/10.3390/curroncol29110674.

References

1. World Health Organization. The Global Breast Cancer Initiative. 2021. Available online: https://www.who.int/multi-media/details/the-global-breast-cancer-initiative-(gbci) (accessed on 3 January 2024).
2. Citgez, B.; Yigit, B.; Capkinoglu, E.; Yetkin, S.G. Management of Breast Cancer during the COVID-19 Pandemic. *Şişli Etfal Hastanesi Tip Bülteni* **2020**, *54*, 132–135. [CrossRef] [PubMed]
3. Tari, D.U.; De Lucia, D.R.; Santarsiere, M.; Santonastaso, R.; Pinto, F. Practical Challenges of DBT-Guided VABB: Harms and Benefits, from Literature to Clinical Experience. *Cancers* **2023**, *15*, 5720. [CrossRef] [PubMed]
4. Freer, P.E. Mammographic breast density: Impact on breast cancer risk and implications for screening. *Radiographics* **2015**, *35*, 302–315. [CrossRef] [PubMed]
5. Heindl, F.; Fasching, P.A.; Hein, A.; Hack, C.C.; Heusinger, K.; Gass, P.; Pöschke, P.; Stübs, F.A.; Schulz-Wendtland, R.; Hartmann, A.; et al. Mammographic density and prognosis in primary breast cancer patients. *Breast* **2021**, *59*, 51–57. [CrossRef] [PubMed]
6. Khan, N.A.J.; Tirona, M. An updated review of epidemiology, risk factors, and management of male breast cancer. *Med. Oncol.* **2021**, *38*, 39. [CrossRef] [PubMed]
7. Graff, S.L.; Principe, J.; Galvin, A.M.; Fenton, M.A.; Strenger, R.; Salama, L.; Bansal, R.; Dizon, D.S.; Begnoche, M.H. Evaluating Patient Experience in a Multidisciplinary Breast Cancer Clinic: A Prospective Study. *J. Women's Health* **2024**, *33*, 39–44. [CrossRef] [PubMed]

Disclaimer/Publisher's Note: The statements, opinions and data contained in all publications are solely those of the individual author(s) and contributor(s) and not of MDPI and/or the editor(s). MDPI and/or the editor(s) disclaim responsibility for any injury to people or property resulting from any ideas, methods, instructions or products referred to in the content.

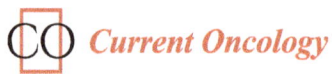

Article

Outcomes of a Multidisciplinary Team in the Management of Patients with Early-Stage Breast Cancer Undergoing Neoadjuvant Chemotherapy at a Community Cancer Center

Prarthna V. Bhardwaj [1,*], Holly Mason [2], Seth A. Kaufman [3], Paul Visintainer [4] and Grace Makari-Judson [1]

1. Division of Hematology—Oncology, University of Massachusetts Chan Medical School—Baystate, 759 Chestnut Street, Springfield, MA 01199, USA
2. Breast Surgery Section, University of Massachusetts Chan Medical School—Baystate, 759 Chestnut Street, Springfield, MA 01199, USA
3. Division of Radiation Oncology, University of Massachusetts Chan Medical School—Baystate, 759 Chestnut Street, Springfield, MA 01199, USA
4. Institute for Healthcare Delivery and Population Science, University of Massachusetts Chan Medical—Baystate, 759 Chestnut Street, Springfield, MA 01199, USA
* Correspondence: prarthna.bhardwaj@baystatehealth.org

Abstract: *Background:* The utilization of neoadjuvant chemotherapy (NAC) remains highly variable in clinical practice. The implementation of NAC requires coordination of handoffs between a multidisciplinary team (MDT). This study aims to assess the outcomes of an MDT in the management of early-stage breast cancer patients undergoing neoadjuvant chemotherapy at a community cancer center. *Methods:* We conducted a retrospective case series on patients receiving NAC for early-stage operable or locally advanced breast cancer coordinated by an MDT. Outcomes of interest included the rate of downstaging of cancer in the breast and axilla, time from biopsy to NAC, time from completion of NAC to surgery, and time from surgery to radiation therapy (RT). *Results:* Ninety-four patients underwent NAC; 84% were White and mean age was 56.5 yrs. Of them, 87 (92.5%) had clinical stage II or III cancer, and 43 (45.8%) had positive lymph nodes. Thirty-nine patients (42.9%) were triple negative, 28 (30.8%) were human epidermal growth factor receptor (HER-2)+, and 24 (26.2%) were estrogen receptor (ER) +HER-2−. Of 91 patients, 23 (25.3%) achieved pCR; 84 patients (91.4%) had downstaging of the breast tumor, and 30 (33%) had axillary downstaging. The median time from diagnosis to NAC was 37.5 days, the time from completion of NAC to surgery was 29 days, and the time from surgery to RT was 49.5 days. *Conclusions:* Our MDT provided timely, coordinated, and consistent care for patients with early-stage breast cancer undergoing NAC as evidenced by time to treatment outcomes consistent with recommended national trends.

Keywords: neoadjuvant chemotherapy; breast cancer; multidisciplinary team; care pathway; breast cancer therapy; breast surgery; breast radiation therapy

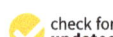

Citation: Bhardwaj, P.V.; Mason, H.; Kaufman, S.A.; Visintainer, P.; Makari-Judson, G. Outcomes of a Multidisciplinary Team in the Management of Patients with Early-Stage Breast Cancer Undergoing Neoadjuvant Chemotherapy at a Community Cancer Center. *Curr. Oncol.* **2023**, *30*, 4861–4870. https://doi.org/10.3390/curroncol30050366

Received: 9 February 2023
Revised: 31 March 2023
Accepted: 4 May 2023
Published: 8 May 2023

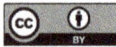

Copyright: © 2023 by the authors. Licensee MDPI, Basel, Switzerland. This article is an open access article distributed under the terms and conditions of the Creative Commons Attribution (CC BY) license (https://creativecommons.org/licenses/by/4.0/).

1. Introduction

Modern breast cancer management has become increasingly complex and specialized over the years. A multidisciplinary approach to cancer care that brings together all pertinent disciplines to discuss optimal care is not only attractive but also promoted in cancer care guidelines [1]. Neoadjuvant chemotherapy (NAC) in breast cancer has historically been reserved for patients with large, inoperable tumors or inflammatory breast cancer, but is now being considered for women with operable disease as well. Larger clinical trials such as EORTC 10902 and NSABP B-18 have shown no differences between the same systemic therapy given pre- or post-surgery on disease-free survival (DFS) and overall survival (OS) [2–4]. However, the purpose of administering chemotherapy prior to surgery is to downstage the tumor and provide information regarding treatment response. Downstaging the tumor may allow less extensive surgery on the breast and axilla, enabling patients to undergo breast conservation surgery instead of mastectomy, improve cosmetic outcomes, and reduce postoperative complications such as lymphedema [5,6]. Several randomized trials have shown that the frequency of mastectomies was decreased using NAC as opposed to adjuvant systemic treatment [2,7].

NAC can also eliminate axillary nodal metastases [7]. While sentinel lymph node biopsy (SLNB) is widely accepted post-NAC for patients who are clinically node-negative at presentation [8], the management of the axilla in patients who present with nodal metastases and appear to downstage with NAC remains controversial. Mamtani et al. determined the ability to avoid axillary lymph node dissections at the time of surgery in nearly 50% of patients with node-positive disease after receiving NAC [6].

NAC is also now being used to tailor adjuvant therapies for patients with human epidermal growth factor receptor (HER-2) positive and triple-negative breast cancers (TNBC) based on the presence or absence of minimal residual invasive disease in the breast or lymph nodes [9,10]. Early response after two to three cycles of NAC is thought to be a predictor of pathologic complete response (pCR) and may therefore serve as a predictor for long-term outcome [11]. Studies have also shown that the rate of pCR in patients with TNBC receiving NAC is significantly higher than that of non-TNBC patients [12,13].

Although there is common consensus on the patient subgroups most likely to benefit from NAC in breast cancer [14,15], its utilization in clinical practice remains highly variable. Candidacy for receiving NAC is carefully determined based on discussions between breast surgeons, medical oncologists, radiation oncologists, pathologists, and radiologists. Optimized care of breast cancer patients undergoing NAC requires coordination within the multidisciplinary care team (MDT) to streamline care through multiple handoffs between specialties to minimize unnecessary delays and provide consistent, continuous, coordinated, and improved care to patients with early-stage breast cancer. MDT and the collegial discussion of patient cases offer the benefits of an optimal approach to therapy in a simple and practical way. In most cases, patients feel more comfortable knowing that their situation has been evaluated and discussed by different health care professionals and the teams caring for them are communicating effectively.

While most of the data regarding patterns of NAC use in early-stage operable breast cancer are available from larger clinical trials and academic institutions, there is a paucity of real-life data describing the contemporary use of NAC in community cancer centers and the feasibility as well as outcomes of the MDT. Our study aims to evaluate the process of this MDT at our institution in the management of early-stage breast cancer patients undergoing neoadjuvant chemotherapy.

2. Methods

This was a retrospective case-series conducted at Baystate Medical Center, a 715-bed academic teaching hospital in Western Massachusetts. We included patients seen at our cancer center between October 2018 and October 2020. All patients diagnosed with early-stage operable and locally advanced breast cancer who have undergone NAC with intent for surgical resection post-treatment at our institution were included in this study. Patients with metastatic breast cancer at the time of diagnosis were excluded. Patients who underwent surgery or radiation therapy at a different facility were also excluded.

2.1. Outcomes

Outcomes included the proportion of pathologic complete response, proportion of downstaging of cancer in the breast, proportion of downstaging in the axilla, proportion of clinical trial enrollment, quality measures including timeliness of referral back to the breast surgeon during NAC, referral back to radiation oncologist, time from biopsy to NAC, time from completion of NAC to surgery, and time from surgery to radiation therapy (RT). Evaluation of our MDT was based on our quality measures or time to treatment outcomes in comparison with national standards, which is the focus of our study.

2.2. Data Collection

The total number of patients diagnosed with Stage I–III breast cancer during the study period presenting to our cancer center was obtained from our breast cancer tumor registry, which tracks all our early-stage breast cancer patients. The patients receiving NAC were obtained from our NAC registry maintained by a breast cancer intake coordinator, a unique list in our password-protected electronic health record (EHR) established for internal quality improvement purposes only.

Patient and tumor characteristics, management aspects, and outcomes measures were obtained from the EHR, Cerner-powered CIS at our institution. These data were entered into Research Electronic Data Capture (REDCap) [16]. A single author entering all the pertinent patient data ensured uniformity in data collection.

For pCR to be designated in this study, there must have been no histologic evidence of invasive cancer, either in the breast or axillary lymph nodes following definitive surgery. The presence of ductal carcinoma in-situ (DCIS) was disregarded, given that this was not thought to affect the systemic risk of recurrence [17].

We defined downstaging as decreasing the size, extent of metastases, and/or lymph node involvement of a tumor using anti-cancer therapy.

2.3. Analysis

As a case series, data analyses were limited to descriptive statistics. No hypothesis testing was conducted. We utilized descriptive statistics, including means, median, and standard deviations (SD) for continuous variables and counts and proportions for categorical variables to summarize patients' demographic and clinical characteristics.

2.4. MDT

To place MDT in context, we have summarized our conceptualization and process of modern MDT-driven care as available at our cancer center in Figure 1. Baystate Health Breast Network involves breast surgeons, medical oncologists, radiation oncologists, pathologists and radiologists who meet quarterly and are responsible for creating guidelines to standardize various breast cancer related practices across the institution. Through this endeavor, guidelines have been created for candidacy for neoadjuvant systemic therapy as described in Supplementary Table S1. All patients who undergo a breast biopsy at our institution are automatically referred to a breast surgeon, who will then determine the timing of referral to a medical oncologist based on their candidacy for neoadjuvant therapy versus upfront surgery. All potential neoadjuvant therapy candidates based on available guidelines are presented at our weekly virtual tumor board conference for a team consensus on best approach to treatment. Once it has been determined that a patient will initiate NAC, they are referred to medical oncology. A breast cancer clinical coordinator oversees the care process during the pre-operative period to ensure that patients are appropriately referred for their labs and scans, and also referred back to the surgeons more than midway through NAC to avoid delays in surgical planning. All patients who are referred to medical oncology are initially referred to radiation oncology as well. Patients are also provided with a handout with all the steps and appointments delineated in their handout at the time of their initial medical oncology visit. Samples of this handout are available in the Supplement.

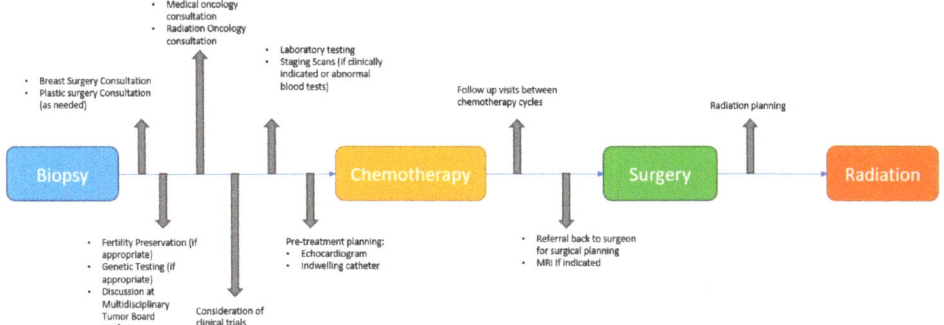

Figure 1. Clinical pathway involving multidisciplinary team-driven care for the management of patients undergoing neoadjuvant chemotherapy for early-stage breast cancer.

3. Results

A total of 54 patients were eventually diagnosed with TNBC stage II, or III between October 2018 and October 2020. Of these patients, 39 (68.4%) were referred to receive NAC. Forty patients were diagnosed with HER-2 positive breast cancer stage II, or III during the study period, of which 28 (66.6%) received NAC. Seventy-eight patients were diagnosed with ER/PR positive HER-2 negative breast cancer stage II or III, of which 24 (30.7%) underwent NAC. This study did not assess the number of patients who may have met the criteria for NAC and were not referred for NAC.

3.1. Patient and Tumor Characteristics

A total of 94 patients underwent NAC. Of these, 84% were White, 12.8% were Black and 3.2% were Asian. This demographic was reflective of all patients presenting to our cancer center with a new diagnosis of breast cancer as available from our breast cancer registry. The mean age was 56.5 years. Of these patients, 87 (92.5%) had clinical stage II or III cancer, and 43 (45.8%) had positive lymph nodes. Thirty-nine patients (42.9%) were triple negative, 18 (19.8%) were ER positive and HER-2 positive, 10 (11.0%) were ER negative and HER-2 positive and 24 (26.2%) were ER positive and HER-2 negative. The most common indications for NAC were to downstage the axilla (42.6%) and for HER-2 tailoring of treatment (25.5%). Several patients had one or more of these indications, as described in Table 1.

Table 1. Patient characteristics.

Patient Characteristics	Overall	Pathological Complete Response
N (%)	94 (100)	23 (24.5)
Age (mean)	56.5 (12.8)	54.4 (12.1)
Race		
White	79 (84.0)	19 (82.6)
Black	12 (12.8)	2 (8.7)
Asian	3 (3.2)	2 (8.7)
Ethnicity		
Hispanic	11 (11.7)	1 (4.3)
Non-Hispanic	82 (88.3)	21 (95.7)
ECOG Performance Status		
0	78 (83.0)	20 (87.0)
1	12 (12.8)	3 (13.0)
2	1 (1.1)	0 (0.0)
Not documented	3 (3.2)	0 (0.0)

Table 1. Cont.

Patient Characteristics	Overall	Pathological Complete Response
Prior Breast Cancer (DCIS or invasive)	11 (12.0)	2 (8.7)
Clinical Stage		
I	5 (5.3)	0 (0.0)
II	66 (70.2)	15 (65.2)
III	21 (22.3)	8 (34.8)
Clinical Tumor Stage		
TI	10 (10.6)	1 (4.3)
T2	60 (63.8)	12 (52.2)
T3	19 (20.2)	9 (39.1)
T4	3 (3.2)	1 (4.3)
Tx	2 (2.1)	0 (0.0)
Clinical Lymph Node Stage		
N0	51 (54.3)	12 (52.1)
N1	38 (40.4)	9 (39.1)
N2	4 (4.3)	1 (4.3)
N3	1 (1.1)	1 (4.3)
ER Receptor Status		
Positive	44 (46.8)	4 (17.4)
Negative	50 (53.2)	19 (82.6)
PR Receptor Status		
Positive	36 (38.3)	2 (8.7)
Negative	58 (61.7)	19 (82.6)
HER-2 Neu Receptor Status		
Positive	28 (29.8)	10 (43.5)
Negative	66 (70.2)	13 (56.5)
Chemotherapy Regimen		
DDAC/T	32 (34.0)	4 (17.4)
DDAC/TC	15 (16.0)	6 (26.1)
TC	9 (9.6)	0 (0.0)
TCHP	22 (23.4)	10 (43.5)
THP	3 (3.2)	1 (4.3)
Time from diagnosis (1st breast biopsy) to NAC (in days)—median (min, max)	37.5 (3, 150) *	41.0 (21, 98)
Indication for NAC		
Less Extensive Surgery	6 (6.4)	3 (13.0)
HER2 tailoring of treatment	24 (25.5)	9 (39.1)
Inoperable to Operable	12 (12.8)	2 (8.7)
Operable Mastectomy to BCS	12 (12.8)	1 (4.3)
Time for genetics	21 (22.3)	6 (26.1)
Time for Surgical Planning	12 (12.8)	3 (13.0)
Lymph Node positive to negative	40 (42.6)	12 (52.2)
Time from completion of NAC to surgery (in days)—median (min, max)	29.0 (9, 118) *	30.0 (13, 48)

Abbreviations: DCIS: Ductal Carcinoma In Situ, DDAC/T: Dose-dense doxorubicin and cyclophosphamide to paclitaxel, DDAC/TC: Dose-dense doxorubicin and cyclophosphamide to paclitaxel and carboplatin, TC: docetaxel and cyclophosphamide, TCHP: docetaxel, carboplatin, trastuzumab and pertuzumab, THP: paclitaxel, trastuzumab and pertuzumab, NAC: Neoadjuvant chemotherapy, ER: Estrogen receptor, HER2: Human Epidermal Growth Factor Receptor 2. * One patient did not follow through with the treatment plan regularly, resulting in delays in treatment.

3.2. Pathological Complete Response

Of the 91 patients who underwent NAC with complete data, 23 (25.3%) achieved a pathologic complete response (pCR). Of these 23 patients, 12 (52.2%) had ER-negative, HER-2-low or negative cancer, 7 (30.4%) had ER-negative HER-2-positive cancer, 3 (13.0%)

had ER-positive HER-2-positive cancer, and 1 (4%) had ER-positive HER-2-negative cancer (Table 2).

Table 2. Pathological Complete Response by Tumor Type.

Tumor Type	Total	RCB 0 [pCR]	RCB I	RCB II	RCB III
N (%)	91 (100.0)	23 (25.3)	19 (20.9)	38 (41.8)	11 (12.1)
ER + HER2 +	18 (19.8)	3 (16.7)	1 (5.6)	12 (66.7)	2 (11.1)
ER + HER2 −	24 (26.4)	1 (4.2)	2 (8.3)	14 (58.3)	7 (29.2)
ER−HER2 +	10 (11.0)	7 (70.0)	3 (30.0)	0 (0.0)	0 (0.0)
ER−HER2 −	39 (42.9)	12 (30.8)	13 (33.3)	12 (30.8)	2 (51.3)

Abbreviations: ER: Estrogen receptor, HER2: Human Epidermal Growth Factor Receptor 2, RCB: Residual Cancer Burden, pCR: Pathologic complete response.

3.3. Other Outcomes

The median time from diagnosis of breast cancer to initiation of NAC was 37.5 days (ranging between 3 and 150 days). Eighty-five (91.4%) patients had downstaging of their breast tumor, and 31 (33%) had axillary downstaging with 53 (57.6%) patients undergoing a lumpectomy while 39 (41.9%) underwent a mastectomy and 22 (23.7%) patients went on to have bilateral mastectomy. A third of patients (33%) had downstaging of axilla based on final surgical pathology (Supplementary Table S2).

All patients followed back with their surgeons before completion of NAC. The median time from completion of NAC to definitive surgery was 29 days (ranging between 9 to 118 days). Of the 78 patients who received adjuvant radiation, all had a radiation oncology consultation before surgery. However, 48 (51.1%) patients returned to see their radiation oncologist before completion of NAC, of which 67.4% were lymph node positive. The median duration of radiation therapy was 33 days (ranging between 12 to 73 days). Five patients (6.4%) underwent radiation therapy for more than two weeks beyond the expected time of completion (i.e., 4–6 weeks based on standard vs. hypo-fractionated RT). The mean time from surgery to radiation therapy was 49.5 days (ranging from 9 to 173 days) (Table 3). Time to treatment outcomes in the context of our MDT have been illustrated in Figure 2.

Table 3. Quality Metrics to assess outcomes of multidisciplinary teams.

	Overall	Clinical Node Positive	Clinical Node Negative
N (%)	94 (100.0)	43 (45.7)	51 (54.3)
Follow up with surgeon prior to completion of NAC—Yes	92 (98.9)	42 (100.0)	50 (98.0)
Follow up with radiation oncology prior to completion of NAC—Yes	48 (51.1)	29 (67.4)	19 (37.3)
Enrollment in clinical trial—Yes	5 (21.7)	3 (21.4)	2 (22.2)
Time from surgery to RT (in days)—median (min, max)	49.5 (9, 173) N = 78	55 (9, 173) N = 43	48 (25, 140) N = 35
Time to complete RT (in days)—median (min, max)	33.0 (12, 73)	39.0 (12, 73)	29.0 (21, 52)
Duration of RT for more than 2 weeks beyond expected time—Yes	5 (6.4)	4 (9.3)	1 (2.9)

Abbreviations: NAC: Neoadjuvant chemotherapy, RT: Radiation therapy. One patient did not follow through with the treatment plan regularly, resulting in delays in treatment.

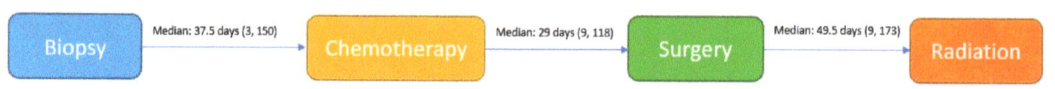

Figure 2. Time to treatment components including time from diagnosis to initiation of neoadjuvant chemotherapy (NAC), time from completion of NAC to surgery, time from surgery to radiation therapy. One patient did not follow through with appointments due to personal conflicts, reflecting the ranges in the median.

4. Discussion

In our study assessing the outcomes of an MDT in managing breast cancer, the median time from completion of NAC to surgery was less than a month. Various studies have established superior overall survival and 5-year recurrence-free survival in patients undergoing surgery within 8 weeks of completion of NAC. There has been a suggested increase in RCB class and a decline in pCR rates after a 4-week interval between chemotherapy and surgery, and worse overall survival after an 8-week interval [18–21]. This observation reinforces the importance of referring patients back to their surgeons in a timely fashion for surgical planning which was noted in our study. All patients saw radiation oncology at least once pre-operatively. Although not all patients were referred back to the radiation oncologist prior to completion of NAC, the mean time from surgery to initiation of radiation therapy was 7 weeks. It is worthy of note that a few patients required second surgeries, including re-excision of margins or complete axillary dissection based on pathology results that delayed the initiation of radiation therapy. Despite this, we were aligned with providing radiation therapy at an optimal recommended interval of within 8 weeks after surgery, which has been associated with better disease-free survival and overall survival [22,23]. The median time from diagnosis of cancer to initiation of NAC was less than 6 weeks. Time to treatment initiation is considered an important metric from a patient perspective, as delays provoke anxiety and are thought to influence long-term outcomes. This perception of longer wait times equating to poorer outcomes may be magnified by the role of mammograms whose prerogative is 'early detection saves lives'; conversely, delays are perceived to result in mortality. Various factors influence the time to start of NAC including additional testing, for e.g., MRI, staging studies, and fertility preservation as indicated. Prior studies have demonstrated no impact on long term patient outcomes so long as NAC is initiated within 8 weeks of diagnosis [24–26].

Overall pCR rates in our patients were noted to be lower than those demonstrated by larger clinical trials however similar or improved compared to other real-world studies [27–29]. Of the patients who achieved pCR, the majority were ER-negative and HER-2-negative, followed by HER-2-positive patients irrespective of ER status. Traditionally, pCR rates are highest in HER-2-positive patients [17]. pCR rates are likely influenced by multiple factors and the small sample size. While assessing treatment regimens used for patients with HER-2 positive disease in our study, a few patients did not receive dual HER-2-based therapies in the neoadjuvant setting. We hypothesize that variable physician prescribing trends during the study period could attribute to lower pCR rates in HER-2-positive patients and hence, the overall population. Despite lack of pCR, most of the patients had at least partial response in the breast and a third had axillary downstaging, resulting in a more conservative axillary approach surgically. Axillary pCR rates remain variable and are affected by age, molecular subtype, tumor grade and Ki-67 [30–32].

Coordinated care through an MDT has previously shown to improve receipt of treatment, adherence to treatment recommendations and overall survival, including in vulnerable cancer populations being treated at safety net hospitals [33–35]. It can level the playing field for patients from various socioeconomic backgrounds and thus, serve as a bridge to overcome disparities in access to care.

Our study had key limitations which include a smaller sample size, given this is a single-institution study. This study did not specifically evaluate how many patients were appropriately referred for neoadjuvant therapies as it was assumed that patients were appropriately referred based on institutional guidelines as referenced in the Supplementary Materials. We did not collect data regarding omission of treatments in subsequent cycles or interruptions in chemotherapy cycles due to various factors, including age, co-morbidities and adverse effects which could have resulted in fewer cycles than intended, resulting in lower overall pCR rates. However, this study can serve as a model for how an MDT can be utilized in ensuring adherence to quality metrics, which can in turn improve long-term patient outcomes.

Although our small sample size did not allow for examining differences in patient subsets, using our standardized clinical pathway model for every new patient with a diagnosis of breast cancer requiring NAC allows high standards for all patients irrespective of race or ethnicity.

5. Conclusions

In our study, the multidisciplinary care process resulted in timely, coordinated, and consistent care for all patients with early-stage breast cancer undergoing NAC. All patients were referred back to the surgeon prior to completion of NAC for surgical planning. The median time to treatment initiation, time from completion of NAC to surgery and time from surgery to radiation were within recommended intervals for optimal long-term patient outcomes. NAC will likely be used in an increasing fashion as the indications expand, especially in smaller cancers that are triple negative and HER-2 positive. Hence, there is a need not only to advance systemic therapies, but also to create a streamlined process to optimize outcomes. To that effect, our multidisciplinary care pathway as described can serve as a model for growing community cancer centers to address disparities in care.

Supplementary Materials: The following supporting information can be downloaded at: https://www.mdpi.com/article/10.3390/curroncol30050366/s1, Table S1: Indications for consideration of neoadjuvant systemic therapy; Table S2: Management after neoadjuvant chemotherapy.

Author Contributions: P.V.B.—Conceptualization, Data Curation, Writing—original draft, H.M.—Conceptualization, Data Curation, Writing—review and editing, Supervision, S.A.K.—Conceptualization, Writing—review and editing, Supervision, P.V.—Formal analysis, Methodology, Writing—review and editing, G.M.-J.—Conceptualization, Investigation, Writing—review and editing, Supervision. All authors have read and agreed to the published version of the manuscript.

Funding: This research received no external funding.

Institutional Review Board Statement: The study was conducted according to the guidelines of the Declaration of Helsinki, and was deemed IRB exempt at Baystate Medical Center as information was recorded by the investigator in such a manner that subjects cannot be identified, directly or through identifiers linked to the subjects.

Informed Consent Statement: Informed consent was waived as there were no direct identifiers of individual patients for this retrospective chart review study.

Data Availability Statement: The data presented in this study are available on request from the corresponding author.

Conflicts of Interest: P.V.B. has stock options with Doximity. Other authors do not have any relevant conflict of interest to disclose.

References

1. Houssami, N.; Sainsbury, R. Breast Cancer: Multidisciplinary Care and Clinical Outcomes. *Eur. J. Cancer Oxf. Engl. 1990* **2006**, *42*, 2480–2491. [CrossRef] [PubMed]
2. Van der Hage, J.A.; van de Velde, C.J.H.; Julien, J.-P.; Tubiana-Hulin, M.; Vandervelden, C.; Duchateau, L. Preoperative Chemotherapy in Primary Operable Breast Cancer: Results From the European Organization for Research and Treatment of Cancer Trial 10902. *J. Clin. Oncol.* **2001**, *19*, 4224–4237. [CrossRef] [PubMed]
3. Wolmark, N.; Wang, J.; Mamounas, E.; Bryant, J.; Fisher, B. Preoperative Chemotherapy in Patients With Operable Breast Cancer: Nine-Year Results From National Surgical Adjuvant Breast and Bowel Project B-18. *JNCI Monogr.* **2001**, *2001*, 96–102. [CrossRef] [PubMed]

4. Mauri, D.; Pavlidis, N.; Ioannidis, J.P.A. Neoadjuvant Versus Adjuvant Systemic Treatment in Breast Cancer: A Meta-Analysis. *JNCI J. Natl. Cancer Inst.* **2005**, *97*, 188–194. [CrossRef]
5. Kaufmann, M.; Hortobagyi, G.N.; Goldhirsch, A.; Scholl, S.; Makris, A.; Valagussa, P.; Blohmer, J.-U.; Eiermann, W.; Jackesz, R.; Jonat, W.; et al. Recommendations From an International Expert Panel on the Use of Neoadjuvant (Primary) Systemic Treatment of Operable Breast Cancer: An Update. *J. Clin. Oncol.* **2006**, *24*, 1940–1949. [CrossRef]
6. Mamtani, A.; Barrio, A.V.; King, T.A.; Van Zee, K.J.; Plitas, G.; Pilewskie, M.; El-Tamer, M.; Gemignani, M.L.; Heerdt, A.S.; Sclafani, L.M.; et al. How Often Does Neoadjuvant Chemotherapy Avoid Axillary Dissection in Patients with Histologically Confirmed Nodal Metastases: Results of a Prospective Study. *Ann. Surg. Oncol.* **2016**, *23*, 3467–3474. [CrossRef] [PubMed]
7. Fisher, B.; Brown, A.; Mamounas, E.; Wieand, S.; Robidoux, A.; Margolese, R.G.; Cruz, A.B.; Fisher, E.R.; Wickerham, D.L.; Wolmark, N.; et al. Effect of Preoperative Chemotherapy on Local-Regional Disease in Women with Operable Breast Cancer: Findings from National Surgical Adjuvant Breast and Bowel Project B-18. *J. Clin. Oncol. Off. J. Am. Soc. Clin. Oncol.* **1997**, *15*, 2483–2493. [CrossRef]
8. Kelly, A.M.; Dwamena, B.; Cronin, P.; Carlos, R.C. Breast Cancer: Sentinel Node Identification and Classification after Neoadjuvant Chemotherapy—Systematic Review and Meta Analysis. *Acad. Radiol.* **2009**, *16*, 551–563. [CrossRef]
9. Masuda, N.; Lee, S.-J.; Ohtani, S.; Im, Y.-H.; Lee, E.-S.; Yokota, I.; Kuroi, K.; Im, S.-A.; Park, B.-W.; Kim, S.-B.; et al. Adjuvant Capecitabine for Breast Cancer after Preoperative Chemotherapy. *N. Engl. J. Med.* **2017**, *376*, 2147–2159. [CrossRef]
10. Von Minckwitz, G.; Huang, C.-S.; Mano, M.S.; Loibl, S.; Mamounas, E.P.; Untch, M.; Wolmark, N.; Rastogi, P.; Schneeweiss, A.; Redondo, A.; et al. Trastuzumab Emtansine for Residual Invasive HER2-Positive Breast Cancer. *N. Engl. J. Med.* **2019**, *380*, 617–628. [CrossRef]
11. Von Minckwitz, G.; Raab, G.; Caputo, A.; Schütte, M.; Hilfrich, J.; Blohmer, J.U.; Gerber, B.; Costa, S.D.; Merkle, E.; Eidtmann, H.; et al. Doxorubicin With Cyclophosphamide Followed by Docetaxel Every 21 Days Compared With Doxorubicin and Docetaxel Every 14 Days As Preoperative Treatment in Operable Breast Cancer: The GEPARDUO Study of the German Breast Group. *J. Clin. Oncol.* **2005**, *23*, 2676–2685. [CrossRef] [PubMed]
12. Ring, A.E.; Smith, I.E.; Ashley, S.; Fulford, L.G.; Lakhani, S.R. Oestrogen Receptor Status, Pathological Complete Response and Prognosis in Patients Receiving Neoadjuvant Chemotherapy for Early Breast Cancer. *Br. J. Cancer* **2004**, *91*, 2012–2017. [CrossRef] [PubMed]
13. Huober, J.; von Minckwitz, G.; Denkert, C.; Tesch, H.; Weiss, E.; Zahm, D.M.; Belau, A.; Khandan, F.; Hauschild, M.; Thomssen, C.; et al. Effect of Neoadjuvant Anthracycline–Taxane-Based Chemotherapy in Different Biological Breast Cancer Phenotypes: Overall Results from the GeparTrio Study. *Breast Cancer Res. Treat.* **2010**, *124*, 133–140. [CrossRef]
14. Coates, A.S.; Winer, E.P.; Goldhirsch, A.; Gelber, R.D.; Gnant, M.; Piccart-Gebhart, M.; Thürlimann, B.; Senn, H.-J.; André, F.; Baselga, J.; et al. Tailoring Therapies—Improving the Management of Early Breast Cancer: St Gallen International Expert Consensus on the Primary Therapy of Early Breast Cancer 2015. *Ann. Oncol.* **2015**, *26*, 1533–1546. [CrossRef]
15. Senkus, E.; Kyriakides, S.; Ohno, S.; Penault-Llorca, F.; Poortmans, P.; Rutgers, E.; Zackrisson, S.; Cardoso, F. Primary Breast Cancer: ESMO Clinical Practice Guidelines for Diagnosis, Treatment and Follow-Up†. *Ann. Oncol.* **2015**, *26*, v8–v30. [CrossRef]
16. Harris, P.A.; Taylor, R.; Thielke, R.; Payne, J.; Gonzalez, N.; Conde, J.G. Research Electronic Data Capture (REDCap)—A Metadata-Driven Methodology and Workflow Process for Providing Translational Research Informatics Support. *J. Biomed. Inform.* **2009**, *42*, 377–381. [CrossRef] [PubMed]
17. von Minckwitz, G.; Untch, M.; Blohmer, J.-U.; Costa, S.D.; Eidtmann, H.; Fasching, P.A.; Gerber, B.; Eiermann, W.; Hilfrich, J.; Huober, J.; et al. Definition and Impact of Pathologic Complete Response on Prognosis After Neoadjuvant Chemotherapy in Various Intrinsic Breast Cancer Subtypes. *J. Clin. Oncol.* **2012**, *30*, 1796–1804. [CrossRef]
18. Sutton, T.L.; Schlitt, A.; Gardiner, S.K.; Johnson, N.; Garreau, J.R. Time to Surgery Following Neoadjuvant Chemotherapy for Breast Cancer Impacts Residual Cancer Burden, Recurrence, and Survival. *J. Surg. Oncol.* **2020**, *122*, 1761–1769. [CrossRef]
19. Sanford, R.A.; Lei, X.; Barcenas, C.H.; Mittendorf, E.A.; Caudle, A.S.; Valero, V.; Tripathy, D.; Giordano, S.H.; Chavez-MacGregor, M. Impact of Time from Completion of Neoadjuvant Chemotherapy to Surgery on Survival Outcomes in Breast Cancer Patients. *Ann. Surg. Oncol.* **2016**, *23*, 1515–1521. [CrossRef]
20. Yoo, T.-K.; Moon, H.-G.; Han, W.; Noh, D.-Y. Time Interval of Neoadjuvant Chemotherapy to Surgery in Breast Cancer: How Long Is Acceptable? *Gland Surg.* **2017**, *6*, 1–3. [CrossRef]
21. Cullinane, C.; Shrestha, A.; Al Maksoud, A.; Rothwell, J.; Evoy, D.; Geraghty, J.; McCartan, D.; McDermott, E.W.; Prichard, R.S. Optimal Timing of Surgery Following Breast Cancer Neoadjuvant Chemotherapy: A Systematic Review and Meta-Analysis. *Eur. J. Surg. Oncol.* **2021**, *47*, 1507–1513. [CrossRef]
22. Silva, S.B.; Pereira, A.A.L.; Marta, G.N.; de Barros Lima, K.M.L.; de Freitas, T.B.; Matutino, A.R.B.; de Azevedo Souza, M.C.L.; de Azevedo, R.G.M.V.; de Viveiros, P.A.H.; da Silva Lima, J.M.; et al. Clinical Impact of Adjuvant Radiation Therapy Delay after Neoadjuvant Chemotherapy in Locally Advanced Breast Cancer. *Breast* **2018**, *38*, 39–44. [CrossRef]
23. Marta, G.N.; AlBeesh, R.; Pereira, A.A.L.; Oliveira, L.J.; Mano, M.S.; Hijal, T. The Impact on Clinical Outcomes of Post-Operative Radiation Therapy Delay after Neoadjuvant Chemotherapy in Patients with Breast Cancer: A Multicentric International Study. *Breast* **2020**, *54*, 46–51. [CrossRef] [PubMed]
24. Livingston-Rosanoff, D.; Hanlon, B.; Marka, N.; Vande Walle, K.; Stankowski-Drengler, T.; Schumacher, J.; Greenberg, C.C.; Neuman, H.; Wilke, L.G. Time to Initiation of Neo-Adjuvant Chemotherapy for Breast Cancer Treatment Does Not Influence Patient Survival: A Study of US Breast Cancer Patients. *Breast J.* **2020**, *26*, 625–629. [CrossRef] [PubMed]

25. Gao, W.; Wang, J.; Yin, S.; Geng, C.; Xu, B. An Appropriate Treatment Interval Does Not Affect the Prognosis of Patients with Breast Cancer. *Holist. Integr. Oncol.* **2022**, *1*, 8. [CrossRef]
26. De Melo Gagliato, D.; Lei, X.; Giordano, S.H.; Valero, V.; Barcenas, C.H.; Hortobagyi, G.N.; Chavez-MacGregor, M. Impact of Delayed Neoadjuvant Systemic Chemotherapy on Overall Survival Among Patients with Breast Cancer. *Oncologist* **2020**, *25*, 749–757. [CrossRef] [PubMed]
27. McFarland, D.C.; Naikan, J.; Rozenblit, M.; Mandeli, J.; Bleiweiss, I.; Tiersten, A. Changes in Pathological Complete Response Rates after Neoadjuvant Chemotherapy for Breast Carcinoma over Five Years. *J. Oncol.* **2016**, *2016*, e4324863. [CrossRef]
28. Kovac, A.; Cankar, K.; Dobovisek, L.; Cavka, L.; Godina, E.; Horvat, V.J.; Rajer, M.; Starman, T.; Matos, E.; Borstnar, S. 207P 10-Year Real-World Outcomes with Neoadjuvant Systemic Therapy in Non-Inflammatory Breast Cancer. *Ann. Oncol.* **2020**, *31*, S324–S325. [CrossRef]
29. De Paula, B.H.R.; Kumar, S.; Morosini, F.M.; Cardoso, D.E.M.C.; de Sousa, C.A.M.; Crocamo, S. Real-World Assessment of the Effect of Impact of Tumor Size on Pathological Complete Response Rates in Triple Negative Breast Cancer after Neoadjuvant Chemotherapy. *Chin. Clin. Oncol.* **2020**, *9*, 78. [CrossRef]
30. Michel, E.; Vincent, L.; Beltjens, F.; Arnould, L.; Ladoire, S.; Coutant, C.; Jankowski, C. Axillary Pathologic Response after Neoadjuvant Chemotherapy and Surgery According to Breast Cancers Subtypes and Survival Impact. *J. Clin. Oncol.* **2022**, *40*, e12595. [CrossRef]
31. Zheng, W.; Zhou, P.; Liu, Y.; Liang, Y.; Wang, Y. Prediction of Axillary Response after Neoadjuvant Chemotherapy in Clinical Node Positive Breast Cancer. *Transl. Cancer Res.* **2021**, *10*, 2822–2830. [CrossRef] [PubMed]
32. Kim, W.H.; Kim, H.J.; Park, H.Y.; Park, J.Y.; Chae, Y.S.; Lee, S.M.; Cho, S.H.; Shin, K.M.; Lee, S.Y. Axillary Pathologic Complete Response to Neoadjuvant Chemotherapy in Clinically Node-Positive Breast Cancer Patients: A Predictive Model Integrating the Imaging Characteristics of Ultrasound Restaging with Known Clinicopathologic Characteristics. *Ultrasound Med. Biol.* **2019**, *45*, 702–709. [CrossRef] [PubMed]
33. Doe, S.; Petersen, S.; Buekers, T.; Swain, M. Does a Multidisciplinary Approach to Invasive Breast Cancer Care Improve Time to Treatment and Patient Compliance? *J. Natl. Med. Assoc.* **2020**, *112*, 268–274. [CrossRef] [PubMed]
34. Kelly, K.N.; Hernandez, A.; Yadegarynia, S.; Ryon, E.; Franceschi, D.; Avisar, E.; Kobetz, E.N.; Merchant, N.; Kesmodel, S.; Goel, N. Overcoming Disparities: Multidisciplinary Breast Cancer Care at a Public Safety Net Hospital. *Breast Cancer Res. Treat.* **2021**, *187*, 197–206. [CrossRef]
35. Kesson, E.M.; Allardice, G.M.; George, W.D.; Burns, H.J.G.; Morrison, D.S. Effects of Multidisciplinary Team Working on Breast Cancer Survival: Retrospective, Comparative, Interventional Cohort Study of 13 722 Women. *BMJ* **2012**, *344*, e2718. [CrossRef]

Disclaimer/Publisher's Note: The statements, opinions and data contained in all publications are solely those of the individual author(s) and contributor(s) and not of MDPI and/or the editor(s). MDPI and/or the editor(s) disclaim responsibility for any injury to people or property resulting from any ideas, methods, instructions or products referred to in the content.

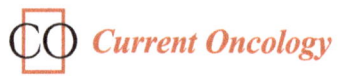

Guidelines

Preoperative Breast Magnetic Resonance Imaging: An Ontario Health (Cancer Care Ontario) Clinical Practice Guideline

Derek Muradali [1,*], Glenn G. Fletcher [2], Erin Cordeiro [3], Samantha Fienberg [4], Ralph George [5], Supriya Kulkarni [1], Jean M. Seely [6], Rola Shaheen [7,8] and Andrea Eisen [9,*]

1. Department of Medical Imaging, University of Toronto, Toronto, ON M5T 1W7, Canada; supriya.kulkarni@uhn.ca
2. Program in Evidence-Based Care, Department of Oncology, McMaster University, Hamilton, ON L8S 4L8, Canada; gfletche@mcmaster.ca
3. Department of Surgery, University of Ottawa, Ottawa, ON K1N 6N5, Canada; ecordeiro@toh.ca
4. Ontario Health (Cancer Care Ontario), Toronto, ON M5G 2L3, Canada; samantha.fienberg@ontariohealth.ca
5. Department of Surgery, University of Toronto, Toronto, ON M5T 1P5, Canada; ralph.george@unityhealth.to
6. Department of Radiology, The Ottawa Hospital, University of Ottawa, Ottawa, ON K1N 6N5, Canada; jeseely@toh.ca
7. Department of Radiology, Queen's University, Kingston, ON K7L 3N6, Canada; rshaheen@prhc.on.ca
8. Diagnostic Imaging, Peterborough Regional Health Centre, Peterborough, ON K9J 7C6, Canada
9. Department of Medical Oncology, Odette Cancer Centre, Sunnybrook Health Sciences Centre, Toronto, ON M4N 3M5, Canada
* Correspondence: derek.muradali@unityhealth.to (D.M.); andrea.eisen@sunnybrook.ca (A.E.)

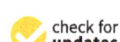

Citation: Muradali, D.; Fletcher, G.G.; Cordeiro, E.; Fienberg, S.; George, R.; Kulkarni, S.; Seely, J.M.; Shaheen, R.; Eisen, A. Preoperative Breast Magnetic Resonance Imaging: An Ontario Health (Cancer Care Ontario) Clinical Practice Guideline. *Curr. Oncol.* **2023**, *30*, 6255–6270. https://doi.org/10.3390/curroncol30070463

Received: 12 May 2023
Revised: 23 June 2023
Accepted: 28 June 2023
Published: 30 June 2023

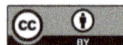

Copyright: © 2023 by the authors. Licensee MDPI, Basel, Switzerland. This article is an open access article distributed under the terms and conditions of the Creative Commons Attribution (CC BY) license (https://creativecommons.org/licenses/by/4.0/).

Abstract: Background: The use of preoperative breast magnetic resonance imaging (MRI) after the diagnosis of breast cancer by mammography and/or ultrasound is inconsistent. Methods: After conducting a systematic review and meta-analysis comparing preoperative breast MRI versus no MRI, we reconvened to prepare a clinical practice guideline on this topic. Results: Based on the evidence that MRI improved recurrence, decreased the rates of reoperations (re-excisions or conversion mastectomy), and increased detection of synchronous contralateral breast cancer, we recommend that preoperative breast MRI should be considered on a case-by-case basis in patients diagnosed with breast cancer for whom additional information about disease extent could influence treatment. Based on stronger evidence, preoperative breast MRI is recommended in patients diagnosed with invasive lobular carcinoma for whom additional information about disease extent could influence treatment. For both recommendations, the decision to proceed with MRI would be conditional on shared decision-making between care providers and the patient, taking into account the benefits and risks of MRI as well as patient preferences. Based on the opinion of the Working Group, preoperative breast MRI is also recommended in the following more specific situations: (a) to aid in surgical planning of breast conserving surgery in patients with suspected or known multicentric or multifocal disease; (b) to identify additional lesions in patients with dense breasts; (c) to determine the presence of pectoralis major muscle/chest wall invasion in patients with posteriorly located tumours or when invasion of the pectoralis major muscle or chest wall is suspected; (d) to aid in surgical planning for skin/nipple-sparing mastectomies, autologous reconstruction, oncoplastic surgery, and breast conserving surgery with suspected nipple/areolar involvement; and (e) in patients with familial/hereditary breast cancer but who have not had recent breast MRI as part of screening or diagnosis.

Keywords: breast cancer; magnetic resonance imaging; practice guideline

1. Introduction

Suspected breast cancer based on clinical examination or screening mammography is generally confirmed by diagnostic mammography (with or without ultrasound) and biopsy. Surgery may be preceded by further advanced imaging of higher sensitivity or diagnostic utility, with contrast-enhanced breast magnetic resonance imaging (CE-MRI, often referred to as MRI) being the most widely used to characterize the locoregional extent of breast cancer.

Breast MRI has a sensitivity for detecting cancer of greater than 90% and as high as 97% to 100% [1–3] in some studies of screening or for preoperative use after diagnosis. Studies published prior to 2000 had suggested poor sensitivity for ductal carcinoma in situ (DCIS); however, with improved equipment and radiologist expertise, this is no longer the case [4–6]. MRI specificity depends on study populations, technical methods, and criteria for interpretation. It is generally greater than 70%, and up to 97% has been reported [1]. The American College of Radiology Breast Imaging Reporting and Data System (BI-RADS) Atlas provides standardized terminology and reporting to assist in interpretation and sets a benchmark for specificity in screening MRI at 85% to 90% [7].

The use of MRI in screening and surveillance is considered standard of care for individuals at higher risk of breast cancer due to genetic factors or previous radiation exposure for another cancer [8,9]. Some recent guidelines include personal history or dense breasts as high-risk factors warranting consideration of an MRI [10,11]. Cancer screening is dealt with in several other guidelines and was not included in the current work.

It has been established that MRI has higher sensitivity than mammography and ultrasound, as illustrated by its incorporation into high-risk screening; however, there is less consensus on whether the additional information provided by preoperative MRI subsequent to the cancer diagnosis improves patient outcomes. Use of breast MRI beyond screening is the topic of guidelines by the European Society of Breast Cancer Specialists (EUSOMA) [12], the European Society of Breast Imaging (EUSOBI) [13], and the Institut national d'excellence en santé et en services sociaux (INESSS; Quebec, Canada) [14], and a practice parameter by the American College of Radiology (ACR) [15]. Also relevant are the Canadian Association of Radiologists imaging guideline [16], which has a section on MRI, and the evidence review/medical policies by Blue Cross/Blue Shield [17]. General breast cancer guidelines such as those by the National Comprehensive Cancer Network (NCCN) [18] also have recommendations on MRI use; several of these have only a few points regarding MRI and may not be based on a review of the primary literature. It was determined that these guidelines either did not cover the most recent studies, had a different focus, or did not conduct a comprehensive review. We therefore conducted a systematic review and meta-analysis [19–21] comparing outcomes such as re-operation rates, recurrence, and survival with versus without preoperative breast MRI, followed by the development of recommendations as reported in this clinical practice guideline.

2. Materials and Methods

2.1. Background

The Program in Evidence-Based Care (PEBC) is an initiative of the Ontario provincial cancer system, Ontario Health (Cancer Care Ontario), supported by the Ontario Ministry of Health. The PEBC produces evidence-based and evidence-informed guidance documents using the methods of the Practice Guidelines Development Cycle [22,23]. This process includes a systematic review, interpretation of the evidence, and draft recommendations by the Working Group; internal review by content and methodology experts; and external review by Ontario clinicians and other stakeholders. PEBC guideline recommendations are based on evidence of the desirable and undesirable effects of an intervention or the accuracy of a test and take into account the certainty of the evidence. PEBC guideline development methods are described in more detail in the *PEBC Handbook* and the *PEBC Methods Handbook* (https://www.cancercareontario.ca/en/guidelines-advice/types-of-cancer/breast, accessed on 1 May 2023).

2.2. Guideline Objective

The primary goal was to make recommendations about whether preoperative breast magnetic resonance imaging (MRI) should be added to conventional imaging (mammography and/or ultrasound) in patients with newly diagnosed breast cancer and to make recommendations about specific indications if evidence allowed.

2.3. Research Question

In patients with newly diagnosed breast cancer, does additional information on the extent of disease obtained by preoperative breast MRI after mammography and/or ultrasound (a) change the type or extent of surgery (breast conserving surgery (BCS), unilateral or bilateral mastectomy), the type or extent of radiation therapy, or the use of adjuvant therapy; or (b) improve patient outcomes such as recurrence, disease-free survival or event-free survival, distant metastasis-free survival, overall survival, rates of re-excision or re-operation, or quality of life?

2.4. Target Population

The target population is patients already diagnosed with breast cancer of any stage for whom additional information on disease location or extent in the breast obtained prior to surgery may influence staging, treatment, or prognosis. The guideline does not address patients diagnosed with breast cancer but without an identified cancerous lesion in the breast (occult breast cancer) or patients undergoing neoadjuvant therapy prior to surgery. Imaging for distant metastasis is the topic of a separate guideline [24].

2.5. Development Process

This guideline is based on a systematic review and meta-analysis originally completed in December 2021 [19]. The systematic review was revised to incorporate study updates until July 2022 and to include additional quality assessment using the Grading of Recommendations, Assessment, Development and Evaluation (GRADE) approach to aid in developing the clinical practice recommendations [20]. An integrated version of the systematic review is also available [21].

The Working Group (the authors of this article) was responsible for reviewing the evidence base, drafting the guideline recommendations, and responding to comments received during the document review process. The Working Group had expertise in radiology, surgery, medical oncology, and health research methodology.

2.6. Literature Search

Embase, MEDLINE, the Cochrane Central Register of Controlled Trials, and the Cochrane Database of Systematic Reviews were searched until 3 July 2019 and updated until 18 January 2021. A targeted search was conducted in July 2022 to identify any additional publications related to the included RCTs and studies identified as ongoing. Studies had to be comparative studies of MRI versus no MRI after a diagnosis of breast cancer and report rates of survival, recurrence, re-excision, reoperation, or mastectomy. One author (GGF) reviewed all studies, and co-authors were consulted in cases of uncertainty regarding inclusion.

Included were 8 randomized controlled trials (RCTs), 1 prospective cohort study, and 42 retrospective studies. The patient population was limited to those with an initial treatment plan of breast conserving surgery in 17 trials (6 RCTs). The retrospective studies included 8 with propensity-matched controls, 4 with historical or equivalent controls, 15 with multivariable/multivariate analysis of data from a single or small number of institutions, and 15 using cancer registry data and multivariable/multivariate analysis. A series of forest plots created using RevMan [25] provide graphical summaries to aid in the interpretation of the tabulated results.

Data was extracted from the included studies. Odds ratios (OR) or hazard ratios (HR) were expressed with a ratio of <1.0, indicating that the experimental group (MRI use) had a more favourable outcome than the control group. The exception to this was the case of synchronous contralateral breast cancer (CBC) detection (identified at the same time or sometimes defined as occurring within 6 months of the index cancer). Higher detection is considered a favourable outcome, but the convention is to report increased detection with HR > 1.0. The risk of bias for randomized studies was assessed per outcome and per study using the Cochrane risk-of-bias (RoB) tool (revised version RoB2) for RCTs and ROBINS-I for non-RCTs, as outlined in the Cochrane Handbook for Systematic Reviews of Interventions [26]. The GRADE approach was used to facilitate recommendation development. The full GRADE evaluation, including risk of bias assessment, summary of findings tables, GRADE profiles, and standardized statements for each outcome, including levels of certainty, has been reported [20]. Both the original review [19] and update [20] should be consulted for further details; the review portions have been merged in a subsequent publication [21].

2.7. Recommendation Development and Review

The Working Group evaluated the systematic review and developed clinical practice recommendations. The document was then reviewed by a Patient- and Caregiver-Specific Consultation Group consisting of five people with personal experience with cancer (patients/survivors/caregivers) who participated as Patient Consultation Group members. The internal review consisted of reviews by an Expert Panel of eight content experts and by the PEBC Report Approval Panel, a three-person panel with methodology expertise. All participants approved of the document; comments were considered by the Working Group in revising the document.

Feedback on the approved draft guideline was obtained from content experts and the target users through two processes. Through the Targeted Peer Review, three individuals with content expertise were identified and asked to review and provide feedback on the guideline document. Through Professional Consultation, relevant care providers and other potential users of the guideline were contacted, and 41 provided feedback on the guideline recommendations through a brief online survey and additional comments. The Working Group considered all feedback in making final revisions.

3. Recommendations and Key Evidence

It has been established that breast MRI can provide additional information on lesion presence, size, location, and distribution; it is less certain in what circumstances this will lead to better patient outcomes. There are both potential benefits and harms to consider (see Table 1), and the relative importance will vary depending on patient and disease characteristics; technical considerations related to equipment and radiology team expertise; and system considerations such as cost, availability of equipment and staff, and wait lists for MRI and other procedures and consultations.

3.1. Recommendation 1
- Preoperative breast MRI **should be considered** on a case-by-case basis in patients diagnosed with breast cancer for whom additional information about disease extent could influence treatment. The ensuing decision of whether to conduct an MRI should be made in consultation with the patient and must take into account the balance of benefits and risks and patient preferences.
- Stronger recommendations for specific situations are provided in Recommendations 2 and 3.

3.1.1. Qualifying Statements for Recommendation 1
- Benefits and harms (see Key Evidence and Table 1) may vary depending on patient and disease characteristics such as breast density, tumour size, tumour stage, number and distribution of tumours (multicentric or multifocal), subtype of cancer, type of surgery being considered or preferred, adjuvant treatment, and patient factors/comorbidities.
- System issues such as MRI availability may result in treatment delays that may modify the decision.
- "Treatment" in the recommendation includes surgery as well as radiation and systemic treatment.

- In patients with a strong preference for mastectomy or with contraindications to BCS, MRI is unlikely to change surgical planning in the ipsilateral breast. Breast MRI may still impact treatment if mammographically occult CBC is detected.
- Contrast-enhanced mammography (contrast-enhanced spectral mammography, contrast-enhanced digital mammography), diffusion-weighted imaging (DWI) MRI, magnetic resonance spectroscopy, or other advanced imaging techniques are known to provide additional information beyond that of conventional imaging and may be suitable instead of or in addition to CE-MRI. Potential adverse effects due to contrast agent and radiation exposure vary among these techniques, whereas many other potential benefits and harms in Table 1 would be relevant. These are mentioned briefly in the systematic review, but the evaluation was outside of scope. They are less widely available, and there is much less evidence regarding their effect on patient outcomes.

Table 1. Potential benefits and harms of preoperative MRI.

Factor	Potential Benefits	Potential Harms
High Sensitivity	• MRI is not impacted by breast density, which limits the sensitivity of mammography. • Higher cancer detection rates with MRI than mammography, with greater ability to detect occult cancer in the ipsilateral breast with multifocal and multicentric disease. • More accurate staging of the contralateral breast reduces the rate of breast cancer detected in follow-up. • Allows the detection of all cancerous lesions at the start so they can be treated at one time instead of having pre-existing cancers only detected on short-term follow-up; this can have cost benefits for patients and the health care system, reduce anxiety, and improve the quality of life of patients. • Confirmation of limited disease may allow for more conservative treatment such as partial breast irradiation (including in patients with previous radiotherapy) or the omission of systemic therapy. • May allow a longer interval between initial treatment and follow-up imaging. • Additional information from MRI reduces the frequency of reoperations to achieve clear margins and reduces the rate of unplanned (salvage) mastectomy subsequent to the initial BCS. This can have cost benefits for patients and the health care system, reduce surgical complications, reduce anxiety, and improve the quality of life of patients. • May confirm or rule out the feasibility of nipple-sparing mastectomy. • In the setting of Paget disease with negative conventional imaging studies, MRI can identify underlying breast malignancy, facilitating proper treatment planning.	• Higher breast biopsy rates, including some lesions that will be negative for cancer (i.e., false-positive by MRI). • Higher mastectomy rates with MRI when disease extent is greater than shown on conventional imaging. • Repeat (short-interval follow-up) MRIs may be required for BI-RADS 3 lesions if an MRI-guided biopsy was not conducted or with benign breast biopsies. • More aggressive surgery or other treatment due to knowledge of additional lesions may not change survival outcomes. • MRI is not necessarily more accurate in estimating tumour size than other imaging; the optimal modality may vary with tumour characteristics.
Specificity	• Specificity is generally greater than 70%, and up to 97% has been reported [1]. MRI specificity depends on study populations, technical methods, and criteria for interpretation.	• Specificity may be lower than mammography in some MRI centres or for some applications. • MRI-detected lesions require biopsy for tissue confirmation and may include false-positive lesions.
Patient Factors	• May reduce the mastectomy rate in patients initially opting for mastectomy due to fear of more extensive disease and not due to clinical factors. • Reduction in anxiety for some patients as they are more confident regarding the appropriateness of treatment planned or received.	• Some patients are not suitable for MRI (anxiety, claustrophobia, MRI does not accommodate body habitus or other patient concerns) or do not want to undergo this procedure. • Increased anxiety for some patients regarding MRI procedures or biopsies, or while waiting for these to occur or results to be reported.
Adverse Effects		• Gadolinium contrast agents may cause allergic reactions ($\approx$0.1% of patients). • Gadolinium retention, especially after multiple MRIs, has been reported in the brain; long-term effects are uncertain but have not been reported to date. Accumulation depends on the type of contrast agent and cumulative exposure. • Nephrogenic systemic fibrosis may occur in patients with acute kidney injury or severe chronic kidney disease; the risk varies with the type and volume of gadolinium contrast agent used.

Table 1. *Cont.*

Factor	Potential Benefits	Potential Harms
Delay in Treatment		• Breast MRI use may potentially lead to delays in treatment due to both MRI scheduling and the characterization of any identified lesions (biopsies and histopathology analysis/reporting). • May increase anxiety for patients while waiting for treatment.
Equity	• Universal access to preoperative MRI would result in more health care equity, provided equivalent facilities and staffing are available.	• Breast MRI, including expertise for interpretation, is not available in all centres, and some patients may need to travel long distances.
Cost	• Better lesion characterization may reduce operative costs by reducing rates of reoperations (direct surgical costs for multiple operations, treating surgical complications, patient time), costs to treat metachronous contralateral breast cancer, and longer-term costs due to decreased recurrence.	• The addition of an MRI and subsequent biopsy of lesions will add to the initial diagnostic cost.

Abbreviations: BCS, breast conserving surgery; BI-RADS, Breast Imaging Reporting and Data System; MRI, magnetic resonance imaging.

3.1.2. Key Evidence for Recommendation 1

The literature review compared patients with and without preoperative MRI and reported the following results:

Recurrence

- Use of MRI is associated with a reduction of recurrence of any type (HR = 0.77, 95% confidence interval [CI] = 0.65 to 0.90) [moderate level of certainty]. Approximate recurrence: 8.2% versus 10.5%; 2.3% less (1% to 3.6% fewer).

Contralateral Cancer

- Use of MRI is associated with an increase in detection of synchronous CBC (prior to initial surgery) (HR = 2.52, 95% CI = 1.75 to 3.62; HR > 1 indicates increased detection with MRI) [moderate level of certainty]. Approximate synchronous CBC detection: 4.7% versus 1.9%; 2.8% more (1.4% to 4.8% more).
- Use of MRI is associated with a slight reduction in metachronous CBC (HR = 0.71, 95% CI = 0.59 to 0.85) [moderate level of certainty]. Approximate metachronous CBC: 1.7% versus 2.4%; 0.7% fewer (0.4% to 1.0% fewer).

Conversion Mastectomy

- Use of MRI is associated with a reduction in the rate of conversion mastectomy OR = 0.76, 95% CI = 0.58 to 0.99) [low level of certainty]. Approximate conversion mastectomy rate: 5.5% versus 7.1%; 1.6% fewer (95% CI = 0.1% to 2.9% fewer).

Positive Margins

- Use of MRI reduced the rate of positive margins in studies with low or low-moderate risk of bias (OR = 0.57, 95% CI = 0.36 to 0.89) [moderate level of certainty]. Approximate rate of positive margins: 6.5% versus 10.9%; 4.4% fewer (95% CI = 1.1% to 6.7% fewer).

Reoperations and Re-Excisions

- Use of MRI is associated with a reduction in the rate of reoperation (OR = 0.73, 95% CI = 0.63 to 0.85) [low level of certainty]. Approximate rate of reoperation: 14.4% versus 18.7%; 4.3% fewer (95% CI = 2.3% to 6.0% fewer).
- Use of MRI is associated with a reduction in the rate of re-excision (OR = 0.63, 95% CI = 0.45 to 0.89) [low level of certainty]. Approximate rate of re-excision: 6.9% versus 10.5%; 3.6% fewer (95% CI = 1.0% to 5.5% fewer).

Mastectomy Rates
- Use of MRI is associated with an increase in the initial mastectomy rate in patients planned (prior to MRI) for BCS (OR = 5.18, 95% CI = 2.37 to 11.29) [very low level of certainty]. Approximate initial mastectomy rate: 5.5% versus 1.1%; 4.4% more (95% CI = 3.6% to 11.5% more). Use of MRI is associated with an increase in the final mastectomy rate (OR = 1.87, 95% CI = 1.23 to 2.85) [very low level of certainty]. Approximate final mastectomy rate: 14% versus 8%; 6% more (95% CI = 1.7% to 11.9% more).
- Studies including all patients diagnosed with breast cancer (not restricted to predetermined BCS) showed that use of MRI is associated with an increase in the initial mastectomy rate (OR = 1.29, 95% CI = 1.09 to 1.35) [low level of certainty]. Approximate initial mastectomy rate: 38.0% versus 32.3%, or 5.8% more (95% CI = 1.9% to 9.9% more). The use of MRI is associated with an increase in the final mastectomy rate (OR = 1.19, 95% CI = 1.06 to 1.33). Approximate final mastectomy rate: 41.8% versus 37.6%, 4.2% more (95% CI = 1.4% to 6.9% more). There was no difference in the final mastectomy rate when the trials using registry data were excluded (OR = 0.98, 95% CI = 0.82 to 1.17).

Other Supporting Studies (Not Part of the Meta-Analysis)
- A meta-analysis of 22 studies by Brennan et al. found the incremental CBC detection rate over conventional imaging to be 4.1% [27]. This is much higher than the cancer rate of 1.4% in the High Risk Ontario Breast Screening Program [28], in which MRI is routinely used.
- Two studies that characterized mammographically occult ipsilateral lesions (>2 cm away or in different quadrants than the index tumour) found that they were larger than the index lesion in approximately 20% of cases [29,30]. In the absence of MRI, such tumours, unless detected coincidentally during the operation of the index tumour, would be untreated surgically.
- Guidelines by The Canadian Association of Radiologists [16], EUSOBI [13,31], and Blue Shield of California/Blue Cross Blue Shield Association [17,32] have similar recommendations.

3.1.3. Justification for Recommendation 1
- We consider the significant reduction in recurrence, probable improvement in disease-free survival and metachronous CBC, and reduction in reoperations (re-excisions and conversion mastectomies) evidence of benefit that outweighs the potential negative effects overall. This recommendation places a higher value on treating cancer in a single operation and avoiding recurrence than on avoiding the discomfort of an MRI and potential additional biopsies.
- While the absolute benefit is small for most outcomes and not always statistically significant, the trend is toward MRI being beneficial for each outcome, and therefore this consistency strengthens the conclusion that preoperative MRI has a positive impact in general.
- While MRI use is associated with an increase in mastectomy rate, the reasons are likely to be multifactorial, including the need to encompass additional foci of cancer, a lack of BCS/oncoplastic surgery expertise for more complex cases, and patient preferences. In retrospective studies (and some of the RCTs), MRI was used for clinical reasons that may not have been recorded or adjusted for but that could be related to mastectomy use. As mastectomy rates may vary by country, region, hospital, and surgeon, and due to patient factors such as age, relationship status, and race/ethnicity, the additional effect of MRI on mastectomy outcomes is difficult to assess.

3.2. Recommendation 2
- Preoperative breast MRI *is recommended* in patients diagnosed with invasive lobular carcinoma (ILC) for whom additional information about disease extent could influence

treatment. The decision of whether to conduct an MRI should be made in consultation with the patient and must take into account the balance of benefits and risks and patient preferences.

3.2.1. Qualifying Statements for Recommendation 2
- Risks and benefits will vary depending on patient and disease characteristics.
- System issues such as MRI availability may result in treatment delays that may modify the decision.

3.2.2. Key Evidence for Recommendation 2

Evidence for Recommendation 1 would apply, in addition to stronger evidence specifically for ILC:
- Use of MRI is associated with a reduction in the rate of conversion mastectomy in patients with ILC (OR = 0.38, 95% CI = 0.25 to 0.56) [high certainty of evidence]. Approximate conversion mastectomy rate in ILC: 5.9% versus 14.2%; 8.3% fewer (5.7% to 10.3% fewer).
- Use of MRI is associated with a reduction in the rate of positive margins in patients with ILC (OR = 0.63, 95% CI = 0.49 to 0.82) [moderate level of certainty]. Approximate rate of positive margins: 18.9% versus 27.0%; 8.1% fewer (3.7% to 11.7%).
- Use of MRI is associated with a large reduction in the rate of reoperation in patients with ILC (OR = 0.30, 95% CI = 0.13 to 0.72) [moderate level of certainty]. Approximate rate of reoperation: 12.3% versus 31.9%; 19.6% fewer (6.77% to 26.1% fewer).
- Lobbes et al. [33] found MRI increased the detection of synchronous CBC in ILC (OR = 4.07, 95% CI = 1.73 to 3.61, $p < 0.001$) (HR > 1 indicates increased detection with MRI).
- A review of the literature by Mann et al. [34] found synchronous CBC detected only by MRI in 7% of patients (95% CI = 4% to 12%). The recommendation is consistent with guidelines by EUSOBI [13], EUSOMA [12], INESSS [14], and The Royal College of Radiologists (London) [35].

3.2.3. Justification for Recommendation 2
- We consider the significant reduction in positive margins resulting in a large reduction in reoperations (including conversion mastectomy), in addition to the benefits in survival and recurrence for all patients (see Recommendation 1), to be evidence of a benefit that outweighs the potential negative effects overall. This recommendation places a higher value on treating cancer in a single operation and avoiding recurrence than on avoiding the discomfort of an MRI and potential additional biopsies. The benefit of MRI is consistent with the results of studies that reported that, compared to invasive ductal carcinoma, ILC has been found to be more difficult to detect by mammography, more likely multifocal, more often occurs with synchronous CBC, and has more involved margins after initial resection [36–41].

3.3. Recommendation 3

Preoperative breast MRI **is recommended**, based on the opinion of the Working Group, in the following situations:
(a) To aid in the surgical planning of BCS in patients with suspected or known multicentric or multifocal disease.
(b) To identify additional lesions in patients with dense breasts.
(c) To determine the presence of pectoralis major muscle/chest wall invasion in patients with posteriorly located tumours or when invasion of the pectoralis major muscle or chest wall is suspected.
(d) To aid in surgical planning for skin/nipple-sparing mastectomies or for autologous reconstruction, oncoplastic surgery, and BCS with suspected nipple/areolar involvement.
(e) Patients with familial/hereditary breast cancer who have not had a recent breast MRI as part of screening or diagnosis.

3.3.1. Qualifying Statement for Recommendation 3

Preoperative breast MRI is recommended in the above situations if additional information about disease extent could influence treatment. The decision of whether to conduct an MRI should be made in consultation with the patient and must take into account the balance of benefits and risks and patient preferences.

3.3.2. Key Evidence for Recommendation 3

Comparative studies meeting the evidence review inclusion criteria were not found. These uses are recommended based on the expert opinion of the authors and are consistent with recommendations in other guidelines [12–14,17,32,35,42,43]. Some of these situations are implicit in Recommendation 1; however, the authors wanted to draw attention to these uses:

(a) Most studies in the literature review [19] either excluded multicentric and multifocal disease or included these in the list of factors used to adjust results in multivariate analysis, indicating these are known to influence outcomes, but with the result that we did not find a direct comparison of outcomes according to MRI use. The presence of multicentric and multifocal disease increases the complexity of surgical planning and in older guidelines was a contraindication to BCS. When the disease is well-characterized, the possibility of BCS may be increased in some cases and ruled out in others, and the likelihood of an incidental finding during surgery decreases. The consensus of the authors is that the increased sensitivity of MRI justifies its use in suspected/known multicentric or multifocal disease if BCS is desired.

(b) Several studies mentioned in the literature review [19] reported that the sensitivity of mammography decreases as breast density increases, while the sensitivity of MRI is high and independent of breast density. The GEMMA (Gadobutrol-Enhanced MR Mammography) trials studied MRI in patients with newly diagnosed and histologically proven breast cancer. In GEMMA1, MRI sensitivity was 83% (independent of density), while the sensitivity of mammography decreased from 79% to 62% as breast density increased [44]. Corresponding results in the GEMMA2 trial were 91% (independent of density) for MRI and 82% (low density) to 64% (high density) for mammography. The Ottawa study of preoperative MRI found additional lesions changing surgical management in 31% of patients with low density (fat density) and 62% with dense breasts [45]. Screening studies reported similar variations in the sensitivity of mammography based on breast density. The Supplemental MRI Screening for Women with Extremely Dense Breast Tissue (DENSE trial) randomized 40,373 women with extremely dense breast tissue and normal screening mammography to either supplemental MRI or only mammography and found MRI reduced interval cancers by 50% in those offered MRI and 80% in those who agreed to have an MRI [46–48]. A systematic review and meta-analysis [49] found that breast density is one of the strongest risk factors for breast cancer.

(c) Tumours near the chest wall may invade the pectoralis major muscle or involve the chest wall, and thus accurate knowledge of tumour extent will influence treatment planning. MRI has been found to have high sensitivity in detecting muscle or chest wall involvement [50–53].

(d) Standard BCS may lead to fair to poor esthetic and functional results [54], and more complex oncoplastic surgery or mastectomy may be more appropriate if the optimal tumour-to-breast ratio for each quadrant is exceeded. Breast MRI or other advanced imaging (e.g., positron emission tomography/computed tomography) may be a prerequisite for extreme oncoplasty [55]. MRI is frequently used prior to nipple-sparing mastectomy, especially in the case of centrally located tumours [56–60]. MRI may rule out nipple involvement such that 2 cm is no longer considered a minimum tumour-to-nipple distance; 5 mm [61] or 1 cm [62–67] may be sufficient.

(e) Hereditary cancer patients have a high risk of synchronous and metachronous CBC. A systematic review reported 10-year CBC rates of 25% to 31% for patients with germline mutations, compared to 4% to 8% for sporadic cases [68].

3.4. Technical Factors for MRI Use

MRI is one of the most sensitive imaging techniques for detecting breast tumours, with the potential to be highly specific. Performance depends on the equipment and MRI techniques used and the expertise of those conducting the analysis. The literature review [19] identified several technical documents and standards for MRI use. Guidance on the performance of CE-MRI and biopsies by the Canadian Association of Radiologists [16], ACR [15,69–79], EUSOBI [13,80], and others may be useful; however, these were not critically reviewed or compared in this evidence summary. Several studies used technical standards for MRI set by the American College of Radiology Imaging Network (ACRIN) 6667 trial [81–84] and EUSOBI, as well as the ACRIN 6698 trial for DWI [85].

Best practice is that additional suspicious lesions detected by preoperative MRI be biopsied or otherwise confirmed if they could alter surgical procedures. Sites performing MRI should have the capacity for an MRI-directed biopsy. This minimizes the need for repeat MRIs and associated costs, delays due to transfer of care (ultimately resulting in a delay in definitive treatment) [86], and the risk of patients not receiving follow-up. Familiarity with the complete process may also result in better expertise in reading and interpreting MRI [87].

4. Discussion

In Ontario, there are currently capacity constraints that affect the availability of MRI. Additional MRI use will add system pressure unless capacity issues are resolved and may increase treatment delays beyond what are considered acceptable in some cases. Availability and accessibility vary among regions. Local availability of breast MRI and projected surgical delays due to the addition of preoperative MRI may be major issues in deciding whether MRI is used. Patients indicated that they would like to be aware of these issues and whether they were modifiable in their situation.

Limited availability and high cost are in part due to the long duration of a full MRI scan (30–45 min). Many studies have investigated whether scan time can be reduced without sacrificing sensitivity and specificity or losing other information. As MRI has been found to be beneficial in screening women at high risk of cancer [88–90], as well as those at intermediate risk [1,11,91], including patients with dense breasts [46], the majority of evidence comes from screening studies or those enriched in cancerous lesions.

The first major study of abbreviated MRI (AB-MRI) in screening by Kuhl et al. was published in 2014 [92]. Women at mildly to moderately increased risk of breast cancer with negative digital mammography underwent a full diagnostic MRI (8 pulse sequences). For AB-MRI, only the first two sequences (precontrast and first postcontrast acquisition) were read. Acquisition time for AB-MRI sequences was 3 min, compared to 17 min for the full protocol. The additional cancer yield was 18.2/1000. Sensitivity was 100%, and specificity was similar to the full protocol (94.3% vs. 93.9%). Based on this work, many other studies of AB-MRI have been conducted. Specificity was lower in some studies (though generally >80%), and variations in protocol, including additional sequences, have been investigated. Adding a T2-weighted sequence and having at least two post-contrast sequences does not increase the scan time by more than 3 to 4 min and allows improved specificity equivalent to the full protocol. Ultrafast MRI involving a fast post-contrast acquisition capturing the inflow of contrast agent may be used on its own or together with abbreviated MRI; in the latter case, it adds information but does not take additional time [93]. AB-MRI has been reported for over 5400 women in 21 studies published from 2014 to 2018 [94], with an overall sensitivity of 94% and a specificity of 90%. A later review identified 41 studies until 2020 involving 15,680 MRI examinations [95]. There is not a common definition of AB-MRI, and it sometimes refers to just the precontrast and postcontrast sequences, sequences less than 7 to 10 min, or any protocol that is significantly shorter than the standard (full) MRI protocol.

The ACR accreditation requirements for breast MRI include a precontrast sequence (T2 weighted/bright fluid series, multi-phase T1-weighted series, and pre-contrast T1; these may be separate or combined), and early postcontrast and delayed postcontrast T1-weighted sequences [96]. Massachusetts General Hospital (Boston, Massachusetts) has used a rapid abridged multiphase (RAMP) breast MRI protocol since 2016 that meets ACR requirements and has a scan time of 10 min [97].

In Ontario, use of the full diagnostic protocol is common and requires 30 to 45 min. Some cancer centres, including those in Ottawa and London, use a shortened protocol that requires a scan time of 12 min and meets Canadian Association of Radiologists [16] and Ontario Breast Screening Program guidelines. As shorter protocols become more standardized and implemented, there is potential for cost reduction and increased patient scans. It is acknowledged that personnel, time for setup, and interpretation of results may be limiting factors until the entire workflow is rebalanced.

4.1. Limitations

This literature review referred to in this guideline included primarily retrospective studies that may have additional confounding factors for which adjustments were not made. While the benefits of MRI use in these studies are generally consistent, the magnitude of the benefit is less certain due to differences in patient populations, study designs, and methods of adjustment for confounders. Comparative studies on the use of MRI versus no MRI that met our inclusion criteria were not found for many of the subgroups of interest, including the use of systemic therapy or radiotherapy. Cost analysis was outside the scope of this work.

4.2. Review and Update

The currency of each document is ensured through periodic review and evaluation of the scientific literature and, where appropriate, the addition of newer literature to the original evidence base. This is described in the *PEBC Document Assessment and Review Protocol*. For the full 1–25 guideline, systematic review, and subsequent updates, please visit the OH (CCO) website at https://www.cancercareontario.ca/en/guidelines-advice/types-of-cancer/breast (accessed on 1 May 2023).

Author Contributions: All authors contributed to the conceptualization and recommendation development. G.G.F. conducted the systematic review and meta-analysis, provided project administration, and prepared initial drafts of the work for discussion and review by all authors. All authors have read and agreed to the published version of the manuscript.

Funding: The Program in Evidence-Based Care (PEBC) is an initiative of the Ontario provincial cancer system, Ontario Health (Cancer Care Ontario), supported by the Ontario Ministry of Health. All work produced by the PEBC is editorially independent from the Ontario Ministry of Health.

Acknowledgments: The Preoperative Breast MRI Guideline Development Group would like to thank Michelle Ghert, Mona el Khoury, Renee Hanrahan, Donna Maziak, Sheila McNair, Amanda Roberts, Jonathan Sussman, Emily Vella, and Xiaomei Yao for providing feedback on draft versions.

Conflicts of Interest: The following interests were disclosed in accordance with the PEBC Conflict of Interest Policy: RG was Co-Principle Investigator for the PET ABC study looking at PET for staging LABC, and JS was site principal investigator for the TMIST (Tomosynthesis Mammography Intervention Screening Trial) in Ottawa, funded by the National Cancer Institute to the Canadian Clinical Trials Group, and received honorariums as a consultant to the Canadian Breast Cancer Network in 2022 and a visiting professor at Queen's University.

References

1. Mann, R.M.; Kuhl, C.K.; Moy, L. Contrast-enhanced MRI for breast cancer screening. *J. Magn. Reson. Imaging* **2019**, *50*, 377–390. [CrossRef]

2. Schoub, P.K. Understanding indications and defining guidelines for breast magnetic resonance imaging. *SA J. Radiol.* **2018**, *22*, a1353. [CrossRef]
3. Orel, S.G.; Schnall, M.D. MR imaging of the breast for the detection, diagnosis, and staging of breast cancer. *Radiology* **2001**, *220*, 13–30. [CrossRef]
4. Lehman, C.D. Magnetic resonance imaging in the evaluation of ductal carcinoma in situ. *J. Natl. Cancer Inst. Monogr.* **2010**, *2010*, 150–151. [CrossRef] [PubMed]
5. Warner, E.; Causer, P.A.; Wong, J.W.; Wright, F.C.; Jong, R.A.; Hill, K.A.; Messner, S.J.; Yaffe, M.J.; Narod, S.A.; Plewes, D.B. Improvement in DCIS detection rates by MRI over time in a high-risk breast screening study. *Breast J.* **2011**, *17*, 9–17. [CrossRef] [PubMed]
6. Kuhl, C.K.; Schrading, S.; Bieling, H.B.; Wardelmann, E.; Leutner, C.C.; Koenig, R.; Kuhn, W.; Schild, H.H. MRI for diagnosis of pure ductal carcinoma in situ: A prospective observational study. *Lancet* **2007**, *370*, 485–492. [CrossRef] [PubMed]
7. Sickles, E.A.; D'Orsi, C.J. ACR BI-RADS®Atlas—Follow-up and Outcome Monitoring. Section II. The Basic Clinically Relevant Audit. In *ACR BI-RADS®Atlas*, 5th ed.; D'Orsi, C.J., Sickles, E.A., Mendelson, E.B., Morris, E.A., Eds.; American College of Radiology: Reston, VA, USA, 2013; [modified 5 Feruary 2014].
8. Ontario Health (Cancer Care Ontario). Guidelines & Advice: Breast Cancer Screening for People at High Risk. 2017. Available online: https://www.cancercareontario.ca/en/guidelines-advice/cancer-continuum/screening/breast-cancer-high-risk (accessed on 21 June 2023).
9. Warner, E.; Messersmith, H.; Causer, P.; Eisen, A.; Shumak, R.; Plewes, D. Magnetic Resonance Imaging Screening of Women at High Risk for Breast Cancer, Version 3. 2021. Available online: https://www.cancercareontario.ca/en/guidelines-advice/types-of-cancer/2051 (accessed on 26 October 2021).
10. Mann, R.M.; Athanasiou, A.; Baltzer, P.A.T.; Camps-Herrero, J.; Clauser, P.; Fallenberg, E.M.; Forrai, G.; Fuchsjäger, M.H.; Helbich, T.H.; Killburn-Toppin, F.; et al. Breast cancer screening in women with extremely dense breasts recommendations of the European Society of Breast Imaging (EUSOBI). *Eur. Radiol.* **2022**, *32*, 4036–4045. [CrossRef]
11. Monticciolo, D.L.; Newell, M.S.; Moy, L.; Lee, C.S.; Destounis, S.V. Breast Cancer Screening for Women at Higher-Than-Average Risk: Updated Recommendations From the ACR. *J. Am. Coll. Radiol.* **2023**, in press. [CrossRef]
12. Sardanelli, F.; Boetes, C.; Borisch, B.; Decker, T.; Federico, M.; Gilbert, F.J.; Helbich, T.; Heywang-Kobrunner, S.H.; Kaiser, W.A.; Kerin, M.J.; et al. Magnetic resonance imaging of the breast: Recommendations from the EUSOMA working group. *Eur. J. Cancer* **2010**, *46*, 1296–1316. [CrossRef]
13. Mann, R.M.; Kuhl, C.K.; Kinkel, K.; Boetes, C. Breast MRI: Guidelines from the European Society of Breast Imaging. *Eur. Radiol.* **2008**, *18*, 1307–1318. [CrossRef]
14. Institut National D'excellence en Santé et en Services Sociaux (INESSS). Main Indications for Breast MRI in the Context of Investigation and Planning of Breast Cancer Treatment. 2018. Available online: https://www.inesss.qc.ca/fileadmin/doc/INESSS/Rapports/Oncologie/IRM_sein/IRM_Cancer-du-sein_EN_VF.pdf (accessed on 26 March 2021).
15. American College of Radiology. ACR Practice Parameter for the Performance of Contrast-Enhanced Magnetic Resonance Imaging (MRI) of the Breast. 2018. Available online: https://www.acr.org/-/media/ACR/Files/Practice-Parameters/MR-Contrast-Breast.pdf?la=en (accessed on 16 March 2020).
16. Appavoo, S.; Aldis, A.; Causer, P.; Crystal, P.; Kornecki, A.; Mundt, Y.; Seely, J.; Wadden, N. CAR Practice Guidelines and Technical Standards for Breast Imaging and Intervention. 2012. Available online: https://car.ca/book/breast-imaging-guidelines/ (accessed on 17 March 2020).
17. Blue Shield of California. 6.01.29—Magnetic Resonance Imaging for Detection and Diagnosis of Breast Cancer. 2020. Available online: https://www.blueshieldca.com/bsca/bsc/public/common/PortalComponents/provider/StreamDocumentServlet?fileName=PRV_MRI_Breast.pdf (accessed on 9 February 2021).
18. Gradishar, W.J.; Moran, M.S.; Abraham, J.; Abramson, V.; Aft, R.; Agnese, D.; Allison, K.H.; Anderson, B.; Burnstein, H.J.; Chew, H.; et al. NCCN Clinical Practice Guidelines in Oncology (NCCN guidelines)®. 2023. Available online: https://www.nccn.org/professionals/physician_gls/pdf/breast-screening.pdf (accessed on 20 June 2023).
19. Eisen, A.; Fletcher, G.G.; Fienberg, S.; George, R.; Holloway, C.; Kulkarni, S.; Seely, J.; Muradali, D. Preoperative Breast Magnetic Resonance Imaging. Program in Evidence-Based Care Evidence Summary No.: 1-25. 2021. Available online: https://www.cancercareontario.ca/sites/ccocancercare/files/assets/pebc1-25es.pdf (accessed on 27 May 2022).
20. Muradali, D.; Fletcher, G.G.; Cordeiro, E.; Fienberg, S.; George, R.; Kulkarni, S.; Seely, J.; Shaheen, R.; Eisen, A. The Preoperative Breast MRI Expert Panel. Preoperative Breast Magnetic Resonance Imaging Guideline. 2023. Available online: https://www.cancercareontario.ca/en/guidelines-advice/types-of-cancer/70786 (accessed on 22 June 2023).
21. Eisen, A.; Fletcher, G.G.; Fienberg, S.; George, R.; Holloway, C.; Kulkarni, S.; Seely, J.; Muradali, D. Breast magnetic resonance imaging for preoperative evaluation of breast cancer. *Can. Assoc. Radiol. J.* **2023**, in press.
22. Browman, G.P.; Newman, T.E.; Mohide, E.A.; Graham, I.D.; Levine, M.N.; Pritchard, K.I.; Evans, W.K.; Maroun, J.A.; Hodson, D.I.; Carey, M.S.; et al. Progress of clinical oncology guidelines development using the Practice Guidelines Development Cycle: The role of practitioner feedback. *J. Clin. Oncol.* **1998**, *16*, 1226–1231. [CrossRef]
23. Browman, G.P.; Levine, M.N.; Mohide, E.A.; Hayward, R.S.; Pritchard, K.I.; Gafni, A.; Laupacis, A. The practice guidelines development cycle: A conceptual tool for practice guidelines development and implementation. *J. Clin. Oncol.* **1995**, *13*, 502–512. [CrossRef] [PubMed]

24. Arnaout, A.; Varela, N.P.; Allarakhia, M.; Grimard, L.; Hey, A.; Lau, J.; Thain, L.; Eisen, A. Baseline staging imaging for distant metastasis in women with stages I, II, and III breast cancer. *Curr. Oncol.* **2020**, *27*, e123–e145. [CrossRef] [PubMed]
25. The Cochrane Collaboration. Review Manager (RevMan). Version 5.4. 2020. Available online: https://training.cochrane.org/online-learning/core-software-cochrane-reviews/revman/revman-5-download (accessed on 6 May 2021).
26. Higgins, J.; Thomas, J.; Chandler, J.; Cumpston, M.; Li, T.; Page, M.; Welch, V. Cochrane Handbook for Systematic Reviews of Interventions Version 6.1. 2020. Available online: https://training.cochrane.org/handbook (accessed on 13 August 2021).
27. Brennan, M.E.; Houssami, N.; Lord, S.; Macaskill, P.; Irwig, L.; Dixon, J.M.; Warren, R.M.; Ciatto, S. Magnetic resonance imaging screening of the contralateral breast in women with newly diagnosed breast cancer: Systematic review and meta-analysis of incremental cancer detection and impact on surgical management. *J. Clin. Oncol.* **2009**, *27*, 5640–5649. [CrossRef] [PubMed]
28. Chiarelli, A.M.; Blackmore, K.M.; Muradali, D.; Done, S.J.; Majpruz, V.; Weerasinghe, A.; Mirea, L.; Eisen, A.; Rabeneck, L.; Warner, E. Performance measures of magnetic resonance imaging plus mammography in the High Risk Ontario Breast Screening Program. *J. Natl. Cancer Inst.* **2020**, *112*, 136–144. [CrossRef]
29. Goodman, S.; Mango, V.; Friedlander, L.; Desperito, E.; Wynn, R.; Ha, R. Are mammographically occult additional tumors identified more than 2 cm away from the primary breast cancer on MRI clinically significant? *Acad. Radiol.* **2019**, *26*, 502–507. [CrossRef]
30. Iacconi, C.; Galman, L.; Zheng, J.; Sacchini, V.; Sutton, E.J.; Dershaw, D.; Morris, E.A. Multicentric cancer detected at breast MR imaging and not at mammography: Important or not? *Radiology* **2016**, *279*, 378–384. [CrossRef]
31. Mann, R.M.; Balleyguier, C.; Baltzer, P.A.; Bick, U.; Colin, C.; Cornford, E.; Evans, A.; Fallenberg, E.; Forrai, G.; Fuchsjager, M.H.; et al. Breast MRI: EUSOBI recommendations for women's information. *Eur. Radiol.* **2015**, *25*, 3669–3678. [CrossRef]
32. Blue Cross Blue Shield Association. 6.01.29—Magnetic Resonance Imaging for Detection and Diagnosis of Breast Cancer. 2019. Available online: https://www.evidencepositioningsystem.com/BCBSA/html/pol_6.01.29.html (accessed on 31 October 2019).
33. Lobbes, M.B.; Vriens, I.J.; van Bommel, A.C.; Nieuwenhuijzen, G.A.; Smidt, M.L.; Boersma, L.J.; van Dalen, T.; Smorenburg, C.; Struikmans, H.; Siesling, S.; et al. Breast MRI increases the number of mastectomies for ductal cancers, but decreases them for lobular cancers. *Breast Cancer Res. Treat.* **2017**, *162*, 353–364. [CrossRef]
34. Mann, R.M.; Hoogeveen, Y.L.; Blickman, J.G.; Boetes, C. MRI compared to conventional diagnostic work-up in the detection and evaluation of invasive lobular carcinoma of the breast: A review of existing literature. *Breast Cancer Res. Treat.* **2008**, *107*, 1–14. [CrossRef] [PubMed]
35. The Royal College of Radiologists. Guidance on Screening and Symptomatic Breast Imaging. 2019. Available online: https://www.rcr.ac.uk/publication/guidance-screening-and-symptomatic-breast-imaging-fourth-edition (accessed on 26 March 2021).
36. Biglia, N.; Maggiorotto, F.; Liberale, V.; Bounous, V.E.; Sgro, L.G.; Pecchio, S.; D'Alonzo, M.; Ponzone, R. Clinical-pathologic features, long term-outcome and surgical treatment in a large series of patients with invasive lobular carcinoma (ILC) and invasive ductal carcinoma (IDC). *Eur. J. Surg. Oncol.* **2013**, *39*, 455–460. [CrossRef] [PubMed]
37. Derias, M.; Subramanian, A.; Allan, S.; Shah, E.; Teraifi, H.E.; Howlett, D. The Role of Magnetic Resonance Imaging in the Investigation and Management of Invasive Lobular Carcinoma-A 3-Year Retrospective Study in Two District General Hospitals. *Breast J.* **2016**, *22*, 384–389. [CrossRef] [PubMed]
38. Dillon, M.F.; Hill, A.D.; Fleming, F.J.; O'Doherty, A.; Quinn, C.M.; McDermott, E.W.; O'Higgins, N. Identifying patients at risk of compromised margins following breast conservation for lobular carcinoma. *Am. J. Surg.* **2006**, *191*, 201–205. [CrossRef]
39. Yeatman, T.J.; Cantor, A.B.; Smith, T.J.; Smith, S.K.; Reintgen, D.S.; Miller, M.S.; Ku, N.N.; Baekey, P.A.; Cox, C.E. Tumor biology of infiltrating lobular carcinoma. Implications for management. *Ann. Surg.* **1995**, *222*, 549–559; discussion 559–561. [CrossRef]
40. Krecke, K.N.; Gisvold, J.J. Invasive lobular carcinoma of the breast: Mammographic findings and extent of disease at diagnosis in 184 patients. *AJR Am. J. Roentgenol.* **1993**, *161*, 957–960. [CrossRef]
41. Veltman, J.; Boetes, C.; van Die, L.; Bult, P.; Blickman, J.G.; Barentsz, J.O. Mammographic detection and staging of invasive lobular carcinoma. *Clin. Imaging* **2006**, *30*, 94–98. [CrossRef]
42. Eastern Health Breast Disease Site Group. Indications for Use of Breast Magnetic Resonance Imaging. 2017. Available online: https://cancercare.easternhealth.ca/health-care-professionals/guidelines/breast-cancer/ (accessed on 26 March 2021).
43. Ditsch, N.; Untch, M.; Thill, M.; Muller, V.; Janni, W.; Albert, U.S.; Bauerfeind, I.; Blohmer, J.; Budach, W.; Dall, P.; et al. AGO recommendations for the diagnosis and treatment of patients with early breast cancer: Update 2019. *Breast Care* **2019**, *14*, 224–245. [CrossRef]
44. Sardanelli, F.; Newstead, G.M.; Putz, B.; Jirakova Trnkova, Z.; Trimboli, R.M.; Abe, H.; Haverstock, D.; Rosenberg, M. Gadobutrol-enhanced magnetic resonance imaging of the breast in the preoperative setting: Results of 2 prospective international multicenter phase III studies. *Investig. Radiol.* **2016**, *51*, 454–461. [CrossRef]
45. Seely, J.M.; Lamb, L.; Malik, N.; Lau, J. The yield of pre-operative breast MRI in patients according to breast tissue density. *Eur. Radiol.* **2016**, *26*, 3280–3289. [CrossRef]
46. Bakker, M.F.; de Lange, S.V.; Pijnappel, R.M.; Mann, R.M.; Peeters, P.H.M.; Monninkhof, E.M.; Emaus, M.J.; Loo, C.E.; Bisschops, R.H.C.; Lobbes, M.B.I.; et al. Supplemental MRI screening for women with extremely dense breast tissue. *N. Engl. J. Med.* **2019**, *381*, 2091–2102. [CrossRef] [PubMed]
47. Klinkenbijl, J.H.G.; van Leeuwen, E.; Verkooijen, H.M. Wat zeggen de uitkomsten van de DENSE-studie? *Ned. Tijdschr. Geneeskd.* **2020**, *164*, D4822. [PubMed]

48. Franz, H.B.G. Profitieren frauen mit extrem dichtem brustgewebe von zusatzlicher MRT? *Geburtshilfe Frauenheilkd.* **2020**, *80*, 460–462. [CrossRef]
49. McCormack, V.A.; dos Santos Silva, I. Breast density and parenchymal patterns as markers of breast cancer risk: A meta-analysis. *Cancer Epidemiol. Biomark. Prev.* **2006**, *15*, 1159–1169. [CrossRef]
50. Samreen, N.; Lee, C.; Bhatt, A.; Carter, J.; Hieken, T.; Adler, K.; Zingula, S.; Glazebrook, K.N. A Clinical Approach to Diffusion-Weighted Magnetic Resonance Imaging in Evaluating Chest Wall Invasion of Breast Tumors. *J. Clin. Imaging Sci.* **2019**, *9*, 11. [CrossRef]
51. Myers, K.S.; Stern, E.; Ambinder, E.B.; Oluyemi, E.T. Breast cancer abutting the pectoralis major muscle on breast MRI: What are the clinical implications? *Br. J. Radiol.* **2021**, *94*, 20201202. [CrossRef]
52. Kazama, T.; Nakamura, S.; Doi, O.; Suzuki, K.; Hirose, M.; Ito, H. Prospective evaluation of pectoralis muscle invasion of breast cancer by MR imaging. *Breast Cancer* **2005**, *12*, 312–316. [CrossRef]
53. Morris, E.A.; Schwartz, L.H.; Drotman, M.B.; Kim, S.J.; Tan, L.K.; Liberman, L.; Abramson, A.F.; Van Zee, K.J.; Dershaw, D.D. Evaluation of pectoralis major muscle in patients with posterior breast tumors on breast MR images: Early experience. *Radiology* **2000**, *214*, 67–72. [CrossRef]
54. Pukancsik, D.; Kelemen, P.; Ujhelyi, M.; Kovacs, E.; Udvarhelyi, N.; Meszaros, N.; Kenessey, I.; Kovacs, T.; Kasler, M.; Matrai, Z. Objective decision making between conventional and oncoplastic breast-conserving surgery or mastectomy: An aesthetic and functional prospective cohort study. *Eur. J. Surg. Oncol.* **2017**, *43*, 303–310. [CrossRef]
55. Silverstein, M.J.; Savalia, N.; Khan, S.; Ryan, J. Extreme oncoplasty: Breast conservation for patients who need mastectomy. *Breast J.* **2015**, *21*, 52–59. [CrossRef]
56. Tousimis, E.; Haslinger, M. Overview of indications for nipple sparing mastectomy. *Gland Surg.* **2018**, *7*, 288–300. [CrossRef] [PubMed]
57. Piato, J.R.; de Andrade, R.D.; Chala, L.F.; de Barros, N.; Mano, M.S.; Melitto, A.S.; Goncalves, R.; Soares Junior, J.M.; Baracat, E.C.; Filassi, J.R. MRI to predict nipple involvement in breast cancer patients. *AJR Am. J. Roentgenol.* **2016**, *206*, 1124–1130. [CrossRef] [PubMed]
58. Yamashita, Y.; Hayashi, N.; Nagura, N.; Kajiura, Y.; Yoshida, A.; Takei, J.; Suzuki, K.; Tsunoda, H.; Yamauchi, H. Long-term oncologic safety of nipple-sparing mastectomy with immediate reconstruction. *Clin. Breast Cancer* **2021**, *21*, 352–359. [CrossRef]
59. Koike-Shimo, A.; Tsugawa, K.; Kawamoto, H.; Kanemaki, Y.; Maeda, I. Oncologic outcome and technical consideration of nipple-sparing mastectomy in breast cancer: The St. Marianna experience with 384 patients. *J. Clin. Oncol.* **2014**, *32*, e12024. [CrossRef]
60. del Riego, J.; Pitarch, M.; Codina, C.; Nebot, L.; Andreu, F.J.; Aparicio, O.; Medina, A.; Martin, A. Multimodality approach to the nipple-areolar complex: A pictorial review and diagnostic algorithm. *Insights Imaging* **2020**, *11*, 89. [CrossRef] [PubMed]
61. Ponzone, R.; Maggiorotto, F.; Carabalona, S.; Rivolin, A.; Pisacane, A.; Kubatzki, F.; Renditore, S.; Carlucci, S.; Sgandurra, P.; Marocco, F.; et al. MRI and intraoperative pathology to predict nipple-areola complex (NAC) involvement in patients undergoing NAC-sparing mastectomy. *Eur. J. Cancer* **2015**, *51*, 1882–1889. [CrossRef] [PubMed]
62. Ryu, J.M.; Nam, S.J.; Kim, S.W.; Lee, S.K.; Bae, S.Y.; Yi, H.W.; Park, S.; Paik, H.J.; Lee, J.E. Feasibility of nipple-sparing mastectomy with immediate breast reconstruction in breast cancer patients with tumor-nipple distance less than 2.0 cm. *World J. Surg.* **2016**, *40*, 2028–2035. [CrossRef]
63. Mariscotti, G.; Durando, M.; Houssami, N.; Berzovini, C.M.; Esposito, F.; Fasciano, M.; Campanino, P.P.; Bosco, D.; Bussone, R.; Ala, A.; et al. Preoperative MRI evaluation of lesion-nipple distance in breast cancer patients: Thresholds for predicting occult nipple-areola complex involvement. *Clin. Radiol.* **2018**, *73*, 735–743. [CrossRef]
64. Gao, Y.; Brachtel, E.F.; Hernandez, O.; Heller, S.L. An analysis of nipple enhancement at breast MRI with radiologic-pathologic correlation. *Radiographics* **2019**, *39*, 10–27. [CrossRef]
65. Seki, H.; Sakurai, T.; Mizuno, S.; Tokuda, T.; Kaburagi, T.; Seki, M.; Karahashi, T.; Nakajima, K.; Shimizu, K.; Jinno, H. A novel nipple-areola complex involvement predictive index for indicating nipple-sparing mastectomy in breast cancer patients. *Breast Cancer* **2019**, *26*, 808–816. [CrossRef]
66. Balci, F.L.; Kara, H.; Dulgeroglu, O.; Uras, C. Oncologic safety of nipple-sparing mastectomy in patients with short tumor-nipple distance. *Breast J.* **2019**, *25*, 612–618. [CrossRef] [PubMed]
67. Frey, J.D.; Salibian, A.A.; Lee, J.; Harris, K.; Axelrod, D.M.; Guth, A.A.; Shapiro, R.L.; Schnabel, F.R.; Karp, N.S.; Choi, M. Oncologic trends, outcomes, and risk factors for locoregional recurrence: An analysis of tumor-to-nipple distance and critical factors in therapeutic nipple-sparing mastectomy. *Plast. Reconstr. Surg.* **2019**, *143*, 1575–1585. [CrossRef] [PubMed]
68. Liebens, F.P.; Carly, B.; Pastijn, A.; Rozenberg, S. Management of BRCA1/2 associated breast cancer: A systematic qualitative review of the state of knowledge in 2006. *Eur. J. Cancer* **2007**, *43*, 238–257. [CrossRef] [PubMed]
69. American College of Radiology. Complete Accreditation Information: Breast MRI. 2020. Available online: https://accreditationsupport.acr.org/support/solutions/articles/11000063266-complete-accreditation-information-breast-mri (accessed on 23 March 2021).
70. American College of Radiology. ACR Appropriateness Criteria®: Monitoring Response to Neoadjuvant Systemic Therapy for Breast Cancer. 2017. Available online: https://acsearch.acr.org/list (accessed on 23 March 2021).

71. American College of Radiology Committee on Quality Assurance in Magnetic Resonance Imaging. Magnetic Resonance Imaging. Quality Control Manual. 2016. Available online: https://www.acr.org/-/media/ACR/NOINDEX/QC-Manuals/MR_QCManual.pdf (accessed on 23 March 2021).
72. American College of Radiology Committee on MR Safety. ACR Manual on MR Safety. Version 1.0. 2020. Available online: https://www.acr.org/Clinical-Resources/Radiology-Safety/MR-Safety (accessed on 23 March 2021).
73. American College of Radiology Committee on Drugs and Contrast Media. ACR Manual on Contrast Media. 2021. Available online: https://www.acr.org/Clinical-Resources/Contrast-Manual (accessed on 13 August 2021).
74. American College of Radiology. ACR Practice Parameter for the Performance of Magnetic Resonance Imaging-Guided Breast Interventional Procedures. 2016. Available online: https://www.acr.org/-/media/ACR/Files/Practice-Parameters/MR-Guided-Breast.pdf?la=en (accessed on 16 March 2020).
75. American College of Radiology. ACR BI-RADS Atlas. Breast Imaging Reporting and Data System. 2013. Available online: https://www.acr.org/Clinical-Resources/Reporting-and-Data-Systems/Bi-Rads (accessed on 13 November 2019).
76. Amurao, M.R.; Einstein, S.A.; Panda, A.; Och, J.G.; Pooley, R.A.; Yanasak, N.E.; American College of Radiology (ACR); American Association of Physicists in Medicine (AAPM). ACR–AAPM Technical Standard for Diagnostic Medical Physics Performance Monitoring of Magnetic Resonance (MR) Imaging Equipment. 2019. Available online: https://www.acr.org/-/media/ACR/Files/Practice-Parameters/mr-equip.pdf?la=en (accessed on 20 September 2019).
77. DeMartini, W.B.; Rahbar, H. Breast magnetic resonance imaging technique at 1.5 T and 3 T: Requirements for quality imaging and American College of Radiology accreditation. *Magn. Reson. Imaging Clin. N. Am.* **2013**, *21*, 475–482. [CrossRef] [PubMed]
78. Edwards, S.D.; Lipson, J.A.; Ikeda, D.M.; Lee, J.M. Updates and revisions to the BI-RADS magnetic resonance imaging lexicon. *Magn. Reson. Imaging Clin. N. Am.* **2013**, *21*, 483–493. [CrossRef]
79. Covington, M.F.; Young, C.A.; Appleton, C.M. American College of Radiology accreditation, performance metrics, reimbursement, and economic considerations in breast MR Imaging. *Magn. Reson. Imaging Clin. N. Am.* **2018**, *26*, 303–314. [CrossRef]
80. Bick, U.; Trimboli, R.M.; Athanasiou, A.; Balleyguier, C.; Baltzer, P.A.T.; Bernathova, M.; Borbely, K.; Brkljacic, B.; Carbonaro, L.A.; Clauser, P.; et al. Image-guided breast biopsy and localisation: Recommendations for information to women and referring physicians by the European Society of Breast Imaging. *Insights Imaging* **2020**, *11*, 12. [CrossRef]
81. Rahbar, H.; Hanna, L.G.; Gatsonis, C.; Mahoney, M.C.; Schnall, M.D.; DeMartini, W.B.; Lehman, C.D. Contralateral Prophylactic Mastectomy in the American College of Radiology Imaging Network 6667 trial: Effect of Breast MR Imaging Assessments and Patient Characteristics. *Radiology* **2014**, *273*, 53–60. [CrossRef]
82. DeMartini, W.B.; Hanna, L.; Gatsonis, C.; Mahoney, M.C.; Lehman, C.D. Evaluation of tissue sampling methods used for MRI-detected contralateral breast lesions in the American College of Radiology Imaging Network 6667 trial. *AJR Am. J. Roentgenol.* **2012**, *199*, W386–W391. [CrossRef]
83. Weinstein, S.P.; Hanna, L.G.; Gatsonis, C.; Schnall, M.D.; Rosen, M.A.; Lehman, C.D. Frequency of malignancy seen in probably benign lesions at contrast-enhanced breast MR imaging: Findings from ACRIN 6667. *Radiology* **2010**, *255*, 731–737. [CrossRef]
84. Lehman, C.D.; Gatsonis, C.; Kuhl, C.K.; Hendrick, R.E.; Pisano, E.D.; Hanna, L.; Peacock, S.; Smazal, S.F.; Maki, D.D.; Julian, T.B.; et al. MRI evaluation of the contralateral breast in women with recently diagnosed breast cancer. *N. Engl. J. Med.* **2007**, *356*, 1295–1303. [CrossRef] [PubMed]
85. Rakow-Penner, R.; Murphy, P.M.; Dale, A.; Ojeda-Fournier, H. State of the art diffusion weighted imaging in the breast: Recommended protocol. *Curr. Radiol. Rep.* **2017**, *5*, 3. [CrossRef]
86. Nessim, C.; Winocour, J.; Holloway, D.P.; Saskin, R.; Holloway, C.M. Wait times for breast cancer surgery: Effect of magnetic resonance imaging and preoperative investigations on the diagnostic pathway. *J. Oncol. Pract.* **2015**, *11*, e131–e138. [CrossRef]
87. Hollingsworth, A.B.; Stough, R.G. Preoperative breast MRI: Barking up the wrong endpoints. *Breast Dis.* **2015**, *26*, 19–25. [CrossRef]
88. Berg, W.A.; Zhang, Z.; Lehrer, D.; Jong, R.A.; Pisano, E.D.; Barr, R.G.; Böhm-Vélez, M.; Mahoney, M.C.; Evans, W.P., 3rd; Larsen, L.H.; et al. Detection of breast cancer with addition of annual screening ultrasound or a single screening MRI to mammography in women with elevated breast cancer risk. *JAMA* **2012**, *307*, 1394–1404. [CrossRef]
89. Berg, W.A.; Blume, J.D.; Adams, A.M.; Jong, R.A.; Barr, R.G.; Lehrer, D.E.; Pisano, E.D.; Evans, W.P., 3rd; Mahoney, M.C.; Hovanessian Larsen, L.; et al. Reasons women at elevated risk of breast cancer refuse breast MR imaging screening: ACRIN 6666. *Radiology* **2010**, *254*, 79–87. [CrossRef] [PubMed]
90. Kuhl, C.; Weigel, S.; Schrading, S.; Arand, B.; Bieling, H.; Konig, R.; Tombach, B.; Leutner, C.; Rieber-Brambs, A.; Nordhoff, D.; et al. Prospective multicenter cohort study to refine management recommendations for women at elevated familial risk of breast cancer: The EVA trial. *J. Clin. Oncol.* **2010**, *28*, 1450–1457. [CrossRef]
91. Mann, R.M.; Cho, N.; Moy, L. Breast MRI: State of the Art. *Radiology* **2019**, *292*, 520–536. [CrossRef]
92. Kuhl, C.K.; Schrading, S.; Strobel, K.; Schild, H.H.; Hilgers, R.D.; Bieling, H.B. Abbreviated breast Magnetic Resonance Imaging (MRI): First postcontrast subtracted images and maximum-intensity projection—A novel approach to breast cancer screening with MRI. *J. Clin. Oncol.* **2014**, *32*, 2304–2310. [CrossRef]
93. Mann, R.M.; van Zelst, J.C.M.; Vreemann, S.; Mus, R.D.M. Is Ultrafast or Abbreviated Breast MRI Ready for Prime Time? *Curr. Breast Cancer Rep.* **2019**, *11*, 9–16. [CrossRef]
94. Heacock, L.; Reig, B.; Lewin, A.A.; Toth, H.K.; Moy, L.; Lee, C.S. Abbreviated breast MRI: Road to clinical implementation. *J. Breast Imaging* **2020**, *2*, 201–214. [CrossRef]

95. Hernandez, M.L.; Osorio, S.; Florez, K.; Ospino, A.; Diaz, G.M. Abbreviated magnetic resonance imaging in breast cancer: A systematic review of literature. *Eur. J. Radiol. Open* **2021**, *8*, 100307. [CrossRef] [PubMed]
96. American College of Radiology. Complete Accreditation Information: MRI and Breast MRI. 2022. Available online: https://accreditationsupport.acr.org/support/solutions/folders/11000012261 (accessed on 14 February 2023).
97. Choudhery, S.; Chou, S.H.S.; Chang, K.; Kalpathy-Cramer, J.; Lehman, C.D. Kinetic Analysis of Lesions Identified on a Rapid Abridged Multiphase (RAMP) Breast MRI Protocol. *Acad. Radiol.* **2020**, *27*, 672–681. [CrossRef] [PubMed]

Disclaimer/Publisher's Note: The statements, opinions and data contained in all publications are solely those of the individual author(s) and contributor(s) and not of MDPI and/or the editor(s). MDPI and/or the editor(s) disclaim responsibility for any injury to people or property resulting from any ideas, methods, instructions or products referred to in the content.

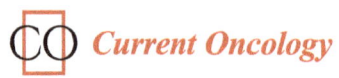

Article

Efficacy and Accuracy of Using Magnetic Seed for Preoperative Non-Palpable Breast Lesions Localization: Our Experience with Magseed

Anna D'Angelo [1,*], Charlotte Marguerite Lucille Trombadori [1], Flavia Caprini [1], Stefano Lo Cicero [1], Valentina Longo [1], Francesca Ferrara [1], Simone Palma [1], Marco Conti [1], Antonio Franco [2], Lorenzo Scardina [2], Sabatino D'Archi [2], Paolo Belli [1] and Riccardo Manfredi [1]

1 Dipartimento di Diagnostica per Immagini, Radioterapia Oncologica ed Ematologia, Fondazione Policlinico Universitario "A. Gemelli", IRCCS, 00168 Rome, Italy
2 Breast Unit, Department of Women, Children and Public Health Sciences, Fondazione Policlinico Universitario Agostino Gemelli IRCCS, 00168 Rome, Italy
* Correspondence: anna.dangelo05@gmail.com

Abstract: In this retrospective study we share our single-center experience using a magnetic seed for the preoperative localization of non-palpable breast lesions. Patients who underwent a preoperative localization with Magseed® (Endomagnetics, Cambridge, UK) placement between 2020 and 2022 were enrolled. Indications to Magseed placement have been established during multidisciplinary meetings prior to surgery and all patients underwent breast-conserving surgery (BCS). 45 patients were included. Magnetic seeds have been introduced under ultrasound guidance in 40 patients (88.9%) and under stereotactic guidance in 5 patients (11.1%). We registered a highly successful placement rate (97.8%), with only one case of migration (2.2%). After BCS, all the magnetic seeds were recovered (100% retrieval rate). The re-excision rate for positive margins was 0%. Our experience, with a highly successful placement and retrieval rate and a re-excision rate equal to 0%, is consistent with the encouraging literature published on Magseed so far, suggesting this technique to be extremely effective. Moreover, our single case of seed migration supports the existing data stating that Magseed migration is rare. In conclusion, despite acknowledging Magseed limitations, we highly value the advantages linked to this technique, and we, therefore, uphold its use.

Keywords: Magseed; breast cancer; preoperative localization; magnetic seed

1. Introduction

Breast cancer (BC) has become the leading cause of global cancer incidence and the fifth leading cause of cancer mortality worldwide [1]. Considering the increasing of BC incidence [1], principally related to improvements in diagnostic techniques and the aging of the population, the detection of non-palpable breast lesions has become increasingly frequent.

For non-palpable BC, the treatment of choice is Breast Conserving Surgery (BCS) [2]. In order to be successful in achieving a complete excision of the lesion, a correct pre-operative localization is required. Thus, accurate and state-of-the-art localization is a pivotal step in the management of a BC patient, with an increasing demand for the development of reliable localization approaches for non-palpable lesions.

Recently, localization techniques have undergone constant improvements. One of the first types of localization technique was the wire guide localization (WGL), still widely used, consisting of locating a wire inside the lesion under ultrasound or mammography guidance. The main limitations of this procedure are the need to perform it on the same day of the surgery, the risk of displacement, and a worse aesthetic result as the breast tissue along the path of the thread must be removed.

Given the above strains, non-wire localization systems have been developed. One of the earliest non-wire systems to be implemented was the Radio-guided Occult Lesion Localization (ROLL) [3] which uses a radioactive marker. However, this localization method requires to be performed on the day of the surgery or a few days before, depending on the half-life of the radioactive molecule. Furthermore, this technique necessitates a nuclear medicine service within the hospital and determines a risk of exposure for both the operator and the patient. Therefore, over the following years, non-wire and non-radioactive localization tools have been implemented, such as the Radio-Frequency Identification tag (RFID), the Savi-Scout and the magnetic seed systems.

The RFID system uses radio frequencies and, despite some limitations [4], is considered safe and effective for non-palpable breast lesions localization, with re-excision rates similar to WGL. It can be deployed inside the lesions the day before surgery. The Savi-Scout system is another non-wire and non-radioactive alternative technique; it uses a micro-impulse infrared radar to localize the lesions and is particularly useful for patients that need MRI examinations during follow-up, without artifacts [5].

Magnetic localization techniques were developed as an alternative to the methods mentioned above [6]. The Magseed® (Endomagnetics, Cambridge, UK), a non-wire and non-radioactive paramagnetic localization tool was approved in 2016 by the Food and Drug Administration (FDA) [7]. It has the crucial advantage that it can be introduced inside the lesion and can remain in place until the time of BCS, despite the first indications that recommend the placement of Magseed up to 30 days before surgery [8]. Hence, the workload of the radiologist before the surgery is reduced as well as delays in surgical theaters due to localization procedures.

Magseed is composed of a seed of 5 × 1 mm inserted within an 18-G sterile needle (Figure 1), and its introduction can be performed either under ultrasound or mammography guidance. Following accurate disinfection of the skin and the injection of local anesthesia, the needle with the magnetic marker is inserted and centered with its distal end as proximal as possible to the target lesion, where the marker is released. A double-view mammography is performed to assess the right placement of the seed. On the day of the surgery, an ultrasound or a mammography examination is performed to evaluate the correct position of the marker, to avoid migration. The magnetic clip is then identified during surgery by the SentiMag® (Endomagnetics, Inc., Cambridge, UK) probe, which generates a magnetic field and magnetizes the seed. During surgery, the distance of the probe from the Magseed is indicated by numerical values displayed on the monitor and with audio feedback. The magnetic seed is considered detectable within a distance that is around 4 cm away from the SentiMag [9].

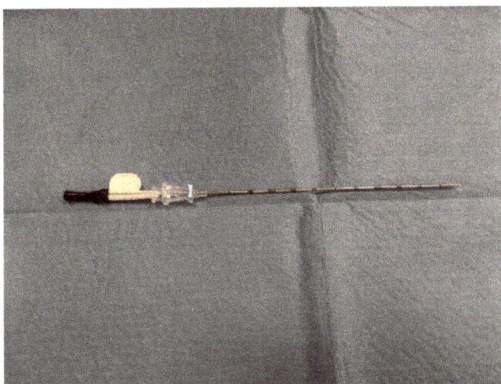

Figure 1. The 18-gauge Magseed introducer.

This retrospective study aimed to share our experience with magnetic seed and to evaluate its efficacy and accuracy for preoperative non-palpable breast lesion localizations.

2. Materials and Methods

2.1. Patients

Our institutional review board approved this single-institution retrospective study. A total of 45 patients who underwent Magseed placement between June 2020 and February 2022 were included. Inclusion criteria were: 18 years old or older, single non-palpable breast lesion and surgery performed in our center. Exclusion criteria were: palpable breast lesions and patients who underwent previous chemotherapy treatment. Each patient enrolled signed informed consent before undergoing the interventional procedure.

2.2. Procedure

The placement of Magseed was decided and approved by a multidisciplinary meeting between breast surgeons, plastic surgeons and radiologists. A total of 45 Magseeds were placed, 40 under ultrasound guidance (88.9%) and 5 under stereotactic placement (11.1%) (Figure 2). Each procedure followed accurate disinfection of the skin (chlorhexidine) and the injection of local anesthetic (Mepicain 2%); after the introduction of the magnetic seed, an ultrasound and a mammogram (two-views mammography, mediolateral oblique, and craniocaudal views) were performed, in order to document the correct position of the marker (Figure 3). On the day of the surgery, a double-view mammography is performed to verify the correct position of the seed (Figure 3).

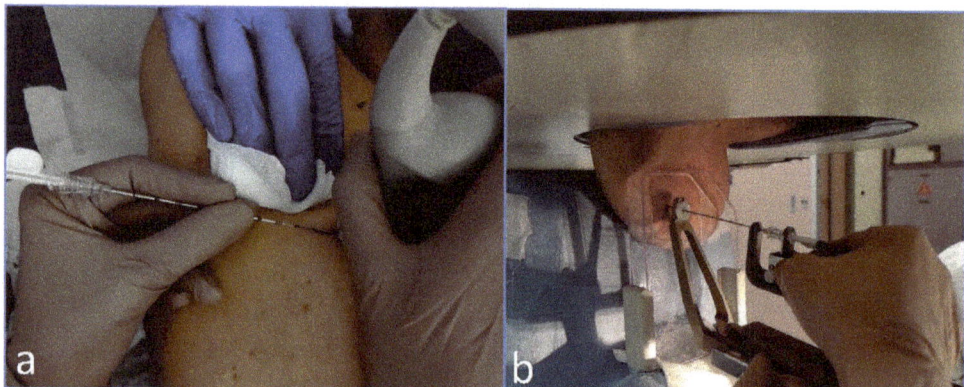

Figure 2. Magseed insertion: ultrasound (**a**) and stereotactic guidance (**b**).

The Magseed was identified during surgery using the SentiMag probe (Figure 4); the audio signal has a frequency that varies according to the intensity of the magnetic field or with the distance of the seed from the probe, helping the surgeon to find the lesion. At the end of the surgery, surgical specimen radiography in craniocaudal view with the tomosynthesis (the routine practice in our center) was performed to assess the presence of the Magseed and to evaluate the distance between the lesion and the close margins (Figures 3f and 4b). If the lesion is detected on the surgical specimen margin at the radiography, intraoperative widening is performed. After that, the surgical specimen was examined by the pathologist for the histological assessment and for the evaluation of margin status ("no ink on tumor") [10].

We evaluated patient demographics, lesions characteristics, Magseed localization features (ultrasound-guided or stereotactic-guided), seed migration, successful Magseed detection and retrieval in the surgical specimen, time of Magseed placement (in minutes) and time between Magseed placement and surgery (in days).

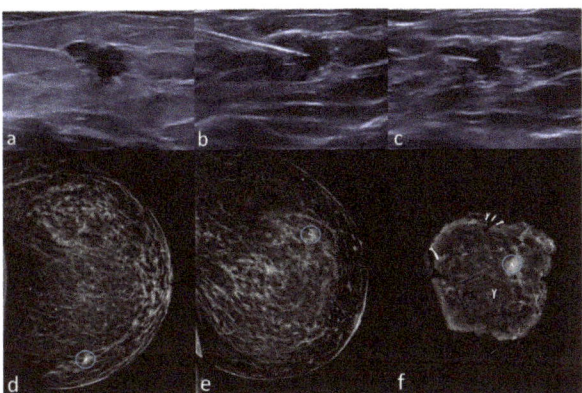

Figure 3. Magseed placement under ultrasound guidance. Preoperative ultrasound localization of a non-palpable, hypoechoic lesion (invasive ductal carcinoma) in the left upper inner quadrant (**a**), and placement of Magseed inside the lesion (**b**,**c**). Preoperative mammogram in two views confirms the correct placement of the Magseed (blue circle, (**d**,**e**)). The surgical specimen shows the presence of both the tumor and Magseed (blue circle, (**f**)).

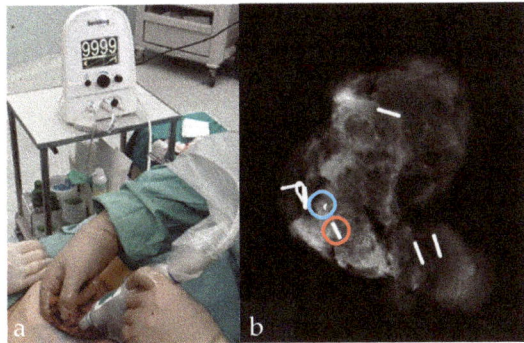

Figure 4. The SentiMag probe (**a**), used intraoperatively to locate the Magseed using a small and transient magnetic field that magnetizes the clip making it recognizable to the probe itself. In (**b**) radiographic examination of the surgical specimen shows the Magseed (red circle) adjacent to the previously clipped lesion (blue circle).

3. Results

A total of 45 patients were included in the study. The mean patient age was 57, 58 years (range 31–80). The preoperative mean size of the breast lesions was 8.8 millimeters (mm) (range 3–18 mm) (Table 1). The patients enrolled in the study underwent BCS. The intraoperative widening and the re-excision rate for positive margins were 0% (Table 1).

Table 1. Clinical and surgical data. Millimeters (mm). Ductal carcinoma in situ (DCIS). Invasive ductal carcinoma (IDC). B3 lesions according to the lexicon BI-RADS®.

Patients Age (Years)	57.58 (range 31–80)
Breast lesions dimension (mm)	8.8 (range 3–18)
Type of surgery: Lumpectomy Quadrantectomy	3 43
Re-excision rate	0%

Table 1. *Cont.*

Intraoperative widening	0%
Post-operative histology:	
DCIS	4 (8.8%)
IDC	35 (77.8%)
B3	6 (13.4%)

The pathological examination found a prevalence of malignant lesions, of which 77.8% were invasive ductal carcinoma (IDC) and 8.8% ductal carcinoma in situ (DCIS), while the remaining 13.4% were B3 lesions [11] (Table 1).

Magseed localization features were reported in Table 2. A total of 40 magnetic seeds were placed under ultrasound guidance (88.9%) and 5 under stereotactic guidance (11.1%) (Table 2). No immediate complications after placement were observed (0.0%) and we obtained a high placement success rate (97.8%) since all markers were correctly positioned, except for one case of migration of the marker placed under stereotactic guidance (2.2%) (Figure 5). All magnetic seeds were recovered in the surgical specimens (100%) (Table 2).

Table 2. Magseed localization data. Days (d). Minutes (min).

Total Magseed Placed	45
Localization modality:	
Ultrasound localization	40 (88.9%)
Stereotactic localization	5 (11.1%)
Seed migration/malpositioning	1 (2.2%)
Successful detection and retrieval	45 (100%)
Time between Magseed placement and surgery (d)	3.46
Time for Magseed placement (min)	5.5

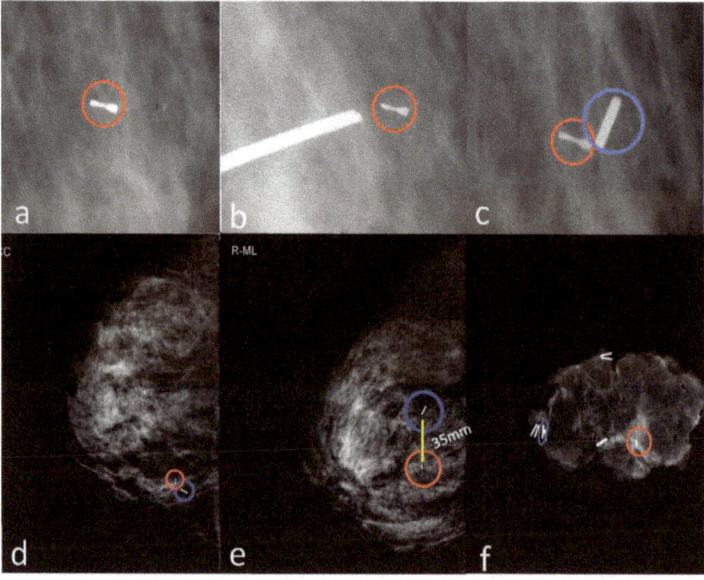

Figure 5. Misplaced Magseed. In (**a**–**c**), the placement of the Magseed (blue circle in (**c**)) under stereotactic guidance in the site of a previous stereotactic biopsy with a metallic clip (the red circles). Preoperative mammography in two views (**d**,**e**) shows a cranial displacement of the Magseed (blue circles in (**e**)) at a distance of 35 millimeters (mm) from the biopsy-clipped lesion (red circles). The surgical specimen radiogram reveals the Magseed (blue circle) and the clipped lesion (red circle) (**f**) correctly removed.

Most of the seeds were placed some days before surgery or the same day of surgery (average time was 3.46 days). On average, Magseed placement took about 5.5 min.

4. Discussion

Magseed represents one of the most promising options for the localization of non-palpable breast lesions. Recent data on its use are unarguably encouraging, proving this technique to be extremely effective.

A recent systematic review by Gera et al. [9] demonstrated the effectiveness of the Magseed in localizing non-palpable breast lesions, particularly as compared to the WGL. Indeed, the results obtained from the analysis of 16 studies, with a highly successful localization and retrieval rate (99.86%) and a relatively low re-excision rate (11.25%), support the use of this technique. In a multicenter clinical retrospective trial, Žatecký́a et al. [12] evaluated a pilot use of the magnetic seed in 34 breast tumors. They reported negative margins after surgery in 29 out of 34 (85.3%) patients. Positive resection margins were found in 4 out of 34 patients (11.8%), and 1 case of seed migration was reported, with a rate of 14.7% (5/34) re-excision rate. Several studies reported no seed migration after perioperative tumor marking [13,14], being this a rare occurrence. The experience of our center is consistent with previous literature with a highly successful localization rate (97.8%); conversely, compared to other studies, our intraoperative widening and re-excision rate are lower (0%), with 0% of positive margins.

As we said above, one of the benefits of the Magseed is the possibility to deploy the seed several days ahead of surgery, enabling a more efficient and flexible organization of the workflow [15]. For this reason, the magnetic seed could be useful in case of a long follow-up, especially during neoadjuvant chemotherapy, despite the well-known signal-void MRI artifact [7]. This limitation significantly affects image quality and can, in some cases, hamper the use of the MRI for the follow-up after therapy. However, contrast-enhanced mammography can be chosen as a good and performing alternative for those patients with wider artifacts. We reported a mean time of 3.46 days between seed deployment and the day of surgery, even if most of the localizations took place on the same day of the surgery. We reported one case (2.2%) of seed migration, which is in line with the literature [14].

One limitation of the magnetic seed is related to the depth of the lesion in the breast, measured as its distance from the skin. As we stated in the introduction, Magseed is considered detectable within a distance of around 4 cm away from the SentiMag, making it harder for deeper lesions to be found [8,15]. However, many studies in literature report that intraoperatively using palpation with the detector, seeds far deeper were detected [9,15]. Given this, it may be preferable for extremely deep lesions to use WGL. Another important aspect that disincentives the use of Magseed is the cost [16]. In our analysis, we have not considered either.

This study has some limitations. The experience was limited to one center, and above all, it included a small cohort of patients. Moreover, we did not analyze some variables (e.g., depth from the skin of the breast lesion and Magseed costs), and the time between Magseed placement and surgery was short (3.46 days), probably affecting the data regarding the seed migration.

5. Conclusions

With the limits mentioned above, our single-center experience is consistent with the data reported in literature, suggesting this technique is effective in the preoperative localization of non-palpable breast lesions.

Future studies including a bigger sample size and a longer time interval between seed placement and surgery are needed to validate our results.

Author Contributions: Conceptualization, A.D. and C.M.L.T.; methodology, S.P. and F.F.; formal analysis, S.L.C., M.C. and S.D.; investigation, S.L.C. and V.L.; resources, R.M.; data curation, F.C. and A.F.; writing—original draft preparation, F.C., L.S. and A.D.; writing—review and editing, C.M.L.T. and A.D.; visualization, P.B. and R.M.; supervision, P.B. and R.M. All authors have read and agreed to the published version of the manuscript.

Funding: This research received no external funding.

Institutional Review Board Statement: The study was conducted in accordance with the Declaration of Helsinki, and approved by the Institutional Review Board of Fondazione Policlinico Universitario "A. Gemelli", IRCCS.

Informed Consent Statement: Informed consent was obtained from all subjects involved in the study.

Data Availability Statement: Not applicable.

Conflicts of Interest: The authors declare no conflict of interest.

References

1. Sung, H.; Ferlay, J.; Siegel, R.L.; Laversanne, M.; Soerjomataram, I.; Jemal, A.; Bray, F. Global Cancer Statistics 2020: GLOBOCAN Estimates of Incidence and Mortality Worldwide for 36 Cancers in 185 Countries. *CA Cancer J. Clin.* **2021**, *71*, 209–249. [CrossRef] [PubMed]
2. Benson, J.R.; Jatoi, I.; Keisch, M.; Esteva, F.J.; Makris, A.; Jordan, V.C. Early Breast Cancer. *Lancet* **2009**, *373*, 1463–1479. [CrossRef]
3. Paganelli, G.; Luini, A.; Veronesi, U. Radioguided occult lesion localization (ROLL) in breast cancer: Maximizing efficacy, minimizing mutilation. *Ann. Oncol.* **2002**, *13*, 1839–1840. [CrossRef]
4. Wazir, U.; Tayeh, S.; Perry, N.; Michell, M.; Malhotra, A.; Mokbel, K. Wireless Breast Localization Using Radio-frequency Identification Tags: The First Reported European Experience in Breast Cancer. *In Vivo* **2020**, *34*, 233–238. [CrossRef]
5. Wazir, U.; Kasem, I.; Michell, M.J.; Suaris, T.; Evans, D.; Malhotra, A.; Mokbel, K. Reflector-Guided Localisation of Non-Palpable Breast Lesions: A Prospective Evaluation of the SAVI SCOUT® System. *Cancers* **2021**, *13*, 2409. [CrossRef] [PubMed]
6. Kurita, T.; Taruno, K.; Nakamura, S.; Takei, H.; Enokido, K.; Kuwayama, T.; Kanada, Y.; Akashi-Tanaka, S.; Matsuyanagi, M.; Hankyo, M.; et al. Magnetically Guided Localization Using a Guiding-Marker System® and a Handheld Magnetic Probe for Nonpalpable Breast Lesions: A Multicenter Feasibility Study in Japan. *Cancers* **2021**, *13*, 2923. [CrossRef] [PubMed]
7. Žatecký, J.; Kubala, O.; Jelínek, P.; Lerch, M.; Ihnát, P.; Peteja, M.; Brát, R. Magnetic marker localisation in breast cancer surgery. *Arch. Med. Sci.* **2020**, *16*, 383–388. [CrossRef]
8. Gray, R.J.; Salud, C.; Nguyen, K.; Dauway, E.; Friedland, J.; Berman, C.; Peltz, E.; Whitehead, G.; Cox, C.E. Randomized Prospective Evaluation of a Novel Technique for Biopsy or Lumpectomy of Nonpalpable Breast Lesions: Radioactive Seed Versus Wire Localization. *Ann. Surg. Oncol.* **2001**, *8*, 711–715. [CrossRef] [PubMed]
9. Gera, R.; Tayeh, S.; Al-Reefy, S.; Mokbel, K. Evolving Role of Magseed in Wireless Localization of Breast Lesions: Systematic Review and Pooled Analysis of 1,559 Procedures. *Anticancer Res.* **2020**, *40*, 1809–1815. [CrossRef] [PubMed]
10. Fleming, F.; Hill, A.; Mc Dermott, E.; O'Doherty, A.; O'Higgins, N.; Quinn, C. Intraoperative margin assessment and re-excision rate in breast conserving surgery. *Eur. J. Surg. Oncol.* **2004**, *30*, 233–237. [CrossRef] [PubMed]
11. Rao, A.A.; Feneis, J.; LaLonde, C.; Ojeda-Fournier, H. A Pictorial Review of Changes in the BI-RADS Fifth Edition. *RadioGraphics* **2016**, *36*, 623–639. [CrossRef] [PubMed]
12. Žatecký, J.; Kubala, O.; Coufal, O.; Kepičová, M.; Faridová, A.; Rauš, K.; Lerch, M.; Peteja, M.; Brát, R. Magnetic Seed (Magseed) Localisation in Breast Cancer Surgery: A Multicentre Clinical Trial. *Breast Care* **2020**, *16*, 383–388. [CrossRef] [PubMed]
13. Harvey, J.R.; Lim, Y.; Murphy, J.; Howe, M.; Morris, J.; Goyal, A.; Maxwell, A.J. Safety and feasibility of breast lesion localization using magnetic seeds (Magseed): A multi-centre, open-label cohort study. *Breast Cancer Res. Treat.* **2018**, *169*, 531–536. [CrossRef] [PubMed]
14. Hersi, A.-F.; Eriksson, S.; Ramos, J.; Abdsaleh, S.; Wärnberg, F.; Karakatsanis, A. A combined, totally magnetic technique with a magnetic marker for non-palpable tumour localization and superparamagnetic iron oxide nanoparticles for sentinel lymph node detection in breast cancer surgery. *Eur. J. Surg. Oncol.* **2019**, *45*, 544–549. [CrossRef] [PubMed]
15. Price, E.R.; Khoury, A.L.; Esserman, L.J.; Joe, B.N.; Alvarado, M.D. Initial Clinical Experience With an Inducible Magnetic Seed System for Preoperative Breast Lesion Localization. *Am. J Roentgenol.* **2018**, *210*, 913–917. [CrossRef] [PubMed]
16. Tayeh, S.; Gera, R.; Perry, N.; Michell, M.; Malhotra, A.; Mokbel, K. The Use of Magnetic Seeds and Radiofrequency Identifier Tags in Breast Surgery for Non-palpable Lesions. *Anticancer Res.* **2020**, *40*, 315–321. [CrossRef] [PubMed]

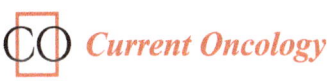

Review

Estrogen-Receptor-Low-Positive Breast Cancer: Pathological and Clinical Perspectives

Christina Panagiotis Malainou, Nikolina Stachika, Aikaterini Konstantina Damianou, Aristotelis Anastopoulos, Ioanna Ploumaki, Efthymios Triantafyllou, Konstantinos Drougkas, Georgia Gomatou * and Elias Kotteas

Oncology Unit, Third Department of Medicine, "Sotiria" General Hospital for Diseases of the Chest, National and Kapodistrian University of Athens, 152 Messogion Avenue, 11527 Athens, Greece; ilkotteas@med.uoa.gr (E.K.)
* Correspondence: georgiagom@med.uoa.gr

Citation: Malainou, C.P.; Stachika, N.; Damianou, A.K.; Anastopoulos, A.; Ploumaki, I.; Triantafyllou, E.; Drougkas, K.; Gomatou, G.; Kotteas, E. Estrogen-Receptor-Low-Positive Breast Cancer: Pathological and Clinical Perspectives. *Curr. Oncol.* 2023, *30*, 9734–9745. https://doi.org/10.3390/curroncol30110706

Received: 23 September 2023
Revised: 30 October 2023
Accepted: 2 November 2023
Published: 4 November 2023

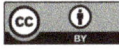

Copyright: © 2023 by the authors. Licensee MDPI, Basel, Switzerland. This article is an open access article distributed under the terms and conditions of the Creative Commons Attribution (CC BY) license (https://creativecommons.org/licenses/by/4.0/).

Abstract: The expression of estrogen receptors (ERs) in breast cancer (BC) represents a strong prognostic and predictive biomarker and directs therapeutic decisions in early and advanced stages. ER-low-positive BC, defined by the immunohistochemical (IHC) expression of ERs from 1% to 9%, constitutes a distinct subset of total BC cases. Guidelines recommend that a low expression of ERs be reported in pathology reports since the benefit of endocrine therapy in patients with ER-low-positive BC is uncertain. Recently, several cohorts, mostly of a retrospective nature, have been published, reporting the clinicopathological characteristics and outcomes of ER-low-positive BC. However, the majority of the data focus on early-stage BC and the use of (neo)adjuvant therapy, and there is a significant lack of data regarding metastatic ER-low-positive BC. Further factors, including tumor heterogeneity as well as the potential loss of ER expression due to endocrine resistance, should be considered. Including patients with ER-low-positive BC in clinical trials for triple-negative breast cancer (TNBC) might improve the understanding of this entity and allow novel therapeutic approaches. The design and conduct of randomized clinical trials regarding this subgroup of patients are greatly anticipated.

Keywords: estrogen receptor; breast cancer; estrogen receptor-low-positive breast cancer; endocrine therapy; triple-negative breast cancer

1. Introduction

Hormone receptors (HR), including estrogen (ER) and progesterone receptors (PR), are expressed in 70–75% of breast cancer (BC) cases and represent one of the cornerstones that direct the therapeutic decisions for patients with BC both in early and metastatic stages [1,2]. The 2020 update of the recommendations of the American Society of Clinical Oncology/College of American Pathology (ASCO/CAP) defines ER-positive BC as samples with 1% or more of tumor nuclei positive for ER expression by validated immunohistochemistry (IHC). Nevertheless, the recommendations outline that a small subset of patients with ER expression between 1 and 10% should be termed ER-low-positive BC and are not likely to benefit from endocrine therapy (ET) [3]. A lack of consensus exists regarding whether the exact 10% expression should be considered ER-low-positive or ER-positive. Hence, the definition of ER-low expression differs in the literature as either 1 to 9% or 1 to 10% [4].

ER-low BC is associated with interesting biological aspects, but it also poses several challenges regarding its management. A low expression of ERs might be observed de novo, or it might develop in the course of the disease [5,6]. In addition, it should be noted that tumors are heterogeneous entities; therefore, the expression of ERs derived from a specific biopsy might not represent the expression in the whole tumor [5]. The optimal management of patients with ER-low BC in early and metastatic settings has not been defined yet. Several recent studies, mostly of a retrospective nature, have described the features of ER-low BC and assessed the benefit of ET, mainly in an adjuvant setting. In the present review, we attempt to summarize the literature and shed light on the biological and clinical perspectives of ER-low BC.

2. Estrogens and ER-Mediated Signaling Pathways

Estrogens, known as female sex hormones, play a crucial role in the development and function of the female reproductive system and secondary sex characteristics. They also affect other systems, such as the cardiovascular, musculoskeletal, central nervous and immune systems [7,8]. Four steroid hormones belong to the estrogen family: estrone, estradiol, estriol and estretrol [7]. Estriol and estretrol are present mainly in the course of pregnancy. Estrone is present during menopause, while estradiol is the predominant form during the reproductive years [9]. Estradiol promotes cell proliferation in the endometrium and mammary gland starting from puberty, while during pregnancy, the dominant forms prepare the mammary gland for milk production [7].

At the cellular level, estrogens act through their receptors, the estrogen receptors a (ERa) and b (ERb), which are part of the nuclear receptor family and are encoded by two different genes, *ESR1* and *ESR2* [7]. Similarly to other nuclear receptors [7], their structure enables them to bind with their ligands but also to DNA and act as transcription factors with the aid of other co-activators and co-repressors [9,10]. The isoforms ERa and ERb are highly similar except for their NH2-terminal domain (NTD), which is involved in gene transcription activation [9].

Estrogens pass through the cellular plasma membrane and interact with their receptors via their ligand binding domain (LBD). From this point, they activate several signaling pathways, which can be divided into genomic and non-genomic based on the ability of the hormone-receptor complex to bind directly to the DNA chain at specific domains, known as estrogen response elements (EREs) [9,11]. Moreover, rapid responses to estrogens have been observed, which do not involve genomic signaling and are known as indirect non-genomic signaling. They are mediated through second messenger production and protein kinase activation pathways, leading to signaling cascades that ultimately regulate gene expression. The most important intracellular cascades involve the phospholipase C/protein kinase C cascade, the mitogen-activated protein kinase (MAPK) pathway, the phosphoinositide 3-kinase (PI3K) pathway and the cyclic adenosine monophosphate (cAMP)/protein kinase A cascade [9,12]. For example, the PI3K/protein kinase B (AKT)/mammalian target of the rapamycin (mTOR) pathway, activated by non-genomic estrogen signaling, has been found to be overactive in up to 70% of BCs and is related to ET resistance after long-term estrogen deprivation [13]. Interestingly, crosstalk between non-genomic and genomic signaling pathways has been described, leading to the regulation of transcription factors by protein-kinase-mediated phosphorylation [11].

Progesterone is another steroid hormone involved in the proliferation and morphogenesis of the luminal epithelium, primarily through paracrine signaling pathways. Progesterone binds to a nuclear receptor, the progesterone receptor (PR) [14]. It should be noted that PR expression depends on estrogen levels since PR is a target gene of an ER [15]. Although the expression of the PR is routinely assessed in BC, the clinical value of PR expression is not so strongly established as it is for ER expression; rather, the presence of an intact and functionally active ER pathway is implied when the PR is expressed [16].

3. ER-Low-Positive BC

3.1. Epidemiology and Clinicopathological Characteristics

Although ER-low-positive BC represents a small subset of all patients with BC, it is important to understand its nature to provide tailored and effective treatment [5]. Lately, several studies have been published reporting the prevalence and characteristics of ER-low BC as well as their response to treatment.

The prevalence of ER-low BC varies from 1.6 to 5.1%, as reported in recent large-scale cohorts (Table 1) [4,17–24]. Interestingly, Makhlouf et al. performed a re-evaluation of ER status in cases considered ER-low-positive at initial evaluation and demonstrated that 45% of these tumors were ER-negative with repeated IHC staining, confirmed by in situ hybridization (ISH) and a quantitative polymerase chain reaction (qPCR). In particular, ER-low-positive samples derived from needle core biopsies were enriched with false-positive ER staining [4]. In the same study, they focused on tumors with precisely 10% ER expression. The results revealed that those cases were significantly lower grade and more PR-positive than tumors with an ER expression of 1–9% and did not show a significant difference from tumors with an ER expression of 11–30% [4].

Table 1. The prevalence of ER-low-positive breast cancer.

Author (Year)	N	Prevalence of ER-Low BC	Reference
Makhlouf (2023)	7559	1.6% (123/7559)	[4]
Moldoveanu (2023)	232,762 [a]	2.0% (4584/232,762)	[17]
Li (2023)	9082	3.29% (299/9082)	[18]
Luo (2022)	5466 [b]	5.1% (277/5466)	[19]
Yoon (2022)	2162 [b]	2.5% (54/2162)	[20]
Park (2021)	5930 [b]	2.0% (117/5930)	[21]
Schrodi (2021)	38,560 [b]	2.0% (861/38,560)	[22]
Fei (2021)	4179	2.3% (97/4179)	[23]
Poon (2020)	1824	3% (54/1824)	[24]

[a] only HER2 (−) [b] only early breast cancer cases. ER: estrogen receptor, BC: breast cancer, HER2: human epidermal growth factor receptor 2.

Regarding the characteristics of patients with ER-low BC, a study showed that ER-high-positive, ER-low-positive and ER-negative BC had no statistical difference related to the age of menarche and body mass index kg/m^2 [25]. Among patients with ER-high-positive BC, there were significantly more white patients compared to ER-low-positive BC (93.9% vs. 82.9%, $p < 0.05$) [25]. Indeed, it appears that a patient's profile is similar between ER-low and triple-negative breast cancer (TNBC), as reported in a multicenter prospective registry between 2011 and 2019. The study showed that demographic and clinical characteristics, including racial and ethnic distribution—it is well-known that TNBC is more prevalent among the African American race—and the prevalence of germline BRCA1/2 mutations were not different between the TNBC and ER-low groups [26].

Several studies have investigated the morphological and immunohistochemical characteristics of ER-low-positive BC in relation to ER-negative and ER-high-positive BC. ER-low BCs are more likely to have a ductal phenotype of a higher histological grade compared to ER-high BCs (83.5% vs. 71.4%, $p = 0.005$) [23]. In another study, ER-low-positive cases were associated with larger tumors, higher grades, more necrosis, more stromal tumor infiltrating lymphocytes (sTILs) and a higher pathologic N stage [24]. In particular, regarding sTILs, the ER-low-positive cases were associated with more sTILs than the ER-high-positive cases, whereas no difference was found between ER-low-positive and ER-negative tumors. A further survival analysis demonstrated that higher sTIL levels are associated with reduced mortality in ER-negative and ER-low-positive BC [24]. Cases of BC with 1–9% ER expression are more likely to have a higher Ki-67 index and are more likely to be PR-negative [27–29]. Moreover, a recent study demonstrated that HER2-low expression was positively associated with the level of ER expression, and ER-low-positive tumors were enriched among HER2 0–2+ tumors [30].

Additionally, studies with further IHC and molecular analyses have demonstrated that vimentin, the epidermal growth factor receptor (EGFR), CPK5/6, and CK14 are highly expressed in ER-low-positive or negative BC and less expressed in ER-high-positive BC [5]. ER-high-positive BCs are more frequently negative for C-kit, p63 and the androgen receptor (AR) compared to ER-low-positive or ER-negative BC [24]. A decrease in vimentin expression was correlated with an increase in ER expression in an older study [31]. In addition, the expression of the *ESR1* gene has been investigated among cases with ER-low-positive BC. Iwamoto et al. reported that the average *ESR1* expression was significantly increased in the ≥10% ER-positive group compared to the 1% to 9% ER expression or ER-negative groups [32]. Consistent findings were reported in a recent study where the average *ESR1* expression was significantly higher in the ER-high-positive cohort than in the ER-low or negative cohort [19]. However, in another study that evaluated the expression levels of a selected set of ER-regulated genes, namely *ESR1*, *PgR*, *GATA3*, *TFF1*, *FOXA1* and *XBP1* along with a panel of three reference genes, the results demonstrated that the tumors in the ER-low group were almost evenly distributed between the ER-high-positive and negative groups [33]. ER-low BCs are more likely to carry a *BRCA1* or *BRCA2* mutation, and this finding indicates the need for genetic counseling and *BRCA* testing in this subset of patients [34]. High frequencies of *TP53* but not *PIK3CA* mutations have been shown in ER-low-positive BC Furthermore, a recent study investigated the prognostic role of H3 lysine nine trimethylation (H3K9me3) in relation to ER status. ER-positive tumors were stratified by ER-low and ER-high-positive tumors, and the prognostic role of H3K9me3 was significant only among the ER-high-positive patients, indicating distinct pathogenicity among the two groups [35].

3.2. Prognosis and (Neo)adjuvant Therapy

Most data on the prognosis of ER-low-positive BC are obtained from retrospective studies mainly involving patients with early BC (Table 2). A large-scale retrospective study from Europe showed that the time to local recurrence, time to lymph node recurrence and time to metastasis among HER2-negative BC were similar in ER-low and ER-negative BC and higher compared to ER-high-positive BC [22]. Notably, in the category of HER2-positive BC, ER-low-positive, ER-negative and ER-high-positive BC did not have significant differences in terms of prognosis. The authors conclude that HER2-negative and concomitantly ER-low-positive BC resemble TNBC [22]. A large cohort from Korea reported consistent findings. In this epidemiological retrospective study, the highest 5-year disease-free survival (DFS) rate was observed in patients in the ER-high/HER2-negative cohort (94.0%), and the lowest 5-year DFS rates were in patients in the TNBC cohort (81.3%) and the ER-low/HER2-negative cohort (85.7%) [21]. The shorter DFS for the TNBC and ER-low/HER2-negative combined cohorts were significantly correlated with higher tumor stage, lymphovascular invasion, greater regional lymph node involvement, and larger tumor size [21]. The patients with ER-low BC had a statistically significant worse DFS and overall survival (OS) compared with patients with ER-positive BC, whereas no differences were reported between the ER-low and ER-negative subgroups in a meta-analysis of retrospective studies that included patients with BC who received neoadjuvant chemotherapy (NAC) [36]. However, it should be noted that a recent study from Norway that included women diagnosed with BC in 1995 or later demonstrated that the cumulative risk of death from BC was 22.3% after five years for ER expression < 1% and 8.3% for both the ER-low-positive and ER expression ≥ 10% groups, meaning that there was no apparent difference in the risk of death from BC between the ER-low-positive and ER expression > 10% groups [37].

An important and relevant question is whether adjuvant ET confers survival benefits in patients with ER-low-positive BC. In 2011, the Early Breast Cancer Trialists' Collaborative Group conducted a patient-level meta-analysis aiming to associate the levels of ER expression with the recurrence reduction with the use of 5-year adjuvant tamoxifen [38]. The results showed a significant benefit in the subgroup analysis even for patients with marginally ER-positive BC (10–19 fmol/mg cytosol protein) from tamoxifen (risk ratio ± standard error, 0.67 ± 0.08) [38]. Nevertheless, several recent retrospective studies have not confirmed this finding. In a retrospective study of 9639 patients with early BC, it was reported that (a) no significant difference was observed in recurrences between patients with ER-low and ER-negative tumors (19.4%) ($p = 0.5$), (b) for patients receiving ET, recurrence rates were higher in patients whose tumors were ER-low-positive compared with those that were ER-positive with ER expression ≥ 10% (17.7% versus 7.7%, $p = 0.02$) and (c) there was no significant difference in total recurrences between the groups of patients who did not receive ET [39]. Another study showed that the 5-year DFS and OS did not significantly differ between ER-negative and ER-low-positive groups, irrespective of receiving endocrine treatment [40]. A lack of benefit from ET in patients with ER-low BC has recently been shown in a meta-analysis, including more than 16,000 patients. This meta-analysis indicated that patients with early BC and ER expression between 1 and 9% gained no significant survival benefit from ET but exhibited a better overall prognosis than patients with ER expression < 1% [41]. Nevertheless, a recent study demonstrated that ET was correlated with increased breast cancer-specific survival in patients with ER-low BC. No significant difference in breast cancer-specific survival was observed between patients who received 2–3 years and >3 years of ET [42]. The potential of a de-escalation strategy was also suggested in a recent propensity-matched analysis, which reported that there was no significant difference in DFS between patients who received 2–3 years and five years of ET (HR, 0.82; 95% CI, 0.51–1.33; p = 0.43), indicating that short-term ET for 2 to 3 years might be an alternative for patients who have ER-low-positive BC [43].

Table 2. Recent studies on prognosis of patients with early-stage ER-low BC.

Author (Year)	Type of Study	Results	Reference
Schrodi (2021)	Retrospective population-based cohort study	Significantly decreased OS of ER-low/HER2(−) compared to ER-positive/HER2(−)	[22]
Park (2021)	Retrospective unicentric cohort	DFS and OS in the ER-low/HER2(−) cohort were more similar to the TNBC cohort than those with ER-high/HER2(−) BC	[21]
Paakkola (2021)	Meta-analysis	Significantly worse DFS and OS of ER-low patients compared to patients with ER-positive BC	[36]
Skjervold (2023)	Retrospective population-based cohort study	No significant difference in prognosis (risk of death from BC) of patients with ER-low BC compared to those with ER-positive BC for patients diagnosed after 1995	[37]

OS: overall survival; ER: estrogen receptor; HER2: human epidermal growth factor 2; DFS: disease-free survival; TNBC: triple-negative breast cancer; BC: breast cancer.

In early-stage ER-positive BC, the decision to offer adjuvant chemotherapy depends on the risk of recurrence, which is assessed with clinicopathological criteria and genomic tests [1]. Assuming that a case of ER-low-positive BC is diagnosed in an early stage, without lymph nodes or with minimal node involvement (1–3 lymph nodes), it is reasonable to ask whether using genomic tests is of the same utility as for ER-high BC [44]. A recent study evaluated the role of the Oncotype Dx Breast Recurrence Score Assay in 38 patients with ER-low-positive BC [45]. The results revealed that the majority of the patients with HER2-negative/ER-low-positive BC had a recurrence score (RS) > 25, and the authors concluded that perhaps genomic tests are of limited use as most patients are likely to benefit from adjuvant chemotherapy [45].

Furthermore, NAC therapy is sometimes indicated in early ER-positive BC in order to downstage the tumor; however, it is well known that patients with ER-positive BC are not likely to achieve a pathologic complete response (pCR), contrary to patients with TNBC and HER2-positive disease. It has been reported that the pCR rate of patients with ER-low BC was intermediate between the pCR rate of patients with ER-high and ER-negative BC following NAC treatment [46]. In another study, among 358 patients receiving NAC, the pCR rates were similar for the TNBC and ER-low-positive groups (49.2% vs. 51.3%, respectively, p = 0.808) [26]. Moreover, in a cohort of 165 patients that received NAC, the pCR rate was comparable between the two groups (38% in the ER-negative group, 44% in the ER-low-positive group, p = 0.498) [47]. Interestingly, Fujii et al. identified 9.5% ER expression as the cut-off percentage below which a pCR was likely [48]. Additionally, when comparing ER-negative, ER-low, and ER-high-positive BC in NAC clinical trial cohorts (n = 2765), the results demonstrated no significant differences in the pCR rates between women with ER-low-positive tumors and women with TNBC [49]. In general, the significant pCR rates in TNBC cases are attributed to the higher cell proliferation rates compared to ER-positive BC [50]. The addition of immunotherapy has also increased the rates of pCR in TNBC, which is mainly relevant for the immunogenic subtypes of the disease [50]. It has been suggested that patients with ER-low and HER2-negative BC could be included in the clinical trials of NAC for TNBC and potentially share the same benefit from the addition of immunotherapy, as discussed below [50].

3.3. Immune Microenvironment and Immunotherapy

Given the remarkable advances in the field of oncology immunotherapeutics, particular interest lies in the potential of immunotherapy in BC. In general, ER-negative tumors are characterized by increased sTIL infiltration, CD8 + T-cells, and a higher expression of immune-related gene sets, resulting in a more inflamed tumor microenvironment, while ER-positive BC is traditionally considered to be an immunologically "cold" tumor [51,52].

The immunological features of HER2-negative BC with low-positive (1–9%) or intermediate-positive (10–50%) ER expression were investigated in a recent study, as compared to TNBC and tumors with high ER expression (>50%) [53]. The results showed that among the groups of BC with an ER expression of 0%, an ER expression of 1–9% and an ER expression of 10–50%, the levels of stromal TILs, CD8 + T cells and PD-L1 positivity were similar [53]. Also, the expression of certain immune-related gene signatures in tumors with an ER expression of 1–9% and an ER expression of 10–50% was analogous to an ER expression of 0% and higher than in tumors with an ER expression of 51–99% and an ER expression of 100% [53]. Although there is currently no data on patients with ER-low BC who received immunotherapy in early or metastatic settings, since ER-low BC biologically mimics TNBC, it has been suggested that those patients could be included in clinical trials of TNBC and potentially derive benefit from immunotherapy [50]. However, it should be noted that TNBC exhibits a great degree of heterogeneity and includes several phenotypes, not all of which are immunogenic [50]. The presumed biological similarities between ER-low-positive BC and TNBC might be limited to particular phenotypes of TNBC and need to be further explored.

4. Knowledge and Research Gaps in ER-Low-Positive BC (Figure 1)
4.1. Early-Stage ER-Low-Positive BC

Accumulating evidence has been published questioning the benefit of adjuvant ET for patients with ER-low-positive BC; however, the data remain contradictory [38,39,41,42]. The retrospective nature of the majority of the studies, the heterogeneous design and the different endpoints limit the drawing of clear conclusions. Notably, at the 17th St. Gallen International Breast Cancer Consensus in 2021, the panel was dichotomized on the optimal ER threshold for endocrine therapy initiation [54]. The duration of ET could also be discussed, with some studies suggesting an alternative option with short-term adjuvant ET [42,43].

Besides adjuvant ET, numerous questions arise concerning the following: (a) when should NAC therapy be proposed for patients with ER-low BC and which is the optimal regimen; (b) should the majority of the patients with ER-low BC receive adjuvant chemotherapy; and (c) what is the role of adjuvant cyclin-dependent kinase (CDK)4/6 inhibitor therapy, which has been recently introduced in high-risk patients with ER-positive BC [44]. The stratification of patients according to ER status, including the ER-low-positive group, in randomized clinical trials might improve the understanding of those questions. In parallel, the introduction of patients with ER-low BC in clinical trials of TNBC may illustrate better tactics for their management. A recent phase II trial (NeoPACT) assessing the addition of pembrolizumab in carboplatin plus docetaxel in patients with TNBC allowed for the inclusion of patients with ER-low BC, who comprised 15% of the study population [55].

4.2. Metastatic ER-Low-Positive BC

There is a significant lack of published real-world cohorts regarding patients with metastatic ER-low-positive BC. The combination of a CDK 4/6 inhibitor plus ET, the current standard of care for ER-positive BC, is theoretically indicated in these cases [2]. However, should these patients be assumed to be mostly endocrine-resistant and more chemo-sensitive? In parallel, the introduction of immunotherapy for metastatic TNBC raises the question of the potential benefit to the biologically similar ER-low-positive BC.

The latest European School of Oncology/European Society of Medical Oncology (ESO/ESMO) consensus guidelines recommend that the 2020 ASCO/CAP acknowledgment that patients with tumors with ER staining between 1% and 10% represent a new reporting category with proximity to ER-negative BC, without solid data concerning the benefit from ET, should also be adopted for patients with metastatic BC with a low ER-positive status [56]. In particular, the guidelines state that patients with ER-low-positive and HER2-negative metastatic BC should not be considered for ET exclusively and could be considered patients with TNBC for clinical trials [56].

4.3. ER Expression Heterogeneity

The identification of low ER expression in a single biopsy might not reflect the expression pattern of the whole tumor mass(es). It has been observed that BC exhibits a degree of genotypic and phenotypic heterogeneity, which could be distinguished into intertumor and intratumor heterogeneity [57]. The expression of ERs could be different between primary and metastatic lesions or in different parts of the same tumor. This phenomenon cannot be currently encompassed in a single pathology report, especially when the biopsy is small [58].

For example, the hormone receptors' conversion in metastatic BCs, either from a positive primary tumor to a negative metastasis or the opposite, has been reported as high as 18.3% for ERs and 40.3% for the PR [59]. Such discordance could mislead the selection of an effective therapy, especially when only one biopsy is available and it may not reflect the phenotype of the whole tumor [58,60]. The latest guidelines recommend considering the use of ET whenever ER expression is positive in at least one biopsy, even in cases of discordance between ER expression in primary and metastatic samples [56]. Identifying and quantifying the heterogeneity is of utmost importance, as it has a significant role in deciding the suitable therapy and predicting the outcome [57]. Perhaps the development, validation and incorporation of liquid biopsies could bypass this obstacle and lead to optimal therapeutic decisions [61,62].

4.4. ER Loss Due to Endocrine Resistance

Endocrine resistance, either primary or secondary, is a major challenge that could occur during the therapy of ER-positive BC [63]. It has been proposed that a proportion of ER-negative and ER-low-positive cells stem from ER-positive cells that lose their ER expression [64]. This alteration could happen spontaneously, due to the selective pressure caused by the absence of estrogen, or even as an adaptive response against specific pharmacological agents [64]. More specifically, it has been shown that a loss of ER expression occurs in approximately 10–20% of the cases during disease progression [63].

The mechanisms involved in the suppression of ER expression include genetic or epigenetic changes in the *ESR1* gene, post-translational modifications or altered receptor tyrosine kinase signaling and cell cycle regulation [63,65,66]. Perhaps the identification of ER-low-positive BC during the disease course could be attributed to ER loss due to endocrine resistance. With an "out-of-the-box" approach, mainly in the pre-clinical research field, we could assume that the finding of ER-low positivity might not preclude ET but rather guide a strategy aiming to reverse this process and re-sensitize the tumor to ET [64].

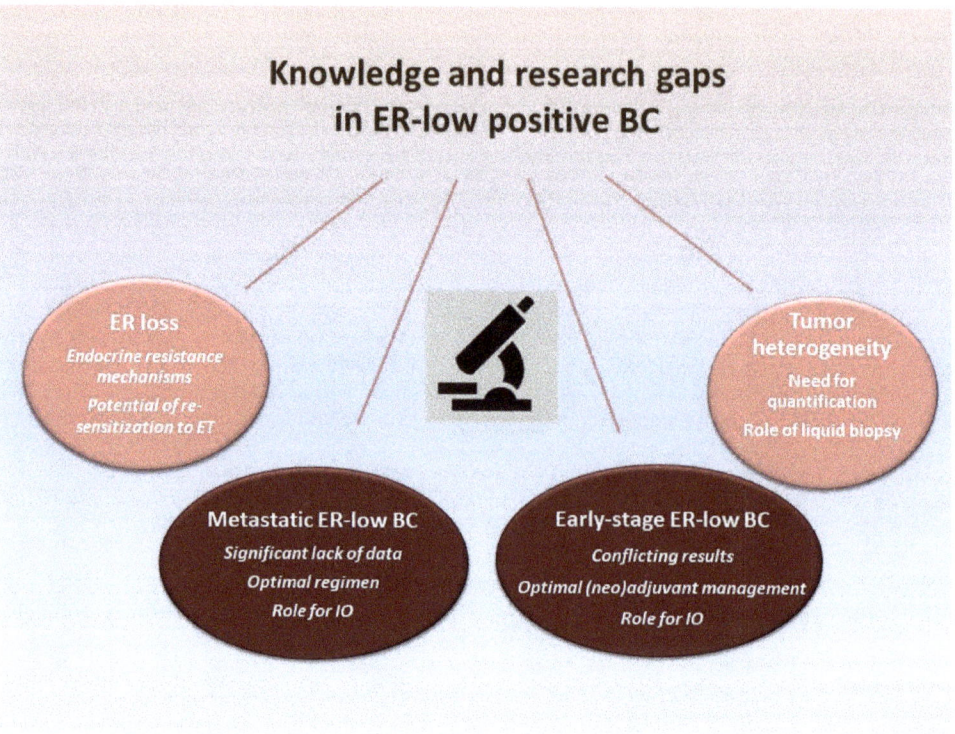

Figure 1. The figure illustrates the research and knowledge gaps regarding ER-low-positive BC. Knowledge and research gaps regarding ER-low-positive BC include the interpretation of conflicting data on early-stage ER-low-positive BC, the significant lack of data on metastatic ER-low BC and incorporating aspects of ER heterogeneity and ER loss due to endocrine resistance. ER: estrogen receptor; BC: breast cancer; ET: endocrine therapy; IO: immunotherapy.

5. Conclusions

ER-low-positive BC comprises a small subgroup of the total BC cases but represents a challenging entity with unclear management. Given the conflicting results leading to uncertainty in clinical practice, the role of biomarkers for predicting the benefit of different therapies should be evaluated, including the expression of PR, HER2 or other immune-related biomarkers, such as the sTILs. The inclusion of those patients in clinical trials for TNBC might provide valuable information regarding better management options; however, the significant heterogeneity of TNBC should be taken into account. Finally, well-designed randomized clinical trials for this well-characterized population are greatly anticipated.

Author Contributions: C.P.M. performed the literature review and wrote the original manuscript, and N.S., A.K.D., A.A., I.P., E.T. and K.D. wrote the revised manuscript and prepared the figure. G.G. and E.K. interpreted the data, critically revised the manuscript and supervised the work. Data authentication is not applicable. All authors have read and agreed to the published version of the manuscript.

Funding: This research received no external funding.

Conflicts of Interest: The authors declare no conflict of interest.

Abbreviations

AKT: Protein Kinase B; AR: Androgen Receptor; ASCO: American Society of Clinical Oncology; BC: Breast Cancer; BRCA1/2: Breast Cancer gene 1/2; cAMP: cyclic Adenosine Monophosphate; CAP: College of American Pathology; CDK: Cyclin-dependent Kinase; CK14: Cytokeratine 14; CPK 5/6: Creatine Phosphokinase; DFS: Disease-Free Survival; DNA: Deoxyribonucleic Acid; EGFR: Epidermal Growth Factor Receptor; ER: Estrogen Receptor; ERE: Estrogen Response Elements; ESMO: European Society of Medical Oncology; ESO: European School of Oncology; ESR1: Estrogen Receptor 1; ET: Endocrine Therapy; FOXA1: Forkhead Box A1; HER2: Human Epidermal Growth Factor Receptor 2; HR: Hormone Receptor; IHC: Immunohistochemistry; IO: Immunotherapy; ISH: In Situ Hybridization; LBD: Ligand-Binding Domain; MAPK: Mitogen-Activated Protein Kinase; mTOR: mammalian Target Of Rapamycin; NAC: Neoadjuvant Chemotherapy; NTD: NH2-Terminal Domain; OS: Overall Survival; P63: Protein 63; pCR: pathologic Complete Response; PD-L1: Programmed Death-Ligand1; PgR: Progesterone Receptor; PI3K: Phosphoinositide-3 Kinase; PIK3CA: Phosphatidylinositol-4,5-Bisphosphate 3-Kinase Catalytic Subunit Alpha; H3K9me3:H3 Lysine 9 Trimethylation; PR: Progesterone Receptor; qPCR: quantative Polymerase Chain Reaction; RS: Recurrence Score; sTILs: stromal Tumor Infiltrating Lymphocytes; TFF1: Trefoil Factor 1; TILs: Tumor-Infiltrating Lymphocytes; TNBC: Triple-Negative Breast Cancer; TP53: Tumor Protein 53; XBP1: X-box Binding Protein 1.

References

1. Cardoso, F.; Kyriakides, S.; Ohno, S.; Penault-Llorca, F.; Poortmans, P.; Rubio, I.T.; Zackrisson, S.; Senkus, E.; ESMO Guidelines Committee. Early breast cancer: ESMO Clinical Practice Guidelines for diagnosis, treatment and follow-updagger. *Ann. Oncol.* **2019**, *30*, 1194–1220. [CrossRef]
2. Gennari, A.; Andre, F.; Barrios, C.H.; Cortes, J.; de Azambuja, E.; DeMichele, A.; Dent, R.; Fenlon, D.; Gligorov, J.; Hurvitz, S.A.; et al. ESMO Clinical Practice Guideline for the diagnosis, staging and treatment of patients with metastatic breast cancer. *Ann. Oncol.* **2021**, *32*, 1475–1495. [CrossRef]
3. Allison, K.H.; Hammond, M.E.H.; Dowsett, M.; McKernin, S.E.; Carey, L.A.; Fitzgibbons, P.L.; Hayes, D.F.; Lakhani, S.R.; Chavez-MacGregor, M.; Perlmutter, J.; et al. Estrogen and Progesterone Receptor Testing in Breast Cancer: ASCO/CAP Guideline Update. *J. Clin. Oncol.* **2020**, *38*, 1346–1366. [CrossRef]
4. Makhlouf, S.; Althobiti, M.; Toss, M.; Muftah, A.A.; Mongan, N.P.; Lee, A.H.S.; Green, A.R.; Rakha, E.A. The Clinical and Biological Significance of Estrogen Receptor-Low Positive Breast Cancer. *Mod. Pathol.* **2023**, *36*, 100284. [CrossRef] [PubMed]
5. Yu, K.D.; Cai, Y.W.; Wu, S.Y.; Shui, R.H.; Shao, Z.M. Estrogen receptor-low breast cancer: Biology chaos and treatment paradox. *Cancer Commun.* **2021**, *41*, 968–980. [CrossRef] [PubMed]
6. Gomatou, G.; Syrigos, N.; Vathiotis, I.A.; Kotteas, E.A. Tumor Dormancy: Implications for Invasion and Metastasis. *Int. J. Mol. Sci.* **2021**, *22*, 4862. [CrossRef]
7. Heldring, N.; Pike, A.; Andersson, S.; Matthews, J.; Cheng, G.; Hartman, J.; Tujague, M.; Strom, A.; Treuter, E.; Warner, M.; et al. Estrogen receptors: How do they signal and what are their targets. *Physiol. Rev.* **2007**, *87*, 905–931. [CrossRef]
8. Tsagkaraki, I.M.; Kourouniotis, C.D.; Gomatou, G.L.; Syrigos, N.K.; Kotteas, E.A. Orbital metastases of invasive lobular breast carcinoma. *Breast Dis.* **2019**, *38*, 85–91. [CrossRef] [PubMed]
9. Fuentes, N.; Silveyra, P. Estrogen receptor signaling mechanisms. *Adv. Protein Chem. Struct. Biol.* **2019**, *116*, 135–170. [CrossRef]
10. Vrtacnik, P.; Ostanek, B.; Mencej-Bedrac, S.; Marc, J. The many faces of estrogen signaling. *Biochem. Med.* **2014**, *24*, 329–342. [CrossRef] [PubMed]
11. Bjornstrom, L.; Sjoberg, M. Mechanisms of estrogen receptor signaling: Convergence of genomic and nongenomic actions on target genes. *Mol. Endocrinol.* **2005**, *19*, 833–842. [CrossRef] [PubMed]
12. Cheskis, B.J.; Greger, J.G.; Nagpal, S.; Freedman, L.P. Signaling by estrogens. *J. Cell. Physiol.* **2007**, *213*, 610–617. [CrossRef] [PubMed]
13. Gomatou, G.; Trontzas, I.; Ioannou, S.; Drizou, M.; Syrigos, N.; Kotteas, E. Mechanisms of resistance to cyclin-dependent kinase 4/6 inhibitors. *Mol. Biol. Rep.* **2021**, *48*, 915–925. [CrossRef] [PubMed]
14. Obr, A.E.; Edwards, D.P. The biology of progesterone receptor in the normal mammary gland and in breast cancer. *Mol. Cell. Endocrinol.* **2012**, *357*, 4–17. [CrossRef]
15. Lashen, A.G.; Toss, M.S.; Mongan, N.P.; Green, A.R.; Rakha, E.A. The clinical value of progesterone receptor expression in luminal breast cancer: A study of a large cohort with long-term follow-up. *Cancer* **2023**, *129*, 1183–1194. [CrossRef]
16. Cui, X.; Schiff, R.; Arpino, G.; Osborne, C.K.; Lee, A.V. Biology of progesterone receptor loss in breast cancer and its implications for endocrine therapy. *J. Clin. Oncol.* **2005**, *23*, 7721–7735. [CrossRef]
17. Moldoveanu, D.; Hoskin, T.L.; Day, C.N.; Schulze, A.K.; Goetz, M.P.; Boughey, J.C. Clinical Behavior, Management, and Treatment Response of Estrogen Receptor Low (1–10%) Breast Cancer. *Ann. Surg. Oncol.* **2023**, *30*, 6475–6483. [CrossRef]

18. Li, M.; Zhou, S.; Lv, H.; Cai, M.; Wan, X.; Lu, H.; Shui, R.; Yang, W. FOXC1 and SOX10 in Estrogen Receptor-Low Positive/HER2-Negative Breast Cancer: Potential Biomarkers for the Basal-like Phenotype Prediction. *Arch. Pathol. Lab. Med.* **2023**. [CrossRef]
19. Luo, C.; Zhong, X.; Fan, Y.; Wu, Y.; Zheng, H.; Luo, T. Clinical characteristics and survival outcome of patients with estrogen receptor low positive breast cancer. *Breast* **2022**, *63*, 24–28. [CrossRef]
20. Yoon, K.H.; Park, Y.; Kang, E.; Kim, E.K.; Kim, J.H.; Kim, S.H.; Suh, K.J.; Kim, S.M.; Jang, M.; Yun, B.; et al. Effect of Estrogen Receptor Expression Level and Hormonal Therapy on Prognosis of Early Breast Cancer. *Cancer Res. Treat.* **2022**, *54*, 1081–1090. [CrossRef]
21. Park, Y.H.; Karantza, V.; Calhoun, S.R.; Park, S.; Lee, S.; Kim, J.Y.; Yu, J.H.; Kim, S.W.; Lee, J.E.; Nam, S.J.; et al. Prevalence, treatment patterns, and prognosis of low estrogen receptor-positive (1% to 10%) breast cancer: A single institution's experience in Korea. *Breast Cancer Res. Treat.* **2021**, *189*, 653–663. [CrossRef] [PubMed]
22. Schrodi, S.; Braun, M.; Andrulat, A.; Harbeck, N.; Mahner, S.; Kiechle, M.; Klein, E.; Schnelzer, A.; Schindlbeck, C.; Bauerfeind, I.; et al. Outcome of breast cancer patients with low hormone receptor positivity: Analysis of a 15-year population-based cohort. *Ann. Oncol.* **2021**, *32*, 1410–1424. [CrossRef] [PubMed]
23. Fei, F.; Siegal, G.P.; Wei, S. Characterization of estrogen receptor-low-positive breast cancer. *Breast Cancer Res. Treat.* **2021**, *188*, 225–235. [CrossRef]
24. Poon, I.K.; Tsang, J.Y.; Li, J.; Chan, S.K.; Shea, K.H.; Tse, G.M. The significance of highlighting the oestrogen receptor low category in breast cancer. *Br. J. Cancer* **2020**, *123*, 1223–1227. [CrossRef] [PubMed]
25. Landmann, A.; Farrugia, D.J.; Zhu, L.; Diego, E.J.; Johnson, R.R.; Soran, A.; Dabbs, D.J.; Clark, B.Z.; Puhalla, S.L.; Jankowitz, R.C.; et al. Low Estrogen Receptor (ER)-Positive Breast Cancer and Neoadjuvant Systemic Chemotherapy: Is Response Similar to Typical ER-Positive or ER-Negative Disease? *Am. J. Clin. Pathol.* **2018**, *150*, 34–42. [CrossRef]
26. Yoder, R.; Kimler, B.F.; Staley, J.M.; Schwensen, K.; Wang, Y.Y.; Finke, K.; O'Dea, A.; Nye, L.; Elia, M.; Crane, G.; et al. Impact of low versus negative estrogen/progesterone receptor status on clinico-pathologic characteristics and survival outcomes in HER2-negative breast cancer. *NPJ Breast Cancer* **2022**, *8*, 80. [CrossRef]
27. He, A.; Zhou, T. Clinicopathological Features and Survival for Low ER-positive Breast-cancer Patients. *Altern. Ther. Health Med.* **2022**, *28*, 36–41.
28. Gloyeske, N.C.; Dabbs, D.J.; Bhargava, R. Low ER+ breast cancer: Is this a distinct group? *Am. J. Clin. Pathol.* **2014**, *141*, 697–701. [CrossRef]
29. Deyarmin, B.; Kane, J.L.; Valente, A.L.; van Laar, R.; Gallagher, C.; Shriver, C.D.; Ellsworth, R.E. Effect of ASCO/CAP guidelines for determining ER status on molecular subtype. *Ann. Surg. Oncol.* **2013**, *20*, 87–93. [CrossRef]
30. Tarantino, P.; Jin, Q.; Tayob, N.; Jeselsohn, R.M.; Schnitt, S.J.; Vincuilla, J.; Parker, T.; Tyekucheva, S.; Li, T.; Lin, N.U.; et al. Prognostic and Biologic Significance of ERBB2-Low Expression in Early-Stage Breast Cancer. *JAMA Oncol.* **2022**, *8*, 1177–1183. [CrossRef]
31. Domagala, W.; Lasota, J.; Bartkowiak, J.; Weber, K.; Osborn, M. Vimentin is preferentially expressed in human breast carcinomas with low estrogen receptor and high Ki-67 growth fraction. *Am. J. Pathol.* **1990**, *136*, 219–227.
32. Iwamoto, T.; Booser, D.; Valero, V.; Murray, J.L.; Koenig, K.; Esteva, F.J.; Ueno, N.T.; Zhang, J.; Shi, W.; Qi, Y.; et al. Estrogen receptor (ER) mRNA and ER-related gene expression in breast cancers that are 1% to 10% ER-positive by immunohistochemistry. *J. Clin. Oncol.* **2012**, *30*, 729–734. [CrossRef] [PubMed]
33. Prabhu, J.S.; Korlimarla, A.; Desai, K.; Alexander, A.; Raghavan, R.; Anupama, C.; Dendukuri, N.; Manjunath, S.; Correa, M.; Raman, N.; et al. A Majority of Low (1–10%) ER Positive Breast Cancers Behave Like Hormone Receptor Negative Tumors. *J. Cancer* **2014**, *5*, 156–165. [CrossRef]
34. Sanford, R.A.; Song, J.; Gutierrez-Barrera, A.M.; Profato, J.; Woodson, A.; Litton, J.K.; Bedrosian, I.; Albarracin, C.T.; Valero, V.; Arun, B. High incidence of germline BRCA mutation in patients with ER low-positive/PR low-positive/HER-2 neu negative tumors. *Cancer* **2015**, *121*, 3422–3427. [CrossRef] [PubMed]
35. Zhou, M.; Yan, J.Q.; Chen, Q.X.; Yang, Y.Z.; Li, Y.L.; Ren, Y.X.; Weng, Z.J.; Zhang, X.F.; Guan, J.X.; Tang, L.Y.; et al. Association of H3K9me3 with breast cancer prognosis by estrogen receptor status. *Clin. Epigenetics* **2022**, *14*, 135. [CrossRef] [PubMed]
36. Paakkola, N.M.; Karakatsanis, A.; Mauri, D.; Foukakis, T.; Valachis, A. The prognostic and predictive impact of low estrogen receptor expression in early breast cancer: A systematic review and meta-analysis. *ESMO Open* **2021**, *6*, 100289. [CrossRef] [PubMed]
37. Skjervold, A.H.; Valla, M.; Bofin, A.M. Oestrogen receptor low positive breast cancer: Associations with prognosis. *Breast Cancer Res. Treat.* **2023**, *201*, 535–545. [CrossRef]
38. Early Breast Cancer Trialists' Collaborative Group; Davies, C.; Godwin, J.; Gray, R.; Clarke, M.; Cutter, D.; Darby, S.; McGale, P.; Pan, H.C.; Taylor, C.; et al. Relevance of breast cancer hormone receptors and other factors to the efficacy of adjuvant tamoxifen: Patient-level meta-analysis of randomised trials. *Lancet* **2011**, *378*, 771–784. [CrossRef]
39. Yi, M.; Huo, L.; Koenig, K.B.; Mittendorf, E.A.; Meric-Bernstam, F.; Kuerer, H.M.; Bedrosian, I.; Buzdar, A.U.; Symmans, W.F.; Crow, J.R.; et al. Which threshold for ER positivity? a retrospective study based on 9639 patients. *Ann. Oncol.* **2014**, *25*, 1004–1011. [CrossRef]
40. Balduzzi, A.; Bagnardi, V.; Rotmensz, N.; Dellapasqua, S.; Montagna, E.; Cardillo, A.; Viale, G.; Veronesi, P.; Intra, M.; Luini, A.; et al. Survival outcomes in breast cancer patients with low estrogen/progesterone receptor expression. *Clin. Breast Cancer* **2014**, *14*, 258–264. [CrossRef]

41. Chen, T.; Zhang, N.; Moran, M.S.; Su, P.; Haffty, B.G.; Yang, Q. Borderline ER-Positive Primary Breast Cancer Gains No Significant Survival Benefit From Endocrine Therapy: A Systematic Review and Meta-Analysis. *Clin. Breast Cancer* **2018**, *18*, 1–8. [CrossRef] [PubMed]
42. Xie, Y.; Yang, L.; Wu, Y.; Zheng, H.; Gou, Q. Adjuvant endocrine therapy in patients with estrogen receptor-low positive breast cancer: A prospective cohort study. *Breast* **2022**, *66*, 89–96. [CrossRef]
43. Cai, Y.W.; Shao, Z.M.; Yu, K.D. De-escalation of five-year adjuvant endocrine therapy in patients with estrogen receptor-low positive (immunohistochemistry staining 1%–10%) breast cancer: Propensity-matched analysis from a prospectively maintained cohort. *Cancer* **2022**, *128*, 1748–1756. [CrossRef] [PubMed]
44. Reinert, T.; Cascelli, F.; de Resende, C.A.A.; Goncalves, A.C.; Godo, V.S.P.; Barrios, C.H. Clinical implication of low estrogen receptor (ER-low) expression in breast cancer. *Front. Endocrinol.* **2022**, *13*, 1015388. [CrossRef] [PubMed]
45. Giordano, J.; McGrath, M.; Harrison, B.; Kantor, O.; Vora, H.; Burstein, H.J.; Tolaney, S.M.; King, T.A.; Mittendorf, E.A. Is there a role for the oncotype DX breast recurrence score genomic assay in estrogen receptor-low positive breast cancer? *J. Clin. Oncol.* **2022**, *40*, 564. [CrossRef]
46. Ding, Y.; Ding, K.; Yu, K.; Zou, D.; Yang, H.; He, X.; Mo, W.; Yu, X.; Ding, X. Prognosis and endocrine therapy selection for patients with low hormone receptor-positive breast cancer following neoadjuvant chemotherapy: A retrospective study of 570 patients in China. *Oncol. Lett.* **2019**, *18*, 6690–6696. [CrossRef]
47. Dieci, M.V.; Griguolo, G.; Bottosso, M.; Tsvetkova, V.; Giorgi, C.A.; Vernaci, G.; Michieletto, S.; Angelini, S.; Marchet, A.; Tasca, G.; et al. Impact of estrogen receptor levels on outcome in non-metastatic triple negative breast cancer patients treated with neoadjuvant/adjuvant chemotherapy. *NPJ Breast Cancer* **2021**, *7*, 101. [CrossRef]
48. Fujii, T.; Kogawa, T.; Dong, W.; Sahin, A.A.; Moulder, S.; Litton, J.K.; Tripathy, D.; Iwamoto, T.; Hunt, K.K.; Pusztai, L.; et al. Revisiting the definition of estrogen receptor positivity in HER2-negative primary breast cancer. *Ann. Oncol.* **2017**, *28*, 2420–2428. [CrossRef]
49. Villegas, S.L.; Nekljudova, V.; Pfarr, N.; Engel, J.; Untch, M.; Schrodi, S.; Holms, F.; Ulmer, H.U.; Fasching, P.A.; Weber, K.E.; et al. Therapy response and prognosis of patients with early breast cancer with low positivity for hormone receptors—An analysis of 2765 patients from neoadjuvant clinical trials. *Eur. J. Cancer* **2021**, *148*, 159–170. [CrossRef]
50. Tarantino, P.; Corti, C.; Schmid, P.; Cortes, J.; Mittendorf, E.A.; Rugo, H.; Tolaney, S.M.; Bianchini, G.; Andre, F.; Curigliano, G. Immunotherapy for early triple negative breast cancer: Research agenda for the next decade. *NPJ Breast Cancer* **2022**, *8*, 23. [CrossRef]
51. Vathiotis, I.A.; Trontzas, I.; Gavrielatou, N.; Gomatou, G.; Syrigos, N.K.; Kotteas, E.A. Immune Checkpoint Blockade in Hormone Receptor-Positive Breast Cancer: Resistance Mechanisms and Future Perspectives. *Clin. Breast Cancer* **2022**, *22*, 642–649. [CrossRef]
52. O'Meara, T.A.; Tolaney, S.M. Tumor mutational burden as a predictor of immunotherapy response in breast cancer. *Oncotarget* **2021**, *12*, 394–400. [CrossRef] [PubMed]
53. Voorwerk, L.; Sanders, J.; Keusters, M.S.; Balduzzi, S.; Cornelissen, S.; Duijst, M.; Lips, E.H.; Sonke, G.S.; Linn, S.C.; Horlings, H.M.; et al. Immune landscape of breast tumors with low and intermediate estrogen receptor expression. *NPJ Breast Cancer* **2023**, *9*, 39. [CrossRef] [PubMed]
54. Burstein, H.J.; Curigliano, G.; Thurlimann, B.; Weber, W.P.; Poortmans, P.; Regan, M.M.; Senn, H.J.; Winer, E.P.; Gnant, M.; Panelists of the St Gallen Consensus Conference. Customizing local and systemic therapies for women with early breast cancer: The St. Gallen International Consensus Guidelines for treatment of early breast cancer 2021. *Ann. Oncol.* **2021**, *32*, 1216–1235. [CrossRef]
55. Sharma, P.; Stecklein, S.; Yoder, R.; Staley, J.; Schwensen, K.; O'Dea, A.; Nye, L.; Elia, M.; Satelli, D.; Crane, G.; et al. Clinical and biomarker results of neoadjuvant phase II study of pembrolizumab and carboplatin plus docetaxel in triple-negative breast cancer (TNBC) (NeoPACT). *J. Clin. Oncol.* **2022**, *40*, 513. [CrossRef]
56. Cardoso, F.; Paluch-Shimon, S.; Senkus, E.; Curigliano, G.; Aapro, M.S.; Andre, F.; Barrios, C.H.; Bergh, J.; Bhattacharyya, G.S.; Biganzoli, L.; et al. 5th ESO-ESMO international consensus guidelines for advanced breast cancer (ABC 5). *Ann. Oncol.* **2020**, *31*, 1623–1649. [CrossRef] [PubMed]
57. Luond, F.; Tiede, S.; Christofori, G. Breast cancer as an example of tumour heterogeneity and tumour cell plasticity during malignant progression. *Br. J. Cancer* **2021**, *125*, 164–175. [CrossRef]
58. Turashvili, G.; Brogi, E. Tumor Heterogeneity in Breast Cancer. *Front. Med.* **2017**, *4*, 227. [CrossRef]
59. Chen, R.; Qarmali, M.; Siegal, G.P.; Wei, S. Receptor conversion in metastatic breast cancer: Analysis of 390 cases from a single institution. *Mod. Pathol.* **2020**, *33*, 2499–2506. [CrossRef]
60. Shi, Y.J.; Tsang, J.Y.; Ni, Y.B.; Tse, G.M. Intratumoral Heterogeneity in Breast Cancer: A Comparison of Primary and Metastatic Breast Cancers. *Oncologist* **2017**, *22*, 487–490. [CrossRef]
61. Reinhardt, F.; Franken, A.; Fehm, T.; Neubauer, H. Navigation through inter- and intratumoral heterogeneity of endocrine resistance mechanisms in breast cancer: A potential role for Liquid Biopsies? *Tumour Biol.* **2017**, *39*, 1010428317731511. [CrossRef] [PubMed]
62. Joseph, C.; Papadaki, A.; Althobiti, M.; Alsaleem, M.; Aleskandarany, M.A.; Rakha, E.A. Breast cancer intratumour heterogeneity: Current status and clinical implications. *Histopathology* **2018**, *73*, 717–731. [CrossRef] [PubMed]
63. Hartkopf, A.D.; Grischke, E.M.; Brucker, S.Y. Endocrine-Resistant Breast Cancer: Mechanisms and Treatment. *Breast Care* **2020**, *15*, 347–354. [CrossRef] [PubMed]

64. Zattarin, E.; Leporati, R.; Ligorio, F.; Lobefaro, R.; Vingiani, A.; Pruneri, G.; Vernieri, C. Hormone Receptor Loss in Breast Cancer: Molecular Mechanisms, Clinical Settings, and Therapeutic Implications. *Cells* **2020**, *9*, 2644. [CrossRef] [PubMed]
65. Rasha, F.; Sharma, M.; Pruitt, K. Mechanisms of endocrine therapy resistance in breast cancer. *Mol. Cell. Endocrinol.* **2021**, *532*, 111322. [CrossRef] [PubMed]
66. Zhang, J.; Zhou, C.; Jiang, H.; Liang, L.; Shi, W.; Zhang, Q.; Sun, P.; Xiang, R.; Wang, Y.; Yang, S. ZEB1 induces ER-alpha promoter hypermethylation and confers antiestrogen resistance in breast cancer. *Cell Death Dis.* **2017**, *8*, e2732. [CrossRef]

Disclaimer/Publisher's Note: The statements, opinions and data contained in all publications are solely those of the individual author(s) and contributor(s) and not of MDPI and/or the editor(s). MDPI and/or the editor(s) disclaim responsibility for any injury to people or property resulting from any ideas, methods, instructions or products referred to in the content.

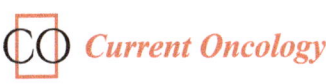

Brief Report

Is There a Role for Risk-Reducing Bilateral Breast Surgery in *BRCA1/2* Ovarian Cancer Survivors? An Observational Study

Daniela Oliveira [1,2,3], Sofia Fernandes [4], Isália Miguel [4,5], Sofia Fragoso [6] and Fátima Vaz [4,5,*]

1. Medical Genetics Unit, Centro Hospitalar e Universitário de Coimbra, 3000-602 Coimbra, Portugal; danielaoliveira@chuc.min-saude.pt
2. University Clinic of Genetics, Faculdade de Medicina, Universidade de Coimbra, 3000-548 Coimbra, Portugal
3. Clinical Academic Center of Coimbra, 3004-561 Coimbra, Portugal
4. Familial Cancer Risk Clinic, Instituto Português de Oncologia de Lisboa Francisco Gentil, 1099-023 Lisboa, Portugal; sffernandes@ipolisboa.min-saude.pt (S.F.); imiguel@ipolisboa.min-saude.pt (I.M.)
5. Medical Oncology Service, Instituto Português de Oncologia de Lisboa Francisco Gentil, 1099-023 Lisboa, Portugal
6. Molecular Pathobiology Research Unit, Instituto Português de Oncologia de Lisboa Francisco Gentil, 1099-023 Lisboa, Portugal; afragoso@ipolisboa.min-saude.pt
* Correspondence: fvaz@ipolisboa.min-saude.pt

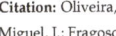

Abstract: Background: Risk-reducing surgeries are an option for cancer risk management in *BRCA1/2* individuals. However, while adnexectomy is commonly recommended in breast cancer (BC) survivors, risk-reducing bilateral breast surgery (RRBBS) is controversial in ovarian cancer (OC) survivors due to relapse rates and mortality. Methods: We conducted a retrospective analysis of *BRCA1/2*-OC survivors, with OC as first cancer diagnosis. Results: Median age at OC diagnosis for the 69 *BRCA1/2*-OC survivors was 54 years. Median overall survival was 8 years, being significantly higher for *BRCA2* patients than for *BRCA1* patients ($p = 0.011$). Nine patients (13.2%) developed BC at a median age of 61 years. The mean overall BC-free survival was 15.5 years (median not reached). Eight patients (11.8%) underwent bilateral mastectomy (5 simultaneous with BC treatment; 3 RRBBS) at a median age of 56.5 years. The median time from OC to bilateral mastectomy/RRBBS was 5.5 years. Conclusions: This study adds evidence regarding a lower BC risk after *BRCA1/2*-OC and higher survival for *BRCA2*-OC patients. A comprehensive analysis of the competing risks of OC mortality and recurrence against the risk of BC should be individually addressed. Surgical BC risk management may be considered for longer *BRCA1/2*-OC disease-free survivors. Ultimately, these decisions should always be tailored to patients' characteristics and preferences.

Keywords: ovarian cancer; breast cancer; hereditary cancer; *BRCA*; risk-reducing bilateral breast surgery

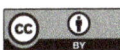

1. Introduction

Women with hereditary breast and ovarian cancer syndrome have an increased risk of developing cancer, mainly breast cancer (BC)—absolute risk > 60% for *BRCA1/2* carriers—and ovarian cancer (OC)—absolute risk of 39–58% for *BRCA1* and 13–29% for *BRCA2* carriers [1].

Currently, breast imaging, such as ultrasound, mammography and/or magnetic resonance imaging (MRI), is widely recommended to detect malignant lesions at an early stage in *BRCA1/2* women [1]. However, the most significant approach to reduce BC risk in *BRCA1/2* carriers is risk-reducing bilateral breast surgery (RRBBS) [2]. Some previous reports stated that there was a BC risk reduction of 90 to 95% in *BRCA1/2* women that underwent RRBBS, although no significative reduction in mortality was observed [3]. Likewise, risk-reducing adnexectomy is strongly recommended, typically between 35 and 40 years, to manage OC risk in *BRCA1/2* women [1]. In addition to a profound decrease in OC incidence, risk-reducing adnexectomy also leads to a substantial reduction in all-cause and OC-related mortality [3]. While risk-reducing adnexectomy is still commonly recommended in *BRCA1/2*-BC survivors, RRBBS is controversial in *BRCA1/2*-OC survivors, due to the high relapse rate and mortality associated with OC. In fact, there is a lack of thorough recommendations concerning BC risk and the role of RRBBS in *BRCA1/2*-OC survivors. In this study, we evaluate the incidence of BC after *BRCA1/2*-OC and report our experience with RRBBS in these patients.

2. Materials and Methods

All consenting women testing positive for *BRCA1* or *BRCA2* were invited to participate in long-term prospective follow-up in the Familial Risk Clinic of IPO Lisboa. Patients are kept under surveillance until death, loss to follow-up or consent withdrawal. For this study, patients with OC as first cancer diagnosis and a *BRCA1/2*-positive test between January 2000 and August 2022 were selected. Women who had had another cancer before OC were excluded. Data before testing were retrospectively collected from available clinical reports. The start of the follow-up period was defined as the date of OC diagnosis. The overall and BC-free survival were calculated using the Kaplan–Meier method. The log-rank test was used to compare survival and BC incidence between different groups. Overall survival was considered as the time from OC diagnosis to the time of death, whereas BC-free survival was defined as the time from OC to BC diagnoses. Statistical analysis was conducted using SigmaPlot software, version 15.0.

3. Results

Over a period of 22 years, a total of 69 women, from 63 different families, were diagnosed with *BRCA1/2*-OC. The median age at OC diagnosis was 54 years (range: 18–85 years). Most patients for whom data were available were diagnosed with epithelial serous OC (75.9%) and at a III or IV FIGO stage (73.7%). Regarding molecular testing, 33 (47.8%) individuals were identified with a germline *BRCA1* variant and 36 (52.2%) with a germline *BRCA2* variant. Of the 36 *BRCA2* patients, 9 (25%) had the founder variant of Portuguese origin *BRCA2*:c.156_157insAlu. Among the 69 patients, 55 (79.7%) had at least one relative with BC, while 14 (20.3%) had no known relatives diagnosed with BC. Among those with positive family history of BC, 38 (69.1%) had an affected first-degree relative (Table 1). In the subgroup of nine patients who developed BC, eight (88.9%) reported positive family history, and only one (11.1%) patient had no family history of BC. Among those eight with a positive family history of BC, half had an affected first-degree relative (Table 2).

The median duration of follow-up for all patients since OC diagnosis was 6 years (range: 1–22 years). In this group, there were a total of 35 deaths from all causes (all-cause mortality rate: 50.7%) throughout the follow-up period. Death occurred at a median age of 59 years (range: 40–89 years), at a median of 4 years (range: 1–16 years) after OC diagnosis, and, in 94.3% of the cases (33 patients), within the first 10 years of follow-up. For the entire cohort, the median overall survival was 8.0 years (mean: 11.6 years), being significantly higher for *BRCA2*-OC patients (median: not reached; mean: 14.3 years) than for *BRCA1*-OC patients (median: 5 years; mean: 8 years) ($p = 0.011$).

Further, one of the 69 patients was lost to follow-up more than two years before death, so she is not considered when assessing BC (or other cancer types) risk in this cohort. A total of nine (13.2%) patients developed BC after the OC at a median age of 61 years (range: 44–68 years). The median BC-free survival could not be calculated via Kaplan–Meier survival analysis because of the small number of patients who were diagnosed with BC after OC, with the mean BC-free survival in the total population being 15.5 years (Figure 1). The difference in BC-free survival between *BRCA1*-OC women (median: not reached; mean: 12.9 years) and *BRCA2*-OC women (median: not reached; mean: 15.9 years) did not reach statistical significance ($p = 0.440$). The difference in the overall survival between *BRCA1/2*-OC women with BC (median: not reached; mean: 16.4 years) and *BRCA1/2*-OC women without BC (median: 8.0 years; mean: 9.9 years) was also not statistically significant ($p = 0.107$).

Table 1. Characterization of the cohort.

CHARACTERISTIC		
	Number of patients	69
	Number of families	63
MOLECULAR RESULT		
	BRCA1	33 (47.8%)
	BRCA2	36 (52.2%)
	BRCA2:c. c.156_157insAlu	9 (25%)
OVARIAN CANCER		
	Median age [range]	54 y [18–85 y]
	FIGO stage	
	I	11 (18.0%)
	II	5 (8.2%)
	III	34 (55.7%)
	IV	11 (18.0%)
	Unknown	8
	Histology	
	Epithelial serous	44 (75.9%)
	Epithelial endometrioid	3 (5.2%)
	Epithelial mucinous	1 (1.7%)
	Epithelial transitional cell	1 (1.7%)
	Mixed epithelial serous and endometrioid	2 (3.4%)
	Mixed epithelial serous and transitional cell	1 (1.7%)
	Poorly differentiated	6 (10.3%)
	Unknown	11
NUMBER OF DEATHS (all causes)		35 (50.7%)
	Median age [range]	59 y [40–89 y]
	Median time after OC [range]	4 y [1–16 y]
	Death within the first 10 years of follow-up	33 (94.3%)
FAMILY HISTORY OF BC		
	Positive—all known relatives	55 (79.7%)
	First-degree relatives	38 (69.1%)
	Negative	14 (20.3%)

Table 2. Characterization of BC diagnosed in the cohort.

BREAST CANCER	9 (13.2%)
Median age [range]	61 y [44–68 y]
Median time after OC [range]	5 y [2–14 y]
RECEPTORS	
ER and PR negative	2 (22.2%)
ER and/or PR positive	7 (77.8%)
Her2 negative	7 (77.8%)
Triple negative	2 (22.2%)
FAMILY HISTORY OF BC	
Positive-all known relatives	8 (88.9%)
First-degree relatives	4 (50.0%)
Negative	1 (11.1%)

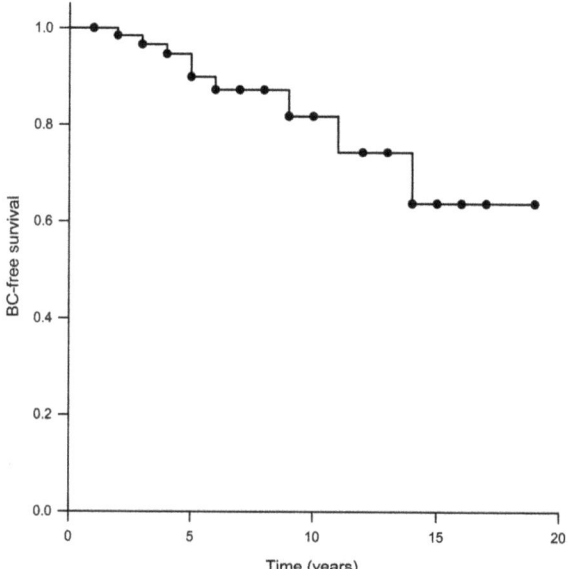

Figure 1. Kaplan–Meier analysis of BC-free survival.

All diagnosed BCs were unilateral, and two of them were triple-negative (both *BRCA1* patients). Of the nine patients with BC, five (55.6%) had a *BRCA1* variant, whereas four (44.4%) had a *BRCA2* variant (two with the Portuguese founder variant). Three out of the nine *BRCA1/2*-OC women with BC died at a median age of 51 years (range: 50–61 years) and at a median time of 7 years after the OC diagnosis (range: 5–9 years). The cause of death of these three patients was unrelated to BC: 1—ovarian cancer progression; 2—refractory leukemia; 3—overdose in a patient in remission of both cancers. The characterization of BC diagnosed in our cohort is detailed in Table 2.

Five (7.4%) patients underwent bilateral mastectomy in a unilateral BC context (Table 3). Bilateral mastectomy was performed at a median age of 54 years (range: 44–69 years) and at a median of 6 years (range: 2–15 years) after the OC diagnosis. Three (4.4%) patients, without personal history of BC, were submitted to RRBBS at a median age of 58 years (range: 55–61 years) (Table 3). The median time from OC diagnosis to RRBBS was 5 years (range: 3–15 years).

Table 3. Characterization of bilateral mastectomy and RRBBS in the cohort.

BILATERAL MASTECTOMY	5 (7.4%)
Median age [range]	54 y [44–69 y]
Median time after OC [range]	6 y [2–15 y]
RRBBS	3 (4.4%)
Median age [range]	58 y [55–61 y]
Median time after OC [range]	5 y [3–15 y]

In this cohort, five other cancers were diagnosed during the follow-up period—a squamous cell carcinoma of the tongue at the age of 51 (one patient), a synchronous high-stage serous carcinoma of the endometrium at the age of 75 (one patient) and basal cell carcinomas of the skin at ages of 59 and 72 (two patients). One patient was diagnosed with acute myeloid leukemia, secondary to chemotherapy for ovarian cancer, at the age of 60 and BC at the age of 61.

4. Discussion

In this study, we observed an incidence of 13.2% of BC in a cohort of 68 *BRCA1/2*-OC women during a median follow-up period of 6 years. The mean BC-free survival in the total population was 15.5 years (median: not reached), with no significant difference for *BRCA1*-OC, as compared to *BRCA2*-OC patients. While we observed a significantly higher overall survival for *BRCA2*-OC patients as compared with *BRCA1*-OC patients, the difference in overall survival between *BRCA1/2*-OC women with BC and *BRCA1/2*-OC women without BC was not found to be statistically significant.

The incidence of BC in our cohort was slightly higher than that reported in previous studies, such as that described by Vencken et al. [4], who identified 8 primary BCs in 79 *BRCA1/2*-OC women (10.1%) during a mean period of 6.7 years, and by Domchek et al. [5], who reported 11% of BCs (18 patients) in a group of 164 during a mean follow-up of 5.8 years. Similarly, Gangi et al. [6] described an incidence of 8.9% of BC (12 women) in 135 patients with a mean follow-up period of 6.6 years, and Fong et al. [7] identified 8.3% (16 patients) in 192 *BRCA1/2*-OC women. More recently, a larger cohort of 502 patients was characterized by Safra et al. [8], who reported a lower incidence (6.2%) of BC in 502 *BRCA1/2*-OC women, with a median follow-up of 5.0 years. The small number of *BRCA1/2*-OC women included in most of the studies, including our own, is a limitation regarding conclusions about the incidence of BC in this specific population. However, caution should also be taken when drawing conclusions, as inclusion criteria and mutational *BRCA1/2* patterns differ among these studies. For example, Safra et al. [8] included women with BC and other cancers diagnosed prior to OC (representing 17.5% and 1.6% of the cohort, respectively) in their cohort. In our study, any type of cancer diagnosed before OC was an exclusion criterion. Another note that must be emphasized is that women who underwent RRBBS were maintained in our cohort, even after prophylactic surgery. Even after RRBBS, there is a remaining BC risk, and, in our registry, patients are kept in surveillance until death, are lost to follow-up or withdraw their consent.

Regarding mutational *BRCA1/2* patterns, our study is the first where the numbers of *BRCA2*-OC women are higher than *BRCA1*-OC patients (*BRCA2*: 52.2% vs *BRCA1*: 47.8%). In all previous studies, *BRCA1*-OC patients represented more than 70% of the cohort [4–8]. As we discuss below, data are conflicting regarding *BRCA1* and *BRCA2* as biomarkers for better survival when compared with sporadic OC. However, a relevant finding in our study is the increased overall survival observed in the *BRCA2*-OC subgroup when compared to *BRCA1*-OC patients (14.3 years vs. 8 years, $p = 0.011$). This observation was previously described in a pooled analysis of 26 studies [9].

Vencken et al. [4] reported a BC risk of 3%, 6% and 11% in *BRCA1/2*-OC survivors in the following 2, 5 and 10 years after OC diagnosis. The same study reported a significantly higher BC risk in unaffected variant carriers during the same follow-up period (6%, 16% and 28%, respectively) [4]. Domchek et al. [5] also reported a less-than-10% risk of developing BC in the 10-year follow-up period (12% for *BRCA1* carriers and 2% for *BRCA2* carriers). In a more recent study, McGee et al. [10] reported a risk of 7.8% of developing BC in a 10-year interval, conditional on OC survival and other causes of death. Despite the fact that data are still limited and larger studies are needed, *BRCA1/2*-OC survivors appear to have a significantly lower risk of developing BC after OC than unaffected individuals. Previous studies suggested several reasons for the apparent lower BC risk in *BRCA1/2*-OC survivors compared to unaffected women. One of the reasons is the premature termination of ovarian function due to salpingo-oophorectomy, usually performed in an OC treatment context [4–6]. In line with that, previous studies reported that risk-reducing adnexectomy reduces the risk of BC in *BRCA1/2* patients, mainly if performed at a premenopausal age [4,5,11,12]. Another aspect that is likely to contribute to a lower rate of BC in this subgroup is the effect of the therapy for OC. Some authors argue that platinum-based chemotherapy usually used for OC treatment could contribute to eradicating submicroscopic breast disease, leading to a lower number of BCs in these patients [4–6].

Although there are conflicting data in the literature, some studies reported that carrying a *BRCA1* or *BRCA2* variant leads to better responses to both platinum- and non-platinum-based chemotherapies, as well as better progression-free and overall survival in OC patients [13]. Nonetheless, McLaughlin et al. [14] demonstrated that *BRCA1* or *BRCA2* variants could be an advantage in OC patients to short-term survival but not to long-term survival. Although there is a trend for increasing OC survival due to recent advances in therapeutic approaches, OC 5-year and 10-year survival rates remain poor (63% and 35%, respectively) [4]. In our study, we report a mortality rate of 50.7% at a median age of 59 years, which is similar to those previously reported (53.2%, 51.1%, 40.7% and 36.3%) [4,6,8,10]. Moreover, most patients in our cohort (74.6%) were diagnosed with a high-stage OC, which is comparable to the 76% reported in Vencken et al. [4] and the most prevalent stage IIIC in Gangi et al. [6]. Currently, patients' outcome is essentially determined by OC mortality rate and the risk of relapse, mainly during the first years after diagnosis. Noteworthily, 94.3% of deaths in our cohort occurred within the first 10 years of follow-up after OC diagnosis. We registered three deaths among *BRCA1/2*-OC women with BC but none were linked to the diagnosis of BC. Similarly, Domchek et al. [5] and Safra et al. [8] also stated that none of the deaths in their cohorts of women with OC and BC were related to BC. In the Fong et al. [7] study, only one patient died of BC.

Taking all data into consideration, we propose that BC after *BRCA1/2*-OC would still require specific surveillance, especially in those women who have better prognosis. Based on simulation studies, McGee et al. [10] concluded that the risk of death from BC after OC is about 1%, and breast MRI screening and RRBBS will have a very small impact on survival. For example, among all *BRCA1/2* women diagnosed with stage III/IV OC at the age of 50, breast MRI screening and RRBBS will reduce, by 1% and 2%, respectively, the chance of dying by the age of 80. However, these effects could be greater if OC was diagnosed at an early age or at lower stages, leading several authors to propose that RRBBS or breast MRI screening should be recommended to all patients diagnosed with stage I or II OC and those patients with stage III or IV OC diagnosed at or before the age of 50 and surviving at least 10 years without relapse [10]. It is of note that in our study, eight patients underwent BC risk-reducing surgery, but for five of these patients, surgery was decided in the context of a BC diagnosis and regarding contralateral BC risk reduction.

We are aware that several limitations of this study, particularly the small cohort and the lack of a control group, should be considered when conclusions are discussed. Data regarding individual treatment and OC relapse were also not included in the current discussion. However, this study adds data to the discussion regarding the risk of developing BC in a population of *BRCA2*-enriched OC survivors. With recent advances in treatment, the number of *BRCA1/2*-OC survivors may increase in the near future, and this information may help clinicians to provide more accurate counseling regarding BC risk and risk management options to these patients. We are looking forward to in-depth future collaborative studies, including larger cohorts, so as to obtain more robust recommendations for this subgroup.

5. Conclusions

During the early period after OC diagnosis, OC mortality and recurrence rates are significantly high, and BC risk appears to be lower than in unaffected *BRCA1/2* individuals. With that in mind, invasive BC risk management could bring an inappropriate burden without significant benefits to these patients. However, with the positive survival impact of new therapeutic advances, we expect a rising number of *BRCA1/2*-OC survivors with health professionals having to face the dilemma of RRBBS in the context of a potentially life-limiting OC diagnosis. We propose a comprehensive analysis of the competing risks of OC mortality and OC recurrence against the risk of BC that should be individually addressed, particularly in those patients with longer disease-free survival. Ultimately, decisions regarding preventive measures should always be tailored to patients' characteristics and preferences.

Author Contributions: Writing—original draft preparation, D.O.; writing—review and editing, S.F. (Sofia Fernandes), I.M., S.F. (Sofia Fragoso) and F.V.; supervision, F.V. All authors have read and agreed to the published version of the manuscript.

Funding: This research received no external funding.

Institutional Review Board Statement: Ethical review and approval were waived for this observational study, since all patients included consented previously in data collection during prospective, non-interventional, follow-up. Data collection during follow-up of patients with a positive genetic testing was approved by the Ethics Committee of our Institute (Comissão de Ética do Instituto Português de Oncologia de Lisboa, EPE). Of note, after implementation of the European 679/2016 Regulation, data collection and consent forms were reviewed and approved by the same Ethics Committee.

Informed Consent Statement: Informed consent was obtained from all subjects involved in the study. All genetic records are protected with restricted access, as per Portuguese law. All forms related to this study were approved by the Ethics Committee of our Institute (Comissão de Ética do Instituto Português de Oncologia de Lisboa, EPE).

Data Availability Statement: Data are contained within the article.

Acknowledgments: We want to thank all patients and their families that contributed to this study.

Conflicts of Interest: The authors declare no conflict of interest.

References

1. National Comprehensive Cancer Network. Genetic/Familial High-Risk Assessment: Breast, Ovarian, and Pancreatic, (version 1.2023). Available online: https://www.nccn.org/professionals/physician_gls/pdf/genetics_bop.pdf (accessed on 30 October 2022).
2. Speight, B.; Tischkowitz, M. When to Consider Risk-Reducing Mastectomy in BRCA1/BRCA2 Mutation Carriers with Advanced Stage Ovarian Cancer: A Case Study Illustrating the Genetic Counseling Challenges. *J. Genet. Couns.* **2017**, *26*, 1173–1178. [CrossRef] [PubMed]
3. Ludwig, K.K.; Neuner, J.; Butler, A.; Geurts, J.L.; Kong, A.L. Risk reduction and survival benefit of prophylactic surgery in BRCA mutation carriers, a systematic review. *Am. J. Surg.* **2016**, *212*, 660–669. [CrossRef] [PubMed]
4. Vencken, P.M.L.H.; Kriege, M.; Hooning, M.; Menke-Pluymers, M.B.; Heemskerk-Gerritsen, B.A.M.; Van Doorn, L.C.; Collée, M.M.; Jager, A.; Van Montfort, C.; Burger, C.W.; et al. The risk of primary and contralateral breast cancer after ovarian cancer in BRCA1/BRCA2 mutation carriers: Implications for counseling. *Cancer* **2013**, *119*, 955–962. [CrossRef]
5. Domchek, S.M.; Jhaveri, K.; Patil, S.; Stopfer, J.E.; Hudis, C.; Powers, J.; Stadler, Z.; Goldstein, L.; Kauff, N.; Khasraw, M.; et al. Risk of metachronous breast cancer after BRCA mutation-associated ovarian cancer. *Cancer* **2013**, *119*, 1344–1348. [CrossRef]
6. Gangi, A.; Cass, I.; Paik, D.; Barmparas, G.; Karlan, B.; Dang, C.; Li, A.; Walsh, C.; Rimel, B.J.; Amersi, F.F. Breast Cancer Following Ovarian Cancer in BRCA Mutation Carriers. *JAMA Surg.* **2014**, *149*, 1306. [CrossRef]
7. Fong, A.; Cass, I.; John, C.; Gillen, J.; Moore, K.M.; Gangi, A.; Walsh, C.; Li, A.J.; Rimel, B.J.; Karlan, B.Y.; et al. Breast Cancer Surveillance Following Ovarian Cancer in BRCA Mutation Carriers. *Am. Surg.* **2020**, *86*, 1243–1247. [CrossRef] [PubMed]
8. Safra, T.; Waissengrin, B.; Gerber, D.; Bernstein-Molho, R.; Klorin, G.; Salman, L.; Josephy, D.; Chen-Shtoyerman, R.; Bruchim, I.; Frey, M.K.; et al. Breast cancer incidence in BRCA mutation carriers with ovarian cancer: A longitudal observational study. *Gynecol. Oncol.* **2021**, *162*, 715–719. [CrossRef] [PubMed]

9. Bolton, K.L. Association Between BRCA1 and BRCA2 Mutations and Survival in Women with Invasive Epithelial Ovarian Cancer. *JAMA* **2012**, *307*, 382. [CrossRef] [PubMed]
10. McGee, J.; Giannakeas, V.; Karlan, B.; Lubinski, J.; Gronwald, J.; Rosen, B.; McLaughlin, J.; Risch, H.; Sun, P.; Foulkes, W.D.; et al. Risk of breast cancer after a diagnosis of ovarian cancer in BRCA mutation carriers: Is preventive mastectomy warranted? *Gynecol. Oncol.* **2017**, *145*, 346–351. [CrossRef] [PubMed]
11. Olopade, O.I.; Artioli, G. Efficacy of Risk-Reducing Salpingo-Oophorectomy in Women with BRCA-1 and BRCA-2 Mutations. *Breast J.* **2004**, *10*, S5–S9. [CrossRef] [PubMed]
12. Domchek, S.M. Association of Risk-Reducing Surgery in BRCA1 or BRCA2 Mutation Carriers with Cancer Risk and Mortality. *JAMA* **2010**, *304*, 967. [CrossRef] [PubMed]
13. Alsop, K.; Fereday, S.; Meldrum, C.; deFazio, A.; Emmanuel, C.; George, J.; Dobrovic, A.; Birrer, M.J.; Webb, P.M.; Stewart, C.; et al. BRCA Mutation Frequency and Patterns of Treatment Response in BRCA Mutation–Positive Women With Ovarian Cancer: A Report From the Australian Ovarian Cancer Study Group. *J. Clin. Oncol.* **2012**, *30*, 2654–2663. [CrossRef] [PubMed]
14. McLaughlin, J.R.; Rosen, B.; Moody, J.; Pal, T.; Fan, I.; Shaw, P.A.; Risch, H.A.; Sellers, T.A.; Sun, P.; Narod, S.A. Long-Term Ovarian Cancer Survival Associated With Mutation in BRCA1 or BRCA2. *JNCI J. Natl. Cancer Inst.* **2013**, *105*, 141–148. [CrossRef] [PubMed]

Disclaimer/Publisher's Note: The statements, opinions and data contained in all publications are solely those of the individual author(s) and contributor(s) and not of MDPI and/or the editor(s). MDPI and/or the editor(s) disclaim responsibility for any injury to people or property resulting from any ideas, methods, instructions or products referred to in the content.

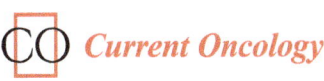

Article

Controlateral Symmetrisation in SRM for Breast Cancer: Now or Then? Immediate versus Delayed Symmetrisation in a Two-Stage Breast Reconstruction

Donato Casella [1], Daniele Fusario [2,*], Dario Cassetti [3], Anna Lisa Pesce [2], Alessandro De Luca [4], Maristella Guerra [5], Roberto Cuomo [6], Diego Ribuffo [7], Alessandro Neri [8] and Marco Marcasciano [9]

1. Department of Medicine, Surgery and Neurosciences, Unit of Breast Cancer Surgery, University of Siena, 53100 Siena, Italy
2. Department of Medicine, Surgery and Neurosciences, Unit of General Surgery and Surgical Oncology, University of Siena, 53100 Siena, Italy
3. Unit of General Surgery, USL Toscana Sud-Est, Valdarno Hospital Santa Maria alla Gruccia, 52025 Arezzo, Italy
4. Department of Surgery, Sapienza Università di Roma, 00185 Rome, Italy
5. Unit of Plastica Surgery, Polo Ospedaliero Santo Spirito ASL/RME, 00193 Rome, Italy
6. Department of Medicine, Surgery and Neurosciences, Unit of Plastic and Reconstructive Surgery, University of Siena, 53100 Siena, Italy
7. Department of Plastic Reconstructive and Aesthetic Surgery, Sapienza Università di Roma, 00185 Rome, Italy
8. Unit of Breast Surgery, USL Toscana Sud-Est, San Donato Hospital, 52100 Arezzo, Italy
9. Unit of Plastic and Reconstructive Surgery, University of Catanzaro "Magna Graecia", 88100 Catanzaro, Italy
* Correspondence: dani.fusario@gmail.com

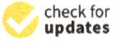

Citation: Casella, D.; Fusario, D.; Cassetti, D.; Pesce, A.L.; De Luca, A.; Guerra, M.; Cuomo, R.; Ribuffo, D.; Neri, A.; Marcasciano, M. Controlateral Symmetrisation in SRM for Breast Cancer: Now or Then? Immediate versus Delayed Symmetrisation in a Two-Stage Breast Reconstruction. *Curr. Oncol.* **2022**, *29*, 9391–9400. https://doi.org/10.3390/curroncol29120737

Received: 14 November 2022
Accepted: 27 November 2022
Published: 30 November 2022

Publisher's Note: MDPI stays neutral with regard to jurisdictional claims in published maps and institutional affiliations.

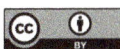

Copyright: © 2022 by the authors. Licensee MDPI, Basel, Switzerland. This article is an open access article distributed under the terms and conditions of the Creative Commons Attribution (CC BY) license (https://creativecommons.org/licenses/by/4.0/).

Abstract: *Introduction:* The timing of contralateral symmetrisation in patients with large and ptotic breasts undergoing a unilateral skin-reducing mastectomy (SRM) is one of the most debated topics in the reconstructive field. There is no evidence to support the advantage of immediate or delayed symmetrisation to help surgeons with this decision. The aim of this study was to investigate the clinical and aesthetic outcomes of immediate symmetrisation. *Methods:* A randomised observational study was conducted on patients who underwent an SRM for unilateral breast cancer. Based on a simple randomisation list, patients were divided into two groups: a delayed symmetrisation group versus an immediate symmetrisation group. The postoperative complications, BREAST-Q outcomes and reoperations were compared. *Results:* Out of a total of 84 patients undergoing an SRM between January 2018 and January 2021, 42 patients underwent immediate symmetrisation and 42 patients had delayed symmetrisation. Three implant losses (7.2%) were observed and we reported three wound dehiscences; one of these was in a contralateral breast reconstruction in the immediate symmetrisation group. The BREAST-Q patient-reported outcome measures recorded better aesthetic outcomes and a high patient satisfaction for the immediate symmetrisation group. *Conclusions:* Simultaneous controlateral symmetrisation is a good alternative to achieve better satisfaction and quality of life for patients; from a surgical point of view, it does not excessively impact on the second time of reconstruction.

Keywords: breast reconstruction; skin-reducing mastectomy; implant-based breast reconstruction; subcutaneous implant positioning; controlateral breast symmetrisation

1. Introduction

In 1991, Toth et al. [1] first described a skin-sparing mastectomy (SSM). By preserving the breast envelope and inframammary fold, a much more satisfactory cosmetic outcome could be achieved during a reconstruction.

Rice and Stickler in 1951 [2] described an "adeno-mammectomy" for benign diseases and Freeman in 1962 [3] presented the term "subcutaneous mastectomy": these are the first descriptions of a nipple-sparing mastectomy (NSM). An NSM is similar to an SSM for the dissection of skin flaps, but considers the NAC.

In patients with large and ptotic breasts that are higher than the second degree according to the Regnault classification [4], it is difficult to approach a mastectomy because an excellent satisfactory aesthetic outcome is hard to obtain [5].

Carlson et al. [6] in 1997 described four types of incision that could be used for an SSM; in particular, the Wise pattern is used for those patients with medium-sized or large ptotic breasts. Therefore, these authors first described a technique that combined a skin-sparing mastectomy with a simultaneous reduction of the breast envelope. For many years, this was not universally known; thus, in 2006, Nava et al. reproposed and renamed this technique the skin-reducing mastectomy (SRM) [7].

Although the results were reassuring, patients with macromastia and ptotic breasts remained a stimulating group to treat; the timing of contralateral symmetrisation remains one of the most debated topics in the breast reconstruction field [8–10].

Nowadays, breast surgeons regularly try to perform a symmetrical and aesthetically pleasing breast reconstruction to achieve a better outcome.

Despite the pros and cons of immediate versus delayed symmetrisation being well-documented, the ideal moment for performing a contralateral surgical procedure remains debated [11].

Currently, immediate symmetrisation is a questioned procedure. On one hand, a few surgeons prefer delayed symmetrisation to reduce the operating times and blood loss, thus potentially decreasing the morbidities. Additionally, important fat necrosis or partial flap losses may impose a change in the plan for reconstructed and contralateral breasts. On the other hand, several surgeons prefer immediate symmetrisation in order to give the patient immediate psychological wellness and increase their quality of life by the immediate reduction of asymmetry and, furthermore, to reduce the number of postoperative expansions needed to the reach the final volume and to avoid another operation.

The purpose of this study was to investigate the clinical and aesthetic outcomes of immediate symmetrisation and to suggest our indication in an attempt to help surgeons with this operative decision.

2. Materials and Methods

This was a randomised observational study conducted on a population of patients with a diagnosis of unilateral breast cancer who underwent an SRM with a prepectoral tissue expander (Mentor CPX4, Mentor Worldwide LLC, Irvine, CA, USA) reconstruction implanted with specific covering devices (TiLoop® Bra, PFM medical, Cologne, Germany) followed by a substitution with a silicon-based implant at a later stage [12,13]. The enrolment started in January 2018 and ended in January 2021 at the Unit of Oncological Breast Surgery, University of Siena.

All women had a confirmed breast cancer diagnosis, were aged 18 years or older, met the criteria suggested by Nava et al. [7] for an SRM (patients with medium to large breasts with breast ptosis and at least grade II from the Regnault classification) and had a Pre-BRA score [14] from five to eight, indicating the implant of a prepectoral tissue expander and a subcutaneous definitive prosthesis from a second-time surgery.

The exclusion criteria were clinical evidence of axillary metastases or skin or chest wall tumour involvement, a body mass index greater than 35 kg/m^2, pregnancy, active smokers, connective tissue disease, diabetes, previous thoracic radiotherapy and previous breast surgery.

All data were collected upon informed consent acceptance and when the patients enrolled had accepted contralateral symmetrisation. We then divided the patients into two groups: one with delayed symmetrisation and one with immediate symmetrisation, based on a simple randomisation list using a dedicated computer program.

The patient data (including the age, body mass index and treatment characteristics as well as the indication for surgery, including the type of cancer, axillary surgery and locoregional or systemic recurrence, surgical complications and aesthetic outcomes) were collected from our specifically designed database.

The study was accomplished according to the ethical standards of the Declaration of Helsinki. Ethics approval was not required because the different timings of contralateral symmetrisation did not require any modifications to the standard therapeutic protocols.

All SRMs were conducted by a Wise pattern incision or a modified Wise pattern incision used to remove the skin overlying or infiltrated by the tumour in the lateral quadrants of the breast, as shown in Figure 1; in all cases, the nipple–areola complex (NAC) was removed at the beginning of the surgical procedure and reimplanted with the free-nipple graft (FNG) technique at the end of the surgical operation.

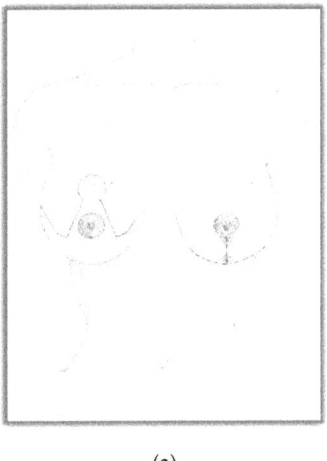 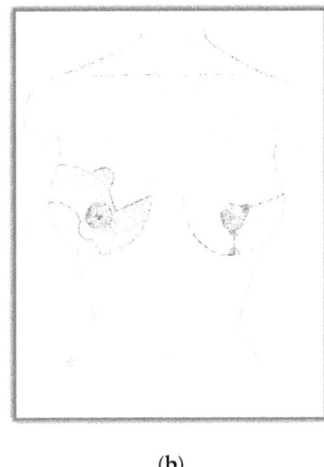

(a) (b)

Figure 1. (a) Wise pattern incision for SRM; (b) modified Wise pattern incision for SRM used to remove the skin overlying or infiltrated by the tumour in the lateral quadrants of the breast.

For the symmetrisation procedure, the patients underwent a reduction mammoplasty performed by a Wise pattern incision.

All the patients underwent an intraoperative sentinel lymph node (SLN) examination by a one-step nucleic acid amplification (OSNA) assay (Sysmex, Kobe, Japan) [15].

A health-related quality of life (HRQOL) evaluation was conducted using the preoperative and postoperative BREAST-Q modules. It has been largely corroborated for research in breast reconstruction and is routinely used at our institutions [16,17].

After a consultation with the oncology and plastic surgeon, the enrolled patients received the preoperative questionnaire 1 month before surgery. The BREAST-Q postoperative modules were administered 1 year after the breast reconstruction. All aspects of the BREAST-Q reconstructive modules (satisfaction with the breasts, satisfaction with the outcome, psychosocial wellbeing, physical wellbeing and sexual wellbeing) were considered [18].

SPSS software version 27.0 (IBM Corp., Armonk, NY, USA) was used for the simple descriptive statistics, accounting for the patient sociodemographic and clinical characteristics as well as the complications and capsular contracture grade.

The BREAST-Q scores for each patient were converted from the survey scores (1 to 5) to a continuous range from 0 to 100 using QScore Scoring Software. A higher score indicated grater satisfaction or a better HRQOL. To verify the normal distribution of the continuous variables, we used the Shapiro–Wilk test; we then analysed the BREAST-Q scores and expert scores as the continuous variables with a Student's t-test. The discrete variables were analysed with the χ^2 test. p-Values less than 0.05 were considered to be statistically significant.

3. Results

We enrolled 84 patients who underwent an SRM with the FNG technique and a prepectoral tissue expander reconstruction implanted with specific covering devices (TiLoop® Bra, PFM medical, Cologne, Germany) between January 2018 and January 2021 in our centre and divided them into two groups using a simple randomisation list. In the first group, 42 patients underwent immediate symmetrisation; in the second group, 42 patients underwent delayed symmetrisation (performed after a median of 9 months).

The characteristics of the study population are collated in Table 1. In the immediate group, the median age was 55.5 years and the average BMI was 24.9; in the delayed group, the median age was 55.8 years and the average BMI was 25.3.

Table 1. Characteristics of the study population.

Characteristics of the Study Population		Immediate Sy.		Delayed Sy.	
		No. of Cases	%	No. of Cases	%
Patients		42		42	
Age		55.5		55.8	
BMI		24.9		25.3	
Histology	Invasive ductal carcinoma	29	69%	28	66.6%
	DCIS	5	11.9%	6	14.2%
	Invasive lobular carcinoma	3	7.2%	4	9.6%
	Invasive ductal carcinoma + DCIS	5	11.9%	4	9.6%
Tumour size	pT1a	1	2.4%	2	4.8%
	pT1b	10	24%	11	26.2%
	pT1c	19	45%	17	40.2%
	pT2	11	26.2%	10	24%
	pT3	1	2.4%	2	4.8%
Pre-BRA	5	7	16.6%	8	19%
	6	14	33.4%	16	38%
	7	12	28.6%	10	24%
	8	9	21.4%	8	19%

The histology most represented was, in both groups, an invasive ductal carcinoma, with 29 cases (69%) in the immediate symmetrisation group and 28 cases (66.6%) in the delayed symmetrisation group.

In the immediate symmetrisation group, we performed an axillary resection on 10 patients (23.8%) with a macrometastasis at the SNL examination with an OSNA, on 4 after a neoadjuvant CHT and on 32 after sentinel lymph node biopsies (76.2%) (Table 2).

In the delayed symmetrisation group, we performed an axillary resection on 11 patients (26.2%) with a macrometastasis at the SNL examination with an OSNA, on 4 after a neoadjuvant CHT and on 26 after sentinel lymph node biopsies (61.9%) (Table 2).

The median follow-up time after surgery was 22 months (from 1 to 4 years). The postoperative morbidity is shown in Table 2. Complications requiring a second operation occurred in seven cases: in the immediate symmetrisation group, we reported two wound dehiscence cases (4.8%)—one on the mastectomy side and one on the symmetrisation side—as well as one seroma (2.4%) and one case of skin-nipple necrosis (2.4%), both on the mastectomy side; in the delayed symmetrisation group, we reported one infection (2.4%), one seroma (2.4%) and one case of skin-nipple necrosis (2.4%). We had to remove the tissue expander in three cases because of implant exposure; one in the immediate symmetrisation group and two in the delayed group. In the case of the removal of the prepectoral tissue expander, in two cases a salvage surgery was performed with a submuscular replacement of the tissue expander with the selective denervation of the pectoralis major muscle [5,6] and in one case the tissue expander was removed and a surgical revision was made supplemented with an antibiotate pulse lavage of the pocket surface and a new definitive implant placement [19].

Table 2. Characteristics of the study population.

Characteristics of the Study Population	Immediate Sy.		Delayed Sy.	
	No. of Cases	%	No. of Cases	%
Axillary dissection (following neoadjuvant CHT)	4	9.50%	4	9.50%
Axillary dissection (without neoadjuvant CHT)	6	14.30%	7	16.70%
Sentinel lymph node biopsy	32	76.20%	31	73.90%

Regarding disease recurrence, we reported one case of locoregional cancer recurrence (2.4%) in the delayed symmetrisation group and one case of systemic recurrence (2.4%) in each group. No statistical difference was found between the two groups. The safety and oncological outcomes are reported in Table 3.

Table 3. Safety and oncological outcomes.

Safety and Oncological Outcomes.		Immediate Sy.				Delayed Sy.	
		No. of Cases	%			No. of Cases	%
Tumour Recurrence	Locoregional	0	0%			1	2.4%
	Systemic	1	2.4%			1	2.4%
	No recurrence	41	97.6%			40	95.2%
				Symmetrisation side			
Complications	Skin-nipple necrosis	1	2.4%	0	0%	0	0%
	Infection	0	0%	0	0%	1	2.4%
	Wound dehiscence	1	2.4%	1	2.4%	1	2.4%
	Seroma	1	2.4%	0	0%	1	2.4%
Implant Loss		1	2.4%			2	4.8%

As shown in Table 4, we reported two cases (4.8%) in each group significative of capsular contractures (Baker III–IV grade) and in these cases we corrected this issue during the surgical procedure of the definitive implant. We observed a rippling in five cases (12%) in both groups 12 months after the primary surgery. Expander rippling was documented in five breasts (11.9%) in the immediate symmetrisation group and four breasts (9.5%) in the delayed symmetrisation group 12 months after the primary surgery.

Table 4. Aesthetic complications.

Aesthetic Complications.		Immediate Sy.		Delayed Sy.	
		No. of Cases	%	No. of Cases	%
Capsular Contracture					
	Grade I	35	83.3%	29	69.0%
	Grade II	5	11.9%	10	23.8%
	Grade III	2	4.8%	1	2.4%
	Grade IV	0		1	2.4%
Rippling		5	11.9%	4	9.5%
Complication Requiring Reoperation		7	16.6%	6	14.3%

Measure of the HRQOL and Aesthetic Outcomes

All the patients answered the five domains of the survey. The results are reported, divided for the two different groups, in Table 5. The survey was administered during a follow-up visit 1 year after surgery. The patients scored a high level of satisfaction about the outcomes within each group.

Table 5. BREAST-Q results.

BREAST-Q	Delayed Sy.	Immediate Sy.	p-Value
Satisfaction: breasts	73 ± 10	78 ± 11.9	0.04 *
Psychosocial wellness	76.6 ± 12	79.2 ± 14.2	0.36
Sexual wellness	60.7 ± 12.9	65.3 ± 14.7	0.13
Physical impact	56.5 ± 13.2	58.8 ± 11.8	0.40
Satisfaction with outcome	73 ± 12.1	75 ± 10.7	0.42

* Statistically significant ($p < 0.05$).

The scores in all the domains were higher in the immediate symmetrisation group, but only the satisfaction with the breasts score had a statistically higher result than the delayed symmetrisation group ($p < 0.05$).

4. Discussion

Although the study of breast cancer and its surgical treatment have paved the way for numerous discoveries in the field of oncology [20], there are still technical innovations in both the demolition and reconstructive fields [21,22].

Breast reconstruction during oncological surgery is, today, a recommended practice that provides optimal aesthetic satisfaction to patients and surgeons [13,17]. In an era where continuous innovations such as 3D printing can aid surgical planning [23,24], the search for new materials can radically change surgical tactics. The introduction of biological and synthetic devices aimed at providing an additional layer between the prosthesis and subcutaneous tissue has contributed to prepectoral reconstructions as a predominant role among the reconstructive techniques, reducing the complication rate and increasing the possibility of refining the shape of the breast with fat grafting [25–27]. Recent studies in the literature report a small complication rate for this technique with the advantage of a more natural aesthetic result compared with submuscular implants [28–34].

In this context, SRMs with an FNG for an immediate breast reconstruction are nowadays a preferred surgical strategy for selected patients [7], allowing both a safe oncological clearance and an improved cosmesis [35,36].

The prepectoral approach requires the placement of the tissue expander and the reconstruction to occur in two stages in a few cases when the vascularisation of the skin is not optimal and patients have risk factors such as diabetes, a history of smoking, obesity and a previous RT treatment [14,37].

In the last decade, the need to achieve increasingly satisfactory aesthetic outcomes has led breast surgeons to consider the treatment of the opposite breast as an important aspect of postmastectomy breast reconstructions [38–40].

This study aimed to demonstrate the improved outcomes that can be derived from the immediate symmetrisation of the healthy breast during an oncoplastic procedure. Currently, there are no indications of this type of surgical strategy in the literature [11]; however, in our experience, it appeared to us that we were able to guarantee patients a better aesthetic aspect due to the symmetry of the two breasts, especially after a procedure such as an SRM where the asymmetry in quite evident.

Giordano et al. [10] demonstrated that performing immediate symmetrisation at the time of a breast reconstruction was a reasonable and safe option in autologous latissimus dorsii breast reconstructions.

We analysed the satisfaction concerning the cosmetic and functional aspects of patients undergoing a unilateral SRM with an FNG and a prepectoral tissue expander reconstruction through a comparison between the results of patients subjected to immediate symmetrisation and the ones who were candidates for delayed symmetrisation.

We did not find significant differences in the analysis of the clinical outcomes between the two groups in the study or between these populations and the ones reported in the literature [19,41–43]. In two cases, a reintervention was required for implant exposure: one in the symmetrisation group and one in the immediate group.

We also reported an acceptable number of patients with aesthetic complications that required a second surgery; in the majority of cases, a lipofilling with a small quantity of fat grafting was sufficient to correct them [27,44,45]. A high-grade capsular contracture was reported only in 4.8% of cases in each group, according to the literature [46].

In the immediate symmetrisation group, compared with the patients with an SRM and an FNG without symmetrisation, there was a higher subjective satisfaction rate as it improved the aesthetic results by reducing negative self-perception.

5. Conclusions

This is, to the best of our knowledge, the first study evaluating immediate symmetrisation during a subcutaneous reconstruction for demolitive surgery. Our findings suggested that immediate symmetrisation was a possible, safe and highly tolerable technique of reconstruction in terms of the aesthetic outcome and the quality of life of the patients. Moreover, immediate symmetrisation did not delay the adjuvant oncological treatments compared with the choice of symmetrisation at the second time of reconstruction.

Furthermore, the consolidated use of covering devices in prepectoral reconstructions in selected patients confirmed how this technique could be applied with a low rate of complications.

This technique, providing patients an aesthetic result in terms of immediate symmetry, allowed us to better manage the waiting times for the second reconstructive surgery whilst still providing an excellent result, even if it was not definitive. Moreover, at the time of the definitive reconstruction, it was possible to evaluate the natural ageing process of the symmetrised breast in order to accordingly adjust the definitive implant of the reconstructed breast. In conclusion, even if not indicated in the literature, it seems to us that the choice of immediate symmetrisation is a viable choice to provide immediate better satisfaction and quality of life for patients and does not excessively impact, from a surgical point of view, on the second time of the reconstruction.

Author Contributions: Conceptualisation, D.C. (Donato Casella) and D.F.; methodology, D.C. (Donato Casella); validation, D.C. (Dario Cassetti), R.C. and M.G.; investigation, A.L.P.; data curation, D.F. and A.L.P.; writing—original draft preparation, D.F.; writing—review and editing, D.C.; visualisation, D.R. and A.D.L.; supervision, A.N.; project administration, M.M. All authors have read and agreed to the published version of the manuscript.

Funding: This research received no external funding.

Institutional Review Board Statement: The study was conducted in accordance with the Declaration of Helsinki. Ethics approval was not required because the different timing of contralateral symmetrisation did not require any modification of the standard therapeutic protocols.

Informed Consent Statement: Informed consent was obtained from all subjects involved in the study.

Data Availability Statement: The data presented in this study are available on request from the corresponding author.

Acknowledgments: We here acknowledge Ottavia Cecchi for her explanatory drawings of the incision.

Conflicts of Interest: Author Donato Casella has received a speaker honorarium from Pfm Medical and TiLOOP Bra manufacturing company. The other authors declare that they have no conflict of interest.

References

1. Toth, B.A.; Lappert, P. Modified Skin Incisions for Mastectomy: The Need for Plastic Surgical Input in Preoperative Planning. *Plast. Reconstr. Surg.* **1991**, *87*, 1048–1053. Available online: https://europepmc.org/article/med/1852020 (accessed on 8 November 2022). [CrossRef] [PubMed]
2. Rice, C.O.; Strickler, J.H. Adeno-Mammectomy for Benign Breast Lesions. *Surg. Gynecol. Obstet.* **1951**, *93*, 759–762. Available online: https://europepmc.org/article/med/14893082 (accessed on 8 November 2022). [PubMed]
3. Freeman, B.S. Subcutaneous Mastectomy for Benign Breast Lesions with Immediate or Delayed Prosthetic Replacement. *Plast. Reconstr. Surg. Transpl. Bull.* **1962**, *30*, 676–682. Available online: https://pubmed.ncbi.nlm.nih.gov/13959443/ (accessed on 8 November 2022). [CrossRef] [PubMed]
4. Regnault, P. Breast Ptosis. Definition and Treatment. *Clin. Plast. Surg.* **1976**, *3*, 193–203. Available online: https://europepmc.org/article/med/1261176 (accessed on 7 July 2022). [CrossRef]
5. Giudice, G.; Maruccia, M.; Nacchiero, E.; Elia, R.; Annoscia, P.; Vestita, M. Dual plane breast implant reconstruction in large sized breasts: How to maximise the result following first stage total submuscular expansion. *JPRAS Open* **2018**, *15*, 74–80. [CrossRef]
6. Carlson, G.W.; Bostwick, J.; Styblo, T.M.; Moore, B.; Bried, J.T.; Murray, D.R.; Wood, W.C. Skin-Sparing Mastectomy Oncologic and Reconstructive Considerations. *Ann Surg.* **1997**, *225*, 570–578. [CrossRef]
7. Nava, M.B.; Cortinovis, U.; Ottolenghi, J.; Riggio, E.; Pennati, A.; Catanuto, G.; Greco, M.; Della Rovere, G.Q. Skin-reducing mastectomy. *Plast. Reconstr. Surg.* **2006**, *118*, 603–610. [CrossRef]
8. Bostwick, J. Reconstruction after mastectomy. *Surg. Clin. N. Am.* **1990**, *70*, 1125–1140. [CrossRef]
9. Salgarello, M.; Visconti, G.; Barone-Adesi, L.; Franceschini, G.; Masetti, R. Contralateral breast symmetrisation in immediate prosthetic breast reconstruction after unilateral nipple-sparing mastectomy: The tailored reduction/augmentation mammaplasty. *Arch. Plast. Surg. Korean Soc. Plast. Reconstr. Surg.* **2015**, *42*, 302–308. [CrossRef]
10. Giordano, S.; Harkkila, S.; Oranges, C.M.; di Summa, P.G.; Koskivuo, I. Immediate Versus Delayed Contralateral Breast Symmetrisation in Breast Reconstruction with Latissimus Dorsi Flap: A Comparative Study. *Breast Care* **2019**, *5*, 272–277. Available online: https://www.karger.com/Article/FullText/502769 (accessed on 8 November 2022).
11. Rizki, H.; Nkonde, C.; Ching, R.C.; Kumiponjera, D.; Malata, C.M. Plastic surgical management of the contralateral breast in post-mastectomy breast reconstruction. *Int. J. Surg.* **2013**, *11*, 767–772. [CrossRef]
12. Lo Torto, F.; Cigna, E.; Kaciulyte, J.; Casella, D.; Marcasciano, M.; Ribuffo, D. National breast reconstruction utilization in the setting of postmastectomy radiotherapy: Two-stage implant-based breast reconstruction. *J. Reconstr. Microsurg.* **2017**, *33*, E3. [CrossRef]
13. Lo Torto, F.; Marcasciano, M.; Kaciulyte, J.; Redi, U.; Barellini, L.; De Luca, A.; Perra, A.; Frattaroli, J.M.; Cavalieri, E.; Di Taranto, G.; et al. Prepectoral breast reconstruction with TiLoop®Bra Pocket: A single center prospective study. *Eur. Rev. Med. Pharmacol. Sci.* **2020**, *24*, 991–999.
14. Casella, D.; Kaciulyte, J.; Lo Torto, F.; Mori, F.L.R.; Barellini, L.; Fausto, A.; Fanelli, B.; Greco, M.; Ribuffo, D.; Marcasciano, M. "To Pre or not to Pre": Introduction of a Prepectoral Breast Reconstruction Assessment Score to Help Surgeons Solving the Decision-Making Dilemma. Retrospective Results of a Multicenter Experience. *Plast. Reconstr. Surg.* **2021**, *147*, 1278–1286. Available online: https://journals.lww.com/plasreconsurg/Fulltext/2021/06000/_To_Pre_or_Not_to_Pre___Introduction_of_a.4.aspx (accessed on 17 October 2022).

15. Tsujimoto, M.; Nakabayashi, K.; Yoshidome, K.; Kaneko, T.; Iwase, T.; Akiyama, F.; Kato, Y.; Tsuda, H.; Ueda, S.; Sato, K.; et al. One-step nucleic acid amplification for intraoperative detection of lymph node metastasis in breast cancer patients. *Clin. Cancer Res.* **2007**, *13*, 4807–4816. [CrossRef]
16. Casella, D.; Di Taranto, G.; Marcasciano, M.; Sordi, S.; Kothari, A.; Kovacs, T.; Lo Torto, F.; Cigna, E.; Calabrese, C.; Ribuffo, D. Evaluation of prepectoral implant placement and complete coverage with Tiloop bra mesh for breast reconstruction: A prospective study on long-term and patient-reported breast-q outcomes. *Plast. Reconstr. Surg.* **2019**, *43*, 1E–9E. [CrossRef]
17. Marcasciano, M.; Frattaroli, J.; Mori, F.L.R.; Lo Torto, F.; Fioramonti, P.; Cavalieri, E.; Kaciulyte, J.; Greco, M.; Casella, D.; Ribuffo, D. The New Trend of Pre-pectoral Breast Reconstruction: An Objective Evaluation of the Quality of Online Information for Patients Undergoing Breast Reconstruction. *Aesthetic Plast. Surg.* **2019**, *43*, 593–599. Available online: https://pubmed.ncbi.nlm.nih.gov/30710175/ (accessed on 22 June 2022). [CrossRef]
18. Casella, D.; Di Taranto, G.; Marcasciano, M.; Sordi, S.; Kothari, A.; Kovacs, T.; Torto, F.L.; Cigna, E.; Ribuffo, D.; Calabrese, C. Nipple-sparing bilateral prophylactic mastectomy and immediate reconstruction with TiLoop®Bra mesh in BRCA1/2 mutation carriers: A prospective study of long-term and patient reported outcomes using the BREAST-Q. *The Breast. Churchill Livingstone* **2018**, *39*, 8–13. [CrossRef]
19. Marcasciano, M.; Kaciulyte, J.; Di Giuli, R.; Marcasciano, F.; Torto, F.L.; Guerra, M.; Dal Prà, G.; Barellini, L.; Mazzocchi, M.; Casella, D.; et al. "Just Pulse it!" Introduction of a Conservative Implant Salvage Protocol to Manage Infection in Pre-Pectoral Breast Reconstruction: Case Series and Literature Review. *J. Plast. Reconstr. Aesthet. Surg.* **2022**, *75*, 571–578. Available online: https://pubmed.ncbi.nlm.nih.gov/34794920/ (accessed on 8 November 2022). [CrossRef]
20. Boccardi, V.; Marano, L.; Rossetti, R.R.A.; Rizzo, M.R.; di Martino, N.; Paolisso, G. Serum CD26 Levels in Patients with Gastric Cancer: A Novel Potential Diagnostic Marker. *BMC Cancer.* **2015**, *15*, 703. Available online: https://bmccancer.biomedcentral.com/articles/10.1186/s12885-015-1757-0 (accessed on 5 November 2022). [CrossRef]
21. Marcasciano, M.; Torto, F.L.; Codolini, L.; Kaciulyte, J.; Luridiana, G.; Cassetti, D.; Barellini, L.; Neri, A.; Ribuffo, D.; Greco, M.; et al. "Hook Shape" Nipple-Sparing Mastectomy and Prepectoral Implant Reconstruction: Technique, Results and Outcomes from a Preliminary Case Series. *Aesthetic Plast. Surg.* **2022**. Available online: https://pubmed.ncbi.nlm.nih.gov/36280606/ (accessed on 8 November 2022).
22. Sisti, A.; Sadeghi, P.; Cuomo, R.; Alvarez, S.M. Pre-Pectoral One-Stage Breast Reconstruction with Anterior Coverage Using Superior Anterior Biological Acellular Dermal Matrix (ADM) and Inferior Anterior Dermal Sling Support. *Medicina* **2022**, *58*, 992. [CrossRef]
23. Huang, Y.-H.; Tuttle, T.M.; Hoven, N. 3D Printed Model for Triple Negative Inflammatory Breast Cancer. *3D Print. Med.* **2022**, *8*, 32. Available online: https://threedmedprint.biomedcentral.com/articles/10.1186/s41205-022-00158-4 (accessed on 7 November 2022). [CrossRef]
24. Marano, L.; Ricci, A.; Savelli, V.; Verre, L.; Di Renzo, L.; Biccari, E.; Costantini, G.; Marrelli, D.; Roviello, F. From Digital World to Real Life: A Robotic Approach to the Esophagogastric Junction with a 3D Printed Model. *BMC Surg.* **2019**, *19*, 153. Available online: https://bmcsurg.biomedcentral.com/articles/10.1186/s12893-019-0621-6 (accessed on 5 November 2022). [CrossRef]
25. Casella, D.; di Taranto, G.; Onesti, M.G.; Greco, M.; Ribuffo, D. A retrospective Comparative Analysis of Risk Factors and Outcomes in Direct-to-Implant and Two-Stages Prepectoral Breast Reconstruction: BMI and Radiotherapy as New Selection Criteria of Patients. *Eur. J. Surg. Oncol.* **2019**, *45*, 1357–1363. Available online: https://pubmed.ncbi.nlm.nih.gov/30827802/ (accessed on 13 July 2022). [CrossRef]
26. Casella, D.; Di Taranto, G.; Torto, F.L.; Marcasciano, M.; Kaciulyte, J.; Greco, M.; Onesti, M.G.; Ribuffo, D. Body Mass Index Can Predict Outcomes in Direct-to-Implant Prepectoral Breast Reconstruction. *Plast. Reconstr. Surg.* **2020**, *145*, 867E–868E. Available online: https://pubmed.ncbi.nlm.nih.gov/32221244/ (accessed on 13 July 2020). [CrossRef]
27. Gentile, P.; Casella, D.; Palma, E.; Calabrese, C. Engineered Fat Graft Enhanced with Adipose-Derived Stromal Vascular Fraction Cells for Regenerative Medicine: Clinical, Histological and Instrumental Evaluation in Breast Reconstruction. *J. Clin. Med.* **2019**, *8*, 504. [CrossRef] [PubMed]
28. Jagsi, R.; Jiang, J.; Momoh, A.O.; Alderman, A.; Giordano, S.H.; Buchholz, T.A.; Kronowitz, S.J.; Smith, B.D. Trends and Variation in Use of Breast Reconstruction in Patients With Breast Cancer Undergoing Mastectomy in the United States. *J. Clin. Oncol. Am. Soc. Clin. Oncol.* **2014**, *32*, 919. Available online: https://pmc/articles/PMC4876312/ (accessed on 17 October 2022). [CrossRef]
29. Snyderman, R.K.; Guthrie, R.H. Reconstruction of the female breast following radical mastectomy. *Plast. Reconstr. Surg.* **1971**, *47*, 565–567. [CrossRef]
30. Radovan, C. Breast reconstruction after mastectomy using the temporary expander. *Plast. Reconstr. Surg.* **1982**, *69*, 195–206. [CrossRef]
31. Reitsamer, R.; Peintinger, F. Prepectoral implant placement and complete coverage with porcine acellular dermal matrix: A new technique for direct-to-implant breast reconstruction after nipple-sparing mastectomy. *J. Plast. Reconstr. Aesthetic Surg.* **2015**, *68*, 162–167. [CrossRef]
32. Casella, D.; Di Taranto, G.; Marcasciano, M.; Torto, F.L.; Barellini, L.; Sordi, S.; Gaggelli, I.; Roncella, M.; Calabrese, C.; Ribuffo, D. Subcutaneous expanders and synthetic mesh for breast reconstruction: Long-term and patient-reported BREAST-Q outcomes of a single-center prospective study. *J. Plast. Reconstr. Aesthetic Surg.* **2019**, *72*, 805–812. [CrossRef]
33. Cuomo, R. Submuscular and Pre-Pectoral ADM Assisted Immediate Breast Reconstruction: A Literature Review. *Medicina* **2020**, *56*, 256. Available online: https://www.ncbi.nlm.nih.gov/pubmed/32466619 (accessed on 11 October 2022). [CrossRef]

34. Cuomo, R. The state of the art about etiopathogenetic models on breast implant associated–anaplastic large cell lymphoma (Bia-alcl): A narrative review. *J. Clin. Med.* **2021**, *10*, 2082. [CrossRef]
35. Caputo, G.G.; Marchetti, A.; Dalla Pozza, E.; Vigato, E.; Domenici, L.; Cigna, E.; Governa, M. Skin-Reduction Breast Reconstructions with Prepectoral Implant. *Plast. Reconstr. Surg.* **2016**, *137*, 1702–1705. Available online: https://journals.lww.com/plasreconsurg/Fulltext/2016/06000/Skin_Reduction_Breast_Reconstructions_with.9.aspx (accessed on 8 November 2022). [CrossRef]
36. Maruccia, M.; Elia, R.; Gurrado, A.; Moschetta, M.; Nacchiero, E.; Bolletta, A.; Testini, M.; Giudice, G. Skin-Reducing Mastectomy and Pre-pectoral Breast Reconstruction in Large Ptotic Breasts. *Aesthetic. Plast. Surg.* **2022**, *44*, 664–672. [CrossRef]
37. Bernini, M.; Calabrese, C.; Cecconi, L.; Santi, C.; Gjondedaj, U.; Roselli, J.; Nori, J.; Fausto, A.; Orzalesi, L.; Casella, D. Subcutaneous direct-to-implant breast reconstruction: Surgical, functional, and aesthetic results after long-term follow-up. *Plast. Reconstr. Surg. Glob. Open* **2015**, *3*, e574. [CrossRef]
38. Losken, A.; Carlson, G.W.; Bostwick, J.; Jones, G.E.; Culbertson, J.H.; Schoemann, M. Trends in Unilateral Breast Reconstruction and Management of the Contralateral Breast: The Emory Experience. *Plast. Reconstr. Surg.* **2002**, *10*, 89–97. Available online: https://europepmc.org/article/med/12087236 (accessed on 7 November 2022). [CrossRef]
39. Nava, M.B.; Rocco, N.; Catanuto, G.; Falco, G.; Capalbo, E.; Marano, L.; Bordoni, D.; Spano, A.; Scaperrotta, G. Impact of contralateral breast reshaping on mammographic surveillance in women undergoing breast reconstruction following mastectomy for breast cancer. *Breast* **2015**, *24*, 434–439. [CrossRef]
40. Falco, G.; Rocco, N.; Bordoni, D.; Marano, L.; Accurso, A.; Buccelli, C.; Di Lorenzo, P.; Capasso, E.; Policino, F.; Niola, M.; et al. Contralateral risk reducing mastectomy in Non-BRCA-Mutated patients. *Open Med.* **2016**, *11*, 238. Available online: https://pmc/articles/PMC5329834/ (accessed on 5 November 2022). [CrossRef]
41. Wagner, R.D.; Braun, T.L.; Zhu, H.; Winocour, S. A systematic review of complications in prepectoral breast reconstruction. *J. Plast. Reconstr. Aesthetic Surg.* **2019**, *72*, 1051–1059. Available online: http://www.jprasurg.com/article/S1748681519301731/fulltext (accessed on 29 October 2022). [CrossRef] [PubMed]
42. Marcasciano, M.; Kaciulyte, J.; Marcasciano, F.; lo Torto, F.; Ribuffo, D.; Casella, D. "No Drain, No Gain": Simultaneous Seroma Drainage and Tissue Expansion in Pre-pectoral Tissue Expander-Based Breast Reconstruction. *Aesthetic Plast. Surg.* **2019**, *43*, 1118–1119. Available online: https://pubmed.ncbi.nlm.nih.gov/29987487/ (accessed on 13 July 2022).
43. Sisti, A.; Grimaldi, L.; Tassinari, J.; Cuomo, R.; Fortezza, L.; Bocchiotti, M.A.; Roviello, F.; D'Aniello, C.; Nisi, G. Nipple-areola complex reconstruction techniques: A literature review. *Eur. J. Surg. Oncol.* **2016**, *42*, 441–465. Available online: https://www.ncbi.nlm.nih.gov/pubmed/26868167 (accessed on 17 October 2022). [CrossRef]
44. Vaia, N.; Lo Torto, F.; Marcasciano, M.; Casella, D.; Cacace, C.; De Masi, C.; Ricci, F.; Ribuffo, D. From the "Fat Capsule" to the "Fat Belt": Limiting Protective Lipofilling on Irradiated Expanders for Breast Reconstruction to Selective Key Areas. *Aesthetic. Plast. Surg.* **2018**, *42*, 986–994. [CrossRef]
45. Cuomo, R.; Giardino, F.R.; Neri, A.; Nisi, G.; Brandi, C.; Zerini, I.; Jingjian, H.; Grimaldi, L. Optimization of Prepectoral Breast Reconstruction. *Breast Care* **2021**, *16*, 36–42. [CrossRef]
46. Marques, M.; Brown, S.A.; Oliveira, I.; Cordeiro, M.N.D.S.; Morales-Helguera, A.; Rodrigues, A.; Amarante, J. Long-term follow-up of breast capsule contracture rates in cosmetic and reconstructive cases. *Plast. Reconstr. Surg.* **2010**, *126*, 769–778. [CrossRef]

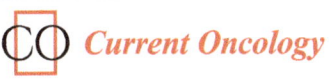

Article

Dose Volume and Liver Function Test Relationship following Radiotheraphy for Right Breast Cancer: A Multicenter Study

Zeliha Güzelöz [1,*], Oğuzhan Ayrancıoğlu [2], Nesrin Aktürk [3], Merve Güneş [2] and Zümre Arıcan Alıcıkuş [2]

1 Department of Radiation Oncology, Health Science University Tepecik Training and Research Hospital, İzmir 35100, Türkiye
2 Department of Radiation Oncology, İzmir Tınaztepe University Galen Hospital, İzmir 35001, Türkiye; oguzhan.ayrancioglu@tinaztepe.com (O.A.); merve.gunes@tinaztepe.com (M.G.); zumre.arican@tinaztepe.edu.tr (Z.A.A.)
3 Department of Radiation Oncology, Katip Çelebi University Atatürk Training and Research Hospital, İzmir 35150, Türkiye; nesrin.akturk@saglik.gov.tr
* Correspondence: z.guzelozcapar@saglik.gov.tr; Tel.: +90-5064019642

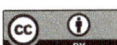

Citation: Güzelöz, Z.; Ayrancıoğlu, O.; Aktürk, N.; Güneş, M.; Alıcıkuş, Z.A. Dose Volume and Liver Function Test Relationship following Radiotheraphy for Right Breast Cancer: A Multicenter Study. *Curr. Oncol.* 2023, *30*, 8763–8773. https://doi.org/10.3390/curroncol30100632

Received: 25 August 2023
Revised: 19 September 2023
Accepted: 22 September 2023
Published: 26 September 2023

Copyright: © 2023 by the authors. Licensee MDPI, Basel, Switzerland. This article is an open access article distributed under the terms and conditions of the Creative Commons Attribution (CC BY) license (https://creativecommons.org/licenses/by/4.0/).

Abstract: Objective: The liver is a critical organ at risk during right breast radiotherapy (RT). Liver function tests (LFTs) such as alanine aminotransferase (ALT), aspartate aminotransferase (AST), and gamma-glutamyl transferase (GGT) serve as biochemical markers for hepatobiliary damage. In this multicenter cross-sectional study, the effects of liver dose–volume on changes in LFTs pre- and post-RT in patients treated for right breast cancer were evaluated. Materials and Methods: Between January 2019 and November 2022, data from 100 patients who underwent adjuvant right breast RT across three centers were retrospectively assessed. Target volumes and normal structures were contoured per the RTOG atlas. Patients were treated with a total dose of 50 Gy in 25 fractions to the CTV, followed by a boost to the tumor bed where indicated. The percentage change in LFT values in the first two weeks post-RT was calculated. Statistics were analyzed with SPSS version 22 software, with significance set at $p < 0.05$. Statistical correlation between liver doses (in cGy) and the volume receiving specific doses (Vx in cc) on the change in LFTs were analyzed using Kolmogorov–Smirnov, Mann–Whitney U test. Results: The median age among the 100 patients was 56 (range: 29–79). Breast-conserving surgery was performed on 75% of the patients. The most common T and N stages were T1 (53%) and N0 (53%), respectively. None of the patients had distant metastasis or simultaneous systemic treatment with RT. A total of 67% of the treatments utilized the IMRT technique and 33% VMAT. The median CTV volume was 802 cc (range: 214–2724 cc). A median boost dose of 10 Gy (range: 10–16 Gy) was applied to 28% of the patients with electrons and 51% with IMRT/VMAT. The median liver volume was 1423 cc (range: 825–2312 cc). Statistical analyses were conducted on a subset of 57 patients for whom all three LFT values were available both pre- and post-RT. In this group, the median values for AST, ALT, and GGT increased up to 15% post-RT compared to pre-RT, and a median liver D_{mean} below 208 cGy was found significant. While many factors can influence LFT values, during RT planning, attention to liver doses and subsequent regular LFT checks are crucial. Conclusion: Due to factors such as anatomical positioning, planning technique, and breast posture, the liver can receive varying doses during right breast irradiation. Protecting patients from liver toxicity secondary to RT is valuable, especially in breast cancer patients with a long-life expectancy. Our study found that, even in the absence of any systemic treatment or risk factors, there was an average increase of nearly 15% in enzymes, indicating acute liver damage post-RT compared with pre-RT. Attention to liver doses during RT planning and regular follow-up with LFTs is essential.

Keywords: right breast; radiotherapy; liver function tests; dose–volume; toxicity

1. Introduction

Breast cancer is the most frequently diagnosed cancer among women worldwide [1]. Adjuvant radiation therapy (RT) plays a pivotal role in the treatment of breast cancer [2,3].

There has been an observed increase in locoregional control in patients undergoing breast-conserving surgery with adjuvant RT and selected patients receiving mastectomy [4,5]. Following breast-conserving surgery, RT to the preserved breast halves the local recurrence rate and lowers breast cancer mortality by approximately one-sixth [5].

The success achieved in locoregional control with RT has also reflected positively in survival rates [4–6]. Variations in local treatments that have a significant impact on local recurrence rates would, under the assumption of no other causes of death, prevent approximately one breast cancer-related death within the next 15 years for every four avoided instances of local recurrence, consequently leading to a decrease in overall mortality over the course of 15 years [5]. Nowadays, due to the diffusion of breast cancer screening programs and advancements in imaging technology, breast cancer diagnoses are being made at younger ages [7,8]. This means that younger-patient populations need to be followed for many years. Advances in both RT and systemic treatments have improved the prognosis of these patients, emphasizing the importance of the quality of life and preservation of normal tissue. Particularly with the increasing young patient population, there has been a growing emphasis on the need for better protection of normal tissues during RT. Protecting these long-surviving patients from acute side effects is just as crucial as minimizing secondary cancer risks in the long term.

For many years, numerous studies have been conducted on radiation-induced liver disease (RILD). Especially in patients undergoing abdominal RT, the liver stands as one of the priority normal tissues to be protected [9]. In right breast RT practices, due to anatomical proximity, the liver is one of the normal tissues at risk. However, the etiology of RILD is multi-factorial, with a central role of veno-occlusive processes and, although as low dose exposure may as well exert some effects, no specific liver dose constraints have been defined in the setting of adjuvant breast irradiation [10].

The liver, being a metabolic organ with vital functions, has liver function tests (LFTs) such as alanine aminotransferase (ALT), aspartate aminotransferase (AST), and gamma-glutamyl transferase (GGT), which are biochemical indicators of hepatobiliary damage for various reasons. The normal ranges for ALT, AST, and GGT are 0–45 IU/L, 0–35 IU/L, and 0–45 IU/L, respectively [10]. In the literature, there are limited studies examining long- and short-term changes in LFTs post-RT [11–14]. Grade 3–4 hepatotoxicity was not identified in these few studies. However, a correlation was found between irradiated liver volume and ALT and ALP tests [11]. A significant increase was detected in IL-6 level [12]. An increase in median AST and ALT values was observed after radiotherapy [13].

In this multicentric cross-sectional study, the aim was to evaluate the impact of liver dose–volume on changes in LFT values before and after RT in patients treated for right breast cancer.

2. Patients and Methods

2.1. Patient Selection

In this study, data from 100 female patients aged 18 and over who underwent RT to the right breast or right chest wall following breast-conserving surgery or mastectomy between January 2019 and November 2022 in three centers with identical RT protocols were retrospectively evaluated. These patients had a diagnosis of invasive breast carcinoma without distant organ metastasis and had pre-radiation therapy (preRT) and post-radiation therapy (postRT) liver function test values (AST, ALT, GGT). Staging was performed according to the American Joint Committee on Cancer tumors, lymph nodes, and distant metastases TNM staging system (8th ed., 2017). Patients diagnosed with stage IV or in situ carcinoma, those who received neoadjuvant chemotherapy, those undergoing concurrent systemic treatment, or those with chronic liver or biliary tract disease were excluded from this study. The study protocol was approved by the national ethics committee (Health Science University Tepecik Training and Research Hospital Ethics Committee approval number: 2023/07-05).

2.2. Radiation Therapy

2.2.1. Simulation

All patients were planned in a supine position using a breast board with arm support. Tomographic slices were acquired at intervals of 3 mm. In the acquired topographies, the entire liver was included in the imaging field.

2.2.2. Contouring of Target Volumes

Target volumes and at-risk normal tissues were contoured on the tomographic slices taken at a 3 mm slice thickness according to the Radiation Therapy Oncology Group (RTOG)/European Organization for Research and Treatment of Cancer (EORTC) guidelines [15]. For patients who underwent breast-conserving surgery, the entire right mammary glandular tissue and skin were determined as breast CTV (clinical target volume). Lumpectomy cavities and seromas were included in the CTV. For patients who underwent mastectomy, the chest wall including the incision scar and skin was contoured. PTV (planning target volume) was obtained by giving a five mm margin to CTV.

2.2.3. Contouring of the Liver

The liver was contoured based on the RTOG upper abdomen normal tissue contouring guidelines [16]. The entire liver in the slice area was contoured in the abdomen window level range. The gallbladder was excluded. The portal vein, branches of the portal vein, and other vessels were included within the liver (except inferior vena cava) contour according to the guidelines [17].

2.2.4. Radiotherapy Prescription and Planning

Patients received a total of 50 Gy RT over 25 fractions of CTV using FIF (field in field)/IMRT (intensity-modulated radiotherapy)/VMAT (volumetric arc therapy) techniques. Where necessary, an additional dose (boost) was given to the tumor bed using either electron or photon energy. The energy of 6–10 MVX was utilized. It was aimed to keep the volume of the right lung receiving 20 Gy below 30%.

2.2.5. Liver Dose–Volume

Assessment from the dose–volume histogram, values for the D_{max} (maximum dose, D_{min} (minimum dose), D_{mean} (mean dose), and (V_x) the volume of the liver (cc) receiving a certain dose (x) were (V_5, V_{10}, V_{20}, V_{30}, V_{40}, and V_{50}) recorded. According to normal tissue dose limitations, the mean dose to the liver was aimed to be below 30–32 Gy [18].

2.3. Laboratory Tests

ALT, AST, and GGT blood values from two weeks before the initial fraction of RT (preRT) and two weeks after the last fraction of RT (postRT) were obtained from hospital and national medical record systems.

2.4. Statistics

The percentage difference (Δ%) for each of the three parameters between preRT and postRT was calculated using the formula Δ% = (postRT − preRT)/preRT × 100. Based on this formula, a positive percentage difference indicated an increase in LFTs after RT, while a negative value indicated a decrease post-RT. The effects of liver doses (cGy) and volumes (Vx) (cc) on Δ% were evaluated. Statistics were analyzed with SPSS© 22 software (Statistical Package for the Social Sciences), with significance set at $p < 0.05$. Statistical correlation between liver doses (in cGy) and the volume receiving specific doses (Vx in cc) on the change in LFTs were analyzed using Kolmogorov–Smirnov, Mann–Whitney U test.

3. Results

The demographic and treatment data of the patients can be seen in Table 1.

Table 1. Demographics and treatment data of patients.

Median Age	56 (29–79)
Median CTV volume	802 (214–2724) cc
Surgery modality	
breast conserving	75%
mastectomy	25%
T Stage	
T1	53%
T2	39%
T3	-
T4	-
Tx	8%
N Stage	
N0	53%
N1	25%
N2	-
N3	-
Nx	22%
RT technics	
FIF/IMRT	67%
VMAT	33%
Deep inspiration breath hold	25%
RT boost dose (median)	10 (10–16) Gy
RT boost	
Electron	28%
IMRT	31%
VMAT	20%
Patient not received boost	21%

CTV: Clinical target volume; RT: Radiotherapy; FIF: Field in field; IMRT: Intensity-modulated radiotherapy; VMAT: Volumetric arc therapy.

After radiotherapy, it was observed that AST values were above the normal range in 12 patients (ranging from 45 to 1107 IU/L), ALT values in 12 patients (ranging from 35 to 365 IU/L), and GGT values in 12 patients (ranging from 49 to 414 IU/L).

No patient received systemic therapy or tamoksifen concurrent with RT. The median liver volume was 1423 cc, with a range of 825–2312 cc. The median D_{min} was 3.4 cGy (range: 0–206.1 cGy), the median D_{max} was 4814 cGy (range: 110–206.1 cGy), and the median D_{mean} was 203 cGy (range: 15–1497 cGy). The observed dose–volume values were as follows: Median V_{50} was 0 cc (range: 0–68), V_{40} was 0.76 cc (range: 0–87.2), V_{30} was 2.14 cc (range: 0–180.7), V_{20} was 6 cc (range: 0–387.7), V_{10} was 11.7 cc (range: 0–949.1), and V_5 was 21.2 cc (range: 0–1352).

For the statistical analyses, 57 patients were included, for whom all three LFTs were completely obtained in both the pre- and post-RT periods. In this patient group, the median CTV volume was 806 cc (range: 214–2519 cc) and the median liver volume was 1457 cc (range: 825–2218 cc). The D_{max}, D_{min}, and D_{mean} dose values are presented in Table 2 and Figure 1, while the liver V_{5-50} dose values are shown in Table 3 and Figure 1.

Table 2. Liver Dosimetric Values (cc) of 57 patients.

Liver Dx	D_{max} (cGy)	D_{min} (cGy)	D_{mean} (cGy)
Dose (median)	5005 (110–5969)	5.8 (0–206.1)	208 (15–1497)

D_{max}: Maximum dose; D_{min} Minimum dose; D_{mean}: Mean dose; cGy centi Gray.

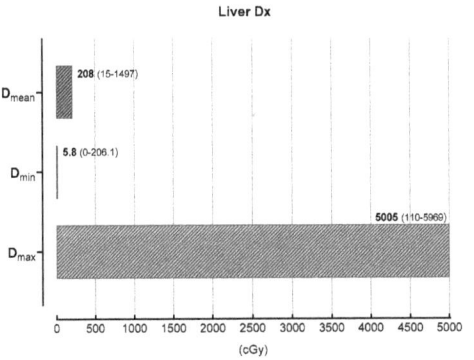 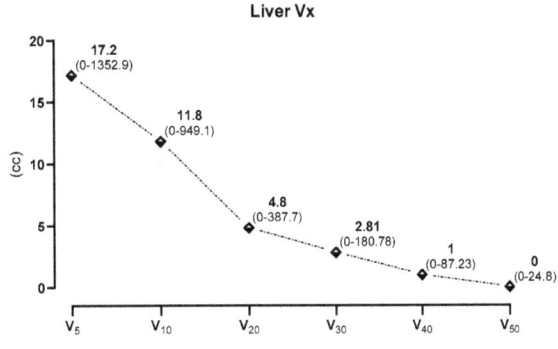

Figure 1. Liver Dosimetric and V_{5-50} Values.

Table 3. Liver V_{5-50} Values (cc) of 57 patients.

Liver V_x	V_5	V_{10}	V_{20}	V_{30}	V_{40}	V_{50}
cc (median)	17.2 (0–1352.9)	11.8 (0–949.1)	4.8 (0–387.7)	2.81 (0–180.78)	1 (0–87.23)	0 (0–24.8)

$V_{5/10/20/30/40/50}$ liver volume receiving 5/10/20/30/40/50 Gy.

The median values and percentage changes in ALT, AST, and GGT tests prior to and following RT are provided in Table 4 and Figure 2.

Table 4. Median and percentage change in liver function test (LFT) values of 57 patients.

Liver Test	Median (U/L)	Median Percentage Change (%)
AST		
preRT	19 (11–35)	13% (−120 to 54.5)
postRT	21 (10–52.32)	
ALT		
preRT	18 (1.97–39)	3.03% (−292 to 46.1)
postRT	20 (8–55)	
GGT		
preRT	20 (12–44)	−6% (−93.18 to 42.86)
postRT	19 (10–85)	

ALT: Alanine aminotransferase; AST: Aspartate aminotransferase; GGT: Gamma-glutamyl transferase; preRT: pre-radiation therapy; postRT: post-radiation therapy.

When examining the effect of liver dose–volume on the percentage change between preRT and postRT in LFT, a statistically significant adverse effect was observed with higher liver D_{mean} ($p = 0.03$) values solely for ALT and for AST with both liver D_{min} ($p = 0.007$) and D_{mean} ($p = 0.023$) values. For GGT, all liver dose–volume values, namely D_{min} ($p = 0.014$), D_{max} ($p = 0.023$), D_{mean} ($p = 0.006$), V_{50} ($p = 0.009$), V_{40} ($p = 0.03$), V_{30} ($p = 0.03$), V_{20}

(p = 0.001), V_{10} (p = 0.02), and V_5 (p = 0.008), were found to be statistically significant. However, the RT technique, CTV volume, the addition of boost, and its technique did not demonstrate a statistically significant effect. The statistically significant values, effect of liver dose–volume and the percentage change are presented in Table 5.

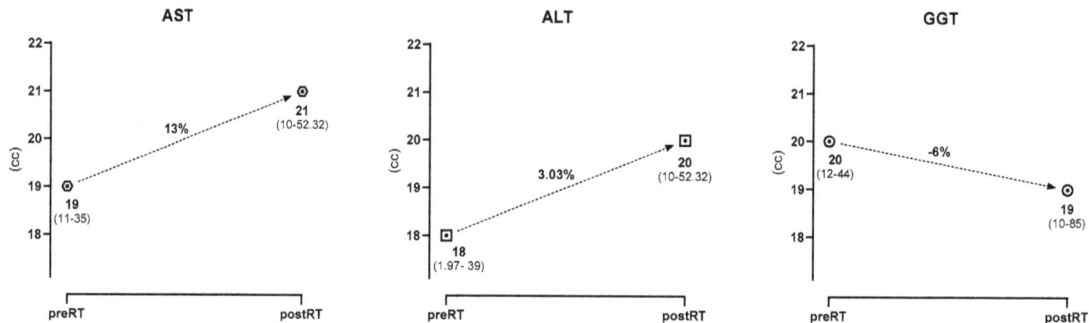

Figure 2. Median and percentage change in liver function test (LFT) values of 57 patients.

Table 5. Significant values of dose–volume and percentage chance on LFT.

Liver Test	Dose–Volume Parameters	p Value
ALT	D_{mean}	0.03
AST	D_{mean}	0.023
	D_{min}	0.007
GGT	D_{mean}	0.006
	D_{min}	0.014
	D_{max}	0.023
	V_{50}	0.009
	V_{40}	0.03
	V_{30}	0.03
	V_{20}	0.01
	V_5	0.02

ALT: Alanine aminotransferase; AST: Aspartate aminotransferase; GGT: Gamma-glutamyl transferase; D_{max}: Maximum dose; D_{min}: Minimum dose; D_{mean}: Mean dose; $V_{5/10/20/30/40/50}$ Liver volume receiving 5/10/20/30/40/50 Gy.

4. Discussion

Radiation in the early phase results in DNA damage, oxidative stress, and an accumulation of free oxygen radicals in the environment, leading to acute inflammation and hepatocellular apoptosis [19]. This scenario creates vascular damage that subsequently results in an increased synthesis of collagen, negatively impacting growth factors, TNF-alpha, TNF-beta, and other elements involved in liver damage regulation and repair [20]. Clinically, this situation is recognized as radiation-induced liver disease (RILD).

Classic RILD is observed between 2 weeks and 4 months post-radiation in patients who have received 30–35 Gy through conventional fractionation of the liver [21]. It arises due to veno-occlusion associated with fibrosis secondary to RT. Its presentation involves an ALP level increased by ≥2 times. With advancements in radiation technology, such as image-guided RT techniques, VMAT plans, IMRT plans, and stereotaxic body radiotherapy, classic RILD has become less common. Instead, non-classic RILD is more frequently observed. In this scenario, even with a lower radiation dose, there can be a rise in LFTs, possibly due to diminished liver regeneration capacity, which may be associated with conditions like cirrhosis or hepatitis [10,21]. In such cases, AST and ALT levels may elevate to ≥5 times [13].

Anatomically, the liver is near the radiation treatment area during breast or chest wall irradiations, particularly on the right side, making it an at-risk organ. Current dose restrictions used in planning RT for right breast cancer recommend a D_{mean} value of 28–32 for the liver [18]. This dose carries a 5% risk of developing RILD [22]. However, when considering the anatomy and the conventional dose of 50 Gy given to the entire breast, this prescribed dose for the liver seems excessively high and is not reflective of reality. Considering the ALARA principle "As Low As Reasonably Achievable", these theoretically appropriate dose limitations pose different challenges in clinical practice. This principle aims at minimizing the risks associated with radiation exposure, thus striving to keep radiation doses in diagnostic and therapeutic processes as low as reasonably achievable. Within the framework of this principle, the use of radiation at necessary therapeutic doses aims to minimize acute and chronic side effects that may occur following RT. Consequently, the objective is to reduce the long-term risk of secondary cancer development attributed to RT.

In studies assessing liver doses in patients diagnosed with breast cancer and treated with right breast irradiation, the mean liver dose was found to be between 1.94 and 4.34 Gy [11,13,14]. The maximum liver dose averages at 26.9 Gy and in some cases reaches as high as 51.7 Gy [14]. There are limited studies in the literature that focus on liver function alterations due to the dose received by the liver during right breast irradiation. You can see these studies in Table 6.

Table 6. Studies examining LFT changes following right breast irradiation.

	The Number of Patients/RT Dose/Timing of Blood Test	Liver Dose	Hepatic Blood Test Results
Lauffer et al. [11]	34 right side 42.5 Gy/16 fr or 50 Gy/25 fr ±16 fr boosts Before and last week of RT	MLV: 1270.2 cc (918.5–2233.2) MLD: 1.94 Gy (0.2–9)	Correlation between irradiated liver volume and ALT ($p = 0.05$) and ALP ($p = 0.006$)
Courtier et al. [12]	52 right side, 100 left side 40 Gy/15 fr Before and during 4 weeks after RT	Mean V_{10}: 226 cm^3 (19%) Mean V_{50}: 92 cm^3 (8%) Mean V_{90}: 62 cm^3 (5%)	V_{10} and IL-6 ($p = 0.001$)
Park et al. [13]	47 right side, 78 left side 42.56–50 Gy/16–25 fr ± 10–14 Gy boost 1 week before vs. 6 months after	$D_{mean\_right\ breast}$ 434.1 cGy $D_{mean\_left\ breast}$ 260.6 cGy V_{10} 3% V_{20} 1% V_{30} 0%	AST_{median}: 23.2 ± 5.3 vs. 29.6 ± 14.6 ALT_{median}: 20.2 ± 7.7 vs. 25.6 ± 20.0
Quintin et al. [14]	27 right side or bilateral, 29 left side Median follow-up 5.4 years	D_{mean} 2.8 Gy (0.3–16.6) D_{max} 26.9 Gy (0.7–51.7)	no grade 3 hepatotoxicity Three patients (6%) with grade 2 delayed hepatotoxicity

RT: Radiotherapy; Gy: Gray; ALT: Alanine aminotransferase; AST: Aspartate aminotransferase; MLV: Mean lung volume; MLD: Mean lung dose; D_{max}: Maximum dose; D_{mean}: Mean dose; $V_{10/20/30/50/90}$ volume of liver irradiated 10/20/30/50/90% of prescription dose.

In our study, unlike in the literature, early changes in LFTs were calculated as a percentage change using a mathematical formula, and the relationship between this value and dose–volume values was evaluated. It was determined that, as the mean dose received by the liver increases, there is a significant increase in ALT and AST values ($p = 0.03$, $p = 0.023$ respectively). Furthermore, it has been shown that the higher the minimum dose the liver receives, the greater the increase in AST value ($p = 0.007$). Therefore, keeping the mean and minimum dose received by the liver as low as possible is seen as one of the essential parameters to avoid LFT increase. A statistically significant decrease in percentage change and GGT values was observed after RT. This could be attributed to the GGT levels not being negatively affected during the acute phase of RT.

In the current study, no significant relationship between percentage difference (Δ%) and a certain volume dose (VxGy) was not detected. In the literature, it is recommended that the liver receives a dose below 30 Gy ($V_{30} < 100\%$). It is argued that a dose above 30 Gy is an indicator of RDIL [17,23–25]. In our study, the median V_{30} value was found to be 2.81 cc, which corresponds to approximately 2% of the median value. We think that, since such a low value was found, there was no clinical change and no relationship was detected with DVH. One of the key points should be the actual clinical impact of low-dose exposure to the liver. The liver is well-know for its ability to regenerate after multiple kinds of damage. Several previous experiences demonstrated that, although RT could result in increased LFT, it did not meet the criteria for RILD [13] and delayed hepatotoxicity was negligible, questioning the definition of liver as an OAR [14]. In a study by Park et al. evaluating LFTs in patients diagnosed with breast cancer undergoing RT, it was reported that 53.6% of the patients had a V_{30} value of 0 and the maximum V_{30} value was 2.6%, and RILD was not observed in any patients. Based on this, it has been suggested to use a liver $D_{mean} \leq 3\text{–}4$ value as the liver normal tissue dose limitation for right breast irradiation and can be considered as a cut-off value [13]. The similar low doses found in our study and absence of changes in LFTs support this thesis.

Survival rates have increased in patients diagnosed with breast cancer due to advancements in RT techniques and progress in systemic treatments. It is possible to observe the long-term stochastic effects of radiation, which are independent of dose, in the patient group monitored with a breast cancer diagnosis. Therefore, the incidence of secondary cancers after breast cancer irradiation during follow-up is higher than that for other types of cancer [26,27]. Even if the results do not manifest clinically as an increase in LFTs, considering the long-term effects of the received radiation, normal tissues should be exposed to the lowest possible radiation dose, as discussed in accordance with the ALARA principle [28]. Radiation-induced cancer is classically defined as a stochastic process, although recent studies developed more complex models; therefore, there is no threshold point and even low doses may increase second neoplasms risk. This phenomenon is relevant especially for long-term survivors and has been extensively investigated for lymphoma and breast cancer patients, mostly focusing on second lung, breast and thyroid malignancies [29–31]. Nonetheless, some studies defined the risk of secondary liver cancer after breast irradiation, with conflicting results: while in some models, the lifetime attributable risk (LAR) for liver cancer induction after breast radiotherapy was extremely low [32], in other experiences high LAR estimates were obtained for liver in case of right-sided targets [33].

Currently, the deep inspiration breath hold (DIBH) is employed as standard in left breast and chest wall irradiation. This technique is used in left breast cancer RT to ensure that cardiac tissues and coronary arteries receive a lower dose [34–36]. The DIBH technique has not yet become standard for right breast or chest wall RT. There are fewer studies on the benefits of the DIBH technique in right breast irradiation. While there are studies that determined that it reduces the dose to the heart, lungs, and liver dosimetrically [37], there are also studies that argue it is effective in reducing liver doses only in cases with hepatomegaly while reducing doses to the heart and LAD (left anterior descending artery) [38]. In the study of Loap and colleagues, although there was no significant change in cardiac structures and the right lung in right breast irradiations using DIBH compared to the free breath technique with VMAT, a significant reduction was observed in the mean liver dose (from 2.54 to 0.87 Gy $p = 0.001$). Therefore, it has been emphasized that, instead of routine use, it should be used in selected patients [39].

Due to its retrospective design, our study inherently possesses some limitations. Despite the availability of 100 patients that met the study criteria, statistical analysis was performed on the 57 patients with data for all three liver function test parameters. None of the patients included in the study received concurrent chemotherapy and tamoxifen alongside RT. Some patients received neoadjuvant or adjuvant chemotherapy. As per our protocol, RT begins approximately 3–4 weeks after chemotherapy. The reason for conducting LFTs just before RT is to assess the reduction in potential toxicity that could occur due to chemotherapy during this period. Furthermore, since the primary focus of our study is on the changes occurring in the acute phase before and after radiation therapy, the effect of chemotherapy has not been separately evaluated. On the other hand, according to the literature, it is known that hormonal therapies used in the post-menopausal period (like letrozole and exemestane) do not have an effect that will reflect on the clinic and tests [40,41]. Although there is a viewpoint that minimal changes in LFTs may not have clinical implications, it is essential to remember that slight elevations in AST, ALT, and GGT due to scattered radiation may indicate potential risks concerning non-RILD and secondary cancers in the long run.

There is a dearth of research in the literature that examines early changes in LFTs after right breast irradiation. We aimed to address this gap. The multicentric design of our study, its evaluation using modern RT techniques, the detailed examination of DVH parameters, and the articulation of LFT changes through a mathematical formula constitute this study's strengths.

5. Conclusions

In conclusion, liver damage can manifest as a spectrum ranging from subtle laboratory abnormalities to severe liver insufficiency. Due to factors such as anatomical positioning, planning technique, and breast posture during right breast irradiation, the liver can receive variable doses. For breast cancer patients with a longer survival expectancy, safeguarding them from potential liver toxicity secondary to RT is of paramount importance. Our findings indicate that, in patients who did not undergo any systemic treatment or had no risk factors, there was an average increase of nearly 15% in enzymes, indicative of acute liver damage post-RT compared with pre-RT. It was deemed significant to maintain liver D_{mean} under 208 cGy. Given the myriad of factors influencing LFT values, our study underscores the necessity for meticulous attention to liver doses during RT planning. We advocate for maintaining the mean dose below 208 cGy and emphasize the importance of regular LFT monitoring during follow-up.

Author Contributions: Conceptualization, Z.A.A. and O.A.; methodology, Z.A.A., Z.G., N.A. and O.A.; software, Z.A.A. and O.A.; validation, Z.A.A. and O.A.; formal analysis, Z.G. and Z.A.A.; investigation, Z.G., N.A., M.G. and O.A.; resources, M.G., Z.G., N.A. and Z.A.A.; data curation, Z.A.A., O.A. and N.A.; writing—original draft preparation, Z.G. and Z.A.A.; writing—review and editing, Z.G. and Z.A.A.; visualization, Z.A.A., Z.G. and N.A.; supervision, Z.A.A.; project administration, Z.A.A., Z.G. and O.A.; funding acquisition, no funding. All authors have read and agreed to the published version of the manuscript.

Funding: This research received no external funding.

Institutional Review Board Statement: The study was designed with the World Medical Association Declaration of Helsinki guidelines, after obtaining local institutional ethics committee approval (No: Tepecik TRH-2023/07-05).

Informed Consent Statement: Informed consent was obtained from all subjects involved in the study.

Data Availability Statement: The data presented in this study are available on the request from the corresponding author.

Conflicts of Interest: The authors declare no conflict of interest.

References

1. Worldwide Cancer Data. Available online: https://www.wcrf.org/cancer-trends/worldwide-cancer-data (accessed on 24 July 2023).
2. Gradishar, W.J.; Moran, M.S.; Abraham, J.; Aft, R.; Agnese, D.; Allison, K.H.; Anderson, B.; Burstein, H.J.; Chew, H.; Dang, C.; et al. Breast Cancer, Version 3.2022, NCCN Clinical Practice Guidelines in Oncology. *J. Natl. Compr. Cancer Netw.* **2022**, *20*, 691–722. [CrossRef] [PubMed]
3. Belkacemi, Y.; Debbi, K.; Loganadane, G.; Ghith, S.; Hadhri, A.; Hassani, W.; Cherif, M.A.; Coraggio, G.; To, N.H.; Colson-Durand, L.; et al. Radiothérapie Adjuvante et Néoadjuvante Des Cancers Du Sein: Mise Au Point Sur Les Données de La Littérature Disponibles En 2020. *Cancer/Radiothérapie* **2020**, *24*, 482–492. [CrossRef] [PubMed]
4. Clarke, M.; Collins, R.; Darby, S.; Davies, C.; Elphinstone, P.; Evans, V.; Godwin, J.; Gray, R.; Hicks, C.; James, S.; et al. Effects of Radiotherapy and of Differences in the Extent of Surgery for Early Breast Cancer on Local Recurrence and 15-Year Survival: An Overview of the Randomised Trials. *Lancet* **2005**, *366*, 2087–2106. [CrossRef] [PubMed]

5. Early Breast Cancer Trialists' Collaborative Group (EBCTCG); Darby, S.; McGale, P.; Correa, C.; Taylor, C.; Arriagada, R.; Clarke, M.; Cutter, D.; Davies, C.; Ewertz, M.; et al. Effect of Radiotherapy after Breast-Conserving Surgery on 10-Year Recurrence and 15-Year Breast Cancer Death: Meta-Analysis of Individual Patient Data for 10,801 Women in 17 Randomised Trials. *Lancet* **2011**, *378*, 1707–1716. [CrossRef]
6. EBCTCG (Early Breast Cancer Trialists' Collaborative Group); McGale, P.; Taylor, C.; Correa, C.; Cutter, D.; Duane, F.; Ewertz, M.; Gray, R.; Mannu, G.; Peto, R.; et al. Effect of Radiotherapy after Mastectomy and Axillary Surgery on 10-Year Recurrence and 20-Year Breast Cancer Mortality: Meta-Analysis of Individual Patient Data for 8135 Women in 22 Randomised Trials. *Lancet* **2014**, *383*, 2127–2135. [CrossRef]
7. Paluch-Shimon, S.; Cardoso, F.; Partridge, A.H.; Abulkhair, O.; Azim, H.A.; Bianchi-Micheli, G.; Cardoso, M.J.; Curigliano, G.; Gelmon, K.A.; Gentilini, O.; et al. ESO-ESMO Fifth International Consensus Guidelines for Breast Cancer in Young Women (BCY5). *Ann. Oncol. Off. J. Eur. Soc. Med. Oncol.* **2022**, *33*, 1097–1118. [CrossRef]
8. Cancer Stat Facts: Female Breast Cancer. Available online: https://seer.cancer.gov/statfacts/html/breast.html (accessed on 24 July 2023).
9. Debbi, K.; Janoray, G.; Scher, N.; Deutsch, É.; Mornex, F. Doses to Organs at Risk in Conformational and Stereotactic Body Radiation Therapy: Liver. *Cancer Radiother.* **2017**, *21*, 604–612. [CrossRef]
10. Kim, J.; Jung, Y. Radiation-Induced Liver Disease: Current Understanding and Future Perspectives. *Exp. Mol. Med.* **2017**, *49*, e359. [CrossRef]
11. Lauffer, D.C.; Miglierini, P.; Kuhn, P.A.; Thalmann, S.U.; Gutierres-Demierre, N.; Khomsi, F.; Tercier, P.-A.; Allal, A.S. Impact of Adjuvant Radiotherapy on Biological and Clinical Parameters in Right-Sided Breast Cancer. *Cancer Radiother.* **2021**, *25*, 469–475. [CrossRef]
12. Courtier, N.; Gambling, T.; Barrett-Lee, P.; Oliver, T.; Mason, M.D. The Volume of Liver Irradiated during Modern Free-Breathing Breast Radiotherapy: Implications for Theory and Practice. *Radiography* **2019**, *25*, 103–107. [CrossRef]
13. Park, H.J.; Cheong, K.-H.; Koo, T.; Lee, M.Y.; Kim, K.J.; Park, S.; Han, T.; Kang, S.-K.; Ha, B.; Yoon, J.-W.; et al. Effects of Radiation Dose on Liver After Free-Breathing Volumetric Modulated Arc Therapy for Breast Cancer. *In Vivo* **2022**, *36*, 1937–1943. [CrossRef] [PubMed]
14. Quintin, K.; Loap, P.; Fourquet, A.; Kirova, Y. Late Hepatic Toxicity after Breast Cancer Intensity-Modulated Radiotherapy Using Helicoidal Tomotherapy. *Cancer Radiother.* **2023**, *27*, 267–272. [CrossRef] [PubMed]
15. Loganadane, G.; Truong, P.T.; Taghian, A.G.; Tešanović, D.; Jiang, M.; Geara, F.; Moran, M.S.; Belkacemi, Y. Comparison of Nodal Target Volume Definition in Breast Cancer Radiation Therapy According to RTOG Versus ESTRO Atlases: A Practical Review From the TransAtlantic Radiation Oncology Network (TRONE). *Int. J. Radiat. Oncol. Biol. Phys.* **2020**, *107*, 437–448. [CrossRef]
16. Jabbour, S.K.; Hashem, S.A.; Bosch, W.; Kim, T.K.; Finkelstein, S.E.; Anderson, B.M.; Ben-Josef, E.; Crane, C.H.; Goodman, K.A.; Haddock, M.G.; et al. Upper Abdominal Normal Organ Contouring Guidelines and Atlas: A Radiation Therapy Oncology Group Consensus. *Pract. Radiat. Oncol.* **2014**, *4*, 82–89. [CrossRef]
17. Alicikus, Z.A.; Aydin, B. Toxicity Management for Upper Abdomen Tumors in Radiation Oncology. In *Prevention and Management of Acute and Late Toxicities in Radiation Oncology*; Springer International Publishing: Cham, Germany, 2020; pp. 171–229.
18. Marks, L.B.; Yorke, E.D.; Jackson, A.; Ten Haken, R.K.; Constine, L.S.; Eisbruch, A.; Bentzen, S.M.; Nam, J.; Deasy, J.O. Use of Normal Tissue Complication Probability Models in the Clinic. *Int. J. Radiat. Oncol. Biol. Phys.* **2010**, *76*, S10–S19. [CrossRef]
19. Robbins, M.E.C.; Zhao, W. Chronic Oxidative Stress and Radiation-Induced Late Normal Tissue Injury: A Review. *Int. J. Radiat. Biol.* **2004**, *80*, 251–259. [CrossRef] [PubMed]
20. Lee, U.E.; Friedman, S.L. Mechanisms of Hepatic Fibrogenesis. *Best Pract. Res. Clin. Gastroenterol.* **2011**, *25*, 195–206. [CrossRef] [PubMed]
21. Koay, E.J.; Owen, D.; Das, P. Radiation-Induced Liver Disease and Modern Radiotherapy. *Semin. Radiat. Oncol.* **2018**, *28*, 321–331. [CrossRef]
22. Pan, C.C.; Kavanagh, B.D.; Dawson, L.A.; Li, X.A.; Das, S.K.; Miften, M.; Ten Haken, R.K. Radiation-Associated Liver Injury. *Int. J. Radiat. Oncol. Biol. Phys.* **2010**, *76*, S94–S100. [CrossRef]
23. Yamada, K.; Izaki, K.; Sugimoto, K.; Mayahara, H.; Morita, Y.; Yoden, E.; Matsumoto, S.; Soejima, T.; Sugimura, K. Prospective Trial of Combined Transcatheter Arterial Chemoembolization and Three-Dimensional Conformal Radiotherapy for Portal Vein Tumor Thrombus in Patients with Unresectable Hepatocellular Carcinoma. *Int. J. Radiat. Oncol.* **2003**, *57*, 113–119. [CrossRef]
24. Liang, S.-X.; Zhu, X.-D.; Xu, Z.-Y.; Zhu, J.; Zhao, J.-D.; Lu, H.-J.; Yang, Y.-L.; Chen, L.; Wang, A.-Y.; Fu, X.-L.; et al. Radiation-Induced Liver Disease in Three-Dimensional Conformal Radiation Therapy for Primary Liver Carcinoma: The Risk Factors and Hepatic Radiation Tolerance. *Int. J. Radiat. Oncol.* **2006**, *65*, 426–434. [CrossRef] [PubMed]
25. Kim, T.H.; Kim, D.Y.; Park, J.-W.; Kim, S.H.; Choi, J.-I.; Kim, H.B.; Lee, W.J.; Park, S.J.; Hong, E.K.; Kim, C.-M. Dose–Volumetric Parameters Predicting Radiation-Induced Hepatic Toxicity in Unresectable Hepatocellular Carcinoma Patients Treated with Three-Dimensional Conformal Radiotherapy. *Int. J. Radiat. Oncol.* **2007**, *67*, 225–231. [CrossRef] [PubMed]
26. Snow, A.; Ring, A.; Struycken, L.; Mack, W.; Koç, M.; Lang, J.E. Incidence of Radiation Induced Sarcoma Attributable to Radiotherapy in Adults: A Retrospective Cohort Study in the SEER Cancer Registries across 17 Primary Tumor Sites. *Cancer Epidemiol.* **2021**, *70*, 101857. [CrossRef]
27. Huang, J.; Mackillop, W.J. Increased Risk of Soft Tissue Sarcoma after Radiotherapy in Women with Breast Carcinoma. *Cancer* **2001**, *92*, 172–180. [CrossRef] [PubMed]

28. Hiniker, S.M.; Donaldson, S.S. ALARA: In Radiation Oncology and Diagnostic Imaging Alike. *Oncology* **2014**, *28*, 247–248. [PubMed]
29. Shi, J.; Liu, J.; Tian, G.; Li, D.; Liang, D.; Wang, J.; He, Y. Association of radiotherapy for stage I-III breast cancer survivors and second primary malignant cancers: A population-based study. *Eur. J. Cancer Prev.* **2023**. Epub ahead of print. [CrossRef]
30. Buglione, M.; Guerini, A.E.; Filippi, A.R.; Spiazzi, L.; Pasinetti, N.; Magli, A.; Toraci, C.; Borghetti, P.; Triggiani, L.; Alghisi, A.; et al. A Systematic Review on Intensity Modulated Radiation Therapy for Mediastinal Hodgkin's Lymphoma. *Crit. Rev. Oncol. Hematol.* **2021**, *167*, 103437. [CrossRef]
31. Grantzau, T.; Overgaard, J. Risk of second non-breast cancer among patients treated with and without postoperative radiotherapy for pri-mary breast cancer: A systematic review and meta-analysis of population-based studies including 522,739 patients. *Radiother. Oncol.* **2016**, *121*, 402–413. [CrossRef]
32. Donovan, E.M.; James, H.; Bonora, M.; Yarnold, J.R.; Evans, P.M. Second cancer incidence risk estimates using BEIR VII models for standard and complex external beam radiotherapy for early breast cancer. *Med. Phys.* **2012**, *39*, 5814–5824. [CrossRef]
33. Santos, A.M.; Marcu, L.G.; Wong, C.M.; Bezak, E. Risk estimation of second primary cancers after breast radiotherapy. *Acta Oncol.* **2016**, *55*, 1331–1337. [CrossRef]
34. Simonetto, C.; Eidemüller, M.; Gaasch, A.; Pazos, M.; Schönecker, S.; Reitz, D.; Kääb, S.; Braun, M.; Harbeck, N.; Niyazi, M.; et al. Does Deep Inspiration Breath-Hold Prolong Life? Individual Risk Estimates of Ischaemic Heart Disease after Breast Cancer Radiotherapy. *Radiother. Oncol.* **2019**, *131*, 202–207. [CrossRef] [PubMed]
35. Dumane, V.A.; Saksornchai, K.; Zhou, Y.; Hong, L.; Powell, S.; Ho, A.Y. Reduction in Low-Dose to Normal Tissue with the Addition of Deep Inspiration Breath Hold (DIBH) to Volumetric Modulated Arc Therapy (VMAT) in Breast Cancer Patients with Implant Reconstruction Receiving Regional Nodal Irradiation. *Radiat. Oncol.* **2018**, *13*, 187. [CrossRef] [PubMed]
36. Swanson, T.; Grills, I.S.; Ye, H.; Entwistle, A.; Teahan, M.; Letts, N.; Yan, D.; Duquette, J.; Vicini, F.A. Six-Year Experience Routinely Using Moderate Deep Inspiration Breath-Hold for the Reduction of Cardiac Dose in Left-Sided Breast Irradiation for Patients with Early-Stage or Locally Advanced Breast Cancer. *Am. J. Clin. Oncol.* **2013**, *36*, 24–30. [CrossRef] [PubMed]
37. Pandeli, C.; Smyth, L.M.L.; David, S.; See, A.W. Dose Reduction to Organs at Risk with Deep-Inspiration Breath-Hold during Right Breast Radiotherapy: A Treatment Planning Study. *Radiat. Oncol.* **2019**, *14*, 223. [CrossRef]
38. Borgonovo, G.; Paulicelli, E.; Daniele, D.; Presilla, S.; Richetti, A.; Valli, M. Deep Inspiration Breath Hold in Post-Operative Radiotherapy for Right Breast Cancer: A Retrospective Analysis. *Rep. Pract. Oncol. Radiother.* **2022**, *27*, 717–723. [CrossRef]
39. Loap, P.; Vu-Bezin, J.; Monceau, V.; Jacob, S.; Fourquet, A.; Kirova, Y. Dosimetric Evaluation of the Benefit of Deep Inspiration Breath Hold (DIBH) for Locoregional Irradiation of Right Breast Cancer with Volumetric Modulated Arctherapy (VMAT). *Acta Oncol.* **2023**, *62*, 150–158. [CrossRef]
40. Mukherjee, A.G.; Wanjari, U.R.; Nagarajan, D.; Vibhaa, K.K.; Anagha, V.; Joshua, P.P.; Tharani, P.T.; Chakraborty, R.; Renu, K.; Dey, A.; et al. Letrozole: Pharmacology, Toxicity and Potential Therapeutic Effects. *Life Sci.* **2022**, *310*, 121074. [CrossRef]
41. Jannuzzo, M.G.; Poggesi, I.; Spinelli, R.; Rocchetti, M.; Cicioni, P.; Buchan, P. The Effects of Degree of Hepatic or Renal Impairment on the Pharmacokinetics of Exemestane in Postmenopausal Women. *Cancer Chemother. Pharmacol.* **2004**, *53*, 475–481. [CrossRef]

Disclaimer/Publisher's Note: The statements, opinions and data contained in all publications are solely those of the individual author(s) and contributor(s) and not of MDPI and/or the editor(s). MDPI and/or the editor(s) disclaim responsibility for any injury to people or property resulting from any ideas, methods, instructions or products referred to in the content.

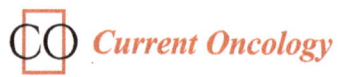

Article

Correlation of High-Sensitivity Cardiac Troponin I Values and Cardiac Radiation Doses in Patients with Left-Sided Breast Cancer Undergoing Hypofractionated Adjuvant Radiotherapy with Concurrent Anti-HER2 Therapy

Katarina Antunac [1,*], Ljiljana Mayer [2], Marija Banovic [3] and Lidija Beketic-Oreskovic [1,4]

1. Division of Oncology and Radiotherapy, University Hospital for Tumours, Sestre Milosrdnice University Hospital Centre, Ilica 197, 10000 Zagreb, Croatia; lidijabeketicoreskovic@gmail.com
2. Department of Medical Biochemistry in Oncology, University Hospital for Tumours, Sestre Milosrdnice University Hospital Centre, Ilica 197, 10000 Zagreb, Croatia; ljiljana.mayer@kbcsm.hr
3. Polyclinic Leptir, Ilica 253, 10000 Zagreb, Croatia; mabanovi@gmail.com
4. Department of Clinical Oncology, School of Medicine University of Zagreb, Salata 3 B, 10000 Zagreb, Croatia
* Correspondence: katarina.antunac@gmail.com

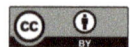

Abstract: Anti HER2 therapy and left breast adjuvant radiation therapy (RT) can both result in cardiotoxicity. The aim of this study was to evaluate the influence of radiation dose on cardiac structures on the values of the early cardiotoxicity marker high-sensitivity cardiac troponin I (hscTnI) in patients with HER2-positive left breast cancer undergoing adjuvant concomitant antiHER2 therapy and radiotherapy, and to establish a correlation between the hscTnI values and cardiac radiation doses. Sixty-one patients underwent left breast hypofractionated radiotherapy in parallel with anti-HER2 therapy: trastuzumab, combined trastuzumab–pertuzumab or trastuzumab emtansine (T-DM1). The hscTnI values were measured prior to and upon completion of radiotherapy. A significant increase in hscTnI was defined as >30% from baseline, with the second value being 4 ng/L or higher. Dose volume histograms (DVH) were generated for the heart, left ventricle (LV) and left anterior descending artery (LAD). The hscTnI levels were corelated with radiation doses on cardiac structures. An increase in hscTnI values was observed in 17 patients (Group 1). These patients had significantly higher mean radiation doses for the heart ($p = 0.02$), LV ($p = 0.03$) and LAD ($p = 0.04$), and AUC for heart and LV ($p = 0.01$), than patients without hscTnI increase (Group 2). The patients in Group 1 also had larger volumes of heart and LV receiving 2 Gy ($p = 0.01$ for both) and 4 Gy ($p = 0.02$ for both). LAD differences were observed in volumes receiving 2 Gy ($p = 0.03$), 4 Gy ($p = 0.02$) and 5 Gy ($p = 0.02$). The increase in hscTnI observed in patients receiving anti-HER2 therapy after adjuvant RT was positively associated with radiation doses on the heart, LV and LAD.

Keywords: HER2-positive breast cancer; adjuvant radiotherapy; radiotherapy dose hypofractionation; cardiotoxicity; high-sensitivity cardiac troponin I; trastuzumab; pertuzumab; trastuzumab emtansine

1. Introduction

Breast cancer adjuvant radiotherapy reduces the risk of disease recurrence (from 35% to 19.3% in 10 years) and the risk of breast cancer death (from 25.2% to 21.4% in 15 years) [1]. However, the incidental exposure of the heart during left breast irradiation increases the risk of ischemic heart disease that starts about 5 years after radiotherapy and continues up to the third decade upon its completion. The ischemic heart disease rate is proportional to the mean dose to the whole heart; it increases linearly by 7.4% per Gray (Gy) and no threshold has been defined [2]. The risk of radiation-induced heart disease is not only dose-dependent but also correlates with the volume of the cardiac structure receiving a certain radiation dose [3]. Therefore, it was shown that the volume of the left ventricle (LV) receiving 5 Gy was the most important prognostic dose-volume parameter for the development of an acute coronary event [4]. A mean dose on the left anterior descending (LAD) artery higher than 5 Gy was associated with an increased requirement for coronary intervention in LAD [5].

Troponin is a contractile apparatus component in both cardiac and skeletal myocytes. Troponin I and T isoforms are highly specific to cardiac myocytes; their detection in serum is a specific marker of cardiac damage [6]. The prognostic value of small changes in high sensitivity cardiac troponins, those below the 99th centile, has been shown in diseases affecting the cardiac muscle, such as coronary disease [7]. Radiation-induced cardiac cell damage could be a consequence of changes in cardiac vasculature and inflammation caused by radiation or could be the direct effect of radiation on the destruction of myocyte membranous structures [8,9].

A meta-analysis of eight randomised trials evaluated whether high-sensitivity cardiac troponin T (hscTnT) can be used as an early diagnostic marker of cancer-treatment-related cardiac dysfunction. A correlation between elevated hscTnT levels and cancer-treatment-related cardiac dysfunction was found and hscTnT testing improved the accuracy of the diagnosis. Still, it was not possible to define exact cut-off values of hscTnT for the early diagnosis of cardiac dysfunction [10].

A correlation between radiation doses on cardiac structures and the increase in troponin I levels during and after radiotherapy has been shown in patients undergoing adjuvant irradiation of the left breast. The patients in this trial did not receive chemotherapy or anti-HER2 therapy [11].

Patients with early HER2-positive breast cancer receive anti-HER2 systemic therapy based on trastuzumab in both neoadjuvant and adjuvant settings. The overall treatment time is usually 1 year and adjuvant radiotherapy of the breast cancer is most often applied concomitantly with anti-HER2 therapy. The most common side effect of trastuzumab is cardiotoxicity, presenting as an asymptomatic decrease in the left ventricular ejection fraction (LVEF), occurring in about one fourth of patients. It mainly occurs during the first three months of the treatment and leads to the treatment discontinuation in about 5% of patients [12]. In 14% of patients receiving trastuzumab, an increase in troponin I levels has been observed A multivariate analysis showed that observed troponin increase was an independent predictor of cardiotoxicity and in these patients LVEF did not recover. Therefore, troponin I elevation can identify patients who are at risk of developing cardiac disfunction that might not be recovered [13].

Little is known about the cardiotoxicity of pertuzumab and trastuzumab emtansine. Pertuzumab is a recombinant humanised monoclonal antibody targeting HER. It is always given in combination with trastuzumab. Its cardiotoxic effect is far less known. An APHINITY trial evaluated the effectiveness and safety of pertuzumab when added to combination of chemotherapy and trastuzumab (dual blockade) in the adjuvant treatment of breast cancer patients. After 6 years of follow up, the incidence of primary cardiac events was less than 1% in both groups of patients. No new safety signals regarding the cardiotoxicity of dual blockade have been detected [14,15]. However, in a meta-analysis of eight randomised controlled trials that included 8420 patients, pertuzumab was associated with an almost two-fold increased risk of heart failure. No other cardiotoxic effects were observed [16].

T-DM1 is a combination of trastuzumab, a HER2 antibody, and emtansine, which is an anti-microtubule agent. Data on its cardiotoxicity are scarce. It was compared to trastuzumab in a KATHERINE trial that enrolled 1486 patients with HER2 breast cancer that did not achieve a complete pathological response on primary systemic therapy. After a median follow up of 41 months, the cardiac events rate was 0.6% in patients receiving trastuzumab and 0.1% in patients receiving T-DM1 [17–19]. In a pooled analysis of seven trials including over 1900 patients receiving T-DM1, the cardiac event rate was about 3%. This included congestive heart failure, LVEF drop, cardiac arrhythmias and cardiac ischemia. In almost 80% of patients, the events resolved upon treatment discontinuation [20]

According to the current position statement of the Cardio-Oncology Study Group of the Heart Failure Association and the Cardio-Oncology Council of the European Society of Cardiology, in patients with breast cancer that should receive anti-HER2 cancer therapies, a baseline cardiovascular risk assessment should be performed, based on previous cardiovascular disease (heart failure or cardiomyopathy, myocardial infarction or CABG, severe valvular heart disease, LVEF value, arrhythmias, stabile angina), cardiac biomarkers (troponin, BNP or NT-proBNP), demographic and cardiovascular risk factors (age, hypertension, diabetes mellitus, chronic kidney disease), current cancer treatment regimen (including anthracyclines before HER2-targeted therapy), previous cardiotoxic cancer treatment (including anthracyclines and chest radiotherapy) and lifestyle risk factors (smoking, obesity) [21].

In patients with breast cancer receiving both anthracyclines and trastuzumab, a measurement of troponin is recommended at baseline, before the commencement of trastuzumab-based therapy and after every four/three/two cycles of trastuzumab according to baseline cardiovascular risk assessment (low/medium/high) [7].

It is not clear whether a heart exposed to trastuzumab is more prone to radiation damage, since the data are equivocal [22,23]. In a retrospective trial of patients undergoing trastuzumab therapy in parallel with radiotherapy of either the right or left breast, radiation doses on the right ventricle (RV), LV and LAD were evaluated. Patients with left-sided breast cancer more often had arrhythmias and cardiac ischemia compared to patients with cancer of the right breast. Also, radiation dose on the RV, LV and LAD was positively correlated with LVEF decline [24].

In this study, we have enrolled patients with HER2-positive left breast cancer undergoing hypofractionated adjuvant left-breast radiotherapy concomitantly with anti-HER2 therapy: trastuzumab, a combination of trastuzumab and pertuzumab or trastuzumab emtansine (T-DM1). Values of high-sensitivity cardiac troponin I (hscTnI), as an early cardiotoxicity biomarker, have been measured prior to and upon completion of radiotherapy. Dose volume histograms (DVH) were generated for cardiac structures and correlated with the increment of hscTnI values in order to define acceptable radiation doses on the heart, left ventricle (LV) and left anterior descending artery (LAD).

2. Materials and Methods

2.1. Patient Population

In this single centre, cohort, prospective, observational trial, 61 female patients with HER2-positive early stage left breast cancer were enrolled. Patients underwent either breast-conserving surgery or mastectomy with axillary lymph node dissection or sentinel lymph node biopsy. Patients were treated with forward intensity-modulated radiotherapy. Clinical target volume consisted of the left breast or chest wall, with or without axillary or supraclavicular lymph nodes. All patients were receiving anti-HER2 therapy: trastuzumab, a combination of trastuzumab and pertuzumab or trastuzumab emtansine (T-DM1) concomitantly with irradiation. Exclusion criteria were myocardial infarction, symptomatic heart failure, chronic atrial fibrillation, malignant cardiac arrhythmias, pacemaker therapy, pulmonary embolism and renal failure.

The study was approved by the Institutional Ethics Committee and all patients signed their informed consent prior to recruitment. It was conducted from January 2022 to April 2023.

2.2. Radiation Therapy

Patients underwent 3D computer tomography treatment simulation during free breathing. Patients were placed on breast board in supine position with arms above their heads. CT slices were 2 mm thick and no intravenous contrast was used. Clinical target volume (CTV) consisted of left breast in 46 patients and left thoracic wall in 15 patients. In 1 patient, both breasts were irradiated. In 31 patients, regional lymph nodes were included in CTV, supraclavicular lymph nodes in 19 patients and both supraclavicular and axillary lymph nodes in 12 patients. Planning target volume (PTV) was created by adding 1 cm margin to account for intra- and inter-fraction movement. DVHs were generated for target volumes, lungs, spinal cord, heart, LV and LAD. In order to avoid interobserver variability, the same radiation oncologist contoured all structures (KA).

Radiation technique was forward intensity-modulated radiotherapy (fIMRT, field-in-field technique). Prescribed dose was 40.05 Gy in 15 fractions of 2.67 Gy over 3 weeks. Patients were irradiated during free breathing. Patient positioning was controlled using electronic portal-imaging device (EPID) prior to first five fractions and, thereafter, prior to every other fraction.

2.3. High-Sensitivity Cardiac Troponin I Analysis

HscTnI was analysed using Architect STAT Troponin I immunoassay (Abbott Laboratories, Abbott Ireland, Longford, Ireland). Serum samples were taken immediately before the first radiation fraction and immediately after the last radiation fraction. All samples were taken in the morning to avoid the influence of possible diurnal changes on hscTnI values. Patient samples were collected into CAT Serum Sep Clot Activator Vacuette with separator gel (Greiner Bio-One) and processed within 2 h of collection. The samples were centrifuged at $3000 \times g$ for 10 min. Analysis were performed on the Abbott Architect i2000 using reagents, calibrators and controls of the same manufacturer. Lowest detection limit was 1 ng/L.

Clinically significant increase was defined as a second value > 30% from the baseline and higher than 4 ng/L. Upon data completion, patients were divided in two groups: Group 1 with clinically significant hscTnI increase and Group 2 without clinically significant hscTnI increase.

2.4. Statistical Analysis

Quantitative data distribution normality was tested using Kolmogorov–Smirnov test. Qualitative features distribution was shown in contingency tables and differences in distribution were analysed using Fisher's exact test. Data were expressed as arithmetic means and standard deviation for normally distributed variables and as medians with interquartile range (IQR) for variables with significant deviation from normal distribution. Differences in distribution of numerical variables were analysed using Mann–Whitney U test and Wilcoxon test. The ROC curve was used to determine the optimal threshold value. Correlation of radiation doses and hscTnI increase was analysed using Spearman's rank correlation test. Data are shown as tables and figures. All statistical analyses are interpreted on a significance level of 5%.

3. Results

3.1. Patients' Characteristics

In total, 61 patients were enrolled in this trial. Their characteristics are shown in Table 1. There was no difference between the groups regarding their age, menopausal status, baseline hscTnI values, frequency of anthracycline based therapy, time since the last anthracycline cycle application, cardiac therapy and ACE inhibitors therapy. Besides ACE inhibitors, cardiac therapy also included angiotensin II receptor blockers, beta blockers, calcium channel blockers, imidazoline receptor agonists, diuretics and anti-aggregation agents.

Table 1. Patients' and treatments' characteristics.

	All N = 61	Group 1 N = 17	Group 2 N = 44	p-Value
Age (x +/− SD)	58 ± 11	55 ± 12.3	59 ± 10.5	0.2767
Premenopausal	16 (26%)	7 (41%)	9 (20%)	0.1018
hscTnI (ng/L) baseline (M,IQR)	4 (2–7)	5 (3–7)	4 (2–7)	0.8336
Anthracycline use	30 (49%)	11 (65%)	19 (43%)	0.1811
Time between anthracycline and RT in days (M,IQR)	208.5 (188–227)	216 (190–245)	208 (185–219)	0.3015
Hormonal therapy	44 (72%)	13 (76.5%)	31 (70%)	0.1811
Tamoxifen	11 (25%)	4 (30.8%)	7 (22.6%)	0.7221
AI (anastrozole, letrozole)	31 (70%)	8 (61.5%)	23 (74.2%)	0.7979
Goserelin + tamoxifen	2 (5%)	1 (7.7%)	1 (3.2%)	0.5208
Clinical target volume				
Left breast	29 (47.5%)	6 (35.4%)	23 (52.3%)	0.6069
Left breast/thoracic wall + lymph nodes	31 (51%)	10 (58.8%)	21 (47.7%)	0.8099
Both breasts	1 (1.55%)	1 (5.8%)	0	-
Cardiac therapy	26 (43%)	8 (47%)	18 (41%)	0.6658
ACE inhibitors	17/61 (28%)	5/17 (29%)	12/44 (27%)	0.8684

During radiotherapy, 72% of all patients received hormonal therapy, 76.5% in the group with hscTnI increase and 70% in the group without hscTnI increase (no difference between the two groups, $p = 0.1811$). Within the group of patients receiving hormonal therapy, 70% were taking aromatase inhibitor (AI, either anastrozole or letrozole), 25% were receiving tamoxifen and 5% a combination of LHRH agonist goserelin and tamoxifen. No difference between the study groups regarding frequency or type of hormonal treatment has been observed.

In 6 patients in Group 1 (35.4%) and 23 patients in Group 2, the clinical target volume consisted of breast only. In 10 patients in Group 1 (58.8%) and 21 patients in Group 2 (47.7%), regional lymph nodes were also involved in CTV. In one patient in Group 1, both left and right breast were irradiated. There was no statistically significant difference between the groups in terms of clinical target volume comprehensiveness.

Data are shown in Table 1.

3.2. Anti-HER2 Treatments' Characteristics

Before the commencement of radiotherapy, patients received either trastuzumab alone (28%), a combination of trastuzumab and pertuzumab (49%), T-DM1 (1%) or combination of trastuzumab and pertuzumab followed by T-DM1 (21%). No difference between the two groups has been shown regarding the type of anti-HER2 regimen or number of cycles of anti-HER2 therapy prior to radiotherapy.

During radiotherapy, patients received either trastuzumab alone (31%), a combination of trastuzumab and pertuzumab (46%) or T-DM1 (23%). Again, no difference between the two groups has been shown regarding the frequency of any anti-HER2 regimen. There was no difference observed between the two groups in terms of the day (fraction) of radiotherapy treatment on which anti-HER2 therapy was administered.

Data are shown in Table 2.

Table 2. Anti-HER2 therapy before and during radiotherapy.

Anti-HER2 Therapy	All N = 61	Group 1 N = 17	Group 2 N = 44	p-Value
Before radiotherapy				
Trastuzumab	17 (28%)	4 (23%)	13 (30%)	1.0000
Trastuzumab/pertuzumab	30 (49%)	9 (53%)	21 (48%)	1.0000
T-DM1	1 (2%)	-	1 (2%)	-
Trastuzumab/pertuzumab T-DM1	13 (21%)	4 (23%)	9 (20%)	1.0000
Number of cycles of anti-HER2 therapy before RT (M,IQR)	7 (5–8)	7 (5–8.25)	7 (5.25–8)	0.9934
During radiotherapy				
Trastuzumab	19 (31%)	4 (23.5%)	15 (34%)	0.7665
Trastuzumab/pertuzumab	28 (46%)	9 (53%)	19 (43%)	0.8024
T-DM1	14 (23%)	4 (23.5%)	10 (23%)	1.0000
RT fraction with anti-HER2 therapy application (M,IQR)	9 (5–12)	10 (4.75–12)	8 (5.5–12)	0.8590

3.3. High-Sensitivity Cardiac Troponin I Values

For the whole study population, the median (IQR) hscTnI values were 4 (2–7) ng/L before radiotherapy and 5 (3–10) ng/L after radiotherapy. A clinically significant increase in hscTnI, defined as a second value > 30% from baseline and higher than 4 ng/L, occurred in 17 patients (Group 1). The median values (IQR) were 4 (2–7) ng/L before RT and 8 (5–11) ng/L after RT. For Group 2, the baseline values were 4 (2–7) ng/L and 3 (2–6) ng/L upon treatment completion (Table 3). The values are shown in Table 1. Data are graphically presented in Figure 1.

Table 3. High-sensitivity cardiac troponin I values.

	All N = 61	Group 1 N = 17	Group 2 N = 44	p-Value
hscTnI (ng/L) baseline (M,IQR)	4 (2–7)	5 (3–7)	4 (2–7)	0.8336
hscTnI (ng/L) after RT (M,IQR)	5 (3–10)	8 (5–11)	3 (2–6)	0.0053

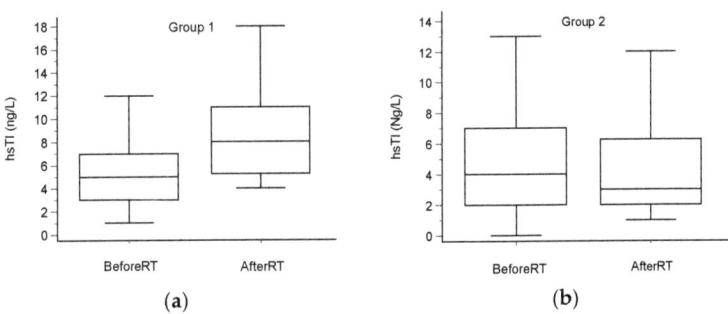

Figure 1. High-sensitivity cardiac troponin I values. Box plot figures to describe hscTnI before and after radiotherapy in (**a**) patients with increase (Group 1, 17 pts) and (**b**) in patients without an increase (Group 2, 44 pts). Borders of the box present Q1 and Q3, middle lines present medians and error bars above and below present maximums and minimums.

3.4. Cardiac Doses

The dose volume histograms for heart, left ventricle (LV) and left anterior descending artery (LAD) for Group 1 and Group 2 are shown in Figure 2. The cardiac doses for both groups are shown in Table 4. Since the risk of cardiac radiation damage correlates with the volume of the cardiac structure receiving a certain radiation dose, besides mean and maximal doses, we have also selected 10 dose volume points for each cardiac structure. For all observed structures, the mean radiation doses were significantly higher in the Group 1 patients with hscTnI increase ($p = 0.02$ for heart, $p = 0.03$ for LV and $p = 0.04$ for LAD). A statistically significant difference between the groups was observed for AUC for heart and left ventricle ($p = 0.01$ for both), for volume of heart receiving 2 Gy and 4 Gy radiation dose ($p = 0.01$ and $p = 0.02$, respectively) and for volume of left ventricle receiving 2 Gy, 4 Gy and 38 Gy radiation doses ($p = 0.01$, $p = 0.02$ and $p = 0.03$, respectively), all values being higher for Group 1. Also, in Group 1, larger volumes of LAD received 2 Gy, 4 Gy and 5 Gy radiation doses ($p = 0.03$, $p = 0.02$ and $p = 0.02$, respectively), compared to Group 2. In conclusion, in the patients in Group 1 who had an increase in hscTnI levels, larger volumes of the heart, LV and LAD received low radiation doses than in patients in Group 2 (patients without hscTnI increase).

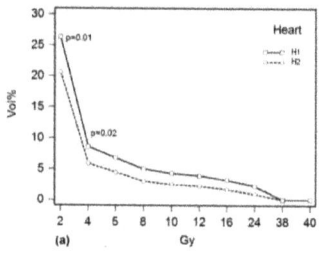

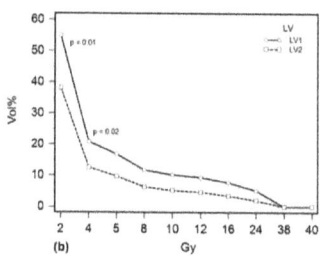

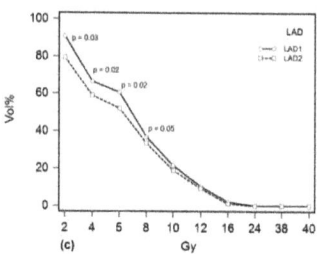

Figure 2. DVH curves for (**a**) heart, (**b**) left ventricle (LV) and (**c**) left anterior descending artery (LAD) in patients with high-sensitivity cardiac troponin I (hscTnI) increase (Group 1, 17 pts) and in patients without hscTnI increase (Group 2, 44 pts).

Table 4. Radiation doses on heart, left ventricle (LV) and left anterior descending artery (LAD) in patients with high-sensitivity cardiac troponin I (hscTnI) increase (Group 1, 17 pts) and in patients without hscTnI increase (Group 2, 44 pts).

Cardiac Structure	Group 1 (N = 17) Median (IQR)	Group 2 (N = 44) Median (IQR)	p Mann–Whitney U
Heart			
Dmean (Gy)	2.4 (1.9–3.9)	1.8 (1.5–2.5)	0.02
Dmax (Gy)	38.3 (35.3–39.6)	37.4 (33.8–38.6)	0.22
V2 (%)	26.3 (21.1–35.2)	20.5 (18.9–23.6)	0.01
V4 (%)	8.6 (6–16)	5.8 (4.4–8.9)	0.02
V5 (%)	6.8 (4–13.8)	4.5 (3.2–7.1)	0.07
V8 (%)	5 (2.3–10.7)	3 (1.5–5)	0.08
V10 (%)	4.3 (1.7–9.5)	2.5 (1–4.2)	0.08
V12 (%)	3.9 (1.3–8.5)	2.1 (0.8–3.7)	0.08
V16 (%)	3.2 (0.8–7)	1.6 (0.5–3)	0.09
V24 (%)	2.2 (0.3–4.4)	0.8 (0.1–4.7)	0.10
V38 (%)	0 (0–0.3)	0 (0–0)	0.27
V40 (%)	0 (0–0.3)	0 (0–0)	0.74
AUC (%)	72.9 (72.1–74.3)	51.4 (51.4–54.3)	0.01
LV			
Dmean (Gy)	4.7 (2.8–6.1)	2.9 (2.3–4.2)	0.03
Dmax (Gy)	38.4 (35.3–39.6)	37.2 (33.5–38.5)	0.13
V2 (%)	54.9 (41.3–62.8)	34.8 (32.3–48.3)	0.01
V4 (%)	20.8 (12.7–27.7)	12.5 (10.4–16.1)	0.02
V5 (%)	16.8 (9–22.8)	9.7 (6.3–15.6)	0.06
V8 (%)	11.7 (5.2–17.5)	6.3 (3.2–10.8)	0.08
V10 (%)	10.2 (3.9–15.7)	5.2 (2.1–9.2)	0.08
V12 (%)	9.3 (3.1–14.4)	4.6 (16–8.1)	0.08
V16 (%)	7.7 (1.8–12.3)	3.7 (0.8–6.5)	0.08
V24 (%)	5.2 (0.7–8.7)	2 (0.2–4.2)	0.09
V38 (%)	0.1 (0–0.6)	0 (0–0)	0.03
V40 (%)	0 (0–0)	0 (0–0)	0.8
AUC (%)	67.8 (67.1–72.9)	51.4 (51.4–52.9)	0.01
LAD			
Dmean (Gy)	6.8 (6.3–19.2)	6.2 (5.1–6.9)	0.04
Dmax (Gy)	22.4 (16–37.8)	19.1 (17.2–25)	0.21
V2 (%)	90.7 (82.2–99.9)	79.2 (71.8–88.9)	0.03
V4 (%)	66.3 (61.8–74.1)	58.8 (48–67.8)	0.02
V5 (%)	60.5 (55.6–70.6)	52 (41.3–63)	0.02
V8 (%)	37 (31.1–55.7)	33.5 (16.3–38.4)	0.05
V10 (%)	21.5 (16.1–53.3)	19.1 (6.6–23.2)	0.07
V12 (%)	10.4 (6.1–51.3)	9.2 (2.5–16.1)	0.08
V16 (%)	2.2 (0–48.2)	1.1 (0.1–3.5)	0.24
V24 (%)	0 (0–44.3)	0 (0–0)	0.16
V38 (%)	0 (0–0)	0 (0–0)	0.19
V40 (%)	0 (0–0)	0 (0–0)	0.54
AUC (%)	63.2 (58.6–68.6)	60 (57.1–63.6)	0.12

LV—left ventricle, LAD—left anterior descending artery, hscTnI—high sensitivity cardiac troponin I, Dmean—mean radiation dose to the structure, Dmax—maximal point radiation dose in the structure, V 40/38/24/16/12/10/8/5/4/2—the volume of structure receiving 40 Gy, 38 Gy, 24 Gy, 16 Gy, 12 Gy, 10 Gy, 8 Gy, 5 Gy, 4 Gy and 2 Gy doses, AUC—area under curve.

Dose volume constraints for hscTnI increase are shown in Table 5.

Table 5. Dose volume constraints for hscTnI increase (ROC curve data).

Radiation Dose (Gy)	Heart Dose-Volume Constraint (%)	LV Dose-Volume Constraint (%)	LAD Dose-Volume Constraint (%)
2	>19.7	>38.7	>86.4
4	>10.2	>12.1	>59.6
5	>8.6	>14.5	>52.4
8	>4.7	>10	>16.7
10	>3.9	>8.2	>7.1
16	>2.6	>7.3	>1.6
38	>0.1	>0.1	>0
40	>0.1	>0.2	≤0

LV—left ventricle, LAD—left anterior descending artery, V 40/38/24/16/12/10/8/5/4/2—the volume of structure receiving 40 Gy, 38 Gy, 24 Gy, 16 Gy, 12 Gy, 10 Gy, 8 Gy, 5 Gy, 4 Gy and 2 Gy radiation dose. Dose-volume constraint—the threshold value for hscTnI value increase.

4. Discussion

Upon completion of left breast radiotherapy, hscTnI levels increased in about one fourth of patients and that increase was correlated with radiation doses on the heart and its structures, LV and LAD suggesting subclinical myocardial damage caused by irradiation. After lower radiation doses, such as those observed in our study, the underlying mechanism is microvasculature damage and inflammatory changes. They lead to focal ischemia resulting in myocyte damage and subsequent troponin release [8]. Based on data from the literature, troponin elevation during cancer treatment is correlated with the later development of cancer-treatment-related cardiac dysfunction that might not recover [10,13,25,26]. Although cut-off values of high-sensitivity cardiac troponin are yet to be defined, its evaluation during cancer treatment can identify patients that require a more thorough follow-up of cardiac function.

In our study, no difference between the groups has been observed regarding patients' age, menopausal status, prior cardiac therapy and the use of ACE inhibitors.

Anthracyclines are cytostatic antibiotics that have been in use in oncology since the 1960s. The risk for developing cardiotoxicity caused by anthracyclines is proportional to their cumulative dose; it occurs in up to 5% of patients with doses of 400 mg/m^2. It can occur years after therapy with anthracyclines and its incidence rises with the time flow from the last application. It is more common in older patients, patients with previous heart conditions, in patients that underwent radiotherapy of the thorax and, in last two decades, in breast cancer patients receiving trastuzumab. The underlying mechanism of anthracycline-caused cardiotoxicity is still not clear. It presents with hypokinetic cardiomyopathy diagnosed by a decrease in left ventricle ejection fraction (LVEF) and eventually leads to heart failure. The early diagnosis and early onset of therapy with ACE inhibitors and beta blockers can result in LVEF improvement. If diagnosed at a later stage, anthracycline-caused cardiotoxicity is usually irreversible and has poor prognosis [27].

Anthracycline-based chemotherapy is known to elevate troponin levels. That elevation is transitional and correlates with the development of cardiotoxicity, including a decline in left ventricular ejection fraction [25,26]. In our study, one half of the patients received anthracycline-based chemotherapy; 65% in Group 1 and 43% in Group 2 ($p = 0.1811$). The median times from the application of the last cycle of anthracycline and the commencement of radiotherapy were 216 days for Group 1 (IQR: 190–245) and 208 days for Group 2 (IQR: 185–219), $p = 0.3015$. In conclusion, no statistically significant difference between the groups in terms of anthracycline use has been observed. Therefore, we did not attribute the hscTnI increase observed in Group 1 to previous anthracycline use.

Trastuzumab itself can also increase troponin levels. As with anthracyclines, troponin increment caused by trastuzumab is transitional and was shown to be predictive of later cardiotoxicity [13]. In our study, no difference between the groups regarding number of anti-HER2 therapy applications prior to radiotherapy has been observed; in both groups, the median number of cycles was 7 (IQR: 5–8.25 for Group 1 and 5.25–8 for Group 2; $p = 0.9934$).

Also, there was no difference regarding the type of anti-HER2 therapy, either before or during radiotherapy. Prior to radiotherapy, patients were receiving trastuzumab, a combination of trastuzumab and pertuzumab, T-DM1 or combination of trastuzumab and pertuzumab followed by T-DM1. During radiotherapy, patients were given either trastuzumab, a combination of trastuzumab and pertuzumab or T-DM1. That is in concordance with most of the literature data showing no difference in cardiotoxicity regarding the type of anti-HER2 treatment [14,15,17–20]. One exception is the meta-analysis of eight randomised controlled trials revealing a higher risk of heart failure associated with pertuzumab [16]. However, although patients in these trials were irradiated concomitantly with anti-HER2 therapy, data on the radiation doses on cardiac structures are lacking.

To exclude the possible acute effect of the application of anti-HER2 therapy during radiotherapy on hscTnI release, we have recorded the radiation fraction with which anti-HER2 therapy was administered. Again, no difference between the groups has been observed. The median radiotherapy fraction values were 10 for Group 1 (IQR: 4.75–12) and 8 for Group 2 (IQR: 5.5–12), $p = 0.859$. Based on the abovementioned, we have excluded the effect of anti-HER2 therapy application on hscTnI levels.

In terms of hormonal therapy, this was prescribed in about three fourths of patients during radiotherapy. About 75% of the patients in each group that were receiving hormonal therapy were given aromatase inhibitor. No difference between the groups has been shown regarding either the use or type of hormonal therapy. Therefore, it is not likely that hormonal therapy might have influenced hscTnI release.

The clinical target volume was either left breast (in the case of breast-conserving surgery), with or without lymph nodes or left thoracic wall with lymph nodes. If included in CTV, lymph nodes were either supraclavicular or both supraclavicular and axillary lymph nodes. The target volumes were determined according to the current guidelines and based on the initial clinical stage of the disease, the type and extent of axillary surgery and the pathohistological report. In one patient in Group 1, both breasts were irradiated upon breast-conserving surgery due to bilateral breast cancer. Although the proportion of patients with lymph nodes included in the target volume was slightly higher in Group 1, 58.8%, compared to 47.7% in Group 2, this was not statistically significant.

The two groups differed only in radiation doses on cardiac structures. The mean heart dose median was 2.4 Gy for Group 1 (IQR: 1.9–3.9) vs. 1.8 Gy for Group 2 (IQR: 1.5–2.5). This is in accordance with the finding that the risk of major cardiac event is proportional to the mean dose to the whole heart and increases linearly by 7.4% per Gray [2]. When analysing DVHs, the measured dose volume points were different for low doses: V2 (volume of heart receiving 2 Gy) and V4 (volume of heart receiving 4 Gy), meaning that, in Group 1 with hscTnI increase, larger volumes of the heart were exposed to more radiation than in Group 2. Though it is still unclear what is more detrimental, a lower dose for a larger volume or a higher dose for a small volume, our data indicate that a low dose applied on a larger volume contributed to acute myocyte damage, resulting in subsequent troponin release.

For the left ventricle and left anterior descending artery, the findings were similar. There was a statistically significant difference for mean doses between the two groups. For LV, the medians were 4.7 for Group 1 (IQR: 2.8–6.1) and 2.9 Gy for Group 2 (IQR: 2.3–4.2). The two groups differed for V2 and V4, but also for V38, with all volumes being larger in Group 1.

LAD is the most anterior part of the heart situated near the clinical target volume. According to data from the literature, the mean dose on LAD higher than 5 Gy was connected with an increased requirement of coronary intervention in LAD years after the completion of radiotherapy [5]. In our study, the median dose on LAD was higher than 5 Gy in both groups: it was 6.8 Gy for Group 1 (IQR: 6.3–19.2) and 6.2 Gy for Group 2 (IQR:

5.1–6.9). The measured dose volume points were different for low doses, with V2, V4 and V5, again, being higher in Group 1 with hscTnI increase.

Radiation-dose-dependent troponin release during irradiation of the left breast has already been described in the literature. High-sensitivity cardiac troponin T was measured prior to, during and after left breast radiotherapy. In patients with increased hscTnT values, higher radiation doses on the whole heart and LV were reported, as well as V15 and V20 for LAD [11]. However, the patients in this trial did not receive chemotherapy prior to irradiation or anti-HER2 therapy either prior to or during irradiation. Lymph nodes were not included in the target volume and, also, fractionation schemes were different than in our study; patients received either 50 Gy in 2 Gy daily fraction over 5 weeks or 42.56 Gy in 2.66 Gy fractions over 3.5 weeks. According to the institutional guidelines based on the data in the literature, the patients in our trial received 40.05 Gy in 2.67 Gy fractions over 3 weeks—a hypofractionated regimen [28,29]. Therefore, the applied radiation dose in our patients was somewhat lower and the overall treatment time was shorter.

Numerous trials did not show any difference in cardiotoxicity between the conventional radiotherapy (CFRT) and hypofractionated radiotherapy (HFRT). In START trials, schedules of 41.6 Gy or 39 Gy in 13 fractions over 5 weeks and 40 Gy in 15 fractions over 3 weeks were compared to the conventional fractionation scheme of 50 Gy in 25 fractions over 5 weeks. After 10 years of follow-up, there was no difference in the frequency of ischemic heart disease between the groups of patients that received HFRT and the patients irradiated with conventional fractionation [29]. Long-term data from a Canadian trial comparing 42.56 Gy in 16 fractions over 22 days with 50 Gy in 25 fractions over 5 weeks are similar; after 12 years of follow-up, few cardiac-related deaths were observed in both groups of patients. There was no increase in cardiac-related deaths in patients who were irradiated with a hypofractionated schedule [30]. In a meta-analysis that was published in 2020, the authors analysed the data from 25 clinical trials that enrolled 3871 postmastectomy patients and compared HFRT with CFRT in terms of both treatment efficacy and toxicity. No difference in late cardiac toxicity between the schedules was observed [31]. In an analysis of the data of 510 breast cancer patients irradiated between 2002 and 2006, either conventionally or with a hypofractionated schedule, cardiac toxicity was evaluated. The rate of ischaemic cardiac disease was low in both group of patients. According to the trial data, the fractionation schedule had no influence on the frequency of cardiotoxicity [32].

The strengths of our study are the clear inclusion criteria that reduce uncertainty and error factors, and the well-balanced subgroups of patients. The limitations could be the possibly confounding effect of anthracycline use, though groups were balanced in this regard and there was a variability of cardiac therapy.

Based on the abovementioned data, we have calculated dose-volume constraints for the whole heart, LV and LAD in order to define the radiation doses above which troponin release as a result of radiation damage can be expected. They should not be considered absolute safe cardiac doses for this patient population, but rather as guidance that might be considered for treatment planning. However, patients with troponin increase should be followed more carefully for the early diagnosis of cardiac dysfunction and timely implementation of cardioprotective treatment strategies in order to improve both oncological and cardiovascular outcomes. It is yet to be explored if this hscTnI increase can predict the future risk of cardiovascular morbidity and mortality in this group of patients.

5. Conclusions

In patients with HER2-positive breast cancer undergoing adjuvant hypofractionated left breast radiotherapy concomitantly with anti-HER2 therapy, high-sensitivity cardiac troponin I is being released, dependent on the radiation dose on the heart and its structures. The results of this study can partially contribute to understanding early cardiotoxicity development and detection.

Author Contributions: Conceptualisation, K.A. and L.B.-O.; methodology, K.A., L.M. and L.B.-O.; formal analysis, K.A. and M.B.; investigation, K.A.; resources, L.M. and L.B.-O.; data curation, K.A. and M.B.; writing—original draft preparation, K.A.; writing—review and editing, L.M., M.B. and L.B.-O.; project administration, K.A. and L.B.-O. All authors have read and agreed to the published version of the manuscript.

Funding: This research received no external funding.

Institutional Review Board Statement: The study was conducted in accordance with the Declaration of Helsinki, and approved by the Institutional Ethics Committee of Sestre Milosrdnice University Hospital Center, Zagreb, Croatia (003-06/21-03/011, 8 April 2021).

Informed Consent Statement: Informed consent was obtained from all subjects involved in the study.

Data Availability Statement: The datasets analysed or generated during the current study are available from the corresponding author upon reasonable request.

Conflicts of Interest: The authors declare no conflict of interest.

Abbreviations

hscTnI	high-sensitivity cardiac troponin I
Gy	Gray
LN	lymph nodes
ROC	receiver operating characteristics
RT	radiation therapy
DVH	dose volume histograms
LAD	left anterior descending artery
LV	left ventricle
LVEF	left ventricular ejection fraction
T-DM1	trastuzumab emtansine
CFRT	conventional fractionated radiotherapy
HFRT	hypofractionated radiotherapy

References

1. Early Breast Cancer Trialists' Collaborative Group (EBCTCG). Effect of radiotherapy after breast-conserving surgery on 10-year recurrence and 15-year breast cancer death: Meta-analysis of individual patient data for 10 801 women in 17 randomised trials. *Lancet* **2011**, *378*, 1707–1716. [CrossRef] [PubMed]
2. Darby, S.C.; Ewertz, M.; McGale, P.; Bennet, A.M.; Blom-Goldman, U.; Brønnum, D.; Correa, C.; Cutter, D.; Gagliardi, G.; Gigante, B.; et al. Risk of ischemic heart disease in women after radiotherapy for breast cancer. *N. Engl. J. Med.* **2013**, *368*, 987–998. [CrossRef] [PubMed]
3. Sardaro, A.; Petruzzelli, M.F.; D'Errico, M.P.; Grimaldi, L.; Pili, G.; Portaluri, M. Radiation-induced cardiac damage in early left breast cancer patients: Risk factors, biological mechanisms, radiobiology, and dosimetric constraints. *Radiother. Oncol.* **2012**, *103*, 133–142. [CrossRef]
4. Van den Bogaard, V.A.; Ta, B.D.; van der Schaaf, A.; Bouma, A.B.; Middag, A.M.; Bantema-Joppe, E.J.; van Dijk, L.V.; van Dijk-Peters, F.B.; Marteijn, L.A.; de Bock, G.H.; et al. Validation and modification of a prediction model for acute cardiac events in patients with breast cancer treated with radiotherapy based on three-dimensional dose distributions to cardiac substructures. *J. Clin. Oncol.* **2017**, *35*, 1171–1178. [CrossRef] [PubMed]
5. Wennstig, A.-K.; Garmo, H.; Isacsson, U.; Gagliardi, G.; Rintelä, N.; Lagerqvist, B.; Holmberg, L.; Blomqvist, C.; Sund, M.; Nilsson, G. The relationship between radiation doses to coronary arteries and location of coronary stenosis requiring intervention in breast cancer survivors. *Radiat. Oncol.* **2019**, *14*, 40. [CrossRef]
6. Garg, P.; Morris, P.; Fazlanie, A.L.; Vijayan, S.; Dancso, B.; Dastidar, A.G.; Plein, S.; Mueller, C.; Haaf, P. Cardiac biomarkers of acute coronary syndrome: From history to high-sensitivity cardiac troponin. *Intern. Emerg. Med.* **2017**, *12*, 147–155. [CrossRef]
7. Pudil, R.; Mueller, C.; Čelutkienė, J.; Henriksen, P.A.; Lenihan, D.; Dent, S.; Barac, A.; Stanway, S.; Moslehi, J.; Suter, T.M.; et al. Role of serum biomarkers in cancer patients receiving cardiotoxic cancer therapies: A position statement from the Cardio-Oncology Study Group of the Heart Failure Association and the Cardio-Oncology Council of the European Society of Cardiology. *Eur. J. Heart Fail.* **2020**, *22*, 1966–1983. [CrossRef]
8. Stewart, F.A. Mechanisms and dose-response relationships for radiation-induced cardiovascular disease. *Ann. ICRP* **2012**, *41*, 72–79. [CrossRef]

9. Wang, H.; Wei, J.; Zheng, Q.; Meng, L.; Xin, Y.; Yin, X.; Jiang, X. Radiation-induced heart disease: A review of classification, mechanism and prevention. *Int. J. Biol. Sci.* **2019**, *15*, 2128–2138. [CrossRef]
10. Lv, X.; Pan, C.; Guo, H.; Chang, J.; Gao, X.; Wu, X.; Zhi, X.; Ren, C.; Chen, Q.; Jiang, H.; et al. Early diagnostic value of high-sensitivity cardiac troponin T for cancer treatment-related cardiac dysfunction: A meta-analysis. *ESC Heart Fail.* **2023**, *10*, 2170–2182. [CrossRef]
11. Skyttä, T.; Tuohinen, S.; Boman, E.; Virtanen, V.; Raatikainen, P.; Kellokumpu-Lehtinen, P.L. Troponin T-release associates with cardiac radiation doses during adjuvant left-sided breast cancer radiotherapy. *Radiat. Oncol.* **2015**, *10*, 141. [CrossRef] [PubMed]
12. Italian Cardio-Oncologic Network. Trastuzumab adjuvant chemotherapy and cardiotoxicity in real-world women with breast cancer. *J. Card. Fail.* **2012**, *18*, 113–119. [CrossRef] [PubMed]
13. Cardinale, D.; Colombo, A.; Torrisi, R.; Sandri, M.T.; Civelli, M.; Salvatici, M.; Lamantia, G.; Colombo, N.; Cortinovis, S.; Dessanai, M.A.; et al. Trastuzumab-induced cardiotoxicity: Clinical and prognostic implications of troponin I evaluation. *J. Clin. Oncol.* **2010**, *28*, 3910–3916. [CrossRef] [PubMed]
14. Von Minckwitz, G.; Procter, M.; de Azambuja, E.; Zardavas, D.; Benyunes, M.; Viale, G.; Suter, T.; Arahmani, A.; Rouchet, N.; Clark, E.; et al. Adjuvant pertuzumab and trastuzumab in Early HER2-positive breast cancer. *N. Engl. J. Med.* **2017**, *377*, 122–131, Erratum in *N. Engl. J. Med.* **2017**, *377*, 702. [CrossRef]
15. Piccart, M.; Procter, M.; Fumagalli, D.; de Azambuja, E.; Clark, E.; Ewer, M.S.; Restuccia, E.; Jerusalem, G.; Dent, S.; Reaby, L.; et al. Abstract GS1-04: Interim overall survival analysis of APHINITY (BIG 4-11): A randomized, multicenter, double-blind, placebo-controlled trial comparing chemotherapy plus trastuzumab plus pertuzumab vs chemotherapy plus trastuzumab plus placebo as adjuvant therapy in patients with operable HER2-positive early breast cancer. *Cancer Res.* **2020**, *80*, GS1-04. [CrossRef]
16. Alhussein, M.M.; Mokbel, A.; Cosman, T.; Aghel, N.; Yang, E.H.; Mukherjee, S.D.; Dent, S.; Ellis, P.M.; Dhesy-Thind, S.; Leong, D.P. Pertuzumab Cardiotoxicity in Patients with HER2-Positive Cancer: A Systematic Review and Meta-analysis. *CJC Open* **2021**, *3*, 1372–1382. [CrossRef] [PubMed]
17. Von Minckwitz, G.; Huang, C.-S.; Mano, M.S.; Loibl, S.; Mamounas, E.P.; Untch, M.; Wolmark, N.; Rastogi, P.; Schneeweiss, A.; Redondo, A.; et al. Trastuzumab emtansine for residual invasive HER2-positive breast cancer. *N. Engl. J. Med.* **2019**, *380*, 617–628. [CrossRef] [PubMed]
18. Loibl, S.; Huang, C.-S.; Mano, M.; Mamounas, T.; Geyer, C.; Untch, M.; von Minckwitz, G.; Thery, J.-C.; Schwaner, I.; Limentani, S.; et al. Adjuvant trastuzumab emtansine (T-DM1) vs. trastuzumab (T) in patients with residual invasive disease after neoadjuvant therapy for HER2+ breast cancer: Subgroup analysis from KATHERINE. *Ann. Oncol.* **2020**, *31* (Suppl. S2), S48. [CrossRef]
19. Mamounas, E.; Untch, M.; Mano, M.; Huang, C.-S., Jr.; Geyer, C.E., Jr.; von Minckwitz, G.; Wolmark, N.; Pivot, X.; Kuemmel, S.; DiGiovanna, M.; et al. Adjuvant T-DM1 versus trastuzumab in patients with residual invasive disease after neoadjuvant therapy for HER2-positive breast cancer: Subgroup analyses from KATHERINE. *Ann. Oncol.* **2021**, *32*, 1005–1014. [CrossRef]
20. Pondé, N.; Ameye, L.; Lambertini, M.; Paesmans, M.; Piccart, M.; de Azambuja, E. Trastuzumab emtansine (T-DM1)-associated cardiotoxicity: Pooled analysis in advanced HER2-positive breast cancer. *Eur. J. Cancer* **2020**, *126*, 65–73. [CrossRef]
21. Lyon, A.R.; Dent, S.; Stanway, S.; Earl, H.; Brezden-Masley, C.; Cohen-Solal, A.; Tocchetti, C.G.; Moslehi, J.J.; Groarke, J.D.; Bergler-Klein, J.; et al. Baseline cardiovascular risk assessment in cancer patients scheduled to receive cardiotoxic cancer therapies: A position statement and new risk assessment tools from the Cardio-Oncology Study Group of the Heart Failure Association of the European Society of Cardiology in collaboration with the International Cardio-Oncology Society. *Eur. J. Heart Fail.* **2020**, *22*, 1945–1960. [CrossRef] [PubMed]
22. Marinko, T.; Dolenc, J.; Bilban-Jakopin, C. Cardiotoxicity of concomitant radiotherapy and trastuzumab for early breast cancer. *Radiol. Oncol.* **2014**, *48*, 105–112. [CrossRef] [PubMed]
23. Cao, L.; Cai, G.; Chang, C.; Yang, Z.-Z.; Feng, Y.; Yu, X.-L.; Ma, J.-L.; Wu, J.; Guo, X.-M.; Chen, J.-Y. Early cardiac toxicity following adjuvant radiotherapy of left-sided breast cancer with or without concurrent trastuzumab. *Oncotarget* **2016**, *7*, 1042–1054. [CrossRef] [PubMed]
24. Abouegylah, M.; Braunstein, L.Z.; El-Din, M.A.A.; Niemierko, A.; Salama, L.; Elebrashi, M.; Edgington, S.K.; Remillard, K.; Napolitano, B.; Naoum, G.E.; et al. Evaluation of radiation-induced cardiac toxicity in breast cancer patients treated with Trastuzumab-based chemotherapy. *Breast Cancer Res. Treat.* **2019**, *174*, 179–185. [CrossRef] [PubMed]
25. Sawaya, H.; Sebag, I.A.; Plana, J.C.; Januzzi, J.L.; Ky, B.; Cohen, V.; Gosavi, S.; Carver, J.R.; Wiegers, S.E.; Martin, R.P.; et al. Early detection and prediction of cardiotoxicity in chemotherapy-treated patients. *Am. J. Cardiol.* **2011**, *107*, 1375–1380. [CrossRef] [PubMed]
26. Cardinale, D.; Sandri, M.T.; Martinoni, A.; Borghini, E.; Civelli, M.; Lamantia, G.; Cinieri, S.; Martinelli, G.; Fiorentini, C.; Cipolla, C.M. Myocardial injury revealed by plasma troponin I in breast cancer treated with high-dose chemotherapy. *Ann. Oncol.* **2002**, *13*, 710–715. [CrossRef] [PubMed]
27. Cardinale, D.; Iacopo, F.; Cipolla, C.M. Cardiotoxicity of Anthracyclines. *Front. Cardiovasc. Med.* **2020**, *7*, 26. [CrossRef] [PubMed]
28. START Trialists' Group; Bentzen, S.M.; Agrawal, R.K.; Aird, E.G.A.; Barrett, J.M.; Barrett-Lee, P.J.; Bentzen, S.M.; Bliss, J.M.; Brown, J.; Dewar, J.A.; et al. The UK standardisation of breast radiotherapy (START) trial B of radiotherapy hypofractionation for treatment of early breast cancer: A randomised trial. *Lancet* **2008**, *371*, 1098–1107. [CrossRef]

29. Haviland, J.S.; Owen, J.R.; Dewar, J.A.; Agrawal, R.K.; Barrett, J.; Barrett-Lee, P.J.; Dobbs, H.J.; Hopwood, P.; Lawton, P.A.; Magee, B.J.; et al. The UK standardisation of breast radiotherapy (START) trials of radiotherapy hypofractionation for treatment of early breast cancer: 10-year follow-up results of two randomised controlled trials. *Lancet Oncol.* **2013**, *14*, 1086–1094. [CrossRef]
30. Whelan, T.J.; Pignol, J.-P.; Levine, M.N.; Julian, J.A.; MacKenzie, R.; Parpia, S.; Shelley, W.; Grimard, L.; Bowen, J.; Lukka, H.; et al. Long-term results of hypofractionated radiation therapy for breast cancer. *N. Engl. J. Med.* **2010**, *362*, 513–520. [CrossRef]
31. Liu, L.; Yang, Y.; Guo, Q.; Ren, B.; Peng, Q.; Zou, L.; Zhu, Y.; Tian, Y. Comparing hypofractionated to conventional fractionated radiotherapy in postmastectomy breast cancer: A meta-analysis and systematic review. *Radiat. Oncol.* **2020**, *15*, 17. [CrossRef]
32. James, M.; Swadi, S.; Yi, M.; Johansson, L.; Robinson, B.; Dixit, A. Ischaemic heart disease following conventional and hypofractionated radiation treatment in a contemporary breast cancer series. *J. Med. Imaging Radiat. Oncol.* **2018**, *62*, 425–431. [CrossRef]

Disclaimer/Publisher's Note: The statements, opinions and data contained in all publications are solely those of the individual author(s) and contributor(s) and not of MDPI and/or the editor(s). MDPI and/or the editor(s) disclaim responsibility for any injury to people or property resulting from any ideas, methods, instructions or products referred to in the content.

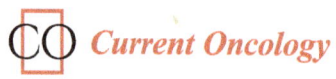

Case Report

Pregnancy in a Young Patient with Metastatic HER2-Positive Breast Cancer—Between Fear of Recurrence and Desire to Procreate

Cristina Marinela Oprean [1,2,3], Andrei Dorin Ciocoiu [2], Nusa Alina Segarceanu [2,3], Diana Moldoveanu [2,3], Alexandra Stan [4], Teodora Hoinoiu [5,6,*], Ioana Chiorean-Cojocaru [7], Daciana Grujic [8], Adelina Stefanut [9], Daniel Pit [6] and Alis Dema [1]

[1] ANAPATMOL Research Center, 'Victor Babes' University of Medicine and Pharmacy of Timisoara, 300041 Timisoara, Romania
[2] Department of Oncology, ONCOHELP Hospital Timisoara, Ciprian Porumbescu Street, No. 59, 300239 Timisoara, Romania
[3] Department of Oncology, ONCOMED Outpatient Unit, Ciprian Porumbescu Street, No. 59, 300239 Timisoara, Romania
[4] Department of Oncology, City Clinical Emergency Hospital of Timisoara, Victor Babes Blvd. No. 22, 300595 Timisoara, Romania
[5] Department of Clinical Practical Skills, "Victor Babes" University of Medicine and Pharmacy, Eftimie Murgu Sq. Nr. 2, 300041 Timisoara, Romania
[6] Center for Advanced Research in Cardiovascular Pathology and Hemostaseology, "Victor Babes" University of Medicine and Pharmacy, 300041 Timisoara, Romania
[7] Department of Obstetrics and Gynaecology, Faculty of Medicine and Pharmacy, "Victor Babes" University of Medicine and Pharmacy, 300041 Timisoara, Romania
[8] Department of Plastic and Reconstructive Surgery, "Victor Babes" University of Medicine and Pharmacy, Eftimie Murgu Sq. Nr. 2, 300041 Timisoara, Romania
[9] Department of Psychology & Sociology, West University, Timisora, Blvd. No. 4, Vasile Pârvan, 300223 Timisoara, Romania
* Correspondence: tstoichitoiu@umft.ro

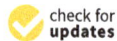

Citation: Oprean, C.M.; Ciocoiu, A.D.; Segarceanu, N.A.; Moldoveanu, D.; Stan, A.; Hoinoiu, T.; Chiorean-Cojocaru, I.; Grujic, D.; Stefanut, A.; Pit, D.; et al. Pregnancy in a Young Patient with Metastatic HER2-Positive Breast Cancer—Between Fear of Recurrence and Desire to Procreate. *Curr. Oncol.* 2023, *30*, 4833–4843. https://doi.org/10.3390/curroncol30050364

Received: 14 April 2023
Revised: 1 May 2023
Accepted: 6 May 2023
Published: 8 May 2023

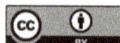

Copyright: © 2023 by the authors. Licensee MDPI, Basel, Switzerland. This article is an open access article distributed under the terms and conditions of the Creative Commons Attribution (CC BY) license (https://creativecommons.org/licenses/by/4.0/).

Abstract: Breast cancer is the most frequent neoplasm among women and the second leading cause of death by cancer. It is the most frequent cancer diagnosed during pregnancy. Pregnancy-associated breast cancer is defined as breast cancer that is diagnosed during pregnancy and/or in the postpartum period. Data about young women with metastatic HER2-positive cancer who desire a pregnancy are scarce. The medical attitude in these clinical situations is difficult and nonstandardized. We present the case of a 31-year-old premenopausal woman diagnosed in December 2016 with a stage IV Luminal HER2-positive metastatic breast cancer (pT2 N0 M1 hep). The patient was initially treated by surgery in a conservative manner. Postoperatively, the presence of liver metastases was found by CT investigation. Consequently, line I treatment (docetaxel 175 mg/m^2 iv; trastuzumab 600 mg/5 mL sq) and ovarian drug suppression (Goserelin 3.6 mg sq at 28 days) was administered. After nine cycles of treatment, the patient's liver metastases had a partial response to the therapy. Despite having a favorable disease evolution and a strong desire to procreate, the patient vehemently refused to continue any oncological treatment. The psychiatric consult highlighted an anxious and depressive reaction for which individual and couple psychotherapy sessions were recommended. After 10 months from the interruption of the oncological treatment, the patient appeared with an evolving pregnancy of 15 weeks. An abdominal ultrasound revealed the presence of multiple liver metastases. Knowing all the possible effects, the patient consciously decided to postpone the proposed second-line treatment. In August 2018, the patient was admitted in the emergency department with malaise, diffuse abdominal pain and hepatic failure. Abdominal ultrasound found a 21-week-old pregnancy which had stopped in evolution, multiple liver metastases and ascites in large quantity. She was transferred to the ICU department where she perished just a few hours later. Conclusions/Discussion: From a psychological standpoint, the patient had an emotional hardship to make the transition from the status of a healthy person to the status of a sick person. Consequently, she entered a process of emotional protection of the positive cognitive distortion type, which favored the decision to abandon treatment and try to complete the pregnancy to the detriment of her own survival. The patient delayed the initiation of oncological treatment in pregnancy until it was too late. The consequence of this delay in treatment led to the death of the mother and fetus. A multidisciplinary team worked to provide this patient with the best medical care and psychological assistance throughout the course of the disease.

Keywords: metastatic breast cancer; pregnancy; trastuzumab; chemotherapy; pregnancy-associated breast cancer; PABC

1. Introduction

Breast cancer is the most common malignancy amongst women. It is the second leading cause of death by cancer [1]. In the US, approximately 11% of 230,000 new cases of invasive breast cancer are diagnosed in women under the age of 45 [2]. In recent years, there has been an increase in the incidence of breast cancer in women under 40 [3]. In the last five decades, since the 1970s, there has been a trend in postponing pregnancies to a more mature age (delaying childbearing) [4]. As the incidence of breast cancer increases with age, more and more women are diagnosed with cancer during pregnancy, and on the other hand, despite being diagnosed with cancer, some women want a child at any cost [5]. Pregnancy-associated breast cancer (PABC) is defined as breast cancer that is diagnosed during pregnancy and/or the postpartum period (Shao 2020). Breast cancer is the most common malignancy diagnosed during pregnancy, with an increase in incidence in recent decades [6]. The incidence of breast cancer in pregnancy is estimated at 1/3000 pregnancies, about 3% of all breast cancers [7–9]. Pregnancy that occurs before or concurrently with a diagnosis of breast cancer is more likely to result in death and decreased disease-free survival [10]. Breast cancer during pregnancy should be treated as much as possible following the recommendations of the guidelines for breast cancer in nonpregnant women. Chemotherapy is contraindicated in the first trimester of pregnancy due to an increased risk of induction of fetal malformation, as it is the period in which oncogenesis is formed [6]. The most common fetal malformations are deafness, gonadal malformations, cardiac complications (arrhythmias, ischemia and thrombocytopenia), or cognitive disabilities [11]. Moreover, administering chemotherapy in the first trimester of the pregnancy carries a 17% risk of inducing a miscarriage [12]. Chemotherapy can be safely administered during the second and third trimesters of pregnancy [5,13]. The use of chemotherapy during the second and third trimesters of pregnancy may be associated in approximately 10–20% of cases with an increase in the number of obstetric and fetal complications, including hypertensive disorders, restriction of intrauterine growth and premature birth [13]. Anthracycline-based chemotherapy is the standard therapy and can be safely administered to pregnant breast cancer patients during the second and third trimesters of pregnancy. Clinical experience in the use of taxanes in this subtype of patient is limited [13,14]. Endocrine therapy as well as anti-HER2 therapy (the monoclonal antibody trastuzumab) should be avoided during pregnancy, and treatment with these agents should be postponed until after birth [6]. Anti-HER2 therapy is associated with an increased risk of anhydramnios (absence of amniotic fluid leading to fetal lung hypoplasia and postpartum respiratory distress or even intrauterine death) [15–17].

Psychological Implications of Breast Cancer Diagnosis

The diagnosis of breast cancer has implications not only on a physical level but also on a psychological level that are closely related to the disease itself but also to the specifics of the treatments applied. Thus, although the efficacy of these treatments has increased over time, one third of patients do not follow an adjuvant treatment, because they refuse it [18]. Understanding the psychological reality of these patients as well as the factors that contribute to refusing or stopping treatment is particularly important.

They may have a reaction of distrust or of denial; they may face a feeling of uncertainty. During this transition period, patients face multiple stressors, and the lack of similar experiences in their own life or in the life of those in their families makes the coping process difficult [19].

Regarding treatment compliance, among the factors that can influence it, we include the existence of depression, the level of medical knowledge, beliefs about treatment and the trust in the medical system [20]. In the case of young women diagnosed with breast cancer, the psychological problem presented above is frequently added to the desire to have children. In general, women's desire to have children can be emotionally grounded or may be the result of society's expectations; it may be based on the desire to please their life partner [21], or it may mean the end of loneliness because the mother has a person who can love her [22]. In addition, the diagnosis of breast cancer can intensify this desire and give it a new symbolic meaning, such as being normal and able to achieve something beautiful, as opposed to death [23]. In the context of breast cancer, young women face a strong sense of injustice derived from the fear of not being able to give birth and the need to change their future plans regarding having a child, which can affect the achievement of life goals [24].

It is also worth noting that young women newly diagnosed with breast cancer report that their most important concerns are children and family, even at the expense of their own survival [25]. A study involving breast cancer survivors and their partners shows that the experience of the disease did not diminish the motivation to have a biological child for either women or their husbands [23].

Data about young women with metastatic HER2-positive cancer who desire a pregnancy are scarce. The medical conduct in these clinical situations is difficult and nonstandardized. Patients need strong emotional support to help them make a decision about procreation and fear of recurrence. To the best of our knowledge, this is the first case report about an unfavorable outcome of a pregnant mother with metastatic HER2-positive breast cancer.

2. Case Presentation

We present the case of a premenopausal, employed, unmarried, urbanite, nulliparous, 31-year-old patient with a negative personal and familial medical history. In December 2015, she was diagnosed clinically and by imaging with a tumor formation in her left breast, in the lower inner quadrant of 25/13/16 mm. The patient delayed the definite diagnosis by performing the biopsy 1 year later, in November 2016. The pathology examination revealed a hormone-dependent (ER = 90, PR = 30%), Ki67 = 30%, HER2 = 3 + (positive) infiltrative ductal breast carcinoma (IDC), G2, with an "in situ" ductal component of the comedo type. The preoperative assessment consisted of performing a bilateral mammogram and a bilateral breast MRI, thus avoiding the diagnosis of liver metastases at the time of diagnosis. The patient was initially clinically staged T2N0, being considered a nonmetastatic disease. On 8 December 2016, a left breast conserving surgery and a sentinel node biopsy was performed. Postoperative histopathological examination confirmed a infiltrative ductal carcinoma with components of "in situ" breast carcinoma; Nsn = 0/2 lymph nodes examined (pT2Nsn0). Immunohistochemistry (IHC) revealed an RE = 80%, RP = 20%, Ki 67 = 30% and HER2 = 3 + (positive) profile. On the CT scan performed during the pretherapeutic assessment on 19 December 2016, two liver metastases of 31 mm and 12 mm were observed in the 4th and 2nd segment (Figure 1). The CA15-3 tumor marker had a value of 86.8 U/mL. First-line treatment with docetaxel 75 mg/m^2 iv, trastuzumab 600 mg/5 mL sq./21 days and medical ovarian suppression (goserelin 3.6 mg sq./28 days) was initiated. The treatment was well tolerated by the patient, with no significant side effects. The CT scan performed in May 2017, after six cycles of treatment, highlighted a partial response: the liver lesion in the 4th segment had decreased dimensions (15 mm vs. 31 mm), and the lesion in segment II was in complete remission (Figure 2). The treatment was continued for three more cycles. The PET-CT performed in July 2017 described a single liver lesion of 22.3 mm in the 2nd segment, intensely metabolically active (SUV = 6.4) (Figure 3).

Transaminases, both after the 6th and 9th cycle, were within normal limits. For the remaining liver injury, the patient performed, in August 2017, two ablation sessions with an MW of 6 and 4 min at 32 W with a temperature set at 96 degrees. Due to the favorable evolution of the disease and the strong desire to have a child, the patient refused to continue any oncological treatment, including ovarian ablation and the recommended hormone therapy (tamoxifen). The psychiatric consultation highlighted an anxious and depressive reaction for which individual and couple psychotherapy sessions were recommended. The patient only attended regular individual psychotherapy sessions, because at that time she had no life partner. Three months later, in January 2018, the CT scan highlighted a progressive disease of the 4th liver segment lesion (from 33 mm to 55 mm) (Figure 4). She was proposed a 2nd-line treatment with the resumption of the ovarian suppression with goserelin, but the patient refused any additional oncological treatment. In July 2018, the patient presented to the clinic after an emergency consultation, being pregnant for 15 weeks and complaining of abdominal pain. Ultrasound revealed multiple hepatic lesions suggestive of metastases. Tumor marker CA 15-3 had a value of 2400 U/mL, and the common liver tests were slightly above the normal limit (AST = 50 U/L; ALAT = 80 U/L, TB = 1.8 mg/dL). Although the patient was informed about the prognosis at this stage of the disease and about the potential vital risks in case of pregnancy, she wanted to keep the pregnancy, being aware of the consequences of this decision on the evolution of the disease and survival. She did not consult with her parents or with her life partner. Psychological counselling was carried out individually only with the patient, who did not want the family present at the counselling sessions. The psychiatric evaluation performed did not find the existence of any psychiatric pathology that would affect her decision making. We proposed the initiation of chemotherapy, but the patient refused, wanting to go abroad for a second-opinion consultation. She hoped that this consultation would give her a lifesaving solution for the clinical situation she was in. At the end of August 2018, the patient was transported to the emergency department with an affected general state, diffuse abdominal pain and liver failure (AST = 6017 U/L, ALT = 782 U/L; TB = 6.67 mg/dL). The abdominal ultrasound that was performed in the OBGYN department revealed a 21-week-old pregnancy halted in evolution, the absence of fetal heartbeat, biometrics corresponding to an 18-week-old pregnancy, amniotic fluid in normal quantity, multiple liver metastases that almost entirely occupied the liver parenchyma and ascites in large quantities. Given the serious general condition and the impossibility of evacuating the pregnancy by surgery (uterine curettage or total hysterectomy) due to the very high risk of anesthetic death, she was transferred to the intensive care unit where she died a few hours later.

The psychological aspects involved in this case are, first of all, the postponement by the patient of the investigations that could specify the diagnosis with certainty. This postponement was justified by the patient on the basis of the belief that it could not be a serious illness considering her young age. With the initiation and then continuation of chemotherapy, its side effects also appeared. Although the patient's body tolerated the medication well, the psychosocial impact of the disease and treatment was considerable. The patient was a very active person and the social and professional limitations resulting from her illness changed not only her life routine but also reduced her access to the situations that could create meaning and significance. These limitations also contributed to the reduction in social support. The patient was the only child in the family, so she thought it was her duty to protect her parents from the negative psychological impact of finding out the diagnosis. Therefore, she presented the situation to her parents in a much better light than it was in reality, and when the treatment was stopped, they thought that it was no longer necessary to continue it. This state of affairs had the consequence of depriving the patient from adequate support from her parents.

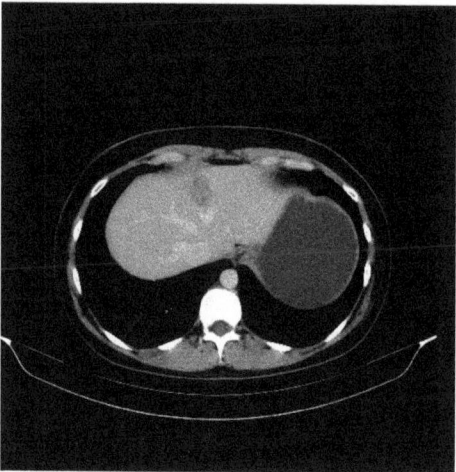

Figure 1. Liver metastasis in 31-year-old women with infiltrative ductal breast carcinoma (IDC), G2, with an "in situ" ductal component of the comedo type. Axial noncontrast abdominal CT image performed in 2016 shows a liver metastasis (31 mm diameter) with an ill-defined area of low attenuation and faint high attenuation.

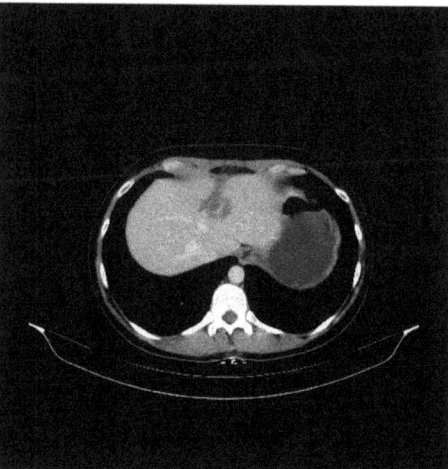

Figure 2. Aspect on the abdominal CT in 2017 after medication with docetaxel 75 mg/m^2 iv, trastuzumab 600 mg/5 mL sq./21 days and medical ovarian suppression (goserelin 3.6 mg sq./28 days) with the liver metastasis (15 mm diameter).

The patient expressed positive beliefs about herself and about her ability to overcome the disease. She also expressed an optimistic view of the course of the disease, believing that it could be stopped even if she interrupted treatment—this view being in fact a way of denying the severity of the disease. Even though she generally acknowledged the severity of the disease, she could not accept that she herself could be in a serious situation.

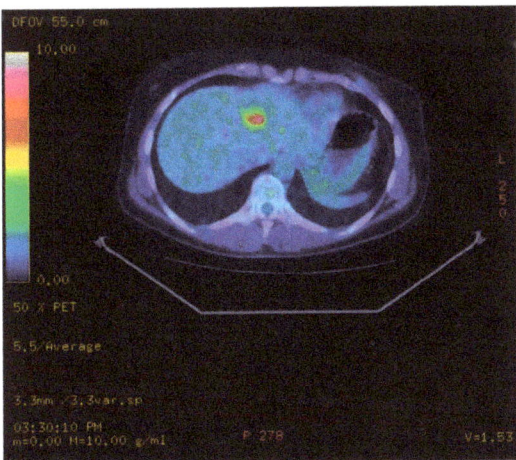

Figure 3. PET/CT scans performed in 2017 showing a single liver lesion of 22.3 mm in the 2nd segment with intense metabolic activity (SUV = 6.4) described as a single liver metastasis.

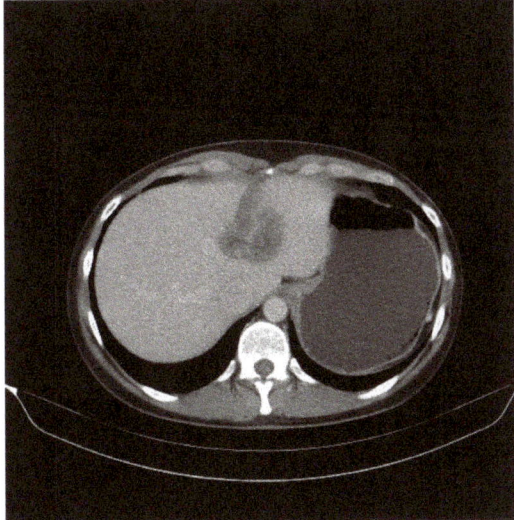

Figure 4. Follow-up abdominal CT performed in 2018 at 6 months after two ablation sessions of the liver metastasis with an MW of 6 and 4 min at 32 W with a temperature set at 96 degrees highlights a progressive disease of the liver metastases at 55 mm diameter.

Although physically the treatment was well tolerated by the patient, she stated that the treatment "does her no good" and that it "changes" her. The way she perceived herself had changed, and she was not satisfied with this new situation. She did not complain about the bodily changes that occurred, but she pointed out the fact that before she was a cheerful, active, full-of-life person, and now she felt deprived of energy and permanently tired. In an attempt to return to her previous condition, once the treatment was stopped, she resumed her professional life, although she could have benefited from another 8 months of medical leave. Involvement in a relationship and then the onset of pregnancy are part of the same attempt to return to her previous life when she was a healthy person.

3. Discussion

Breast cancer, malignant melanoma, cervical cancer, lymphoma and acute leukemia are the most common cancers diagnosed in pregnancy. The occurrence of pregnancy in a patient with metastatic or recurrent disease is a rare and difficult clinical situation. There are few publications in the literature that present these clinical situations. The vast majority of published cases present clinical situations in which the evolution was favorable and the pregnancy was completed. Mauricio Burotto presents such a case in a patient with metastatic malignant melanoma [26]. Clinical cases with successful outcome have also been published: pregnancy in a patient with recurrent ovarian angiosarcoma [27], pregnancy in a patient with recurrent and high-grade metastatic osteosarcoma [28]. Isolated cases have been published in the literature on pregnant patients treated with trastuzumab. Thus, Michelle A. Fanare described a case of HER2-positive metastatic breast cancer in a 27-week-pregnant woman treated with trastuzumab and vinorelbine weekly. Although she suffered an anhydramnios as a side effect, the patient managed to give birth to a healthy baby [16]. One of our explanations would be that since this patient was 27 weeks pregnant, the exposure to trastuzumab during pregnancy was not long-lasting. In our patient, anti-HER2 therapy may not have been a treatment option, requiring longer-term exposure to trastuzumab and probably with more severe side effects. Most likely, our treatment option would have been the use of anthracyclines or taxanes (especially considering the good response to taxanes we had at the first administration), while the use of trastuzumab would have been postponed until after birth.

Pregnancy associated with breast cancer is defined differently in different clinical trials, and this difference explains the inhomogeneous results related to the prognosis of these patients. A recent meta-analysis of 54 articles with 76 included clinical trials that analyzed the prognosis of patients with pregnancy associated with breast cancer concluded that this clinical situation is associated with poor prognosis. However, whether PABC has a worse prognostic is controversial [29]. A meta-analysis published in 2016 showed an increased risk of death in women with PABC compared with non-PABC [10]. Other recent studies found no significant difference in the prognostic of PABC compared with women with non-PABC [30–33]. Case-control studies found that the prognosis is more unfavorable in breast cancer in pregnancy, but when analyzing the data on the TNM stage of the disease, it was observed that the prognosis is not significantly different [34]. For patients who received chemotherapy during pregnancy, the survival data were comparable to those of nonpregnant patients [35,36]. Most children exposed to chemotherapy during intrauterine life have no significant complications [37].

In the case of our patient, the initiation of oncological treatment during pregnancy was postponed until it was too late, which required a multidisciplinary collaboration between the oncologist and obstetrician for the relative benefits of the fetus. Clinical trials have shown that chemotherapy can be safely administered in the second and third trimesters, starting at week 16 of pregnancy. In the selection of treatment, the criteria involve the time of diagnosis, hormonal status and trimester of pregnancy [12]. One of the open questions would be "if we had started chemotherapy, would the patient have managed to complete the pregnancy?" Among the negative prognostic factors present in this case, we mention pregnancy, stage of the disease (patient with metastatic disease at onset), progressive disease at the time of pregnancy, young age and overexpression of HER2. We can assume that if we had initiated chemotherapy, there would have been a chance that the patient would have completed the pregnancy. Unfortunately, the consequence of the delay of the oncological treatment resulted in the death of the fetus and the mother.

The cause of fetal death in utero may be due to hypoxia due to placental detachment with disseminated intravascular coagulation [38] or placental metastases that may affect the fetal circulation if they exceed the villous space of the placenta or may not affect the fetus if they remain at that level [39]. Other causes can be intrauterine growth restrictions or even fetal malformation. Placental metastases are rarely described in the literature, occurring in approximately 17% of cases (4 cases out of 24) [40].

If we refer to the psychological implications associated with this case, we note that finding a diagnosis of a potentially fatal disease can greatly change a person's assumptions about the world and about themself. Reconstructing the worldview requires both emotional and cognitive processing, at a time when the enormity of the threat and emotions can be overwhelming [41]. Young patients newly diagnosed with breast cancer report this passage through various emotional states, which they describe as an "emotional rollercoaster" [19]. From a cognitive perspective, people can resort to three different processes to keep negative emotions aside: cognitive avoidance, emotional avoidance and cognitive distortion. Cognitive avoidance refers to concentrating attention voluntarily or automatically elsewhere to avoid thoughts or images that create distress. Emotional avoidance is a dissociative mechanism by which the person is able to talk about stressful, serious events without having emotional reactions. The last type of avoidance—cognitive distortion—refers to the tendency to operate within a positive bias expressed, for example, by overestimating the probability of experiencing positive events [42].

In the case presented in this study, the hypothesis is that in trying to protect herself emotionally from the implications of the severe diagnosis she was facing, the patient resorted to cognitive distortion. The patient's beliefs about herself before the disease outlined the image of a strong, active person with multiple resources, able to face adversity. These beliefs, which are the basis of an optimistic vision, and which support a fighting spirit against the disease, can make an easy and imperceptible transition to an optimism that is not objectively sustained. This transition was probably made when she gave up treatment, considering the personal resources available to her ensured her success in dealing with the disease. It is also possible that this transition was triggered by the news of encouraging treatment results, known to be the mechanism involved in cognitive distortion through which a person filters a certain category of information (in this case, the negative ones) and focuses on other categories of information (in this case positive). However, the consequence of excluding negative information can be extremely harmful, because it leads to a reduction in the perception of the threat and to the endangerment of the person. Another aspect that can be observed in this case is the fact that the extremely positive assumptions about herself that existed before the diagnosis was made were not changed after the diagnosis or during the treatment. The discrepancy between self-image and the reality of the disease, in which there were aspects that were out of her personal control, created an emotional discomfort expressed by the patient. However, this discomfort was solved not by updating her self-image by integrating the fact that there are situations that are not under one's control but by the positive cognitive distortion of reality as we described previously. An explanatory hypothesis for this way of resolving the internal conflict may be that the acceptance of the personal lack of control in the context of the disease would have led to an intensified perception of the disease threat at a level that the patient would not have been able to cope with. This loss of control and the feeling of being trapped in a system that dictates what to do is reported in the literature by young patients diagnosed with breast cancer [19].

In the present case, the protective attitude that the patient adopted towards the family also draws attention. Although the family was informed of the diagnosis, the situation presented was better than the real one. This position may also be based on the positive beliefs about oneself presented above and is also observed in other young patients with breast cancer [19].

Even in the case of women with early stage breast cancer, the usual medical recommendation is to wait at least two years after the end of the treatment before becoming pregnant, due to the fact that most recurrences occur during this time [42]; when the pregnancy occurred, our patient decided to try to complete it. Despite the risks to her own health, she made the decision, saying that she "wants to leave something behind", which suggests the possible motivation for a symbolic immortality, as evidenced in the literature [23].

4. Conclusions

Pregnancy generally appears to be safe for fetuses, newborns and mothers, without requiring the need for some long-term clinical trials to provide more and more reliable information to doctors and patients [43]. We are, in fact, faced with an enormous challenge. Pregnancy after cancer is an area still being explored and is a fascinating stimulus of knowledge to dedicate oneself to oncology and women's health.

Our conclusion is that in the present case, an important role from a psychological point of view was played by the patient's difficulty to make the transition from the status of a healthy person to the status of a sick person, as well as not updating her self-image according to the new context. This had, as a consequence, an entry into emotional protection processes, such as positive cognitive distortion, which favored the decision to abandon the treatment and the attempt to complete the pregnancy at the expense of her own survival. The patient delayed the initiation of oncological treatment in pregnancy until it was too late. The consequence of this delay in treatment led to the death of the mother and fetus. A multidisciplinary team was committed to providing this patient with the best medical care and psychological assistance throughout the course of the disease. Maybe a strong family and social support, together with more intensive psychological intervention, would have made the evolution of this case different.

Author Contributions: Conceptualization, C.M.O.; writing supervision, C.M.O.; writing—review and editing, T.H.; validation, C.M.O.; methodology: A.D.C. and D.M.; data curation, A.D.C. and I.C.-C.; software, N.A.S. and D.P.; investigation, N.A.S., A.D.C. and D.G.; formal analysis, D.M. and A.S. (Alexandra Stan); validation, A.S. (Adelina Stefanut); visualization, A.S. (Alexandra Stan) and D.P.; supervision, T.H., A.S. (Adelina Stefanut), A.S. (Alexandra Stan) and A.D.; project administration, A.D. All authors have read and agreed to the published version of the manuscript.

Funding: This research received no external funding.

Institutional Review Board Statement: The Institutional Review Board (IRB) of the ONCOHELP Hospital approved the former retrospective study No. 2253/14/12/2021.

Informed Consent Statement: Written informed consent was obtained from the patient for publication of this case report and any accompanying images. A copy of the written consent is available for review.

Data Availability Statement: The data presented in this study are available on request from the corresponding author. The data are not publicly available.

Conflicts of Interest: The authors declare no conflict of interests.

References

1. Kelsey, J.L. Breast Cancer Epidemiology: Summary and Future Directions. *Epidemiol. Rev.* **1993**, *15*, 256–263. [CrossRef] [PubMed]
2. Rosenberg, S.; Newman, L.; Partridge, A. Breast Cancer in Young Women. *JAMA Oncol.* **2015**, *1*, 877–878. [CrossRef] [PubMed]
3. Merlo, D.F.; Wg, A.; Ceppi, M.; Filiberti, R.; Bocchini, V.; Znaor, A.; Gamulin, M.; Primic-Žakelj, M.; Bruzzi, P.; Bouchardy, C.; et al. Breast cancer incidence trends in European women aged 20–39 years at diagnosis. *Breast Cancer Res. Treat.* **2012**, *134*, 363–370. [CrossRef] [PubMed]
4. Mathews, T.J. Delayed Childbearing: More Women Are Having Their First Child Later in Life. 2021. Available online: https://pubmed.ncbi.nlm.nih.gov/19674536/ (accessed on 21 October 2021).
5. Peccatori, F.A.; Azim, J.H.A.; Orecchia, R.; Hoekstra, H.J.; Pavlidis, N.; Kesic, V.; Pentheroudakis, G. Cancer, pregnancy and fertility: ESMO Clinical Practice Guidelines for diagnosis, treatment and follow-up. *Ann. Oncol.* **2013**, *24*, vi160–vi170. [CrossRef] [PubMed]
6. Loibl, S.; Schmidt, A.; Gentilini, O.; Kaufman, B.; Kuhl, C.; Denkert, C.; Von Minckwitz, G.; Parokonnaya, A.; Stensheim, H.; Thomssen, C.; et al. Breast Cancer Diagnosed During Pregnancy. *JAMA Oncol.* **2015**, *1*, 1145–1153. [CrossRef]
7. Loibl, S.; Von Minckwitz, G.; Gwyn, K.; Ellis, P.; Blohmer, J.U.; Schlegelberger, B.; Keller, M.; Harder, S.; Theriault, R.L.; Crivellari, D.; et al. Breast carcinoma during pregnancy. *Cancer* **2006**, *106*, 237–246. [CrossRef]
8. Anderson, J.M. Mammary cancers and pregnancy. *BMJ* **1979**, *1*, 1124–1127. [CrossRef]
9. Navrozoglou, I.; Vrekoussis, T.; Kontostolis, E.; Dousias, V.; Zervoudis, S.; Stathopoulos, E.; Zoras, O.; Paraskevaidis, E. Breast cancer during pregnancy: A mini-review. *Eur. J. Surg. Oncol. (EJSO)* **2008**, *34*, 837–843. [CrossRef]

10. Hartman, E.K.; Eslick, G.D. The prognosis of women diagnosed with breast cancer before, during and after pregnancy: A meta-analysis. *Breast Cancer Res. Treat.* **2016**, *160*, 347–360. [CrossRef]
11. Alfasi, A.; Ben-Aharon, I. Breast Cancer during Pregnancy—Current Paradigms, Paths to Explore. *Cancers* **2019**, *11*, 1669. [CrossRef]
12. Durrani, S.; Akbar, S.; Heena, H. Breast Cancer During Pregnancy. *Cureus* **2018**, *10*, e2941. [CrossRef] [PubMed]
13. Fedro, A.P.; Matteo, L.; Giovanna, S.; Lino, D.P.; Giovanni, C.-P. Biology, staging, and treatment of breast cancer during pregnancy: Reassessing the evidences. *Cancer Biol. Med.* **2018**, *15*, 6. [CrossRef] [PubMed]
14. Theriault, R.; Hahn, K. Management of breast cancer in pregnancy. *Curr. Oncol. Rep.* **2007**, *9*, 17–21. [CrossRef]
15. Mir, O.; Berveiller, P.; Ropert, S.; Goffinet, F.; Pons, G.; Treluyer, J.-M.; Goldwasser, F. Emerging therapeutic options for breast cancer chemotherapy during pregnancy. *Ann. Oncol.* **2007**, *19*, 607–613. [CrossRef] [PubMed]
16. Fanale, M.A.; Uyei, A.R.; Theriault, R.L.; Adam, K.; Thompson, R.A. Treatment of Metastatic Breast Cancer with Trastuzumab and Vinorelbine During Pregnancy. *Clin. Breast Cancer* **2005**, *6*, 354–356. [CrossRef]
17. Nave, O.; Elbaz, M.; Bunimovich-Mendrazitsky, S. Analysis of a breast cancer mathematical model by a new method to find an optimal protocol for HER2-positive cancer. *Biosystems* **2020**, *197*, 104191. [CrossRef]
18. Bickell, N.A.; Lepar, F.; Wang, J.J.; Leventhal, H. Lost Opportunities: Physicians' Reasons and Disparities in Breast Cancer Treatment. *J. Clin. Oncol.* **2007**, *25*, 2516–2521. [CrossRef]
19. Coyne, E.; Borbasi, S.A. Living the experience of breast cancer treatment: The younger women's perspective. *Aust. J. Adv. Nurs.* **2009**, *26*, 6–13.
20. Miranda, C.; De Resende, C.; Melo, C.; Costa, A.; Friedman, H. Depression before and after uterine cervix and breast cancer neoadjuvant chemotherapy. *Int. J. Gynecol. Cancer* **2002**, *12*, 773–776. [CrossRef]
21. Zabin, L.; Huggins, G.; Emerson, M.; Cullins, V. Partner Effects on a Woman's Intention to Conceive: 'Not with This Partner'. *Fam. Plan. Perspect.* **2000**, *32*, 39. [CrossRef]
22. Wesley, Y.; Scoloveno, M. Perception of self, motherhood and gender attitudes among black women. In *Gender Roles*; Lee, J.W., Ed.; Nova Science Publishers Inc.: Hauppauge, NY, USA, 2005; pp. 33–51.
23. Braun, M.; Hasson-Ohayon, I.; Perry, S.; Kaufman, B.; Uziely, B. Motivation for giving birth after breast cancer. *Psycho-Oncol.* **2005**, *14*, 282–296. [CrossRef] [PubMed]
24. Siegel, K.; Gluhoski, V.; Gorey, E. Age-Related Distress Among Young Women with Breast Cancer. *J. Psychosoc. Oncol.* **1999**, *17*, 1–20. [CrossRef]
25. Northouse, L. The impact of breast cancer on patients and husbands. *Cancer Nurs.* **1989**, *12*, 278–284. [CrossRef]
26. Burotto, M.; Gormaz, J.G.; Samtani, S.; Valls, N.; Silva, R.; Rojas, C.; Portiño, S.; de la Jara, C. Viable Pregnancy in a patient with metastatic melanoma treated with double checkpoint immunotherapy. *Semin. Oncol.* **2018**, *45*, 164–169. [CrossRef] [PubMed]
27. Jha, S.; Chan, K.; Poole, C.J.; Rollason, T. Pregnancy following recurrent angiosarcoma of the ovary—A case report and review of literature. *Gynecol. Oncol.* **2005**, *97*, 935–937. [CrossRef] [PubMed]
28. Sathi, B.K.; Khurana, M.; Gruner, B. Recurrent metastatic high-grade osteosarcoma: Disease stabilization and successful pregnancy outcome following aggressive multimodality treatment. *Indian J. Med. Paediatr. Oncol.* **2018**, *39*, 530–532. [CrossRef]
29. Shao, C.; Yu, Z.; Xiao, J.; Liu, L.; Hong, F.; Zhang, Y.; Jia, H. Prognosis of pregnancy-associated breast cancer: A meta-analysis. *BMC Cancer* **2020**, *20*, 746. [CrossRef]
30. Iqbal, J.; Amir, E.; Rochon, P.; Giannakeas, V.; Sun, P.; Narod, S.A. Association of the Timing of Pregnancy with Survival in Women with Breast Cancer. *JAMA Oncol.* **2017**, *3*, 659–665. [CrossRef]
31. Ploquin, A.; Pistilli, B.; Tresch, E.; Frenel, J.; Lerebours, F.; Lesur, A.; Loustalot, C.; Bachelot, T.; Provansal, M.; Ferrero, J.; et al. 5-year overall survival after early breast cancer diagnosed during pregnancy: A retrospective case-control multicentre French study. *Eur. J. Cancer* **2018**, *95*, 30–37. [CrossRef]
32. Boudy, A.-S.; Naoura, I.; Selleret, L.; Zilberman, S.; Gligorov, J.; Richard, S.; Thomassin-Naggara, I.; Chabbert-Buffet, N.; Ballester, M.; Bendifallah, S.; et al. Propensity score to evaluate prognosis in pregnancy-associated breast cancer: Analysis from a French cancer network. *Breast* **2018**, *40*, 10–15. [CrossRef]
33. Choi, M.; Han, J.; Yang, B.R.; Jang, M.-J.; Kim, M.; Kim, T.-Y.; Im, S.-A.; Lee, H.-B.; Moon, H.-G.; Han, W.; et al. Prognostic Impact of Pregnancy in Korean Patients with Breast Cancer. *Oncologist* **2019**, *24*, e1268–e1276. [CrossRef] [PubMed]
34. Rodriguez, A.O.; Chew, H.; Cress, R.; Xing, G.; McElvy, S.; Danielsen, B.; Smith, L. Evidence of Poorer Survival in Pregnancy-Associated Breast Cancer. *Obstet. Gynecol.* **2008**, *112*, 71–78. [CrossRef] [PubMed]
35. Litton, J.K.; Warneke, C.L.; Hahn, K.M.; Palla, S.L.; Kuerer, H.M.; Perkins, G.H.; Mittendorf, E.A.; Barnett, C.; Gonzalez-Angulo, A.M.; Hortobágyi, G.N.; et al. Case Control Study of Women Treated with Chemotherapy for Breast Cancer During Pregnancy as Compared with Nonpregnant Patients with Breast Cancer. *Oncologist* **2013**, *18*, 369–376. [CrossRef] [PubMed]
36. Amant, F.; Von Minckwitz, G.; Han, S.; Bontenbal, M.; Ring, A.E.; Giermek, J.; Wildiers, H.; Fehm, T.; Linn, S.C.; Schlehe, B.; et al. Prognosis of Women with Primary Breast Cancer Diagnosed During Pregnancy: Results From an International Collaborative Study. *J. Clin. Oncol.* **2013**, *31*, 2532–2539. [CrossRef]
37. Cardonick, E.; Dougherty, R.; Grana, G.; Gilmandyar, D.; Ghaffar, S.; Usmani, A. Breast Cancer During Pregnancy. *Cancer J.* **2010**, *16*, 76–82. [CrossRef]
38. Smith, W.; Smith, K. Aggressive Metastatic Breast Cancer to the Placenta Causing Placental Abruption. *Rem. Publ. LLC* **2019**, *3*, 1109.

39. Vetter, G.; Zimmermann, F.; Bruder, E.; Schulzke, S.; Hösli, I.; Vetter, M. Aggressive Breast Cancer during Pregnancy with a Rare Form of Metastasis in the Maternal Placenta. *Geburtshilfe Frauenheilkd.* **2014**, *74*, 579–582. [CrossRef]
40. Potter, J.F.; Schoeneman, M. Metastasis of maternal cancer to the placenta and fetus. *Cancer* **1970**, *25*, 380–388. [CrossRef]
41. Harvey, P.; Moorey, S.; Greer, S. *Cognitive Behaviour Therapy for People with Cancer*; Oxford University Press: Oxford, UK, 2002; 220p, ISBN 0198508662.
42. Averette, H.E.; Mirhashemi, R.; Moffat, F.L. Pregnancy after breast carcinoma. *Cancer* **1999**, *85*, 2301–2304. [CrossRef]
43. Lambertini, M.; Viglietti, G. Pregnancies in young women with diagnosis and treatment of HER2-positive breast cancer. *Oncotarget* **2019**, *10*, 803–804. [CrossRef]

Disclaimer/Publisher's Note: The statements, opinions and data contained in all publications are solely those of the individual author(s) and contributor(s) and not of MDPI and/or the editor(s). MDPI and/or the editor(s) disclaim responsibility for any injury to people or property resulting from any ideas, methods, instructions or products referred to in the content.

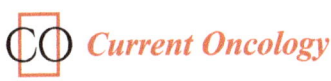 *Current Oncology*

Systematic Review

Assessing Psychological Morbidity in Cancer-Unaffected *BRCA1/2* Pathogenic Variant Carriers: A Systematic Review

Anna Isselhard [1,*], Zoë Lautz [1], Kerstin Rhiem [2] and Stephanie Stock [1]

[1] Institute of Health Economics and Clinical Epidemiology, University Hospital Cologne, 50935 Cologne, Germany
[2] Center for Hereditary Breast and Ovarian Cancer and Center for Integrated Oncology (CIO), Medical Faculty, University Hospital, 50937 Cologne, Germany
* Correspondence: anna.isselhard@uk-koeln.de

Abstract: Female *BRCA1/2* pathogenic variant carriers have an increased lifetime risk for breast and ovarian cancer. Cancer-unaffected women who are newly diagnosed with this pathogenic variant may experience psychological distress because of imminent health threat. No comprehensible review on psychological morbidity in cancer-unaffected *BRCA1/2* pathogenic variant carriers is currently available. This review aims to give an overview about all available the studies in which psychological outcomes have been assessed in cancer-unaffected *BRCA1/2* pathogenic variant carriers, whether as a primary outcome or secondary measurement. A systematic search across four databases (Web of Science, PubMed, ScienceDirect, and EBSCO) was conducted. Studies had to report on cancer-unaffected pathogenic variant carriers (exclusively or separately) and use a validated measure of psychological morbidity to be eligible. Measures were only included if they were used in at least three studies. The final review consisted of 45 studies from 13 countries. Distress measures, including anxiety and cancer worry, were most often assessed. Most studies found a peak of distress immediately after genetic test result disclosure, with a subsequent decline over the following months. Only some studies found elevated distress in carriers compared to non-carriers in longer follow-ups. Depression was frequently investigated but largely not found to be of clinical significance. Quality of life seemed to be largely unaffected by a positive genetic test result, although there was some evidence that younger women, especially, were less satisfied with their role functioning in life. Body image has been infrequently assessed so far, but the evidence suggested that there may be a decrease in body image after genetic test result disclosure that may decrease further for women who opt for a prophylactic mastectomy. Across all the outcomes, various versions of instruments were used, often limiting the comparability among the studies. Hence, future research should consider using frequently used instruments, as outlined by this review. Finally, while many studies included cancer-unaffected carriers, they were often not reported on separately, which made it difficult to draw specific conclusions about this population.

Keywords: BRCA1; BRCA2; breast cancer; anxiety; distress; cancer worry; patient experience

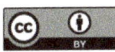

Citation: Isselhard, A.; Lautz, Z.; Rhiem, K.; Stock, S. Assessing Psychological Morbidity in Cancer-Unaffected *BRCA1/2* Pathogenic Variant Carriers: A Systematic Review. *Curr. Oncol.* **2023**, *30*, 3590–3608. https://doi.org/10.3390/curroncol30040274

Received: 31 January 2023
Revised: 8 March 2023
Accepted: 14 March 2023
Published: 25 March 2023

Copyright: © 2023 by the authors. Licensee MDPI, Basel, Switzerland. This article is an open access article distributed under the terms and conditions of the Creative Commons Attribution (CC BY) license (https://creativecommons.org/licenses/by/4.0/).

1. Introduction

BRCA1 and *BRCA2* are tumor suppressor genes that encode proteins, which are responsible for repairing disruptions in damaged DNA that could otherwise result in tumor formation [1,2]. Inheriting a pathogenic variant in either of the two genes leads to erroneous DNA repair and, subsequently, a high risk for breast and ovarian cancer in women [1–3]. For breast cancer, the lifetime risk is roughly five to seven times higher for *BRCA1/2* pathogenic variant carriers compared to women in the general population [3]. For ovarian cancer, the risk is roughly 20 times higher for *BRCA2* and 40 times higher for *BRCA1* pathogenic variant carriers [3]. Albeit independent, a pathogenic variant in either gene is inherited from parent to offspring in autosomal dominant heredity. Therefore, cancer-unaffected members of families with a known *BRCA1/2* pathogenic variant are generally offered genetic counseling and testing [4]. Likewise, index patients of families with a high incidence of breast and ovarian cancers with unknown pathogenic variant status may be offered genetic counseling and testing based on a familial risk assessment. Upon reasonable probability of carrying a pathogenic variant, a blood sample is preferentially drawn from a cancer patient (index patient) and tested. The test result may be positive (individual is a *BRCA1/2* pathogenic variant carrier), negative (individual is a *BRCA1/2* pathogenic variant non-carrier in a *BRCA1/2*-positive family), non-informative (no pathogenic variant was detected in a particular gene), or inconclusive (no pathogenic variant in *BRCA1/2* was found, but a variant of unknown significance (VUS) was) [5]. Pathogenic variant carriers are confronted with difficult decisions in the case of a positive genetic test result on how to deal with their personal cancer risk. Women without previous breast or ovarian cancer history have to make difficult decisions on which risk-reducing strategy to adopt. For breast cancer, this may mean a risk-reducing bilateral mastectomy or participation in intensified surveillance programs [6–8]. While a risk-reducing bilateral mastectomy may reduce breast cancer incidence for carriers of both pathogenic variants, as well as mortality for *BRCA1* pathogenic variant carriers [8,9], worsening of body image and sexual satisfaction have been reported, even with immediate reconstruction [10–13]. On the other hand, breast surveillance is less invasive and can provide survival benefits [14] but cannot reduce breast cancer risk. Both of these options might, therefore, induce distress and worsen psychological wellbeing, as both options come with significant downsides [15]. For ovarian cancer, the only option for effective risk management is a prophylactic bilateral salpingo-oophorectomy [16–18]. For surgical options in particular, female carriers must decide whether to opt for them at all and at what point in their life depending on age-dependent risk, since surgical procedures impact the possibility of bearing or breastfeeding children.

Consequently, undergoing genetic testing, receiving a positive genetic test result, and sharing the test results friends and families may influence levels of psychological morbidity [19,20]. Some women go as far as describing genetic test result disclosure as traumatic [21]. Various studies have assessed psychological wellbeing and morbidity in *BRCA1/2* pathogenic variant carriers, both qualitatively [19,21–24] and quantitatively [25–27]. Previous reviews have attempted to condense the evidence available [12,20,26,28–31]. However, these reviews (1) have focused on the efficacy of psychosocial interventions [28,29], (2) have focused on the psychological effects of different risk-management strategies [12,31], (3) have only included cancer-affected *BRCA1/2* carriers [30], or (4) have reported men and women or cancer-unaffected and cancer-affected *BRCA1/2* pathogenic variant carriers combined [20,26]. This is problematic, as there appears to be a non-negligible difference between cancer-affected compared to cancer-unaffected pathogenic variant carriers [26,32].

To the best of our knowledge, no comprehensive systematic review about the psychological morbidity that female cancer-unaffected *BRCA1/2* pathogenic variant carriers experience after genetic test result disclosure is available thus far. Therefore, the aim of this review is to fill this gap in the literature and explore the short- and long-term psychological consequences of receiving a positive genetic test result for *BRCA1* or *BRCA2* in women without a personal cancer history. To reach these aims, this review sets out to answer two questions:

- How is the psychological morbidity in cancer-unaffected *BRCA1/2* pathogenic variant carriers, both immediately after genetic test result disclosure and long-term?
- Which instruments are frequently employed to assess these psychological morbidities?

2. Materials and Methods

The 2020 Preferred Reporting Items for Systematic Reviews and Meta-Analyses (PRISMA) guidelines were utilized for this review [33]. Four bibliographic databases (Web of Science, PubMed, ScienceDirect, and EBSCO) were systematically searched for studies published from 1997 to January 2023. The search terms included the following keywords, and PubMed medical subject headings (MeSHs) were included individually and in combination depending on the database: *BRCA*, *BRCA1/2*, psychosocial impact, psychosocial distress, coping, anxiety, depression, mental health, psychological adjustment, and mental disorder. The review was not prospectively registered, but the authors will provide protocol upon request.

2.1. Eligibility Criteria

Studies were deemed eligible if they were written in English and if they fulfilled the criteria, as determined by the PICOS framework [34,35].

- Participants: the review focused on cancer-unaffected female adults (age $\geq$ 18 years) with a confirmed pathogenic variant in either *BRCA1* or *BRCA2*.
- Intervention: no special intervention was specified.
- Comparison: studies that compared BRCA pathogenic variant carriers with women who received negative or inconclusive BRCA genetic test results, as well as studies that compared cancer-affected vs. cancer-unaffected pathogenic variant carriers were also included.
- Outcomes: the review included short-term and long-term psychological consequences that were measured with validated instruments.
- Study design: only quantitative studies, irrespective of study design (randomized or non-randomized trials, longitudinal cohort, cross-sectional, or case control), were included; qualitative studies were excluded from the present review.

2.2. Exclusion Criteria

Exclusion criteria consisted of studies not written in English, books, qualitative studies, literature reviews, case reports, or letters to the editor. Studies were also excluded if there was no reporting of psychological consequences or if studies did not specifically identify the population as (1) female, (2) cancer-unaffected, and (3) definitive *BRCA1/2* pathogenic variant carriers. Therefore, studies grouping results for cancer-unaffected with cancer-affected pathogenic variant carriers, carriers with non-carriers, or female with male carriers or those not defining the pathogenic variant as BRCA1/2 were excluded. Additionally, to provide the most value, studies were only included if they measured psychological morbidity with a validated questionnaire that at least three studies used.

2.3. Data Extraction, Data Synthesis, and Quality Assessment

After removal of duplicates, a stepwise approach was undertaken: first, two authors screened titles and abstracts independently (AI and ZL). Conflicts in screening were resolved by discussion. If the disagreement could not be solved quickly, the record went through a full-text review. Next, two authors (AI and ZL) independently screened the full-text articles. Disagreements during this process were solved by discussion. The included studies were analyzed according to the predefined PICOS criteria (see Section 2.1). For each included study, one author (ZL) extracted the following information: full reference, study design, duration of follow-up, and participant characteristics (sample size, age, BRCA1/2 pathogenic variant status, and psychological outcome). Information extraction was overseen and quality-controlled by one author (AI). The findings were divided and grouped into the outcomes utilized within the studies. The goal of this review was a descriptive data analysis and synthesis of evidence. We, therefore, clustered outcomes with their respective validated instruments.

The quality of the included studies was assessed with the AXIS tool [36]. This tool was developed for non-experimental research and includes 20 discrete-choice questions that may be answered with yes or no (e.g., "Was the target population clearly defined?" or "Was ethical approval or consent of participants attained?"). Two reviewers (AI and ZL) rated each item independently and resolved disagreements in the process via discussion. A point was assigned for an item if methodological quality was met, resulting in a score from 0 to 20 for each study, with higher scores indicating higher study quality. The full AXIS assessment can be found in Supplementary Material File S1.

3. Results

The full flow-chart for the review process is displayed in Figure 1. The initial search yielded 810 records. After duplicates were removed, 478 records were screened for eligibility, and 264 records went through full-text review. Additionally, five records were identified by hand search. Forty-five studies met the eligibility criteria and were included in this review. The total number of participants from all the included studies was $n = 2442$, with an age range of 18–83. Overall, the studies showed good quality (see quality assessment 3.5), with some exceptions. Some studies only partially reported outcomes separately for cancer-affected versus cancer-unaffected pathogenic variant carriers. All the studies included in the review are shown in Table 1.

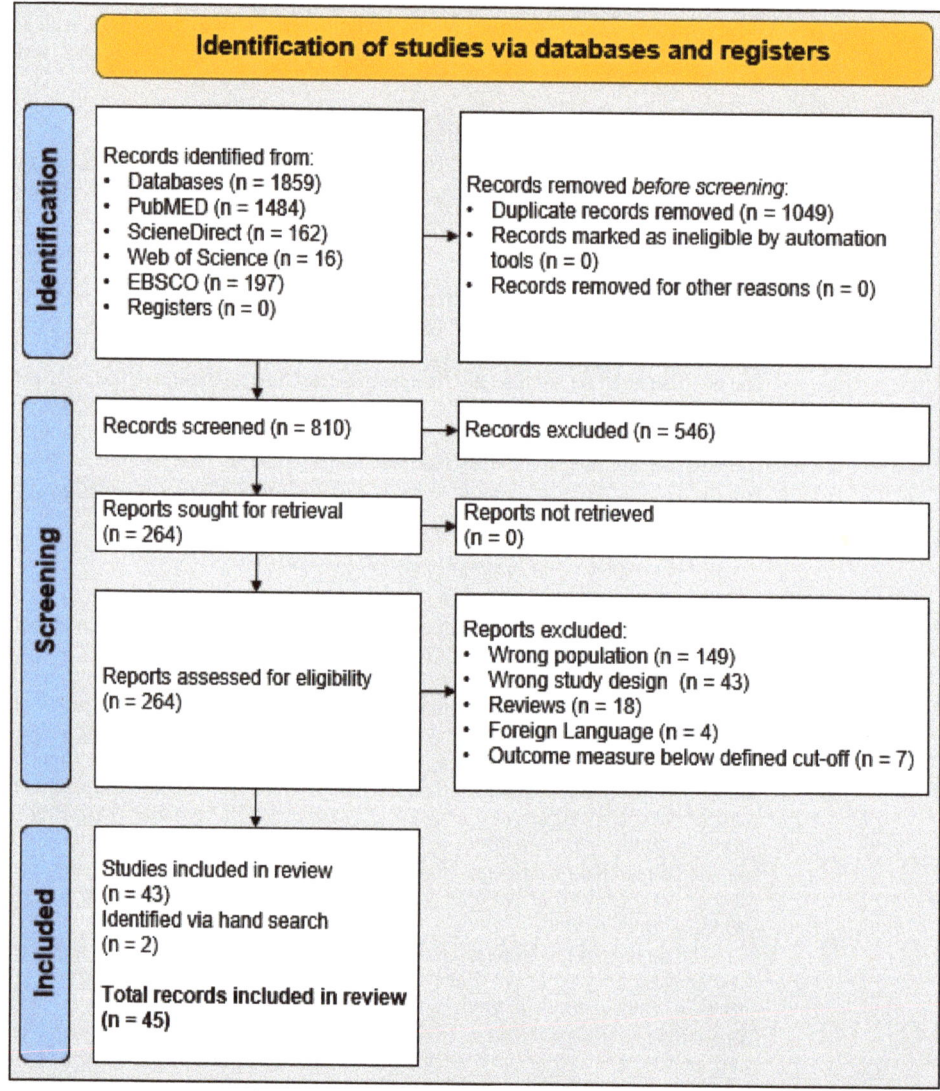

Figure 1. PRISMA flow chart for the identification of studies.

Table 1. Descriptive data of the studies (n = 45) and measures used.

First Author, Year	Country	Participant Characteristics [1]	Study Design, Follow-Up Length	BHS	BIQ	BSI	CES-D	CWS	HADS	IES	GHQ	SF-12/36	STAI
Borreani et al., 2014 [37]	Italy	n = 27 Age range: 26–75	Longitudinal, 15 months					✓	✓			✓	
Brand et al., 2021 [38]	Germany	n = 48 Age mean: 40	Cross-sectional					✓					
Buchanan et al., 2017 [39]	U.S.	n = 97 Age range: 25–40+	Cross-sectional							✓		✓	✓
Carpenter et al., 2014 [40]	U.S.	n = 26 Age mean: 42.9	Experimental							✓			
Claes et al., 2005 [41]	Belgium	n = 34 Age range: 19–61	Longitudinal, 1 year							✓			✓
Croyle et al., 1997 [42]	U.S.	n = 13 Age range: 19–83	Longitudinal, 2 years							✓			✓
Dagan and Gil, 2004 [43]	Israel	n = 36 Age mean: 54.1	Retrospective			✓							
Dagan and Shochat, 2009 [44]	Israel	n = 17 Age mean: 51.4	Case control			✓		✓				✓	
Dorval et al., 2006 [45]	Canada	n = 19 Age mean: 48	Longitudinal, 36 months							✓			
Ertmanski et al., 2009 [46]	Poland	n = 56 Age range: 18–56+	Longitudinal, 1 year							✓			✓
Finch et al., 2013 [47]	Canada	n = 59 Age range: 35–69	Longitudinal, 1 year			✓				✓		✓	
Foster et al., 2007 [48]	U.K.	n = 53 Age range: 23–72	Longitudinal, 3 years					✓			✓		
Geirdal and Dahl, 2008 [49]	Norway	n = 68 Age mean: 42	Cross-sectional	✓					✓				
Geirdal et al., 2005 [50]	Norway	n = 68 Age mean: 42	Cross-sectional						✓	✓	✓		
Gopie et al., 2013 [51]	Netherlands	n = 44 Age mean: 37.1	Longitudinal, 21.7 months		✓					✓	✓	✓	
Graves et al., 2012 [52]	U.S.	n = 47 Age mean: 54.1	Longitudinal, 5 years			✓				✓			✓

Table 1. Cont.

First Author, Year	Country	Participant Characteristics [1]	Study Design, Follow-Up Length	BHS	BIQ	BSI	CES-D	CWS	HADS	IES	GHQ	SF-12/36	STAI
Isern et al., 2008 [53]	Sweden	n = 27, Age range: 25–51	Longitudinal, 42 months						✓				
Isselhard et al., 2023 [54]	Germany	n = 130, Age range: 24–60	Cross-sectional						✓	✓		✓	
Julian-Reynier et al., 2010 [55]	France	n = 244, Age range: <30–50+	Longitudinal, 60 months		✓					✓			
Kinney et al., 2005 [56]	U.S.	n = 19, Age range: <40–50+	Longitudinal, 1 year				✓	✓		✓			✓
Landau et al., 2015 [57]	Israel	n = 56, Age mean: 49.6	Intervention, 12 weeks			✓		✓					
Lapointe et al., 2013 [58]	France	n = 221, Age range: 20–60	Longitudinal, 2 years				✓			✓			
Lodder et al., 2001 [59]	Netherlands	n = 25, Age range: 19–68	Longitudinal, 1–3 weeks						✓	✓			
Lodder et al., 2002 [60]	Netherlands	n = 26, Age mean: 38.8	Longitudinal, 12 months		✓				✓	✓			
Low et al., 2008 [61]	U.S.	n = 7, Age mean: 44.7	Longitudinal, 6 months							✓			
Madalinska et al., 2007 [62]	Netherlands	n = 160, Age range: 35–50+	Longitudinal, 12 months					✓		✓		✓	
Maheu et al., 2012 [63]	France	n = 217, Age range: <35–50+	Longitudinal, 2 years				✓			✓			
Maheu et al., 2014 [64]	France	n = 232, Age mean: 40.7	Longitudinal, 12 months				✓			✓			
Meiser et al., 2002 [65]	Australia	n = 30, Age mean: 40	Longitudinal, 12 months							✓			✓
Metcalfe et al., 2012 [66]	Canada	n = 22, Age range: 25–70	Longitudinal, 2 years							✓			
Metcalfe et al., 2017 [67]	Canada	n = 150, Age range: 25–60	RCT, 12 months							✓			
Metcalfe et al., 2020 [68]	Canada	n = 576, Age range: 25–55	Cross-sectional							✓			

Table 1. *Cont.*

First Author, Year	Country	Participant Characteristics [1]	Study Design, Follow-Up Length	BHS	BIQ	BSI	CES-D	CWS	HADS	IES	GHQ	SF-12/36	STAI
O'Neill et al., 2009 [69]	U.S.	$n = 14$ Age range: 27–68	Longitudinal, 1 year							✓			
Reichelt et al., 2004 [70]	Norway	$n = 80$ Age mean: 43.9	Longitudinal, 6 weeks	✓					✓	✓	✓		
Reichelt et al., 2008 [71]	Norway	$n = 58$ Age mean: 45.4	Longitudinal, 18 months	✓					✓	✓			
Schwartz et al., 2002 [72]	U.S.	$n = 35$ Age mean: 45	Longitudinal							✓			
Shochat and Dagan, 2010 [73]	Israel	$n = 17$ Age mean: 51.4	Cross-sectional			✓		✓					
Smith et al., 2008 [74]	U.S.	$n = 20$ Age range: 22–70	Longitudinal, 6 months				✓			✓		✓	✓
Spiegel et al., 2011 [75]	U.S.	$n = 51$ Age range: 25–60	Longitudinal, 6 months					✓	✓				
Van Dijk et al., 2006 [76]	Netherlands	$n = 22$ Age range: <30–50+	Longitudinal, 6 months					✓		✓			
Van Egdom et al., 2020 [77]	Netherlands	$n = 96$ Age mean: 41.4	Cross-sectional						✓				
Van Oostrom et al., 2003 [78]	Netherlands	$n = 23$ Age mean: 41.9	Longitudinal, 4–6 years		✓			✓	✓	✓			
Van Oostrom et al., 2007 [79]	Netherlands	$n = 49$ Age mean: 42.3	Longitudinal, 12 months					✓	✓	✓			
Van Roosmalen et al., 2004 [80]	Netherlands	$n = 68$ Age mean: 37.6	Longitudinal, 2 weeks				✓			✓			✓
Watson et al., 2004 [81]	U.K.	$n = 91$ Age range: 23–72	Longitudinal, 12 months					✓		✓	✓		

[1] Sample size n refers to number of cancer-unaffected female *BRCA1/2* carriers in the sample and does not represent total sample size.

3.1. Study Characteristics

The studies were published from 1997 to January 2023. Most studies included participants from the U.S. (10 studies), the Netherlands (9 studies), Canada (5 studies), Norway, France, and Israel (4 studies each). Other countries included Italy, Belgium, Poland, the U.K., Sweden, France, and Australia. Most studies employed a (prospective) longitudinal cohort design (thirty-two studies), ranging in follow-up from one week to six years after test result disclosure. Additionally, studies with cross-sectional designs (eight studies) and randomized controlled intervention designs (two studies), as well as one experimental, one retrospective, and one case-control study, were included. Study populations had high heterogeneity in their sample sizes, from $n = 7$ to $n = 576$ cancer-unaffected pathogenic variant carriers. The age ranges in the studies were between 18 and 83 years old. In total, 11 measures were examined within this review (see Table 2).

Table 2. General outcomes and respective measures included in this review.

General Outcome	Specific Measure
Distress	Impact of Event Scale (IES) [82,83]
	Hospital Anxiety and Depression Scale (HADS) [84]
	Cancer Worry Scale (CWS) [85,86]
	Spielberger State-Trait Anxiety Inventory (STAI) [87]
	Brief Symptom Inventory (BSI) [88]
	General Health Questionnaire (GHQ) [89]
Depression	Hospital Anxiety and Depression Scale (HADS) [84]
	Beck's Hopelessness Scale (BHS) [90]
	Center for Epidemiologic Studies Depression Scale (CES-D) [91]
Other	Short Form Health Survey (SF-36/SF-12) [92,93]
	Body Image Questionnaire (BIQ) [60]

3.2. Distress Measures

The anxiety subscale of the Hospital Anxiety and Depression Scale (HADS) [84], the Cancer Worry Scale (CWS) [85,86], the Spielberger State-Trait Anxiety Inventory (STAI) [87], the Brief Symptom Inventory (BSI) [88], the General Health Questionnaire (GHS-28) [89], and the Impact of Event Scale (IES) [82] were characterized as psychological distress parameters.

3.2.1. Impact of Event Scale

By far the most used questionnaire to measure distress was the IES, which was used by 34 studies [39–42,45–47,50–52,54–56,58–72,74,76,78–81]. The IES consists of two subscales for intrusion and avoidance. The revised IES-R additionally has a hyperarousal subscale. Twenty-eight studies used the original version of the questionnaire (IES), whereas three studies used the revised version (IES-R) [54,61,79], and three studies used the intrusion subscale only [62,70,71]. While cut-off values have been reported for different populations, they vary by version used and have been criticized for providing little clinical significance. Fourteen studies report higher IES scores in carriers compared to non-carriers within six months of test result disclosure [42,45,58,59,61,63,65,69,70,72,74,76,80,81]. Of these studies, five reported that distress remained significantly higher in carriers for up to one year after disclosure [58,65,72,76,81]. Contrarily, one study reported that, while carriers experienced higher distress immediately after genetic test result disclosure, there was no significant difference in the distress of non-carriers after 6 months [63]. Two long-term follow-ups with an average time of five years since genetic test result disclosure similarly found no difference between carriers and non-carriers [52,78]. One study reported that, even though distress was higher in carriers, carriers experienced a decrease from before to immediately after test result disclosure, indicating that knowing the test result regardless of the outcome may provide relief [42]. However, this was the only study with this particular result. In fact, four other studies found increases from before to immediately after test result disclosure in carriers [60,65,66,79]. Longitudinal studies among carriers suggested a decrease in distress anywhere between 6 months and two years after disclosure [60,66,67,79]. Higher distress was associated with higher adherence to recommendations about risk-reducing strategies [39] and, among those strategies, higher likelihood to opt for a bilateral mastectomy [60] or a salpingo-oophorectomy [55,62]. Five other studies reported significant decreases in distress after undergoing such risk-reducing surgeries [47,51,66,68,79]. Higher scores were significantly associated with general psychological distress [54] and with receiving a psychological consultation [64], providing some evidence for the real-world validity of the IES. In terms of validity, however, one author pointed to the importance of the definition of the "event" in question: test result disclosure or cancer itself [45]. In fact, one study found differences between carriers and non-carriers in distress when the IES was framed for ovarian cancer but not when it was framed for breast cancer [41]. Therefore, precise wording is important for the interpretation and comparability of results.

3.2.2. Hospital Anxiety and Depression Scale—Anxiety Subscale

Twelve studies assessed anxiety with the anxiety subscale of the HADS (HADS-A) [37,49,50,53,54,59,60,70,71,75,77,78]. Among the studies that compared anxiety in carriers with anxiety in non-carriers, two studies reported differences [59,60]. Both studies were written by the same authors and presumably reported on the same population, with one being focused on anxiety 1–3 weeks after test result disclosure [59] and the other being a one year follow-up [60]. The first of the two studies showed that non-carriers experienced a reduction in anxiety from before genetic testing to shortly after test result disclosure, whereas carriers showed an increase in anxiety [59]. A subgroup analyses based on high and low baseline anxiety was performed and identified a diverging pattern of results: pathogenic variant carriers with high pre-test anxiety remained highly anxious after receiving test results, whereas non-carriers with high pre-test anxiety showed a decrease in anxiety. Further, pathogenic variant carriers with low pre-test anxiety showed an increase in anxiety, whereas non-carriers with low pre-test anxiety showed unchanged levels of anxiety post-test. The second study showed that, at 1 year after receiving test results, anxiety levels for carriers and non-carriers were similar and that those with clinically high scores shortly after test result disclosure remained anxious at 1 year after disclosure [60]. Indeed, many studies found that pre-test anxiety levels were a good predictor of anxiety longitudinally [37,60,75,78]. One study specifically showed that, even after 5 years, current anxiety was best predicted by anxiety pregenetic test result disclosure, regardless of carrier status [78]. The authors of this particular study reported that anxiety in carriers spiked to just sub-clinical levels right after genetic test result disclosure but returned to the level of non-carriers after six months. They noted an increase in anxiety 5 years after genetic post-result disclosure that was present for carriers and non-carriers alike [78]. In contrast to these findings, two other studies found scores well below the clinical threshold for carriers and showed that anxiety scores in carriers were lower compared to women from high-risk families with an absence of demonstrated pathogenic variants [49,50]. Roughly half of the studies included percentages of potential clinical cases (HADS-A score ≥ 8) and reported that roughly one-in-four to one-in-five-carriers (19–24%) showed clinical anxiety [49,53,54,59,60,70,71]. One study reported almost half (49%) of participants scoring in the clinical anxiety range [75]. However, this higher occurrence may have been found because the sample in this study consisted of carriers who were or were not recalled after a suspicious MRI report in intensified breast cancer screening. The anxiety might, therefore, be a result of this recall and not of the genetic test result itself, as the recalled group showed significantly higher anxiety than the non-recalled group. It was shown that, even among recalled carriers, the scores returned to below baseline 6 months after genetic test result disclosure. Three studies were identified that compared carriers opting for different preventive options (risk-reducing surgery vs. surveillance) [37,60,77]. One study reported scores on the higher end of the normal range for both women who opted for surveillance and women who opted for surgery, with women in the surveillance group showing marginally, but not significantly, higher scores [37]. Another study showed a contrary result, with carriers who opted for prophylactic mastectomy showing significantly higher anxiety compared to carriers opting for surveillance [60]. A reduction in anxiety from immediately after test result disclosure to 1 year after result disclosure was reported regardless of preventive option but was steeper for women who opted for a mastectomy. Finally, one study compared women opting for surveillance or bilateral prophylactic mastectomy with immediate breast reconstruction and found no difference in anxiety between the two [77].

3.2.3. Cancer Worry Scale

Thirteen studies measured cancer worry utilizing different versions of the CWS [37,38,44,48,56,57,62,73,75,76,78,79,81]. There was high heterogeneity in the versions used, with one study using a single-item version [76], two studies using a three-item version [37,56], five studies using a four-item version [38,44,73,75,79], two studies using a five-item version [62,78], and two studies using a revised six-item version [48,81]. One study did not specify which version was used [57]. Two studies did not report results relevant to the population [56,57]. Three studies identified no difference in cancer worry in carriers when compared to non-carriers from high-risk families [48,73,78]. In contrast, eight studies identified increased cancer worry, each with unique comparators [37,38,44,62,75,76,79,81]. Three studies compared carriers with non-carriers from high-risk families and found higher cancer worry in those with pathogenic variants for up to one year after genetic test result disclosure [44,79,81]. One of these studies further specified that, especially, carriers under the age of 35 experienced higher levels of cancer worry compared to carriers over 50 years one month after genetic test result disclosure [81]. This difference, however, was no longer significant at one year after genetic test result disclosure. This may be indicative of the complexity of decision making in premenopausal women immediately after genetic test result disclosure. Two other studies provided additional evidence for this by displaying an increase in cancer worry for up to one month after disclosure, with a subsequent decline in cancer worry at six months after genetic test result disclosure [76,79]. Another study compared carriers opting for different preventive strategies (prophylactic surgery vs. intensified breast cancer screening) [62]. The results revealed that, specifically, the surgery group showed an increase in cancer worry symptoms. Further, in another study [75] there was an increase in cancer worry over time. However, the study compared carriers who were recalled after a first MRI with women who were not recalled. Although there was no difference in cancer worry symptoms at the first MRI appointment, there was a significant increase in cancer worry symptoms in the recalled group. The non-recalled group did not exhibit this pattern, indicating that imminent cancer diagnosis may be relevant to the genesis of higher cancer worry.

3.2.4. Spielberger State-Trait Anxiety Inventory

Nine studies measured anxiety using the STAI [39,41,42,46,52,56,65,74,80], eight of which used the state anxiety subscale only. Only one study used both the state and the trait subscales [46]. While this study found no increase in state anxiety right after result disclosure, as well as at one year after, women with the highest trait anxiety also experienced the highest spike in state anxiety after genetic test result disclosure [46]. No specific outcome was reported in one study [52]. Three studies found that non-carriers experienced significantly less state anxiety after genetic test result disclosure, whereas carriers remained at a stable level or experience slightly more anxiety [41,56,65]. In fact, two studies found significantly higher state anxiety in carriers compared to non-carriers at 1–2 weeks after genetic test result disclosure [42,80]. Another study found higher state anxiety at three months after genetic test result disclosure in carriers compared to non-carriers but no longer at six months [74]. Likewise, another study found no differences between carriers and non-carriers at 4 months and 12 months after genetic test result disclosure [65]. One study found that anxiety was not related to adherence to recommended risk management [39].

3.2.5. Brief Symptom Inventory

Six studies assessed psychological distress via the BSI [43,44,47,52,57,73]. Different versions were used, with 1 study utilizing the 53-item version [43], 2 studies utilizing the 48-item version [44,73], 2 studies utilizing the 18-item version [47,57], and 1 study using the anxiety subscale only [52]. For one study, no outcome was specified [52]. Scoring schemes and subsequent cut-off values varied depending on the version used. One study found subclinical levels in carriers after genetic test result disclosure and no change at a three month follow-up [57]. Two studies did not identify an increase in distress in carriers compared to non-carriers from high-risk families [44,57,73]. Conversely, two other studies found that the scores of the somatization subscale were increased in carriers compared to non-carriers of all age groups [43], as well as in premenopausal carriers compared to postmenopausal carriers [47]. High scores on the somatization subscale represent a high focus on physical dysfunction (e.g., pain, fatigue, dizziness, numbness, or tingling) that may, in turn, cause psychological distress. Identifying differences in psychological distress was not related to the version of the BSI used.

3.2.6. General Health Questionnaire

Four studies assessed generalized psychological distress via the GHQ-28 [48,50,70,81]. A score ≥ 5 indicates clinically significant distress [89]. All the included studies reported below this cut-off score, albeit some only marginally [48,81]. Two studies found lower psychological distress in identified carriers compared to untested members of high-risk families [50,70]. Two other studies reported an increase in psychological distress from before genetic testing to 12 months [81] or 3 years after result disclosure [48]. Even though the reported means did not tangent the cut-off score, one of these studies reported that almost 20% of the study participants scored above the cut-off score three years after genetic test result disclosure [48]. Another study identified that carriers aged 35–49 experienced significantly higher psychological distress than high-risk non-carriers 1 month after genetic test result disclosure [81].

3.2.7. Summary Distress Outcomes

In conclusion, many studies found a slight elevation in distress outcomes shortly after genetic test result disclosure. The majority of the studies reported that up to one-fourth of carriers experienced symptoms of anxiety disorder after genetic test result disclosure, irrespective of the instrument used. Longitudinal studies suggested that, even though anxiety symptoms peaked after genetic test result disclosure, they usually declined to the level of non-carriers over time. However, carriers with high pre-test anxiety may experience clinical anxiety, even at longer follow-ups. Some studies provided limited evidence for age dependence, with younger women showing higher distress than older women, especially immediately after genetic test result disclosure. Furthermore, there was some degree of evidence to suggest that those with higher distress were more likely to opt for surgery, albeit the causative nature of this relationship remains unclear. Therefore, sensitive screening tools to identity this subgroup may be beneficial to alleviate long-term distress and prevent the manifestation of anxiety disorders. Finally, some studies showed that carriers showed lower anxiety compared to untested women, suggesting that receiving a definitive test result, regardless of if a pathogenic variant was in fact found, may provide a relief in anxiety.

3.3. Depression

The depression subscale of the Hospital Anxiety and Depression Scale (HADS-D) [84], the Center for Epidemiologic Studies Depression Scale (CES-D) [91], and the Beck Hopelessness Scale (BHS) [90] were characterized as measures of depression.

3.3.1. Hospital Anxiety and Depression Scale—Depression Subscale

Ten studies assessed depression with the HADS-D [37,50,53,54,59,70,71,75,77,78]. Analogous to the anxiety subscale, a score ≥ 8 indicates signs of clinical depression. All the studies reported means well below this cut-off. Among the studies that reported a percentage of cases, the numbers ranged from 2–12.5% of possible clinical depression cases, indicating that depression was as prevalent as in the general population [50,53,54,59,75]. In fact, two studies found that the depression scores in carriers were significantly lower than in the healthy population [50,70]. One of these studies compared collected data from carriers with published normative data [70], whereas one study simultaneously collected data from carriers, non-carriers, and controls and found that carriers had fewer depressive symptoms compared to the other two groups [50]. Furthermore, two other studies found no difference between carriers and non-carriers in terms of depression [53,78]. One study that compared carriers and non-carriers from before to after genetic test result disclosure found an increase from before to after genetic test result disclosure for carriers and the opposite effect for non-carriers [59]. Two studies compared the depression scores of women opting for surveillance vs. risk-reducing surgeries and found no difference [37,77]. Finally, one study found that carrier depression scores were not affected by recall after a suspicious MRI [75], suggesting that depression was not influenced by imminent danger of cancer.

3.3.2. Center for Epidemiologic Studies Depression Scale

Seven studies assessed depression utilizing the CES-D [55,56,58,63,64,74,80], of which all but two reported outcomes relevant to the population [56,64]. Different cut-off scores have been put forward, ranging from scores ≥ 16 to ≥ 23 indicating a clinical case of depression. One study identified higher depressive symptoms in carriers compared to the general female population at baseline, with 21.3% of women scoring in the clinical depression range (scores ≥ 23) [55]. Three studies found increases from before to after genetic test result disclosure [58,74,80]. One of these studies reported means over the cut-off score of 16 at one week and three months after genetic test result disclosure, with no difference between carriers and non-carriers [74]. Similarly, another study found no differences between carriers and non-carriers but identified an increase in depression from pre-test result disclosure to 15 days after, with a subsequent decrease to pre-test levels after one year [58]. One study looked at risk management behaviors and found that women with fewer depressive symptoms were more likely to conduct regular breast self-examination [63].

3.3.3. Beck Hopelessness Scale

Three studies assessed hopelessness and associated suicidal ideation using the BHS [50,70,71]. A score between 4 and 8 generally indicates mild hopelessness, whereas a score of ≥ 9 suggests more severe hopelessness that predicts the presence of at least some suicidal ideation. Two of the studies reported mean scores in the higher end of the normal range [50,70]. One study did not specify the mean for the sample but reported a significant association to psychological distress in general [71].

3.3.4. Summary Depression Outcomes

The patterns of the results from these depression measures suggested that carriers did not show increased depressive symptoms following test disclosure, and some studies remarkably even identified levels of depression that were lower than those in the normal population. Of these depression measures, the CES-D appeared to be the most sensitive in detecting depression in *BRCA1/2* carriers. However, even studies using this instrument showed that depressive symptomology decreased over time, and no lasting effects were found. Only one study showed that depression scores remained above pre-test levels for up to two years. Studies using the other questionnaires indicated that hopelessness or suicidal ideation were generally not a clinical problem in this population.

3.4. Other Psychological Outcomes

Quality of life and body image were categorized as other psychological outcomes that were frequently investigated. Quality of life was assessed using the Short Form Health Survey (SF) [92,93], while body image was assessed using the Body Image Questionnaire (BIQ) [60] following recommendations from Cull on sexual function in cancer patients [94].

3.4.1. Short Form Health Survey

Eight studies assessed quality of life with some version of the SF questionnaire, with four studies utilizing the original SF-36 [44,51,53,74], three studies utilizing the SF-12 [37,39,47], and one study using two subscales of the SF-36 [62]. One study did not report outcomes relevant to the population [53]. The original SF-36 has eight subscales (vitality, physical functioning, bodily pain, general health perceptions, physical role functioning, emotional role functioning, social role functioning, and mental health) that may be summarized into a physical and a mental composite score. Two studies compared quality of life in carriers with non-carriers [44,74]. One study found lower quality of life in some domains, especially in premenopausal women (emotional role functioning, physical role functioning, and physical functioning) [44], whereas the other found no differences [74]. The other studies assessed quality of life in terms of risk management strategies. One study found that higher physical functioning was associated with higher adherence to recommended risk management strategies, but higher mental functioning was not [39]. In terms of opting for one strategy over the other, one study found no difference in quality of life between carriers opting for surgery or surveillance [37], whereas one study found that carriers with lower general health perceptions were more likely to opt for a salpingo-oophorectomy [62]. After risk-reducing surgeries, one study found lower physical quality of life six months after bilateral mastectomy but higher mental quality of life [51], whereas another study found no differences in either composite score after salpingo-oophorectomy [47].

3.4.2. Body Image Questionnaire

Four of the studies included body image as measured by the BIQ [51,55,60,78]. Two of the studies found that body image satisfaction was lower in carriers compared to non-carriers [51,78]. Longitudinally, body image satisfaction of carriers further declined as time after genetic test result disclosure passed [51,78]. One study found that body image satisfaction was unrelated to prophylactic mastectomy uptake [55]. However, two studies showed that undergoing prophylactic mastectomy, mostly combined with immediate reconstruction, may result in lower body image [51,60]. One study specified that those with lower BMI and higher cancer distress at baseline showed lower body image after finishing reconstruction, whereas higher general physical health predicted better body image over time [51]. However, it is unknown how long ago these study participants were found to carry a pathogenic variant and how that might have impacted results.

3.4.3. Summary Other Outcomes

Quality of life seemed to be largely unaffected by a positive genetic test result, although there was some evidence that especially younger women were less satisfied with their role functioning in life. It seems plausible that this was related to distress, which was also found to be slightly more prominent in premenopausal women (see Section 3.2.7). In terms of body image, the results were extremely heterogeneous and only provided limited insight. From the studies identified, it could be concluded that body image may decrease slightly after genetic test result disclosure but was generally unrelated to further decision making.

3.5. Quality Assessment

All the studies included in this review met at least 11 of 20 AXIS points (range: 11–20). The overall quality of the studies was adequate: most of the studies clearly stated the aims of the study, identified a clearly defined target group per inclusion criteria, and included a good description of the basic data with justified conclusions. All but four studies discussed the limitations of the study and the results. Nonetheless, the included studies have some methodological weaknesses: most of the studies did not justify their sample size or did not run a priori power analyses. Additionally, although most studies took a sample from an appropriate frame with an appropriate sampling method, more than half (60%) of the 45 studies expressed concerns about the representativeness or indicated that a bigger sample size would have been desirable. Only 19 studies included information about non-responders, with 10 of these identifying differences between responders and non-responders. A common difference identified was that non-responders were less likely to have a partner, which is a factor to be considered in interpreting results. All AXIS results can be seen in Supplementary Material File S1.

4. Discussion

To the best of our knowledge, this is the first time a systematic review investigated not only the psychological outcomes of cancer-unaffected BRCA1/2 pathogenic variant carriers, but also the instruments that were used to assess these outcomes. Due to the high heterogeneity of measures used by the different studies, it was challenging to draw comprehensive conclusions about all the psychological outcomes. The differences in the design and analyses in the presented studies may underlie this non-conclusive pattern of results.

The psychological outcomes that were most often assessed were distress, anxiety, and cancer worry. Most studies showed an increase in those outcomes, mainly cancer worry and anxiety, after genetic test result disclosure. This appeared to be slightly more prominent in premenopausal women under the age of 50 [44,47,81]. This seems logical considering family planning and breastfeeding decisions for women of childbearing age. In fact, qualitative studies with premenopausal BRCA1/2 pathogenic variant carriers have confirmed that family planning often competes with risk-reducing surgical procedures [22,95]. This may in turn increase anxiety and distress in this younger group. Longitudinally, most studies showed a steady decline in the months after genetic test result disclosure and a complete return to baseline roughly after one year. Only a few studies reported higher frequency of distress one year after genetic test result disclosure. In terms of decision making, it seemed that women deciding for prophylactic surgeries experienced slightly higher levels of distress. This may be the reason why these women opted for risk-reducing surgeries in the first place. In terms of depressive symptomatology and quality of life, merely mild or no negative outcomes at all were identified. Regarding body image, no conclusive results could be drawn due to the small number of studies using a validated measure. Two reviews on various body image outcomes showed that decreased body image and changes in sexuality were common after prophylactic mastectomy [96,97]. However, a recent review reported that sexual health remained understudies in the context of BRCA1/2 testing [98].

Limitations and Recommendations for Future Research

While this review was the first review to systematically investigate the effects of BRCA1/2 pathogenic variant carrier status on psychological outcomes, there are a few limitations that need to be addressed. Firstly, the oldest study included in the review was published 1997, and many others were published in the early 2000s. Breast and ovarian cancer risk may have been communicated differently in those years compared to today, as they were not as well-researched and long-term data were not yet available. This may, in turn, influence the level of psychological morbidity. Secondly, the majority of the studies in the review were conducted in the United States or Europe and investigated mainly well-educated white women. Studies that specifically looked at minorities were very few. Only one study in the review examined an African-American population [56]. Thus, further and larger studies investigating such underrepresented groups are necessary. Moreover, we suspect that at least a few studies reported on the same population over several years, which may taint the results. Two studies reported from Rambam Health Care Campus in Israel [43,44]; two further studies reported baseline and follow-up data from a sample at Rotterdam University Hospital in the Netherlands [59,60]; four studies reported from Oslo University Hospital in Norway within a close timeframe [49,50,70,71]; and finally, four studies utilized the GENESPO study cohort from France [55,58,63,64]. We were unable to exclude the possibility that more studies reported on these or other populations across different publications. Lastly, most studies reported on small study populations, with the majority of the studies including less than 100 cancer-unaffected carriers. This may impact the generalizability of our results.

As discussed above, there have been attempts to condense results from various outcome sources (e.g., integrative reviews on body image [96,97]), but the consequent and continuous use of established and validated instruments is often lacking. Future research could improve data on psychological morbidity in cancer-unaffected *BRCA1/2* pathogenic variant carriers by (1) using validated measures, (2) not conflating cancer-unaffected with cancer-affected carriers or cancer-unaffected carriers with the general population when reporting results, (3) reporting precisely how long carriers knew of their risk status when reporting results, and (4) diversifying the sample populations. Additionally, while *BRCA1/2* pathogenic variants have been known the longest and are well-studied because they are also found comparatively frequently in individuals at risk, several other pathogenic variants in less frequently identified genes exist that have similarly high risks associated with them, such as *PALB2* [99]. Future research should address these pathogenic variants equally in researching psychological morbidity in the hereditary cancer field.

Supplementary Materials: The following supporting information can be downloaded at: https://www.mdpi.com/article/10.3390/curroncol30040274/s1, Supplementary Material File S1: AXIS Report.

Author Contributions: Conceptualization, A.I. and S.S.; methodology, A.I.; software, Z.L.; validation, A.I., Z.L. and S.S.; formal analysis, A.I. and Z.L.; investigation, A.I. and Z.L.; resources, S.S.; data curation, A.I. and Z.L.; writing—original draft preparation, A.I.; writing—review and editing, Z.L., K.R. and S.S.; visualization, Z.L.; supervision, S.S.; project administration, A.I. All authors have read and agreed to the published version of the manuscript.

Funding: This research received no external funding.

Conflicts of Interest: The authors declare no conflict of interest.

References

1. Friedenson, B. The BRCA1/2 pathway prevents hematologic cancers in addition to breast and ovarian cancers. *BMC Cancer* **2007**, *7*, 152. [CrossRef]
2. Tutt, A.; Ashworth, A. The relationship between the roles of BRCA genes in DNA repair and cancer predisposition. *Trends Mol. Med.* **2002**, *8*, 571–576. [CrossRef] [PubMed]
3. Kuchenbaecker, K.B.; Hopper, J.L.; Barnes, D.R.; Phillips, K.-A.; Mooij, T.M.; Roos-Blom, M.-J.; Jervis, S.; van Leeuwen, F.E.; Milne, R.L.; Andrieu, N. Risks of breast, ovarian, and contralateral breast cancer for BRCA1 and BRCA2 mutation carriers. *JAMA* **2017**, *317*, 2402–2416. [CrossRef]
4. Evans, G.; Binchy, A.; Shenton, A.; Hopwood, P.; Craufurd, D. Comparison of proactive and usual approaches to offering predictive testing for BRCA1/2 mutations in unaffected relatives. *Clin. Genet.* **2009**, *75*, 124–132. [CrossRef] [PubMed]
5. Lerman, C.; Shields, A.E. Genetic testing for cancer susceptibility: The promise and the pitfalls. *Nat. Rev. Cancer* **2004**, *4*, 235–241. [CrossRef] [PubMed]
6. Bick, U.; Engel, C.; Krug, B.; Heindel, W.; Fallenberg, E.M.; Rhiem, K.; Maintz, D.; Golatta, M.; Speiser, D.; Rjosk-Dendorfer, D. High-risk breast cancer surveillance with MRI: 10-year experience from the German consortium for hereditary breast and ovarian cancer. *Breast Cancer Res. Treat.* **2019**, *175*, 217–228. [CrossRef]
7. Hartmann, L.C.; Sellers, T.A.; Schaid, D.J.; Frank, T.S.; Soderberg, C.L.; Sitta, D.L.; Frost, M.H.; Grant, C.S.; Donohue, J.H.; Woods, J.E.; et al. Efficacy of Bilateral Prophylactic Mastectomy in BRCA1 and BRCA2 Gene Mutation Carriers. *J. Natl. Cancer Inst.* **2001**, *93*, 1633–1637. [CrossRef]
8. Heemskerk-Gerritsen, B.A.; Menke-Pluymers, M.B.E.; Jager, A.; Tilanus-Linthorst, M.M.; Koppert, L.B.; Obdeijn, I.M.; van Deurzen, C.H.; Collee, J.M.; Seynaeve, C.; Hooning, M.J. Substantial breast cancer risk reduction and potential survival benefit after bilateral mastectomy when compared with surveillance in healthy BRCA1 and BRCA2 mutation carriers: A prospective analysis. *Ann. Oncol.* **2013**, *24*, 2029–2035. [CrossRef] [PubMed]

9. Heemskerk-Gerritsen, B.A.M.; Jager, A.; Koppert, L.B.; Obdeijn, A.I.-M.; Collée, M.; Meijers-Heijboer, H.E.J.; Jenner, D.J.; Oldenburg, H.S.A.; van Engelen, K.; de Vries, J.; et al. Survival after bilateral risk-reducing mastectomy in healthy BRCA1 and BRCA2 mutation carriers. *Breast Cancer Res. Treat.* **2019**, *177*, 723–733. [CrossRef]
10. den Heijer, M.; Seynaeve, C.; Timman, R.; Duivenvoorden, H.J.; Vanheusden, K.; Tilanus-Linthorst, M.; Menke-Pluijmers, M.B.E.; Tibben, A. Body image and psychological distress after prophylactic mastectomy and breast reconstruction in genetically predisposed women: A prospective long-term follow-up study. *Eur. J. Cancer* **2012**, *48*, 1263–1268. [CrossRef]
11. Domchek, S.M. Risk-reducing mastectomy in BRCA1 and BRCA2 mutation carriers: A complex discussion. *JAMA* **2019**, *321*, 27. [CrossRef]
12. Glassey, R.; Ives, A.; Saunders, C.; Musiello, T. Decision making, psychological wellbeing and psychosocial outcomes for high risk women who choose to undergo bilateral prophylactic mastectomy—A review of the literature. *Breast* **2016**, *28*, 130–135. [CrossRef]
13. Altschuler, A.; Nekhlyudov, L.; Rolnick, S.J.; Greene, S.M.; Elmore, J.G.; West, C.N.; Herrinton, L.J.; Harris, E.L.; Fletcher, S.W.; Emmons, K.M.; et al. Positive, negative, and disparate—Women's differing long-term psychosocial experiences of bilateral or contralateral prophylactic mastectomy. *Breast J.* **2008**, *14*, 25–32. [CrossRef] [PubMed]
14. Evans, D.G.; Kesavan, N.; Lim, Y.; Gadde, S.; Hurley, E.; Massat, N.J.; Maxwell, A.J.; Ingham, S.; Eeles, R.; Leach, M.O.; et al. MRI breast screening in high-risk women: Cancer detection and survival analysis. *Breast Cancer Res. Treat.* **2014**, *145*, 663–672. [CrossRef] [PubMed]
15. Hesse-Biber, S. The Genetic Testing Experience of BRCA-Positive Women: Deciding Between Surveillance and Surgery. *Qual. Health Res.* **2014**, *24*, 773–789. [CrossRef]
16. Finch, A.; Evans, G.; Narod, S.A. BRCA carriers, prophylactic salpingo-oophorectomy and menopause: Clinical management considerations and recommendations. *Women's Health* **2012**, *8*, 543–555. [PubMed]
17. Marchetti, C.; de Felice, F.; Palaia, I.; Perniola, G.; Musella, A.; Musio, D.; Muzii, L.; Tombolini, V.; Panici, P.B. Risk-reducing salpingo-oophorectomy: A meta-analysis on impact on ovarian cancer risk and all cause mortality in BRCA 1 and BRCA 2 mutation carriers. *BMC Women's Health* **2014**, *14*, 150. [CrossRef] [PubMed]
18. Xiao, Y.-L.; Wang, K.; Liu, Q.; Li, J.; Zhang, X.; Li, H.-Y. Risk Reduction and Survival Benefit of Risk-Reducing Salpingo-oophorectomy in Hereditary Breast Cancer: Meta-analysis and Systematic Review. *Clin. Breast Cancer* **2019**, *19*, e48–e65. [CrossRef]
19. MacDonald, D.J.; Sarna, L.; Weitzel, J.N.; Ferrell, B. Women's perceptions of the personal and family impact of genetic cancer risk assessment: Focus group findings. *J. Genet. Counsel.* **2010**, *19*, 148–160. [CrossRef]
20. Lombardi, L.; Bramanti, S.M.; Babore, A.; Stuppia, L.; Trumello, C.; Antonucci, I.; Cavallo, A. Psychological aspects, risk and protective factors related to BRCA genetic testing: A review of the literature. *Support Care Cancer* **2019**, *27*, 3647–3656. [CrossRef]
21. Dean, M. "It's not if I get cancer, it's when I get cancer": BRCA-positive patients'(un) certain health experiences regarding hereditary breast and ovarian cancer risk. *Soc. Sci. Med.* **2016**, *163*, 21–27. [CrossRef]
22. Possick, C.; Kestler-Peleg, M. BRCA and Motherhood: A Matter of Time and Timing. *Qual. Health Res.* **2019**, *30*, 825–835. [CrossRef]
23. Glassey, R.; Hardcastle, S.J.; O'Connor, M.; Ives, A.; kConFab Investigators; Saunders, C. Perceived influence of psychological consultation on psychological well-being, body image, and intimacy following bilateral prophylactic mastectomy: A qualitative analysis. *Psycho.-Oncol.* **2018**, *27*, 633–639. [CrossRef] [PubMed]
24. Douglas, H.A.; Hamilton, R.J.; Grubs, R.E. The Effect of BRCA Gene Testing on Family Relationships: A Thematic Analysis of Qualitative Interviews. *J. Genet. Counsel.* **2009**, *18*, 418–435. [CrossRef] [PubMed]
25. Meiser, B. Psychological impact of genetic testing for cancer susceptibility: An update of the literature. *Psycho.-Oncol.* **2005**, *14*, 1060–1074. [CrossRef]
26. Hamilton, J.G.; Lobel, M.; Moyer, A. Emotional distress following genetic testing for hereditary breast and ovarian cancer: A meta-analytic review. *Health Psychol.* **2009**, *28*, 510–518. [CrossRef]
27. Graves, K.D.; Wenzel, L.; Schwartz, M.D.; Luta, G.; Wileyto, P.; Narod, S.A.; Peshkin, B.N.; Marcus, A.; Cella, D.; Emsbo, S.P.; et al. Randomized Controlled Trial of a Psychosocial Telephone Counseling Intervention in BRCA1 and BRCA2 Mutation Carriers. *Cancer Epidemiol. Biomark. Prev.* **2010**, *19*, 648–654. [CrossRef]
28. Boghosian, T.; McCuaig, J.M.; Carlsson, L.; Metcalfe, K.A. Psychosocial Interventions for Women with a BRCA1 or BRCA2 Mutation: A Scoping Review. *Cancers* **2021**, *13*, 1486. [CrossRef]
29. Jeffers, L.; Reid, J.; Fitzsimons, D.; Morrison, P.J.; Dempster, M. Interventions to improve psychosocial well-being in female BRCA-mutation carriers following risk-reducing surgery. *Cochrane Database Syst. Rev.* **2019**, *10*. [CrossRef] [PubMed]
30. Ringwald, J.; Wochnowski, C.; Bosse, K.; Giel, K.E.; Schäffeler, N.; Zipfel, S.; Teufel, M. Psychological Distress, Anxiety, and Depression of Cancer-Affected BRCA1/2 Mutation Carriers: A Systematic Review. *J. Genet. Counsel.* **2016**, *25*, 880–891. [CrossRef] [PubMed]
31. Finch, A.; Narod, S.A. Quality of life and health status after prophylactic salpingo-oophorectomy in women who carry a BRCA mutation: A review. *Maturitas* **2011**, *70*, 261–265. [CrossRef]
32. Kautz-Freimuth, S.; Redaèlli, M.; Rhiem, K.; Vodermaier, A.; Krassuski, L.; Nicolai, K.; Schnepper, M.; Kuboth, V.; Dick, J.; Vennedey, V.; et al. Development of decision aids for female BRCA1 and BRCA2 mutation carriers in Germany to support preference-sensitive decision-making. *BMC Med. Inform. Decis. Mak.* **2021**, *21*, 180. [CrossRef] [PubMed]

33. Page, M.J.; McKenzie, J.E.; Bossuyt, P.M.; Boutron, I.; Hoffmann, T.C.; Mulrow, C.D.; Shamseer, L.; Tetzlaff, J.M.; Akl, E.A.; Brennan, S.E.; et al. The PRISMA 2020 statement: An updated guideline for reporting systematic reviews. *BMJ* **2021**, *372*, n71. [CrossRef] [PubMed]
34. da Costa Santos, C.M.; de Mattos Pimenta, C.A.; Nobre, M.R.C. The PICO strategy for the research question construction and evidence search. *Rev. Lat. Am. Enferm.* **2007**, *15*, 508–511. [CrossRef] [PubMed]
35. Amir-Behghadami, M.; Janati, A. Population, Intervention, Comparison, Outcomes and Study (PICOS) design as a framework to formulate eligibility criteria in systematic reviews. *Emerg. Med. J.* **2020**, *37*, 387. [CrossRef]
36. Downes, M.J.; Brennan, M.L.; Williams, H.C.; Dean, R.S. Development of a critical appraisal tool to assess the quality of cross-sectional studies (AXIS). *BMJ Open* **2016**, *6*, e011458. [CrossRef]
37. Borreani, C.; Manoukian, S.; Bianchi, E.; Brunelli, C.; Peissel, B.; Caruso, A.; Morasso, G.; Pierotti, M.A. The psychological impact of breast and ovarian cancer preventive options in BRCA1 and BRCA2 mutation carriers. *Clin. Genet.* **2014**, *85*, 7–15. [CrossRef]
38. Brand, H.; Speiser, D.; Besch, L.; Roseman, J.; Kendel, F. Making Sense of a Health Threat: Illness Representations, Coping, and Psychological Distress among BRCA1/2 Mutation Carriers. *Genes* **2021**, *12*, 741. [CrossRef]
39. Buchanan, A.H.; Voils, C.I.; Schildkraut, J.M.; Fine, C.; Horick, N.K.; Marcom, P.K.; Wiggins, K.; Skinner, C.S. Adherence to Recommended Risk Management among Unaffected Women with a BRCA Mutation. *J. Genet. Counsel.* **2017**, *26*, 79–92. [CrossRef] [PubMed]
40. Carpenter, K.; Eisenberg, S.; Weltfreid, S.; Low, C.A.; Beran, T.M.; Stanton, A.L. Characterizing biased cancer-related cognitive processing: Relationships with BRCA1/2 genetic mutation status, personal cancer history, age, and prophylactic surgery. *Health Psychol.* **2014**, *33*, 1003–1011. [CrossRef]
41. Claes, E.; Evers-Kiebooms, G.; Denayer, L.; Decruyenaere, M.; Boogaerts, A.; Philippe, K.; Legius, E. Predictive Genetic Testing for Hereditary Breast and Ovarian Cancer: Psychological Distress and Illness Representations 1 Year Following Disclosure. *J. Genet. Counsel.* **2005**, *14*, 349–363. [CrossRef]
42. Croyle, R.; Smith, K.; Botkin, J.; Baty, B.J.; Nash, J. Psychological Responses to BRCA1 Mutation Testing: Preliminary Findings. *Health Psychol. Off. J. Div. Health Psychol. Am. Psychol. Assoc.* **1997**, *16*, 63–72. [CrossRef] [PubMed]
43. Dagan, E.; Gil, S. BRCA1/2 Mutation Carriers. *J. Psychosoc. Oncol.* **2004**, *22*, 93–106. [CrossRef]
44. Dagan, E.; Shochat, T. Quality of life in asymptomatic BRCA1/2 mutation carriers. *Prev. Med.* **2009**, *48*, 193–196. [CrossRef]
45. Dorval, M.; Drolet, M.; LeBlanc, M.; Maunsell, E.; Dugas, M.J.; Simard, J. Using the Impact of Event Scale to Evaluate Distress in the Context of Genetic Testing for Breast Cancer Susceptibility. *Psychol. Rep.* **2006**, *98*, 873–881. [CrossRef]
46. Ertmański, S.; Metcalfe, K.A.; Trempała, J.; Głowacka, M.D.; Lubiński, J.; Narod, S.A.; Gronwald, J. Identification of Patients at High Risk of Psychological Distress After BRCA1 Genetic Testing. *Genet. Test. Mol. Biomark.* **2009**, *13*, 325–330. [CrossRef] [PubMed]
47. Finch, A.; Metcalfe, K.A.; Chiang, J.; Elit, L.; McLaughlin, J.; Springate, C.; Esplen, M.J.; Demsky, R.; Murphy, J.; Rosen, B.; et al. The impact of prophylactic salpingo-oophorectomy on quality of life and psychological distress in women with a BRCA mutation. *Psycho-Oncol.* **2013**, *22*, 212–219. [CrossRef] [PubMed]
48. Foster, C.; Watson, M.; Eeles, R.; Eccles, D.; Ashley, S.; Davidson, R.; Mackay, J.; Morrison, P.J.; Hopwood, P.; Evans, G.; et al. Predictive genetic testing for BRCA1/2 in a UK clinical cohort: Three-year follow-up. *Br. J. Cancer* **2007**, *96*, 718–724. [CrossRef] [PubMed]
49. Geirdal, A.Ø.; Dahl, A.A. The relationship between coping strategies and anxiety in women from families with familial breast–ovarian cancer in the absence of demonstrated mutations. *Psycho-Oncol.* **2008**, *17*, 49–57. [CrossRef] [PubMed]
50. Geirdal, A.Ø.; Reichelt, J.G.; Dahl, A.A.; Heimdal, K.; Mæhle, L.; Stormorken, A.; Møller, P. Psychological distress in women at risk of hereditary breast/ovarian or HNPCC cancers in the absence of demonstrated mutations. *Fam. Cancer* **2005**, *4*, 121–126. [CrossRef]
51. Gopie, J.P.; Mureau, M.A.M.; Seynaeve, C.; ter Kuile, M.M.; Menke-Pluymers, M.B.E.; Timman, R.; Tibben, A. Body image issues after bilateral prophylactic mastectomy with breast reconstruction in healthy women at risk for hereditary breast cancer. *Fam. Cancer* **2013**, *12*, 479–487. [CrossRef]
52. Graves, K.D.; Vegella, P.; Poggi, E.A.; Peshkin, B.N.; Tong, A.; Isaacs, C.; Finch, C.; Kelly, S.; Taylor, K.L.; Luta, G.; et al. Long-Term Psychosocial Outcomes of BRCA1/BRCA2 Testing: Differences across Affected Status and Risk-Reducing Surgery Choice. *Cancer Epidemiol. Biomark. Prev.* **2012**, *21*, 445–455. [CrossRef] [PubMed]
53. Isern, A.E.; Tengrup, I.; Loman, N.; Olsson, H.; Ringberg, A. Aesthetic outcome, patient satisfaction, and health-related quality of life in women at high risk undergoing prophylactic mastectomy and immediate breast reconstruction. *J. Plast. Reconstr. Aesthetic Surg.* **2008**, *61*, 1177–1187. [CrossRef]
54. Isselhard, A.; Lautz, Z.; Töpper, M.; Rhiem, K.; Schmutzler, R.; Vitinius, F.; Fischer, H.; Berger-Höger, B.; Steckelberg, A.; Beifus, K.; et al. Coping Self-Efficacy and Its Relationship with Psychological Morbidity after Genetic Test Result Disclosure: Results from Cancer-Unaffected BRCA1/2 Mutation Carriers. *Int. J. Environ. Res. Public Health* **2023**, *20*, 1684. [CrossRef] [PubMed]
55. Julian-Reynier, C.; Bouhnik, A.-D.; Mouret-Fourme, E.; Gauthier-Villars, M.; Berthet, P.; Lasset, C.; Fricker, J.-P.; Caron, O.; Gesta, P.; Luporsi, E.; et al. Time to prophylactic surgery in BRCA1/2 carriers depends on psychological and other characteristics. *Genet. Med.* **2010**, *12*, 801–807. [CrossRef] [PubMed]

56. Kinney, A.Y.; Bloor, L.E.; Mandal, D.; Simonsen, S.E.; Baty, B.J.; Holubkov, R.; Seggar, K.; Neuhausen, S.L.; Smith, K. The impact of receiving genetic test results on general and cancer-specific psychologic distress among members of an African-American kindred with a BRCA1 mutation. *Cancer* **2005**, *104*, 2508–2516. [CrossRef]
57. Landau, C.; Lev-Ari, S.; Cohen-Mansfield, J.; Tillinger, E.; Geva, R.; Tarrasch, R.; Mitnik, I.; Friedman, E. Randomized controlled trial of Inquiry-Based Stress Reduction (IBSR) technique for BRCA1/2 mutation carriers. *Psycho-Oncol.* **2015**, *24*, 726–731. [CrossRef]
58. Lapointe, J.; Dorval, M.; Nogués, C.; Fabre, R.; Julian-Reynier, C.; GENEPSO Cohort. Is the psychological impact of genetic testing moderated by support and sharing of test results to family and friends? *Fam. Cancer* **2013**, *12*, 601–610. [CrossRef]
59. Lodder, L.; Frets, P.G.; Trijsburg, R.W.; Meijers-Heijboer, H.; Klijn, J.G.M.; Duivenvoorden, H.J.; Tibben, A.; Wagner, A.; van der Meer, C.A.; van den Ouweland, A.M.; et al. Psychological impact of receiving a BRCA1/BRCA2 test result. *Am. J. Med. Genet.* **2001**, *98*, 15–24. [CrossRef]
60. Lodder, L.; Frets, P.G.; Trijsburg, R.W.; Meijers-Heijboer, H.; Klijn, J.G.M.; Seynaeve, C.; van Geel, A.N.; Tilanus, M.M.A.; Bartels, C.C.M.; Verhoog, L.C.; et al. One Year Follow-Up of Women Opting for Presymptomatic Testing for BRCA1 and BRCA2: Emotional Impact of the Test Outcome and Decisions on Risk Management (Surveillance or Prophylactic Surgery). *Breast Cancer Res. Treat.* **2002**, *73*, 97–112. [CrossRef]
61. Low, C.A.; Bower, J.E.; Kwan, L.; Seldon, J. Benefit Finding in Response to BRCA1/2 Testing. *Ann. Behav. Med.* **2008**, *35*, 61–69. [CrossRef] [PubMed]
62. Madalinska, J.B.; van Beurden, M.; Bleiker, E.M.; Valdimarsdottir, H.; Lubsen-Brandsma, L.; Massuger, L.F.; Mourits, M.J.; Gaarenstroom, K.N.; van Dorst, E.B.; van der Putten, H.; et al. Predictors of Prophylactic Bilateral Salpingo-Oophorectomy Compared With Gynecologic Screening Use in BRCA1/2 Mutation Carriers. *J. Clin. Oncol.* **2007**, *25*, 301–307. [CrossRef] [PubMed]
63. Maheu, C.; Apostolidis, T.; Petri-Cal, A.; Mouret-Fourme, E.; Gauthier-Villars, M.; Lasset, C.; Berthet, P.; Fricker, J.-P.; Caron, O.; Luporsi, E.; et al. French women's breast self-examination practices with time after undergoing BRCA1/2 genetic testing. *Fam. Cancer* **2012**, *11*, 269–278. [CrossRef] [PubMed]
64. Maheu, C.; Bouhnik, A.-D.; Nogués, C.; Mouret-Fourme, E.; Stoppa-Lyonnet, D.; Lasset, C.; Berthet, P.; Fricker, J.-P.; Caron, O.; Luporsi, E.; et al. Which factors predict proposal and uptake of psychological counselling after BRCA1/2 test result disclosure? *Psycho-Oncol.* **2014**, *23*, 420–427. [CrossRef] [PubMed]
65. Meiser, B.; Butow, P.N.; Friedlander, M.; Barratt, A.; Schnieden, V.; Watson, M.; Brown, J.; Tucker, K. Psychological impact of genetic testing in women from high-risk breast cancer families. *Eur. J. Cancer* **2002**, *38*, 2025–2031. [CrossRef]
66. Metcalfe, K.A.; Mian, N.; Enmore, M.; Poll, A.; Llacuachaqui, M.; Nanda, S.; Sun, P.; Hughes, K.S.; Narod, S.A. Long-term follow-up of Jewish women with a BRCA1 and BRCA2 mutation who underwent population genetic screening. *Breast Cancer Res. Treat.* **2012**, *133*, 735–740. [CrossRef]
67. Metcalfe, K.A.; Dennis, C.-L.; Poll, A.; Armel, S.; Demsky, R.; Carlsson, L.; Nanda, S.; Kiss, A.; Narod, S.A. Effect of decision aid for breast cancer prevention on decisional conflict in women with a BRCA1 or BRCA2 mutation: A multisite, randomized, controlled trial. *Genet. Med.* **2017**, *19*, 330–336. [CrossRef]
68. Metcalfe, K.A.; Price, M.A.; Mansfield, C.; Hallett, D.C.; Lindeman, G.J.; Fairchild, A.; Posner, J.; Friedman, S.; Snyder, C.; Lynch, H.T.; et al. Predictors of long-term cancer-related distress among female BRCA1 and BRCA2 mutation carriers without a cancer diagnosis: An international analysis. *British J. Cancer* **2020**, *123*, 268–274. [CrossRef]
69. O'Neill, S.M.; Rubinstein, W.S.; Sener, S.F.; Weissman, S.M.; Newlin, A.C.; West, D.K.; Ecanow, D.B.; Rademaker, A.W.; Edelman, R.R. Psychological impact of recall in high-risk breast MRI screening. *Breast Cancer Res. Treat.* **2009**, *115*, 365–371. [CrossRef]
70. Reichelt, J.G.; Heimdal, K.; Møller, P.; Dahl, A.A. BRCA1 testing with definitive results: A prospective study of psychological distress in a large clinic-based sample. *Fam. Cancer* **2004**, *3*, 21–28. [CrossRef]
71. Reichelt, J.G.; Møller, P.; Heimdal, K.; Dahl, A.A. Psychological and cancer-specific distress at 18 months post-testing in women with demonstrated BRCA1 mutations for hereditary breast/ovarian cancer. *Fam. Cancer* **2008**, *7*, 245–254. [CrossRef]
72. Schwartz, M.D.; Peshkin, B.N.; Hughes, C.; Main, D.; Isaacs, C.; Lerman, C. Impact of BRCA1/BRCA2 Mutation Testing on Psychologic Distress in a Clinic-Based Sample. *J. Clin. Oncol.* **2002**, *20*, 514–520. [CrossRef] [PubMed]
73. Shochat, T.; Dagan, E. Sleep disturbances in asymptomatic BRCA1/2 mutation carriers: Women at high risk for breast–ovarian cancer. *J. Sleep Res.* **2010**, *19*, 333–340. [CrossRef]
74. Smith, A.W.; Dougall, A.L.; Posluszny, D.M.; Somers, T.J.; Rubinstein, W.S.; Baum, A. Psychological distress and quality of life associated with genetic testing for breast cancer risk. *Psycho-Oncol.* **2008**, *17*, 767–773. [CrossRef]
75. Spiegel, T.N.; Esplen, M.J.; Hill, K.A.; Wong, J.; Causer, P.A.; Warner, E. Psychological impact of recall on women with BRCA mutations undergoing MRI surveillance. *Breast* **2011**, *20*, 424–430. [CrossRef] [PubMed]
76. van Dijk, S.; Timmermans, D.; Meijers-Heijboer, H.; Tibben, A.; van Asperen, C.J.; Otten, W. Clinical Characteristics Affect the Impact of an Uninformative DNA Test Result: The Course of Worry and Distress Experienced by Women Who Apply for Genetic Testing for Breast Cancer. *J. Clin. Oncol.* **2006**, *24*, 3672–3677. [CrossRef] [PubMed]
77. van Egdom, L.S.E.; de Kock, M.A.; Apon, I.; am Mureau, M.; Verhoef, C.; Hazelzet, J.A.; Koppert, L.B. Patient-Reported Outcome Measures may optimize shared decision-making for cancer risk management in BRCA mutation carriers. *Breast Cancer* **2020**, *27*, 426–434. [CrossRef]

78. van Oostrom, I.; Meijers-Heijboer, H.; Lodder, L.; Duivenvoorden, H.J.; van Gool, A.R.; Seynaeve, C.; van der Meer, C.A.; Klijn, J.G.M.; van Geel, B.N.; Burger, C.W.; et al. Long-Term Psychological Impact of Carrying a BRCA1/2 Mutation and Prophylactic Surgery: A 5-Year Follow-Up Study. *J. Clin. Oncol.* **2003**, *21*, 3867–3874. [CrossRef]
79. van Oostrom, I.; Meijers-Heijboer, H.; Duivenvoorden, H.J.; Bröcker-Vriends, A.H.J.T.; van Asperen, C.J.; Sijmons, R.H.; Seynaeve, C.; van Gool, A.R.; Klijn, J.G.M.; Tibben, A. The common sense model of self-regulation and psychological adjustment to predictive genetic testing: A prospective study. *Psycho-Oncol.* **2007**, *16*, 1121–1129. [CrossRef]
80. van Roosmalen, M.S.; Stalmeier, P.; Verhoef, L.; Hoekstra-Weebers, J.; Oosterwijk, J.C.; Hoogerbrugge, N.; Moog, U.; van Daal, W. Impact of BRCA1/2 testing and disclosure of a positive test result on women affected and unaffected with breast or ovarian cancer. *Am. J. Med. Genet.* **2004**, *124*, 346–355. [CrossRef]
81. Watson, M.; Foster, C.; Eeles, R.; Eccles, D.; Ashley, S.; Davidson, R.; Mackay, J.; Morrison, P.J.; Hopwood, P.; Evans, G.; et al. Psychosocial impact of breast/ovarian (BRCA 1/2) cancer-predictive genetic testing in a UK multi-centre clinical cohort. *Br. J. Cancer* **2004**, *91*, 1787–1794. [CrossRef] [PubMed]
82. Horowitz, M.; Wilner, N.; Alvarez, W. Impact of Event Scale: A measure of subjective stress. *Psychosom. Med.* **1979**, *41*, 209–218. [CrossRef] [PubMed]
83. Weiss, D.S. The impact of event scale: Revised. In *Cross-Cultural Assessment of Psychological Trauma and PTSD*; Springer: Berlin/Heidelberg, Germany, 2007; pp. 219–238.
84. Snaith, P.; Zigmond, A.S. Hospital anxiety and depression scale (HADS). In *Handbook of Psychiatric Measures*; American Psychiatric Association: Washington, DC, USA, 2000; pp. 547–548.
85. Lerman, C.; Trock, B.; Rimer, B.K.; Jepson, C.; Brody, D.; Boyce, A. Psychological side effects of breast cancer screening. *Health Psychol. Off. J. Div. Health Psychol. Am. Psychol. Assoc.* **1991**, *10*, 259–267. [CrossRef]
86. Lerman, C.; Daly, M.; Masny, A.; Balshem, A. Attitudes about genetic testing for breast-ovarian cancer susceptibility. *J. Clin. Oncol.* **1994**, *12*, 843–850. [CrossRef]
87. Spielberger, C.D.; Gonzalez-Reigosa, F.; Martinez-Urrutia, A.; Natalicio, L.F.; Natalicio, D.S. The State-Trait Anxiety Inventory. *Interam. J. Psychol.* **1971**, *5*, 3–4.
88. Derogatis, L.R.; Melisaratos, N. The Brief Symptom Inventory: An introductory report. *Psychol. Med.* **1983**, *13*, 595–605. [CrossRef]
89. Goldberg, D.P.; Hillier, V.F. A scaled version of the General Health Questionnaire. *Psychol. Med.* **1979**, *9*, 139–145. [CrossRef]
90. Beck, A.T.; Weissman, A.; Lester, D.; Trexler, L. The measurement of pessimism: The Hopelessness Scale. *J. Consult. Clin. Psychol.* **1974**, *42*, 861. [CrossRef]
91. Sheehan, T.J.; Fifield, J.; Reisine, S.; Tennen, H. The Measurement Structure of the Center for Epidemiologic Studies Depression Scale. *J. Personal. Assess.* **1995**, *64*, 507–521. [CrossRef]
92. Ware, J.E.; Sherbourne, C.D. The MOS 36-item short-form health survey (SF-36). I. Conceptual framework and item selection. *Med. Care* **1992**, *30*, 473–483. [CrossRef]
93. Ware, J.E.; Kosinski, M.; Keller, S.D. A 12-Item Short-Form Health Survey: Construction of Scales and Preliminary Tests of Reliability and Validity. *Med. Care* **1996**, *34*, 220–233. [CrossRef] [PubMed]
94. Cull, A.M. The assessment of sexual function in cancer patients. *Eur. J. Cancer* **1992**, *28*, 1680–1686. [CrossRef]
95. Donnelly, L.S.; Watson, M.; Moynihan, C.; Bancroft, E.; Evans, D.; Eeles, R.; Lavery, S.; Ormondroyd, E. Reproductive decision-making in young female carriers of a BRCA mutation. *Hum. Reprod.* **2013**, *28*, 1006–1012. [CrossRef]
96. McGaughey, A. Body Image After Bilateral Prophylactic Mastectomy: An Integrative Literature Review. *J. Midwifery Women's Health* **2006**, *51*, e45–e49. [CrossRef]
97. Torrisi, C. Body Image in BRCA-Positive Young Women Following Bilateral Risk-Reducing Mastectomy: A Review of the Literature. *Front. Psychol.* **2021**, *12*, 5592. [CrossRef] [PubMed]
98. Yusufov, M.; Bober, S.L. Sexual Health in the Era of Cancer Genetic Testing: A Systematic Review. *Sex. Med. Rev.* **2020**, *8*, 231–241. [CrossRef] [PubMed]
99. Antoniou, A.C.; Casadei, S.; Heikkinen, T.; Barrowdale, D.; Pylkäs, K.; Roberts, J.; Lee, A.; Subramanian, D.; de Leeneer, K.; Fostira, F.; et al. Breast-Cancer Risk in Families with Mutations in PALB2. *N. Engl. J. Med.* **2014**, *371*, 497–506. [CrossRef] [PubMed]

Disclaimer/Publisher's Note: The statements, opinions and data contained in all publications are solely those of the individual author(s) and contributor(s) and not of MDPI and/or the editor(s). MDPI and/or the editor(s) disclaim responsibility for any injury to people or property resulting from any ideas, methods, instructions or products referred to in the content.

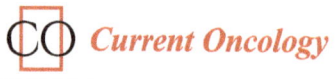

Article

Intimate Partner Violence against Mastectomized Women: Victims' Experiences

Franciéle Marabotti Costa Leite [1,*], Andreia Gomes Oliveira [2], Bruna Lígia Ferreira de Almeida Barbosa [3], Mariana Zoboli Ambrosim [4], Neiva Augusta Viegas Vasconcellos [4], Paulete Maria Ambrósio Maciel [4], Maria Helena Costa Amorim [4], Lorena Barros Furieri [4] and Luís Carlos Lopes-Júnior [1,*]

[1] Graduate Program in Public Health, Health Sciences Center, Federal University of Espírito Santo (UFES), Vitoria 29075-910, ES, Brazil
[2] Prefeitura Municipal de Vitória, Vitoria 29050-945, ES, Brazil
[3] Western New South Wales Primary Health Network-WNSWPHN, Dubbo, NSW 2830, Australia
[4] Nursing Department, Federal University of Espírito Santo (UFES), Vitoria 29075-910, ES, Brazil
* Correspondence: francielemarabotti@gmail.com (F.M.C.L.); lopesjr.lc@gmail.com (L.C.L.-J.); Tel.: +55-27-3335-7280 (F.M.C.L. & L.C.L.-J.)

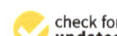

Citation: Leite, F.M.C.; Oliveira, A.G.; Barbosa, B.L.F.d.A.; Ambrosim, M.Z.; Vasconcellos, N.A.V.; Maciel, P.M.A.; Amorim, M.H.C.; Furieri, L.B.; Lopes-Júnior, L.C. Intimate Partner Violence against Mastectomized Women: Victims' Experiences. *Curr. Oncol.* **2022**, *29*, 8556–8564. https://doi.org/10.3390/curroncol29110674

Received: 18 September 2022
Accepted: 2 November 2022
Published: 10 November 2022

Publisher's Note: MDPI stays neutral with regard to jurisdictional claims in published maps and institutional affiliations.

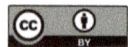

Copyright: © 2022 by the authors. Licensee MDPI, Basel, Switzerland. This article is an open access article distributed under the terms and conditions of the Creative Commons Attribution (CC BY) license (https://creativecommons.org/licenses/by/4.0/).

Abstract: Exposure to situations of domestic violence during the treatment for breast cancer may compromise the treatment and quality of life of women patients, so it is essential that health professionals act in tracking this phenomenon in the approach to and care of women with breast cancer. The purpose of this study was to examine experiences of violence against women by their intimate partners after mastectomy. This is an exploratory descriptive study, with a qualitative approach, carried out in the Rehabilitation Program for Mastectomized Women in a Brazilian reference hospital for oncological treatment. Semi-structured interviews were conducted with 16 mastectomized women. For data analysis, a content analysis technique was performed. The women interviewed were predominantly brown, with a minimum age of 44 years and maximum of 72 years. They presented with low education, were married, and had a mean period of five years of breast cancer diagnosis. The participants reported that after mastectomy, they experienced episodes of violence at a time when they were extremely vulnerable due to the various cancer treatments. Three major thematic categories emerged from interview data across the data collection: (1) experiences of psychological violence, (2) experiences of physical violence, and (3) experiences of sexual violence. Psychological violence took the form of humiliation and contempt for their condition. Physical violence involved assault and sexual violence in the form of forced sex by coercion. Violence was a phenomenon present after mastectomy, practiced in the domestic environment by the intimate partner. We emphasize the importance of health professionals in screening for this issue by listening to and welcoming women, recording cases, exposing this situation, and contributing to prevention.

Keywords: breast neoplasms; violence against women; mastectomy; violence

1. Introduction

A global public health problem, cancer places a high psychosocial and economic burden on individuals, families, and health systems [1]. The projections of the World Health Organization for the period 2018 to 2040 are 29.5 million new cases for all types of cancer across all ages and both sexes [2]. Among the chronic noncommunicable diseases, malignant neoplasms are the second leading cause of death in developed countries and are among the top three causes of death in adults in developing countries [3,4].

The latest report on the global burden of cancer, using the GLOBOCAN 2020 estimates of cancer incidence and mortality produced by the International Agency for Research on Cancer, which focuses on geographical variability in 185 countries worldwide, anticipated an incidence of 19.3 million new cases of cancer and 10 million deaths for 2020 [4]. The report pointed out that the most frequently diagnosed cancer and the main cause of death from cancer vary substantially between countries and within each country, depending on the degree of economic development, social factors, and lifestyle [4]. Breast cancer is the most common cancer among women globally. In 2018, there were 2.1 million new cases, equivalent to 11.6% of all estimated cancers. This value corresponds to an estimated risk of 55.2/100,000 [4,5].

According to data from the latest estimate made by the National Cancer Institute José Alencar Gomes da Silva (INCA), 625,000 new cases of cancer are expected to occur in Brazil for each year of the triennium 2020–2022 [6]. Specifically for women, 66,280 new cases of breast cancer are anticipated for each year of that triennium, which corresponds to an estimated risk of 61.61 new cases per 100,000 women. Excluding non-melanoma skin tumors, female breast cancer is the most common in all Brazilian regions, with an estimated risk of 81.06/100,000 in the Southeast region [6]. In the state of Espírito Santo, for the triennium 2020–2022, 790 cases of female breast cancer per 100,000 inhabitants are forecast [6].

The treatment of breast cancer has made substantial advances in recent years, resulting in the increase in the overall and relative survival rate of patients with this neoplasm. A good prognosis for breast cancer is directly related to early diagnosis, the rapid initiation of treatment, and technological advances in therapy, such as measures for early detection; personalized care; multidisciplinary, interdisciplinary, and specialized teams; combined protocols; target-molecular therapy; and the progress of clinical and translational research in oncology [7–13]. Currently, the 5-year relative survival rate for breast cancer can vary from 72% to 100% depending on staging, early detection, and type of treatment received in a timely manner and in specialized centers [6,7,10].

The diagnosis and treatment of breast cancer damage women's daily lives, especially in relation to their sexuality, femininity, and body image [13]. In that sense, the psychological suffering women go through transcends the suffering of the disease itself, since it is linked to representations and meanings attributed to the disease throughout the history and culture and enters dimensions of the feminine being, interfering many times in the woman's interpersonal relationships [14].

In this context, the family is very important, and the revelation of a diagnosis of cancer, although not always unexpected, is a difficult experience that causes feelings of deep sadness. Each family member reacts in a different way, with feelings of shock, fear, anguish, sadness, or even insecurity due to the stigma attributed to cancer as a painful and incurable disease [15].

It is therefore important to highlight that a healthy family relationship can help provide women with a favorable environment in which to face breast cancer, since any demonstration of care and attention coming from the children and the partner are only beneficial [16]. Reinforcing this statement, a recent study on the perceptions of breast cancer and its repercussions on daily life shows that breast cancer leads to significant changes in a couple's lives and that mutual support is essential for better coping with the pathology, followed by family support [17].

It is important to highlight that women generally receive the diagnosis of breast cancer without their partners. This scenario is maintained throughout the treatment, perpetuating a condition in which the husband is sidelined in all the phases, from the diagnosis to the end of the treatment. This situation hinders the emotional support for the woman, since the partner collaborates in the process of psychological adaptation to the breast cancer [18].

The participation of the partner in all the stages is fundamental, since it will lead to an understanding of the process, enabling the partner to contribute to the reduction in the negative repercussions of breast cancer in the sexual, psychological, and social spheres [18,19].

A recent systematic review on exposure to violence among breast cancer patients showed how much this phenomenon causes harm to the victim [19]. Women diagnosed with breast cancer are victims of violence, have a higher occurrence of depression, as well as have damage to their physical, emotional, and functional well-being, which contributes to a worse prognosis of the neoplasm. In addition, it is important to highlight the underreporting of violence in the group of women with breast cancer, as this topic is still a taboo among patients, making it even more difficult to reveal it [19].

Exposure to situations of domestic violence during the treatment for breast cancer may compromise the treatment and quality of life of women patients, so it is essential that health professionals act in tracking this phenomenon in the approach to and care of women with breast cancer [19].

Hence, this study aimed to examine women's experience of violence against them by their intimate partner after mastectomy.

2. Materials and Methods

2.1. Ethical Approval

The research project was approved by the Research Ethics Committee (CEP) of the Federal University of Espírito Santo under number 2,207,822. All ethical criteria were met, respecting the recommendations of Resolution 466/2012, which refers to research involving human beings.

2.2. Study Design

This was a descriptive study with a qualitative approach, conducted in a Rehabilitation Program for Mastectomized Women (PREMMA), which operates in a Brazilian reference hospital for oncological treatment in the municipality of Vitória, Espírito Santo state, in the Southeast Region of Brazil.

2.3. Participants and Recruitment

The participants were 16 women diagnosed with breast cancer who had submitted to mastectomy, following the criterion of data saturation, which occurs when no new element is found, and the addition of new information is no longer necessary because it does not change the understanding of the phenomenon studied. This is a criterion that allows the validity of a data set to be established in qualitative studies [20].

2.4. Data Collection

The women were invited to participate in the research after receiving care from the nursing sector offered by the Program. It is important to highlight that only those who signed the Informed Consent Form were admitted into the study, after the purpose of the study had been explained to them and they had been advised of their freedom to withdraw at any time. Only the researcher and the interviewee participated in data collection.

The interviewers were female, health professionals, who were not part of PREMMA and who have extensive experience in studies with a qualitative approach.

The interviews were carried out with the application of semi-structured interviews that required sociodemographic data and the following guiding question: "After breast cancer, did you experience violence from your intimate partner?" A pilot study was conducted with ten women in order to verify the suitability of the instruments for conducting the research. The data from this pilot study were not included in this research.

At the end of the interview, each participant received a folder explaining the phenomenon of violence against women and the networks of protection.

2.5. Data Analysis

The characterization data (age, education, marital status, family income, and time of diagnosis) of the participants were recorded and analyzed by obtaining measures of raw and relative frequency. The data concerning the women's reports were recorded, transcribed, and analyzed according to the content analysis technique proposed by Bardin [21]. This analysis includes a set of systematic procedures to describe the content of messages in order to enable inference of knowledge related to the conditions of production/reception of these messages, covering the steps of pre-analysis, exploration of the material, treatment of results, and interpretation [21]. The narratives of the women interviewed were categorized into three thematic units on the basis of their experience of violence: (1) experiences of psychological violence, (2) experiences of physical violence, and (3) experiences of sexual violence. In order to preserve the anonymity of the women interviewed, the code I was used for "interviewee" followed by a number; thus, I1 was used to refer to interviewee number 1.

3. Results

Sixteen mastectomized women participated in the study. The minimum age was 44 years and the maximum 72. Most had an incomplete elementary school education, a partner, and a family income of 1 to 2 minimum wages; the mean time of diagnosis was five years (Table 1).

Table 1. Participants' characteristics. Vitória, Espírito Santo, Brazil, 2018.

Codification	Age	Education *	Marital Status	Family Income **	Time of Diagnosis (Years)
I1	52	2	Married	1	1
I2	64	3	Divorced	1	3
I3	62	1	Married	1	10
I4	68	4	Married	3	9
I5	47	1	Married	2	3
I6	47	1	Married	2	7
I7	45	1	Married	1	<1
I8	47	1	Stable union	1–2	1
I9	52	1	Married	3–4	4
I10	55	1	widow	2	4
I11	44	1	Married	3	<1
I12	56	3	Married	1–2	10
I13	72	3	Married	2	15
I14	49	1	Single	2	5
I15	46	3	Married	1	<1
I16	55	1	Married	1–2	6

I = Interviewee; * Illiterate = 1, Incomplete Elementary = 2, Complete Elementary = 3, Higher Education = 4; ** In Brazilian minimum wage. Brazilian minimum wage corresponds to USD 231.73 (quote on 15 September 2022).

The interviewed women's statements were grouped into three thematic categories depending on their experience of violence: (1) experiences of psychological violence, (2) experiences of physical violence, and (3) experiences of sexual violence.

The analysis of the data related to the guiding question: "After the breast cancer, did you start to experience situations of violence on the part of your intimate partner?" The interviewees' narratives revealed that 50.0% experienced psychological violence, 30% experienced physical violence, and 20.0% experienced sexual violence.

3.1. Experiences of Psychological Violence

With regard to the experience of psychological violence, the comment of I1, married and diagnosed a year ago with breast cancer, indicate the presence of this problem practiced by the intimate partner, who sees the treatment as unnecessary, relating cancer to death.

[...] Sometimes inside the house he would say: there, you are taking treatment for nothing, you are really going to die [...] (I1).

For I12, diagnosed 10 years ago, the diagnosis of breast cancer and the surgery generated changes in the relationship with her partner, as she reported:

[...] From the moment he (the husband) found out I had cancer, that I had breast surgery, he changed completely. He kept saying things to humiliate me, like, "Oh, you are not my wife, I have no wife like that, thin, bald, without both breasts" (pause for crying) [...] (I12).

Breast cancer is a stigmatizing disease, which places female body image, especially after a mastectomy, in opposition to the parameters imposed by society, of what is expected of the female body. I3 reported having been deprecated as "mutilated." A statement such as this reveals the degree of psychological violence by the intimate partner as a result of the breast removal surgery.

[...] I was totally despised when I was "mutilated," right. Mutilated in the breasts... The first time I took off my blouse near him, he said that if he had known that "they were going to" cut me like that, he would have done it himself. (pause)... sometimes I was changing my clothes and he called me a "cripple" [...] (I3).

Participant I8 used resources based on coping and focused on emotion to deal with psychological violence; that is, she "pretended" not to be experiencing such a situation.

[...] What struck me most in all this was the contempt. The worst thing he did was that. I pretended not to hear, but it hurt. It hurts. Sometimes, if it was a stranger, it wouldn't hurt me so much [...] (I8).

3.2. Experiences of Physical Violence

In this category, there were reports of physical aggression by the intimate partner, with incidents that ranged from a pinch, a push, or a punch to the use of a knife as a weapon. Despite the physical vulnerability due to the treatment, there was confrontation with and mastery over fear of the situation in pursuit of the preservation of their physical integrity, with the intervention of neighbors, as shown in the reports:

[...] He pinched me and pushed me. I faced him and said that I am not afraid, I am not afraid of dying, I am not afraid of anything [...] (I1).

[...] There was a moment when he pulled the wig off my head and burned the wig [...] (I8).

[...] He came out of his room with a knife, when I went to get up, he came to punch me I got up and he came with the knife [...] (I12).

The interviewees expressed indignation when questioning the justice of the application of the Maria da Penha Law, given the payment of bail for the release of the aggressor.

[...] I didn't have the physical strength to fight with him. Then it got to the point where he beat me and the neighbors "got involved" and he "went" to jail, but when he got there, he paid bail and got out because to justice, a life is nothing, it's nothing [...] (I12)

3.3. Experiences of Sexual Violence

Reports of sexual practices without consent, which characterizes sexual violence, were present. It was reported by women who, because of fear or economic dependence, felt coerced by their intimate partner to submit to a sexual act.

[...] He came to "get me" and go up against me by force. He said either I gave in or he would not buy anything else for the house [...] (I1).

[...] I slept with my room locked, but three times he broke the door down and forced me to have sex. I did it for fear of him doing something worse than what he was already doing to me, understand? [...] (I12)

[...] I had sex out of fear [...] (I6).

4. Discussion

This study aimed to uncover the violence against women practiced by their intimate partners after mastectomy. The analysis of the statements revealed three thematic categories: (1) experiences of psychological violence, (2) experiences of physical violence, and (3) experiences of sexual violence.

Intimate partner violence (IPV) is a public health concern. A study conducted with users of primary care in the municipality of Vitória, Espírito Santo, Brazil, revealed the prevalence of psychological, physical, and sexual violence perpetrated against women by their intimate partners in the last 12 months: 25.3% (95% CI 22.6–28.2), 9.9% (95% CI 8.1–11.9), and 5.7% (95% CI 4.3–7.3), respectively [22]. The data indicate that this is a topical problem in Brazil, not only because of its magnitude, given the significant number of women affected, but also because of the social problems generated by gender violence, which implies the weakened autonomy of women affected by a relationship of domination and control by their partner [23].

A study conducted with women with breast cancer revealed that psychological violence was the most prevalent, with the partner cited as the main aggressor and the house the most frequent place in which the violence was perpetrated [24]. As noted in the present research, expressions of humiliation and feelings of fear and low self-esteem, as well as contempt exhibited by the intimate partners, reinforce how much psychological violence is present in the daily lives of women who have undergone mastectomies, with the partner as the most commonly cited aggressor.

It is important to emphasize that the experience of violence involves a range of feelings, often ambiguous and contradictory. The victims live between fear, anger, indignation, and surprise in relation to the aggressive actions of their partners, but the violence is perceived as negative [25]. Even so, the naturalization of violence, especially within the domestic space, is legitimized by male domination. This violence, marked by power over and oppression of women, leads us to reflect on the definitions and typology of violence against women emphasized by the Maria da Penha Law in Brazil; this reflection could facilitate a (re)conceptualization of violence in the unequal power relations that circumscribe the cruel dynamics in affective and marital relationships [26].

The breakup of a violent relationship can take years, given that many women continue with their partners due to financial dependence, fear of dying, waiting for a change in their partner's behavior, the shame of assuming the failure of the relationship, or emotional dependence [27]. In the absence of economic factors, aspects such as intimacy and the centrality of the relationship can function to prevent the termination of the relationship [28]. Many women fail to report violence because they have the perception that they are not entitled to autonomy over their lives, because they believe they are guilty of the violence suffered, or because they do not even realize they are in a violent relationship [29].

A study conducted with 553 women diagnosed with breast, cervical, or colorectal cancer showed that domestic violence negatively influenced all health indicators related to cancer, suggesting that the identification of IPV and other stressors can provide important information to health professionals in order to contribute to the better planning of assistance, disruption of violence, and improvement in the well-being of these women [30].

The present study noted the experience of sexual violence in the reports of participants who highlighted coerced sexual practices, committed without consent, or motivated by fear of their partner. These results show how fundamental it is that health professionals take into consideration the complex interaction between the cultural, relational, and subjective aspects of the sexual experience after breast cancer in order to provide better care in the context of oncological assistance [31–40].

Provision of comprehensive care to women with breast cancer experiencing violence requires the construction of a network of services to confront that violence, this network being one of the most important and challenging strategies for dealing with a problem that is complex and multifaceted, so that the network contributes to the strengthening of victims and professionals, and so that they will feel supported and encouraged to act [41].

It is worth considering as a limitation of this study the fact that it did not investigate whether the women had already experienced tensions that interfered with their relationships prior to the disease. However, this does not prevent us from concluding that there is a need for professionals to assist these women and to provide holistic care capable of uncovering previous or current cases of violence, which are often omitted by women because they feel inhibited, ashamed, or too insecure to report what has happened, in order to contribute to their comprehensive care and record their cases, playing an important role in their care and the prevention of this phenomenon.

5. Conclusions

This is one of the few studies that we know of that has approached violence against woman in a context of the great vulnerability that is the experience of mastectomy resulting from a diagnosis of breast cancer. It was observed that the physical, sexual, and psychological violence practiced by their intimate partners may be present in this phase, considered a time of great need for family and social support.

The results of this study reaffirm the importance of health professionals in the care of women with breast cancer, and especially those in situations of violence. Health professionals have a role of immense relevance not only in the reception of victims, but also and especially in the recording of this problem, giving women the opportunity of inclusion in a network of protection and care and thereby enabling the removal of this phenomenon. It is important to emphasize that it is essential that women be assisted by a multidisciplinary and interprofessional team, given the complexity of violence and the demands that arise in different bio-psycho-social areas resulting from the experience of this serious public health phenomenon that is violence against women.

Author Contributions: Conceptualization, F.M.C.L. and M.H.C.A.; methodology, F.M.C.L.; software, F.M.C.L. and M.H.C.A.; validation, A.G.O., B.L.F.d.A.B., M.Z.A., N.A.V.V., P.M.A.M., M.H.C.A., L.B.F. and L.C.L.-J.; formal analysis, P.M.A.M., M.H.C.A., L.B.F. and L.C.L.-J.; investigation, F.M.C.L., A.G.O., B.L.F.d.A.B. and M.H.C.A.; resources, F.M.C.L.; data curation, A.G.O., B.L.F.d.A.B., M.Z.A., N.A.V.V., P.M.A.M., M.H.C.A., L.B.F. and L.C.L.-J.; writing—original draft preparation, F.M.C.L., M.H.C.A. and L.C.L.-J.; writing—review and editing, F.M.C.L., M.H.C.A. and L.C.L.-J.; visualization, A.G.O., B.L.F.d.A.B., M.Z.A., N.A.V.V., P.M.A.M., M.H.C.A., L.B.F. and L.C.L.-J.; supervision, F.M.C.L., M.H.C.A. and L.C.L.-J.; project administration, F.M.C.L. All authors have read and agreed to the published version of the manuscript.

Funding: This research received no external funding.

Institutional Review Board Statement: The study was conducted in accordance with the Declaration of Helsinki and approved by the Research Ethics Committee of the Federal University of Espírito Santo (UFES), under number 2,207,822.

Informed Consent Statement: Verbal informed consent was obtained from all subjects involved in the study prior to conducting the semi-structured interviews.

Data Availability Statement: Data is available from the corresponding author upon reasonable request.

Conflicts of Interest: The authors declare no conflict of interest.

References

1. Siegel, R.L.; Miller, K.D.; Fuchs, H.E.; Jemal, A. Cancer statistics, 2022. *CA Cancer J. Clin.* **2022**, *72*, 7–33. [CrossRef] [PubMed]
2. World Health Organization. Cancer Management. Geneva: WHO. 2021. Available online: https://www.who.int/cancer/en/ (accessed on 2 August 2022).
3. Torre, L.A.; Siegel, R.L.; Ward, E.M.; Jemal, A. Global Cancer Incidence and Mortality Rates and Trends—An Update. *Cancer Epidemiol. Biomark. Prev.* **2016**, *25*, 16–27. [CrossRef] [PubMed]
4. Sung, H.; Ferlay, J.; Siegel, R.L.; Laversanne, M.; Soerjomataram, I.; Jemal, A.; Bray, F. Global Cancer Statistics 2020: GLOBOCAN Estimates of Incidence and Mortality Worldwide for 36 Cancers in 185 Countries. *CA Cancer J. Clin.* **2021**, *71*, 209–249. [CrossRef] [PubMed]
5. Ferlay, J.; Colombet, M.; Soerjomataram, I.; Mathers, C.; Parkin, D.M.; Piñeros, M.; Znaor, A.; Bray, F. Estimating the global cancer incidence and mortality in 2018: GLOBOCAN sources and methods. *Int. J. Cancer* **2019**, *144*, 1941–1953. [CrossRef] [PubMed]

6. Brasil. Instituto Nacional de Câncer José Alencar Gomes da Silva. Coordenação de Prevenção e Vigilância. Estimativa 2020: Incidência de câncer no Brasil. 2019. Available online: https://www.inca.gov.br/sites/ufu.sti.inca.local/files/media/document/estimativa-2020-incidencia-de-cancer-no-brasil.pdf (accessed on 1 April 2022).
7. Lopes-Júnior, L.C.; Lima, R.A.G. Cancer care and interdisciplinary practice. *Cad. Saude Publica* **2019**, *35*, e00193218. [CrossRef]
8. Lopes Júnior, L.C. The era of precision medicine and its impact on nursing: Paradigm shifts? *Rev. Bras. Enferm.* **2021**, *74*, e740501. [CrossRef]
9. Lopes-Júnior, L.C.; Olson, K.; de Omena Bomfim, E.; Pereira-da-Silva, G.; Nascimento, L.C.; de Lima, R.A. Translational research and symptom management in oncology nursing. *Br. J. Nurs.* **2016**, *25*, S12–S14. [CrossRef]
10. Abrahão, C.A.; Bomfim, E.; Lopes-Júnior, L.C.; Pereira-da-Silva, G. Complementary therapies as a strategy to reduce stress and stimulate immunity of women with breast cancer. *J. Evid. Based Integr. Med.* **2019**, *24*, 2515690X19834169. [CrossRef]
11. Lopes-Júnior, L.C. Personalized Nursing Care in Precision-Medicine Era. *SAGE Open Nurs.* **2021**, *7*, 23779608211064713. [CrossRef]
12. Amorim, M.H.C.; Lopes-Júnior, L.C. Psychoneuroimmunology and nursing research: Discovery, paradigm shifts, and methodological innovations. *Acta Paul. Enferm.* **2021**, *34*, e-EDT1.
13. Oliveira, F.B.M.; Santana e Silva, F.; Prazeres, A.S.B. Impacto do câncer de mama e da mastectomia na sexualidade feminina. *Rev. Enferm. UFPE on line* **2017**, *11*, 2533–2540.
14. Silva, L.C. Breast cancer and psychological suffering: Female-related aspects. *Psicol. Estud.* **2008**, *13*, 231–237. [CrossRef]
15. Oliveski, C.C.; Girardon-Perlini, N.M.O.; Cogo, S.B.; Cordeiro, F.R.; Martins, F.C.; Paz, P.P. Experience of families facing cancer in palliative care. *Text. Context. Enferm.* **2021**, *30*, e20200669. [CrossRef]
16. Vale, C.C.S.O.; Dias, I.C.; Miranda, K.M. Breast cancer: The impact of mastectomy on women's psyche. *Mental* **2017**, *11*, 527–545.
17. Ferreira, D.B.; Farago, P.M.; Reis, P.E.D.; Funghetto, S.S. Our life after breast cancer: Perceptions and repercussions from the perspective of the couple. *Rev. Bras. Enferm* **2011**, *64*, 536–544. [CrossRef]
18. Finck, C.; Barradas, S.; Zenger, M.; Hinz, A. Quality of life in breast cancer patients: Associations with optimism and social support. *Int. J. Clin. Health Psychol.* **2018**, *18*, 27–34. [CrossRef]
19. Aygin, D.; Bozdemir, H. Exposure to violence in breast cancer patients: Systematic review. *Breast Cancer* **2019**, *26*, 29–38. [CrossRef]
20. Nunes, N.L.C.; Vignuda, S.T.; Santos, O.I.C.; Moraes, J.R.M.M.; Aguiar, R.C.B.; Silva, L.F. Saturação teórica em pesquisa qualitativa: Relato de experiência na entrevista com escolares. *Rev. Bras. Enferm.* **2018**, *71*, 228–233.
21. Bardin, L. *Análise de Conteúdo*; Edições: São Paulo, Brazil, 2016; Volume 70.
22. Leite, F.M.C.; Amorim, M.H.C.; Wehrmeister, F.C.; Gigante, D.P. Violence against women, Espírito Santo, Brazil. *Rev. de Saúde Pública* **2017**, *33*, 511–512. [CrossRef]
23. Chacham, A.S.; Jayme, J.G. Violência de gênero, desigualdade social e sexualidade: As experiências de mulheres jovens em Belo Horizonte. *Civ.-Rev. de Ciências Sociais* **2016**, *16*, 1–19. [CrossRef]
24. Luvisaro, B.M.O.; Gradim, C.V.C. Violence against Women with Breast Neoplasms. *J. Pharmacy Pharmacol.* **2016**, *4*, 639–648.
25. Moura, M.A.; Oliveira, P.R.F. A percepção das mulheres vítimas de lesão corporal dolosa. *Esc. Anna. Nery* **2000**, *4*, 257–267.
26. Guimarães, M.C.; Pedroza, R.L.S. Violência contra a mulher: Problematizando definições teóricas, filosóficas e jurídicas. *Psicol. Soc.* **2015**, *27*, 256–266. [CrossRef]
27. Brasil. *Secretaria Especial de Políticas para as Mulheres. Enfrentando a Violência contra a Mulher*; Secretaria Especial de Políticas para as Mulheres: Brasília, Brazil, 2005; 64p.
28. Giordano, P.C.; Soto, D.; Manning, W.D.; Longmore, M.A. The characteristics of romantic relationships associated with teen dating violence. *Soc. Sci. Res.* **2010**, *9*, 863–874. [CrossRef] [PubMed]
29. Pazo, C.G.; Aguiar, A.C. Sentidos da violência conjugal: Análise do banco de dados de um serviço telefônico anônimo. *Physis* **2012**, *22*, 253–273. [CrossRef]
30. Coker, A.L.; Follingstad, D.; Garcia, L.S.; Williams, C.M.; Crawford, T.N.; Bush, H.M. Association of intimate partner violence and childhood sexual abuse with cancer-related well-being in women. *J. Womens Health* **2012**, *21*, 1180–1188. [CrossRef]
31. Vieira, E.M.; Santos, D.B.; Santos, M.A.; Giami, A. Vivência da sexualidade após o câncer de mama: Estudo qualitativo com mulheres em reabilitação. *Rev. Latino-Am. Enferm.* **2014**, *22*, 408–414. [CrossRef]
32. Vaziri, S.H.; Lotfi Kashani, F. Sexuality after breast cancer: Need for guideline. *Iran. J. Cancer Prev.* **2012**, *5*, 10–15.
33. Maleki, M.; Mardani, A.; Ghafourifard, M.; Vaismoradi, M. Changes and challenges in sexual life experienced by the husbands of women with breast cancer: A qualitative study. *BMC Womens Health* **2022**, *22*, 326. [CrossRef]
34. Carroll, A.J.; Baron, S.R.; Carroll, R.A. Couple-based treatment for sexual problems following breast cancer: A review and synthesis of the literature. *Support. Care Cancer* **2016**, *24*, 3651–3659. [CrossRef]
35. Santos, D.B.; Santos, M.A.; Vieira, E.M. Sexuality and breast cancer: A systematic literature review. *Saúde Soc.* **2014**, *23*, 1342–1355.
36. Brajkovic, L.; Sladic, P.; Kopilaš, V. Sexual Quality of Life in Women with Breast Cancer. *Health Psychol. Res.* **2021**, *9*, 24512. [CrossRef]
37. Ooi, P.S.; Draman, N.; Muhamad, R.; Yusoff, S.S.M.; Noor, N.M.; Haron, J.; Hadi, I.S.A. Sexual Dysfunction Among Women With Breast Cancer in the Northeastern Part of West Malaysia. *Sex. Med.* **2021**, *9*, 100351. [CrossRef]
38. Dinapoli, L.; Colloca, G.; Di Capua, B.; Valentini, V. Psychological Aspects to Consider in Breast Cancer Diagnosis and Treatment. *Curr. Oncol. Rep.* **2021**, *23*, 38. [CrossRef]
39. Lopes-Júnior, L.C. Cancer symptom clusters: From the lab bench to clinical practice. *Rev. Bras. Enferm.* **2022**, *75*, e2022v75n5inov.

40. Lopes-Júnior, L.C.; Tuma, M.C.; Amorim, M.H.C. Psychoneuroimmunology and oncology nursing: A theoretical study. *Rev. Esc. Enferm. USP* **2021**, *55*, e20210159. [CrossRef]
41. Hasse, M.; Vieira, E.M. How health professional assist women experiencing violence? A triangulated data analysis. *Saúde Debate* **2014**, *38*, 482–493.

MDPI
St. Alban-Anlage 66
4052 Basel
Switzerland
www.mdpi.com

Current Oncology Editorial Office
E-mail: curroncol@mdpi.com
www.mdpi.com/journal/curroncol

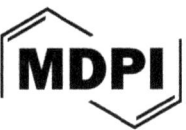

Disclaimer/Publisher's Note: The statements, opinions and data contained in all publications are solely those of the individual author(s) and contributor(s) and not of MDPI and/or the editor(s). MDPI and/or the editor(s) disclaim responsibility for any injury to people or property resulting from any ideas, methods, instructions or products referred to in the content.

www.ingramcontent.com/pod-product-compliance
Lightning Source LLC
LaVergne TN
LVHW070602100526
838202LV00012B/543